SKIN INFECTIONS

Diagnosis and Treatment

EDITED BY

John C. Hall
University of Missouri–Kansas City School of Medicine

Brian J. Hall
St. Louis University School of Medicine

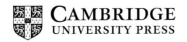

CAMBRIDGE
UNIVERSITY PRESS

CAMBRIDGE UNIVERSITY PRESS
Cambridge, New York, Melbourne, Madrid, Cape Town, Singapore, São Paulo, Delhi

Cambridge University Press
32 Avenue of the Americas, New York, NY 10013-2473, USA

www.cambridge.org
Information on this title: www.cambridge.org/9780521897297

First published 2009

Printed in the United States of America

A catalog record for this publication is available from the British Library.

Library of Congress Cataloging in Publication data
    Skin infections : diagnosis and treatment / [edited by] John C. Hall, Brian J. Hall.
       p. ; cm.
    Includes bibliographical references and index.
    ISBN 978-0-521-89729-7 (hardback)
    1. Skin – Infections.   I. Hall, John C., 1947–   II. Hall, Brian J. (Brian John), 1981–
    III. Title.   [DNLM: 1. Skin Diseases, Infectious – diagnosis.   2. Skin Diseases,
    Infectious – therapy. WR 220 S6279 2009]
    RL201.S57   2009
    616.5–dc22
    2009001262

ISBN 978-0-521-89729-7 hardback

SKIN INFECTIONS
Diagnosis and Treatment

This is the first textbook linking the two disciplines of dermatology and infectious diseases. As the number of elderly, AIDS, transplant, and cancer surviving patients continues to rapidly increase worldwide, all medical personnel need to be able to rapidly recognize and treat infections. The skin is the most easily accessed and monitored of all organs and is often the first sign of infection. Knowledge of the integument's link to infection is a must for the modern medical nurse, nurse practitioner, medical student, resident, and practitioner. To accomplish these goals, the text features authors from around the world who are considered experts in their various fields. The book is organized into types of infections, locations in the integument, specific subpopulations of patients at risk, and regional variations of infections.

John C. Hall, M.D., is an associate staff in dermatology at the University of Missouri–Kansas City School of Medicine. He is also on primary staff in the Department of Medicine (subspecialty dermatology) at St. Luke's Hospital in Kansas City, Missouri, and on staff in dermatology at the Kansas City Free Health Clinic.

Brian J. Hall, M.D., is a pathology resident at St. Louis University School of Medicine.

For Charlotte,
Shelly, Kim, Tony, and Tori

Contents

List of Contributors   page vii
Acknowledgments   xi

INTRODUCTION   1
John C. Hall
**TECHNIQUES IN DIAGNOSING
DERMATOLOGIC MANIFESTATIONS OF
INFECTIOUS DISEASES**   2
Francisco G. Bravo and Salim Mohanna
**PRINCIPLES OF MANAGEMENT OF
DERMATOLOGIC INFECTIONS IN THE SKIN**   8
John C. Hall

PART I   COMMON INFECTIONS
1 **COMMON BACTERIAL INFECTIONS**   17
   Tammie Ferringer
2 **COMMON VIRAL INFECTIONS**   23
   *Alejandra Varela, Anne Marie Tremaine,
   Aron Gewirtzman, Anita Satyaprakash,
   Natalia Mendoza, Parisa Ravanfar, and
   Stephen K. Tyring*
3 **COMMON FUNGAL INFECTIONS**   42
   Aditya K. Gupta and Elizabeth A. Cooper

PART II   LESS COMMON INFECTIONS
4 **CUTANEOUS TUBERCULOSIS**   59
   Bhushan Kumar and Sunil Dogra
5 **LEPROSY**   76
   Arturo P. Saavedra and Samuel L. Moschella
6 **ATYPICAL MYCOBACTERIA**   88
   *Francesca Prignano, Caterina Fabroni,
   and Torello Lotti*
7 **ARTHROPOD-BORNE INFECTION**   92
   Dirk M. Elston
8 **DEEP FUNGAL INFECTIONS**   96
   *Evandro Ararigbóia Rivitti and
   Paulo Ricardo Criado*
9 **PARASITOLOGY**   117
   Francisco G. Bravo and Salim Mohanna

**PART III   INFECTIONS IN
SELECTED ECOSYSTEMS**
10 **INFECTIONS IN THE DESERT**   135
    Joseph C. Pierson and David J. DiCaudo
11 **INFECTION IN THE TROPICS**   150
    *Marcia Ramos-e-Silva, Paula Pereira Araújo,
    and Sueli Coelho Carneiro*

12 **AQUATIC DERMATOLOGY**   167
    Domenico Bonamonte and Gianni Angelini

**PART IV   INFECTIONS IN SELECTED
PATIENT POPULATIONS**
13 **SKIN INFECTIONS IN HIV PATIENTS**   185
    Joseph S. Susa and Clay J. Cockerell
14 **INFECTIONS IN ORGAN
    TRANSPLANT PATIENTS**   195
    *Daniela Kroshinsky, Jennifer Y. Lin,
    and Richard Allen Johnson*
15 **CANCER PATIENTS AND SKIN INFECTIONS**   206
    John C. Hall
16 **SKIN INFECTIONS IN PEDIATRIC PATIENTS**   211
    Michelle R. Wanna and Jonathan A. Dyer
17 **SKIN INFECTIONS IN THE ELDERLY**   233
    Noah S. Scheinfeld
18 **SKIN INFECTIONS IN ATHLETES**   238
    Brian B. Adams
19 **SKIN INFECTIONS IN DIABETES MELLITUS**   246
    Nawaf Al-Mutairi

**PART V   INFECTIONS OF SPECIFIC
SKIN-ASSOCIATED BODY SITES**
20 **INFECTIONS OF THE SCALP**   255
    *Shannon Harrison, Haydee Knott,
    and Wilma F. Bergfeld*
21 **INFECTIONS OF THE NAIL UNIT**   268
    *Gérald E. Piérard, Claudine
    Piérard-Franchimont, and Pascale Quatresooz*
22 **INFECTIONS OF THE MUCOUS MEMBRANES**   275
    *Julia S. Lehman, Alison J. Bruce, and
    Roy S. Rogers, III*

PART VI   SPECIAL DISEASE CATEGORIES
23 **INFECTIONS IN SKIN SURGERY**   303
    *Jean-Michel Amici, Anne-Marie Rogues,
    and Alain Taïeb*
24 **VENEREAL DISEASES**   309
    *Travis Vandergriff, Mandy Harting,
    and Ted Rosen*
25 **LIFE-THREATENING SKIN INFECTIONS:
    SKIN SIGNS OF IMPORTANT BACTERIAL
    INFECTIOUS DISEASES**   322
    Lisa A. Drage

Index   329

Contributors

BRIAN B. ADAMS, MD, MPH
Associate Professor of Dermatology
Director of Sports Dermatology Clinic
Chief of Dermatology, VAMC Cincinnati
University of Cincinnati
Cincinnati, OH

NAWAF AL-MUTAIRI, MD, FRCPC
Associate Professor
Faculty of Medicine
Kuwait University
Safat, Kuwait

JEAN-MICHEL AMICI, MD
Service de Dermatologique
Groupe Hospitalier Saint-Andre
Bordeaux Cedex, France

GIANNI ANGELINI, MD
Professor of Clinical Dermatology
Head of the Dermatology Clinic
Department of Internal Medicine, Immunology
and Infectious Diseases
University of Bari, Italy

PAULA PEREIRA ARAÚJO, MD
Former Post-Graduation Student, Sector of Dermatology
University Hospital, Federal University of Rio de Janeiro
Rio de Janeiro, Brazil

WILMA F. BERGFELD, MD
Head of Dermatology and Pathology
Department of Dermatology
Cleveland Clinic Foundation
Cleveland, OH

KUMAR BHUSHAN, MD
Department of Dermatology, Venereology and Leprology
Postgraduate Institute of Medical Education and Research
Chandigarh, India

DOMENICO BONAMONTE, MD
Research Fellow
Department of Internal Medicine, Immunology
and Infectious Diseases
Dermatologic Clinic
University of Bari
Bari, Italy

FRANCISCO G. BRAVO, MD
Associate Professor of Dermatology and Pathology
Facultad de Medicina Alberto Huardo
Instituto de Medicina Tropical Alexander von Humbold
Universidad Peruano Cayetano Heredia
Lima, Peru

ALISON J. BRUCE, MBChB
Consultant, Department of Dermatology
Mayo Clinic
Associate Professor of Dermatology
College of Medicine, Mayo Clinic
Rochester, MN

SUELI COELHO CARNEIRO, MD, PhD
Dermatologist, Sector of Dermatology
University Hospital, Federal University of Rio de Janeiro
Associate Professor, Sector of Dermatology
University Hospital, State University of Rio de Janeiro
Rio de Janeiro, Brazil

CLAY J. COCKERELL, MD
Professor of Dermatology and Pathology
University of Texas Southwestern Medical Center
Dallas, TX

ELIZABETH A. COOPER, B.E.Sc., H.B.Sc.
Mediprobe Research, Inc.
London, Ontario, Canada

PAULO RICARDO CRIADO, MD
Dermatologist, Division of Dermatology
Hospital das Clinicas
School of Medicine
San Paulo University, Brazil
San Paulo, Brazil

DAVID J. DiCAUDO, MD
Associate Professor
Department of Dermatology and Pathology
Mayo Clinic
Scottsdale, AZ

SUNIL DOGRA, MD, DNB
Assistant Professor
Department of Dermatology, Venereology and Leprology
Postgraduate Institute of Medical Education and Research
Chandigarh, India

LISA A. DRAGE, MD
Assistant Professor of Dermatology
Mayo Clinic
Rochester, MN

JONATHAN A. DYER, MD
Assistant Professor of Dermatology and Child Health
University of Missouri School of Medicine
Columbia, MO

DIRK M. ELSTON, MD
Director, Department of Dermatology
Geisinger Medical Center
Danville, PA

CATERINA FABRONI, MD
Specialist in Dermatology and Venereology
Department of Dermatological Sciences
Florence University
Florence, Italy

TAMMIE FERRINGER, MD
Associate
Departments of Dermatology and Pathology
Geisinger Medical Center
Danville, PA

ARON GEWIRTZMAN, MD
Center for Clinical Studies
Houston, TX

ADITYA K. GUPTA, MD, PhD
Mediprobe Research, Inc.
London, Ontario, Canada
Professor of Dermatology
Sunnybrook Health Sciences Center
University of Toronto
Toronto, Ontario, Canada

BRIAN J. HALL, MD
Resident
Department of Pathology
St. Louis University School of Medicine
St. Louis, MO

JOHN C. HALL, MD
Associate Professor of Dermatology
University of Missouri–Kansas City
St. Luke's Hospital
Kansas City Free Health Clinic
Kansas City, MO

SHANNON C. HARRISON, MBBS, MMed, FACD
Clinical Research Fellow
Department of Dermatology
Cleveland Clinic Foundation
Cleveland, OH

MANDY HARTING, MD
Assistant Professor
Department of Dermatology
Baylor College of Medicine
Houston, TX

RICHARD ALLEN JOHNSON, MDCM
Department of Dermatology
Massachusetts General Hospital
Harvard Medical School
Boston, MA

HAYDEE KNOTT
Department of Dermatology
Cleveland Clinic Health Sciences Center
Cleveland, OH

DANIELA KROSHINSKY, MD
Department of Dermatology
Massachusetts General Hospital
Harvard Medical School
Boston, MA

JULIA S. LEHMAN, MD
Resident of Dermatology
Mayo School of Graduate Medical Education
Rochester, MN

JENNIFER Y. LIN, MD
Dermatologist
Department of Dermatology
Brigham and Women's Hospital
Harvard Medical School
Boston, MA

TORELLO LOTTI, MD
Chairman
Department of Dermatological Sciences
Florence University
Florence, Italy

NATALIA MENDOZA, MD, MSc
Center for Clinical Studies
Houston, TX

SALIM MOHANNA, MD
Clinical Research Associate
Instituto de Medicina Tropical Alexander von Humbold
Universidad Peruano Cayetano Heredia
Lima, Peru

SAMUEL L. MOSCHELLA, MD
Clinical Professor (Emeritus) of Dermatology
Harvard Medical School
Staff Dermatologist
Lahey Clinic
Burlington, MA

GÉRALD E. PIÉRARD, MD, PhD
Professor and Head of the Dermatopathology Department
University Hospital of Liège
Liège, Belgium

CLAUDINE PIÉRARD-FRANCHIMONT, MD, PhD
Associate Professor, Chief of Laboratory
Dermatopathology Department
University Hospital of Liège
Liège, Belgium

JOSEPH C. PIERSON, MD
Dermatopathologist, Anatomic and Clinic Pathologist
Uniformed Services University of Health Sciences
Bethesda, MD
United States Military Academy
West Point
New York, NY

FRANCESCA PRIGNANO, MD, PhD
Assistant Professor
Department of Dermatological Sciences
Florence University
Florence, Italy

PASCALE QUATRESOOZ, MD, PhD
Master of Conference, Chief of Laboratory
Dermatopathology Department
University Hospital of Liège
Liège, Belgium

MARCIA RAMOS-E-SILVA, MD, PhD
Associate Professor and Head, Sector of Dermatology
University Hospital, Federal University of Rio de Janeiro
Rio de Janeiro, Brazil

PARISA RAVANFAR, MD, MBA, MS
Dermatology Clinic Research Fellow
Center for Clinical Studies
Houston, TX

EVANDRO ARARIGBÓIA RIVITTI, MD
Dermatologist and Chairman of
Department of Dermatology
School of Medicine
San Paulo University, Brazil
San Paulo, Brazil

ROY S. ROGERS III, MD
Professor of Dermatology
Mayo Medical School
Consultant in Dermatology
Mayo Clinic
Rochester, MN

ANNE-MARIE ROGUES, MD, PhD
Service d'Hygiene Hospitaliere
Groupe Hospitaliere Pellegrin
Bordeaux, France

TED ROSEN, MD
Professor of Dermatology
Baylor College of Medicine
Chief of Dermatology
Michael E. DeBakey VA Medical Center
Houston, TX

ARTURO P. SAAVEDRA, MD, PhD
Instructor in Dermatology
Harvard Medical School
Boston, MA

ANITA SATYAPRAKASH
Dermatology Clinic Research Fellow
Center for Clinical Studies
Houston, TX

NOAH S. SCHEINFELD, MD, JD
Assistant Clinical Professor
Department of Dermatology
Columbia University
New York, NY

JOSEPH S. SUSA, DO
Assistant Clinical Professor
Department of Dermatology
University of Texas Southwestern Medical Center
Dallas, TX

ALAIN TAÏEB, MD, PhD
Head
Department of Dermatology and Pediatric Dermatology
University Hospitals of Bordeaux
National Reference Center for Rare Skin Disorders
Bordeaux Cedax, France

ANNE MARIE TREMAINE, MD
Clinical Research Fellow
Center for Clinical Studies
Houston, TX

STEPHEN K. TYRING, MD, PhD, MBA
Clinical Professor of Dermatology
University of Texas Health Science Center
Houston, TX

TRAVIS VANDERGRIFF, MD
Department of Dermatology
Baylor College of Medicine
Houston, TX

ALEJANDRA VARELA, MD
University of Texas Health Science Center
Houston, TX

MICHELLE R. WANNA, MD
Resident Physician, Dermatology
University of Missouri School of Medicine
Columbia, MO

Acknowledgments

My wife, Charlotte, gave me all the encouragement anyone could ask.

The late Richard Q. Crotty, MD, gave me the chance to be a dermatologist. The late Clarence S. Livingood, MD, taught me to be true to my science and my patients. The late David Gibson, MD, and Ken Watson, DO, led my way in dermatopathology. My office manager, Christa Czysz, has kept me afloat. My nurses, Brandi DelDebbio and Kelly Hudgens, and my office staff, Kelly Howell and Jennifer Phillips, have helped in enumerable ways.

A special thanks is due to my son, Brian J. Hall, MD, for endless hours helping edit and organize this text. The incredible group of authors in this book will speak for themselves through these pages. It would be an honor to be half the physician these dermatologists have proven to be.

INTRODUCTION

John C. Hall

A comprehensive melding of the fields of dermatology and infectious diseases is long overdue. It is the skin that is often the first sign of infection and the easiest organ to quickly access with an educated eye, culture, scraping, and histopathologic evaluation. It is the observation of the skin that can hold the chance for the earliest diagnosis and thus the most timely attempts at therapy. This same observation can guide the clinician through the maze of enumerable, often confusing, and sometimes costly follow-up confirmatory tests. Let us now, in these pages, take this opportunity the integument has given us to lead us through the ever-increasingly important field of infectious diseases.

TECHNIQUES IN DIAGNOSING DERMATOLOGIC MANIFESTATIONS OF INFECTIOUS DISEASES

Francisco G. Bravo and Salim Mohanna

GETTING THE SAMPLE

A vital step toward making the right diagnosis when dealing with infectious diseases is ordering the appropriate test. That implies having a certain idea of the range of possible organisms involved and directing your workup toward ruling in or out a specific agent. Of course, there will be cases where a more blind approach is in order and a large range of diagnostic possibilities should be considered. In those situations, smears and cultures for bacterial, mycobacterial, and fungal microorganisms are indicated. Also viral diseases should be considered in specific situations, such as febrile patients with disseminated maculopapular or vesicular rashes. However, just for practical purposes, it is better to take a syndromic approach, considering a range of possibilities regarding the etiology of the lesions and then, selecting the appropriate test. Let us take an example such as a patient with a sporotrichoid pattern of lesions. If the diagnosis to confirm is sporotrichosis, a fungal culture will be very sensitive and very specific. Pyogenic bacteria such as *Staphylococcal aureus* can also produce such a pattern. In these cases, a Gram stain and routine culture will be helpful. But, if the patient likes fishing, swimming, or diving besides gardening an atypical mycobacterial infection (*M. marinum*) also has to be listed in the differential. In such cases, a biopsy, acid-fast stain, and mycobacterial culture should also be considered, although recognizing this is a difficult diagnosis to make because of the low sensitivity of each individual test. In the same line of thought, the same patient just came back from a trip to the Amazon: leishmaniasis is then another possibility. In leishmaniasis, there is no test with high sensitivity, so a panel approach is indicated (direct exam, culture, intradermal reaction, histopathology, and PCR, when available). Nocardia, another disease capable of giving such a pattern, can only be detected if the laboratory takes special precautions while culturing. Then, it is better to direct our workup toward a specific diagnosis. Of course, that also implies having some knowledge regarding the sensitivity and specificity of each test for a specific etiological agent.

Nobody other than the clinician will know best where to take the sample from. Unfortunately for regulatory or administrative reasons, the task is commonly left to a technician.

As a rule, purulent or oozing secretions are considered excellent samples and should be regularly submitted for direct examination with Gram, fungal, and acid-fast staining. Abscesses should be punctured and the pus submitted under sterile conditions. Taking a biopsy of an abscess is usually not rewarding, but clinically if there is a thick wall surrounding the cavity, it may reveal a granulomatous infiltrate when biopsied.

Solid lesions, such as those suspicious for granulomatous diseases, are better studied submitting the tissue for culture; even then, the appropriate area should be sampled. In mycetoma, for example, unless the biopsy is taken from areas containing granules, the yield of histology and culture will be very low.

When dealing with dry, scaly lesions, such as in tinea cases, the scraping is very sensitive. However, in hairy areas (scalp, beard), getting some hairs may reveal the presence of spores in the absence of superficial hyphae. This is usually the case when a tinea barbae has been previously treated blindly with a topical antifungal. In cases where there is a possibility of tinea incognita, it is advisable to microscopically examine the proximal portion of the hairs. When dealing with white onychomycosis, scrape the surface. If the subungeal area is affected, the detritus under the nail are most likely to reveal the hypha or spore. Nail clippings are considered good samples, even suitable for histological study. The diagnosis of microscopic ectoparasites, such as scabies, requires taking the sample from the most commonly affected areas. Blindly scrapping off different areas is not very rewarding. In contrast, scrapping a whole scabies burrow will frequently reveal the presence of the mites, eggs, or feces.

Moist ulcers can be swabbed and the secretions submitted for direct examination and culture; dry ulcers can be sampled by touch preparation. Aspirating the fluid under the border of the ulceration with a micropipette is useful for leishmania; in leprosy, examining the fluid obtained by slitting the ear lobe under pressure is an excellent method to visualize the mycobacteria.

TECHNIQUES

Smears

Direct examination of material obtained from lesions is a vital first step to orient the clinician toward a specific etiology. Gram and acid-fast stains are now routinely performed by laboratory technicians, and the techniques themselves are beyond the scope of this book. However, the results provided are of vital importance. Gram stain is regularly done in urethral secretions to look for *Neisseria gonorrhoeae*; its absence in the presence of neutrophils is indicative of nongonococcal chlamydial urethritis. Acid-fast staining of smears from leprosy patients may help establish the bacterial load.

Some tests are more easily done, on a daily basis, at dermatology offices around the world. Examples of such tests are potassium hydroxide (KOH) preparations and the Tzanck test. The KOH preparation is usually done using a 5% to 40% concentration. The idea is that the reaction will dissolve most of the normal host cells, sparing the infectious agent. The condenser of the microscope is lowered, to facilitate observation by light contrast. The test is done on skin scrapings to detect the presence of hyphae in dermatophytes or candida. Yeast of invasive fungi such as *Blastomyces* and *Paracoccidioides* can also be detected by this method in purulent secretions. Hairs and nails can also be examined under the microscope in a similar manner. The same preparation can be used to examine scrapings while looking for scabies mites and *Demodex*. A variation on the theme is adding colored stains to facilitate viewing of fungal structures. Using mineral oil instead of KOH may allow the assessment of viability and motility of ectoparasitic mites. Instead of regular scraping, one can use adhesive tape to take the sample, a technique especially useful when dealing with rapidly moving targets, such as the face of a small child. Surprisingly, a similar technique will allow detection of large fungal structures, such as the agents of chromoblastomycosis and lobomycosis when the tape is applied on top of the clinical lesion. This is possible because of the phenomenon of transepidermal elimination of the microorganisms. Tzanck test implies the examination of cells at the base of an unroofed blister in suspected cases of Herpes simplex or Herpes Zoster infection. Once air dried, the slide is stained with Wright, Giemsa, or methylene blue. The goal is to detect multinucleated giant keratinocytes that are indicative of herpetic infections. A more sophisticated technique utilizes an immunofluorescent antibody against the virus, allowing species-specific identification.

Touch preparation of a genital ulcer can be examined under dark field for the presence of treponemal spirochetes. The same preparations, if stained as a PAP smear may allow detection of the presence of multiple intracellular bacteria in cases of granuloma inguinale. Touch preparation of the bottom of a large ulcer with undermined borders and acid-fast staining will be extremely useful in detecting large amount of mycobacterium in a Buruli ulcer (Table T-1).

Culture

The purpose of cultures is isolation of the infectious agent to comply with one of the Koch postulates. If the diagnosis is uncertain, samples should be sent for bacterial, fungal, viral and acid-fast bacterial cultures. Culturing requires special media, depending on the microorganism suspected (see Table T-2). One has to keep in mind that certain areas of the body are heavily contaminated, such as the mouth and perianal region. The skin, by no means an aseptic organ, can be colonized by different bacteria and fungi. The result of cultures should be interpreted appropriately, with correlation to the clinical lesion. Some culture media are designed to facilitate the growth of the microorganism (such as the Thayer-Martin media for gonococcal infection or oxygen depleted systems for anerobes). Others, such as the Mycosel, will restrict the growth of saprophytic fungi while allowing the growth of dermatophytes. Most bacteria will grow in a matter of days; some, such as Brucella, may require weeks in specially designed media (such as Ruiz Castañeda). *Candida* will also grow fast, even on bacterial culture media, in days. Regular fungi, cultured in Sabouraud's agar may grow as fast as in 1 week (*Sporothrix*), 2 weeks (dermatophytes), or 4 weeks (*Histoplasma* and *Actinomyces*). Mycobacteria may be fast growers (*M. fortuitum*, *M. chelonae*, or *M. abscessus*) or take several weeks (*M. tuberculosis* and *M. ulcerans*), with additional specific temperature requirements.

Table T-1: Selected Microorganism with Special Culture Requirements

H. influenza	Chocolate agar with factors V and X
N. gonorrhea	Thayer-Martin media
B. pertussis	Bordet-Gengou agar
C. diphtheriae	Tellurite plate, Loffler's medium, blood agar
M. tuberculosis	Lowenstein-Jensen agar
Lactose-fermenting enterics	MacConkey's agar (pink colonies)
Legionella	Buffered charcoal yeast extract agar
F. tularensis	Blood or chocolate cystine agar
Leptospira	Fletcher's or Stuart's medium with rabbit serum
Fungi	Sabouraud's agar

Table T-2: Special stains

Giemsa	*Borrelia, Plasmodium*, trypanosomes, *Chlamydia, Leishmania*
PAS	Stains glycogen, mucopolysaccharides; good for fungi
Ziehl-Neelsen	Acid-fast bacteria and *Nocardia*
India ink	*Cryptococcus neoformans*
Silver stain	*Fungi, PCP, Legionella, Bartonella, Klebsiella granulomatis*

Surprisingly enough, even in the 21st century, some famous pathogens are still unable to be isolated in culture media. *Treponema pallidum, Mycobacterium leprae,* and *Loboa Loboi* are three examples. The isolation of virus by culture is not routinely done (except for herpes simplex and varicella-zoster viruses). Modern diagnosis relies more on molecular techniques or serologic assays.

Intradermal reactions

Intradermal reactions are widely used to support the diagnosis of some dermatological and nondermatological diseases. They are mainly indicated for the detection of type I (immediate hypersensitivity) and type IV (delayed hypersensitivity) reactions toward exogenous or endogenous antigens. Intradermal reactions for the diagnosis of infectious diseases are indicated to detect previous contact with the agent as revealed by delayed hypersensitivity to the whole organisms or their antigens.

The intradermal reaction is a localized inflammatory reaction with marked proliferation of lymphocytes, monocytes, and small numbers of neutrophiles, with a tendency toward cellular accumulations arround small vessels. The induration results from fibrin formation.

The principle of an intradermal reaction is the inoculation of an antigen into the superficial layer of the dermis through a fine-bore needle with its bevel pointing upward. The quantity injected may vary from 0.01 to 0.1 mL, but 0.1 mL is universally used. Although the test could be done at any site, the proximal part of the flexor aspect of the forearm is conventionally used. Corticosteroids or immunosuppressive agents should be discontinued before testing for intradermal reactions because they may inhibit the delayed hypersensitivity reaction. Intradermal reactions for the detection of delayed hypersensitivity are read at 48 hours, although they can be read as early as 12 hours and as late as 4 days. The size of the induration is more important than erythema when interpreting delayed hypersensitivity reactions.

The tuberculin test (also called PPD [purified protein derivative], Pirquet test, or Mantoux test) is a diagnostic tool used to detect latent infection or recent infection (as shown by conversion from negative to positive) and as part of the diagnosis of tuberculous disease. A standard dose of tuberculin is injected intradermally on the flexor aspect of the forearm and a reading is taken after 48 hours. The reaction is read by measuring the diameter of induration in millimeters. The interpretation of the test result will depend on all relevant clinical circumstances. An induration measuring more than 10 mm in diameter is considered to be a positive response while that measuring less than 5 mm is considered negative. A positive test indicates past or present infection with *M. tuberculosis* or vaccination with bacillus Calmette-Guérin (BCG). An induration of more than 15 mm is unlikely to be due to BCG vaccination and is strong evidence in favor of active tuberculosis. In the absence of specific risk factors for tuberculosis, an induration between 6 and 10 mm is more likely to be due to previous BCG vaccination or infection with environmental mycobacteria than to tuberculosis infection. When there is a higher probability of tuberculosis, such as recent contact with an infectious case, a high occupational risk or residence in a high prevalence country, an induration of 6 mm or more is more likely to be due to tuberculosis. Anergy is present in AIDS patients. Other factors that can weaken the reaction include severe tuberculous disease, renal failure, diabetes, immunosuppressive drugs, and old age. Initial skin tests may have a booster effect on reactions to subsequent doses. More sophisticated tests based on interferon production by stimulated cells are also available. Intradermal reactions for atypical mycobacteria have also been prepared. They include PPD-Y for *Mycobacterium kansasii*, Scrofulin for *Mycobacterium scrofulaceum*, and Burulin for *Mycobacterium ulcerans*.

The leishmanin test was first done by Montenegro in 1926, in Brazil. This test (also called the Montenegro test) is indicative of the delayed hypersensitivity reaction to leishmania, which plays a major role in disease resolution and wound healing. It usually becomes positive early in the course of cutaneous or mucocutaneous leishmaniasis (except in diffuse cutaneous leishmaniasis) and only after recovery from visceral leishmaniasis. It is highly sensitive for cutaneous leishmaniasis. The test is considered positive when induration is more than 5 mm in diameter after 48 to 72 hours. The test is not species specific. A negative test may be attributed to an anergic state, decreased cell mediated immunity, early treatment, or presence of an unusual serotype of leishmania, whereas a positive test favors active disease if the patient is not a resident of the area. The same positive reaction does not have the same relevance for natives and current residents.

The lepromin test classifies the stage of leprosy based on the reaction and differentiates tuberculoid leprosy, (in which there is a positive delayed reaction at the injection site) from lepromatous leprosy (in which there is no reaction despite the active infection). The test is not diagnostic since normal uninfected persons may react. Two types of antigens are available: Mitsuda lepromin, an autoclaved suspension of tissue (whole bacilli) obtained from experimentally infected armadillos; and Dharmendra lepromin, a purified chloroform-ether extracted suspension of *M. leprae* (fractionated bacilli with a soluble protein component). The response after intradermal injection is typically biphasic, with an early Fernandez reaction (in the form of a tuberculin reaction with Dharmendra antigen) and a late Mitsuda reaction (in the form of erythematous, papular nodules with Mitsuda antigen).

Other important tests used for diagnostic aid, or to evaluate the cellular immune response in patients suspected of having reduced cell-mediated immunity, or in epidemiological studies include the anthraxin test, the onchocerca skin test, the candidin test, the coccidioidin or spherulin test, the histoplasmin test, and the trichophytin test. Finally, there are some tests of historical importance only, as they are no longer used for diagnostic purposes: Lymphogranuloma venereum (Frei's test), Chancroid (Ito Reenstierna test), Bartonellosis (Foshay test) and Scarlet fever (Dick's test).

Serology

Some tests are based on the detection of the infectious agent antigens in serum or by the detection of the circulating antibodies generated by the host. Agglutination tests (latex agglutination test) are based on the capturing the antibody from a suspected patient with whole bacteria or antigen absorbed to latex particles. The presence of circulating antibodies will then be detected by the agglutination phenomenon. *N. meningitidis* and *Cryptococcus* can be detected by latex agglutination. The complement fixation (CF) test measures complement-consuming (complement-fixing) antibody in the serum or CSF of the patient. The serum to be tested is mixed with known quantities of complement plus the antigen targeted by the antibodies to be measured. The degree of complement fixation indicates the amount of antibody in the specimen. CF is used for diagnosis of some viral and fungal infections, particularly coccidioidomycosis.

Enzyme immunoassays are based on detection of antibody binding to a substrate linked to an enzyme. They are very sensitive and for that reason, commonly used for screening. They include the enzyme immunoassay (EIA) and the enzyme-linked immunosorbent assay (ELISA). ELISA is available for *Chlamydia* infections, herpes virus, and human immunodeficiency virus (HIV). On the other hand, Western blot test detects the specific antibodies by measuring its union to antigens fixed to a membrane by blotting. It is quite specific and commonly used as a confirmatory test in tandem with ELISA as the screening test (i.e. in HIV, HTLV-1, and *Borrelia burgdorferi*).

Other examples of humoral responses that can be tested include the treponemal serology test (including VDRL, RPR, and the most specific FTA-Abs), as well as antibodies against *Borrelia*, *Legionella*, *Bartonella*, and *Leptospira*. Also many viral infections, such as hepatitis A, B and C, Epstein-Barr virus (EBV), dengue, CMV, coxsackie, and parvovirus can be tested. Rising titers of four times the normal baseline over a 2-week period are especially useful in viral diseases with occasional skin involvement. Even parasitic diseases such as enteric amebiasis, cysticercosis, and fasciolasis, as well as toxocariasis and toxoplasmosis can be studied via serology.

Molecular biology

The current concept in the use of molecular biology techniques is based on the detection of DNA and RNA material from specific organisms, providing an extremely reliable method of diagnosis with high specificity and sensitivity. The current method can rely either on the amplification of the material and posterior identification (polymerase chain reaction) or on the direct detection of the material in tissues (in situ hybridization).

Polymerase chain reaction (PCR) consists of denaturalization of nuclear material (DNA), with posterior addition of complementary primers and synthesis of new chains by adding an enzyme such as a polymerase. By using repeated cycles of high and low temperatures one can obtain an amplification of nuclear material (amplicon) until reaching amounts detectable by gel eletrophoresis or enzyme assay base using color detection. Real time PCR is a more sophisticated method, whereas the newly synthesized amplicons can be detected as they are produced by using immunofluorescent methods. Ligase-based method (LCR) amplifies the probe rather than the microorganism's nuclear material. Some methods, like transcription-mediated amplification (TMA) and nucleid acid sequence-based amplification (NASBA), rely on the amplification of RNA material, which is usually more abundant than DNA. The current application for those techniques includes several pathogens listed in Table T-3. For example, both PCR and TMA are FDA approved for the diagnosis of pulmonary and extrapulmonary tuberculosis. By this technique, some researchers have been able to demostrate the presence of bacillus in cutaneous tuberculosis and tuberculids. These findings are, however, not consistent with other similar studies. The variable sensitivity and specificity of the method may be related to tissue inhibitors or fixation methods. PCR is also available for the second and third most common mycobacteriosis around the world, which are, *Mycobacterium leprae* and *Mycobacterium ulcerans*. The PCR technique has been very helpful in the study and discovery of new bartonella species as well.

Several viruses are suitable for PCR testing, with some variations in methodology such as the multiplex reverse transcriptase PCR used in varicella zoster infections. The cause–effect relation between HHV-8 and Kaposi's sarcoma has been demostrated by PCR. The role of different HPV in cutaneous neoplasia, such as HPV-16 in verrucous carcinoma of the foot and HPV-6 and -11 in anogenital verrucous carcinoma have been possible by this amplification method. PCR allows not only identification but also quantification of viral loads in in HIV infections. In some parasitic diseases such as leishmaniasis, the PCR techniques are considered quite sensitive and quite specific. The gene targets include 18S-rRNA, small subunit rRNA, mini-exon gene repeat, β-tubulin gene, transcriber spacer regions, and microsatellite DNA of the kinetoplast. The sensitivity is so high that it may allow detection of as little as half a parasite. Many fungal infections can now be precisely identified, as is the case for mycetomas by *Madurella mycetomatis*.

Another useful technique now available is in situ hybridization (ISH). It is based on the detection of nucleic acid material from different microorganisms directly in tissues, even if they are fixed in formalin. Fluorescent ISH (FISH) is a more sophisticated

Table T-3: Skin infectious diseases where PCR can be a useful diagnostic technique

Bacterial pathogens

  Mycobacterium tuberculosis

  M. leprae

  M. ulcerans

  Rickettsia rickettsii

  R. prowazekii

  Baronella henselae

Spirochetes

  Treponema pallidum

  Borrelia burgdorferi

Virus

  Herpes simplex 1 and Herpes simplex 2

  Varicela zoster virus

  Human herpesvirus 8

  Human papillomavirus

  HIV

  Hepatitis C virus

  Parvovirus B19

  Epstein-Barr virus

Parasites

  Leishmania infantum

  Leishmania braziliensis

  Balamuthia mandrillaris

Fungi

  Aspergillus fumigatus

  Aspergillus versicolor

  Aspergillus flavus

  Blastomyces dermatitides

  Cryptococcus neoformans

  Candida albicans

  Candida dubliniensis

  Coccidioides immitis

  Histoplasma capsulatum

  Sporothrix schenckii

  Madurella mycetomatis

  Various dermatophytes

Modified from Sra KK, Torres G, Rady P, Hughes TK, Payne DA, Tyring SK. Molecular diagnosis of infectious diseases in dermatology. J Am Acad Dermatol. 2005 Nov;53(5):749–65.

Table T-4: Infectious Agents that can be Identified by ISH

Varicella Zoster

Molluscum contagiosum

HIV

HPV

EBV

Hepatitis C virus

HHV-8

Mycobacterium tuberculosis

Mycobacterium leprae

Leishmania spp.

Candida albicans

Cryptococcus neoformans

Modified from Sra KK, Torres G, Rady P, Hughes TK, Payne DA, Tyring SK. Molecular diagnosis of infectious diseases in dermatology. *J Am Acad Dermatol* 2005;53(5):749–765.

method that is used not only to identify infectious agents but also in gene mapping and chromosome analysis. ISH has been used to confirm the presence of HPV in epidermodysplasia verruciformis and EBV in hydroa-like lymphomas. Table T-4 details infectious agents that can be identified by ISH.

The development of DNA microarray technology, also known as DNA chip technology, will allow testing for multiple microorganisms or genetic defects, all at once. In this method, DNA from a clinical sample is first amplified by PCR, converted to RNA or more DNA, mixed with fluorescent dyes, and then applied over a plate containing many different oligonucleotides or cDNA libraries. After the hybridization between sample material and fixed probes on the plates takes place, stimulation by laser will light up the hybridized labeled probes. The total image then obtained will reflect the DNA or RNA contents in the original sample and compare them to control arrays. This technique has allowed identification of M. tuberculosis variants with gene mutations conferring resistance to isoniazid and rifampin. As more of these sophisticated methods become available, our understanding of disease mechanisms and the interactions between humans and pathogens will be complemented by knowledge about microorganism genetic variations, drug resistance, and disease epidemiology.

Skin biopsy as a diagnostic technique

While dealing with cutaneous infectious diseases the accessibility of skin as a source of sampling makes the biopsy an important diagnostic tool. Like any other method, one can determine the sensitivity and specificity of the biopsy for diagnostic purposes. Specificity can be very high, as in a case of molluscum contagiosum or rhinoscleroma, or very low, such as in a grossly superinfected ulcer, where one can see many bacterial colonies on the surface. The sensitivity can be very high, in a case of South

American blastomycosis (paracoccidioidomycosis), or very low in a case of sporotrichosis.

Biopsies can be considered suggestive of, compatible with, or diagnostic of a specific infectious disease. How we use these terms, although subjective, may be based on the frequency of specific histological patterns seen associated with a specific agent, or the findings of the microorganism itself in the histological cuts. We think the term "suggestive" should be used if the histological pattern is commonly seen in a condition unsuspected by the clinician. The term "compatible with" should be used if the pattern seen coincides with one of the entities considered in the differential listed by the clinician, although the microorganism itself is not seen. The term "diagnostic of" should imply visualizing the agent itself, and carries the most certainty. Biopsies also allow establishing the inflammatory or neoplastic nature of a lesion.

The prevalence of a specific cell in a pattern will also direct our diagnosis:. For example a plasma cell–rich liquenoid infiltrate with histiocytes will be in favor of a spirochete-induced disease (either syphilis or borreliosis). Vacuolated histiocytes accompanied by a lymphoplasmacytic infiltrate are commonly seen in leishmaniasis, rhinoscleroma, and granuloma inguinale. Suppurative granulomas are indicative of mycobacteria and deep fungal infection. A dense perivascular and interstitial, superficial and deep inflammatory infiltrate rich in eosinophils, with extension into the subcutaneous tissue, is suggestive of a deep larva migrans or gnathostomiasis.

An important fact obtained from the skin biopsy is the granulomatous nature of an infiltrate. Many chronic infectious diseases are characteristically granulomatous. Granulomas can be divided into five types: tuberculous, suppurative, foreign body, palisaded, or sarcoidal. It should be mentioned that tuberculous granulomas are not exclusively seen in tuberculosis but in several other entities. Caseation necrosis is a more reliable sign of tuberculosis, but in its absence, other diagnostic possibilities for tuberculoid granulomas may include leishmaniasis, tuberculoid leprosy, and sporotrichosis. Even caseation necrosis may not be that specific as it can be seen in nontuberculous processes such as rosacea.

Suppurative granulomas, containing neutrophils in the center, are commonly seen in deep fungal infections such as North American blastomycosis, paracoccidioidomycosis, chromoblastomycosis, and sporotrichosis, as well as in some atypical mycobacterioses. A pseudocarcinomatous hyperplasia may be seen on top of the granuloma. Stellate necrosis in a granuloma is suggestive of cat scratch disease. Sarcoidal granulomas can be seen in sarcoidosis but also as a reaction to foreign materials such as silica and beryllium. Rarely, leprosy and paracoccidioidomycosis can be quite sarcoidal in appearance.

The diagnosis by histological patterns of the inflammatory diseases of the skin, as was outlined by Dr. Ackerman, can also be applied to these infections. There are some patterns that are quite specific for certain diseases like rhinoscleroma, bartonellosis, lepromatous leprosy, and Buruli ulcer.

In rhinoscleroma there is a diffuse infiltrate that occupies all of the dermis. The infiltrate is made up of foamy histiocytes, arranged in mantles. Plasma cells are intermixed in the infiltrates. Some of these cells accumulate such an amount of immunoglobulin within their cytoplasm that they develop into eosinophilic globules, so-called Russell bodies. Occasionally, rod-shaped bacteria will be seen within some of the histiocytes. These represent the causal agent, *Klebsiella rhinoscleromatis*.

The cutaneous lesions of bartonellosis (including verruga peruana and bacillary angiomatosis) are characterized by a dome-shaped silhouette. Below a flattened epidermis there is a capillary vascular proliferation, with a background of histiocytes intermingled with small neutrophilic abscesses. Occasionally in cases of bacillary angiomatosis, there is a purple material in the intercellular space representing aggregates of bartonellas. The combination of histiocytes, vascular proliferation, and neutrophilic abscesses should be considered suggestive of infection by this group of bacteria.

Lepromatous leprosy is characterized by a proliferation of foamy histiocytes at the level of the reticular dermis, either in a diffuse or linear form, following vascular or neural structures. Commonly a zone of uninvolved papillary dermis separated from the epidermis may be seen (which is referred to as the Grenz Zone). Basophilic globi represent clumps of intracellular mycobacteria. Buruli ulcer, an infection induced by *M. ulcerans*, will produce a pattern of necrotizing panniculitis with a sparse or absent inflammatory infiltrate, and innumerable acid-fast bacilli will be present as well. This pattern of bacteria-rich necrotizing panniculitis is not seen in any other mycobacterioses like tuberculosis or leprosy.

Depending on how easily the causative microorganism can be seen, skin biopsies can be divided into three categories: biopsies of high, medium, and low sensitivity.

The first category is those biopsies that have a high diagnostic sensitivity. They are diagnostic when the causal agent is seen either in routine (H&E) or slides stained for microorganisms. Examples in this category include molluscum contagiosum, *K. rhinoescleromatis*, and deep fungal agents such as *P. braziliensis* (South American blastomycosis), *L. loboi* (lobomycosis), *C. neoformans*, *C. immitis*, *B. dermatitides*, *H. capsulatum*, and the agents of chromoblastomycosis. Easily detectable as well are the sulphur grains of actinomycosis, eumycetomas, and actinomycetomas. The acid-fast stain allows the detection of innumerable bacilli in lepromatous leprosy and Buruli ulcer. PAS and Gomori stains typically reveal large amounts of hyphae in mucormycosis or in immunosuppresed patients with invasive aspergillosis.

The second category includes entities with biopsies of medium diagnostic sensitivity. In such cases the infectious agent is not always visible in the routine cuts. Agents occasionally seen in skin biopsies include leishmaniasis, free living amebas, bartonellas in cases of bacillary angiomatosis (with Warthin-Starry stain), and dermatophytes. In leishmaniasis the number of visible parasites is related to the different evolutionary stages and the degree of immunity developed by the host. In early lesions the *Leishmania* spp. are seen intracellulary inside macrophages close to the epidermis. In cases of poor immune response (the so-called diffuse cutaneous leishmaniasis), the parasites are observed in great numbers as intracellular forms. In long-standing cases, the infiltrate is made of lymphocytes and plasma cells, and the possibility of finding parasites is small. If present, they are scarce, and they can easily be confused with fragments of plasma cells. So, in leishmania cases the specificity of the biopsy diminishes as a method of diagnosis. It is better to take a panel approach, including intradermal leishmanin tests, direct examination and culture, and where available, PCR studies. In syphilis cases, an inmunoperoxidase stain is now available that can facilitate the identification of treponemes in tissue cuts.

The last category is of those biopsies with very little diagnostic sensitivity, where the microorganism is particularly difficult to visualize, even with special stains. This includes parasites causing cutaneous larvae migrans, gnathostomiasis, fungi such as *Sporotrichum*, and bacteria such as the bartonellas of verruga peruana. Also difficult to see are *M. tuberculosis*, *M. marinum*, and the *M. leprae* in cases of tuberculoid leprosy. In sporotrichosis, diagnosis is based on culture isolation, which is by far the method of greatest sensitivity. In tuberculosis, the direct examination and culture also have a low sensitivity. Commonly, just a tuberculous granulomatous inflammation is seen. It is in this group of diseases that PCR technology appears very promising. Special stains such as rodamine or immunoperoxidases such as anti-BCG may allow better detection.

In summary, the biopsy of skin is of variable utility from a diagnostic point of view. The diagnosis can be suggested by a specific pattern, but absolute certainty is only obtained when the causal agent can be seen. The clinician should consider these limitations. Rather than depending only on special stains, the pathologist should familiarize himself or herself with the histological pattern of the disease, as well as with the frequency the causal organisms are seen in routine cuts. The new techniques of immunoperoxidase and PCR will indeed play a role in those entities where routine H&E-stained biopsies have the lowest sensitivity.

SUGGESTED READINGS

Nagar R, Pande S, Khopkar U. Intradermal tests in dermatology-I: tests for infectious diseases. *Indian J Dermatol Venereol Leprol* 2006;72(6):461–465.

Nelson K. Tuberculin testing to detect latent tuberculosis in developing countries. *Epidemiology* 2007;18(3):348–349.

Sadeghian G, Momeni A, Siadat AH, Usefi P. Evaluation of leishmanin skin test and its relationship with the clinical form and duration of cutaneous leishmaniasis. *Dermatol Online J* 2006;12(7):3.

Sra KK, Torres G, Rady P, Hughes TK, Payne DA, Tyring SK. Molecular diagnosis of infectious diseases in dermatology. *J Am Acad Dermatol* 2005;53(5):749–765.

PRINCIPLES OF MANAGEMENT OF DERMATOLOGIC INFECTIONS IN THE SKIN

John C. Hall

As with all of medicine, correct therapy depends on a correct diagnosis, which is established through clinical and laboratory (see chapter on *techniques in diagnosing manifestations of infections*) observations.

The progress of an infection can be more carefully monitored in the skin than in any other organ due to ease of clinical observation. The four primary signs of acute infection are color, warmth, tenderness (and/or pain) and swelling. Additional signs include induration, erosion or ulceration, vesiculation, pustulation, linear streaking along lymphatics, lymphadenopathy, asymmetry, vasculitic appearance, necrosis, and progression. This progression can be visually monitored and marking the edge with an indelible marker can help demonstrate the spread or regression of the edge of the infection. These clinical signs can all be less apparent in the growing population of immunocompromised patients who do not mount the typical immune response. On the contrary, immunocompromised patients may have worse clinical signs that appear at a faster rate than those seen in nonimmunocompromised individuals.

Probably the best example of the importance of these principles in all of medicine is illustrated in the case of necrotizing fasciitis, the sine qua non of importance for the skin and infectious diseases. Each chapter will have a brief history about the disease or diseases covered at the beginning as well as a reminder of potential pitfalls and myths at the end. The pitfalls and myths section will help to serve as a summary of where it is easy to go wrong clinically and where you want to go right. Necrotizing fasciitis will be used as a brief sample of how each chapter will be laid out in the book.

HISTORY

Necrotizing fasciitis is thought to be first named and described in detail by Joseph Jones, who was a historian and leading medical officer in the Confederate army during the Civil War of the United States. He kept copious records of hundreds of patients seen during the civil war including many injured soldiers at Andersonville prison in Georgia, which was ill equipped in resources and physical room to keep the overabundance of captured Union troops who often died of malnutrition, disease, and starvation. The original designation for this illness was "hospital gangrene." Fournier, a respected French dermatologist was credited with describing a group of patients with this form of cellulitis in the groin, mainly in men, 1883 and hence the designation "Fournier's gangrene." In 1924, Meleny ("Meleney's ulcer") recognized that this condition rapidly became a fatal systemic disease. Wilson coined the term "necrotizing fasciitis" in 1952. Five cases were reported in Gloucestershire, England, between June 1 and June 30, 1994 and two of theses cases were seen in patients who had an operation in the same operating theater. This led to the idea that it was a highly contagious "flesh-eating" bacterial infection. No other such cluster of patients has ever been reported, however.

CLINICAL DIAGNOSIS

The commonest predisposing condition is diabetes (seen in 40 to 50%), especially when associated with dialysis. Other associated underlying diseases are traumatic wounds, AIDS, metastatic cancer (with or without chemotherapy), varicella (especially in children which is sometimes called varicella gangrenosum), postoperatively and rarely post delivery. The abdomen, perineum, and extremities are the commonest areas affected.

Fever is present in at least two-thirds of patients with hypotension and in at least a third of cases. Altered sensorium is present in approximately one-fourth of patients and crepitus in 10%.

Pain and anesthesia have both been reported at the site of erythema, which rapidly becomes edematous and bluish. Gangrene develops within 5 days or less and may or may not be covered with a bulla. Mortality can range from 25% to 50%, especially if treatment is delayed. An unexplained association with the oral use of nonsteroidal anti-inflammatory agents has been reported in some cases.

LABORATORY DIAGNOSIS

A several fold increase in creatinine phosphokinase can be helpful in differentiating necrotizing fasciitis from erysipelas or other more benign types of cellulitis. Culture most often shows group A β-hemolytic streptococci (including strains causing toxic shock) when there is a single agent present. *Klebsiella* is probably the second most common. Community-acquired methicillin-resistant *Staphylococcus aureus* has also been reported as a pathogen. There is a trend toward more polymicrobic infections. Necrotic tissue for culture may be helpful in determining the causative bacteria, but awaiting this report can be fatal for the patient.

TREATMENT

Poor prognosis is associated with increased age (especially greater than 60 years old), female gender, delay of first debridement, extent of infection, increased creatinine, increased lactate, anemia, thrombocytopenia, and extent of other organ system involvement.

Early extensive surgical debridement is mandatory (magnetic resonance imaging may help tell the extent of debridement necessary) and may have to be repeated multiple times.

Immediate intravenous broad-spectrum antibiotic therapy with adequate coverage for streptococci, staphylococci, as well as gram-negative organisms is also important. This can be modified when cultures are obtained. Hyperbaric oxygenation and high-dose intravenous IgG immunoglobulin have been advocated as being beneficial by some authors.

PITFALLS AND MYTHS

This skin infection illustrates the importance of early decision making based on clinical data. Laboratory data may be confirmatory but may be acquired too late to save the patient's life. Overtreatment of a less serious infection is preferable to undertreatment of necrotizing fasciitis. The difficult patient is the one with a paucity of symptoms, (i.e. patients exhibiting no pain and little generalized toxicity). Do not assume that a relatively asymptomatic patient is not gravely ill and will stay symptom free for very long. Hospitalization is quite helpful since significant changes in the patient's condition can occur over hours. This disease is usually more extensive than first suspected (see Fig. Principles.1).

Do not let cultures that do not show streptococci or are polymicrobic dissuade you from the diagnosis. When reviewing the medical literature remember that multiple names may have been used for the same condition. "Progressive ischemic gangrene" is one example.

Clinical judgment and close observation are of no small importance. Remember that in any skin infection the great advantage is that the skin can be easily seen and followed as no other organ. Use your skill of careful surveillance.

While awaiting laboratory confirmation of a clinical diagnosis there are a subgroup of patients (such as those discussed already with necrotizing fasciitis) that are so ill that empiric therapy needs to be started before actual identification of the offending organism is established (see Table Principles.1).

With infections in dermatology, unlike many other specialties, there is often an opportunity to use topical instead of oral, intramuscular, subcutaneous, or intravenous therapy. The advantages of topical versus systemic treatment of cutaneous infections is discussed in Table Principles.2. Combination therapy in serious disease is often the best choice.

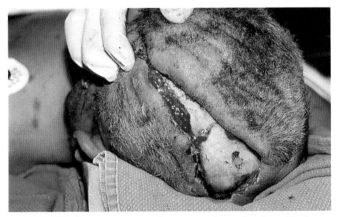

Figure Principles.1 Necrotizing fasciitis on the scalp of an elderly man with MRI showing extension well into the neck and shoulders. Culture was positive for β-hemolytic streptococci. The patient survived in large part due to repeated aggressive surgeries.

Table Principles.1 Conditions Where Empiric Therapy Is Needed

Blueberry muffin baby with generalized papules, pustules, or purpura at birth (always cover for herpes simplex virus until diagnosis is confirmed) and consider the TORCH (toxoplasmosis, others {HIV, syphilis, varicella}, rubella, cytomegalovirus, herpes simplex) complex

Necrotizing Fasciitis (always cover for streptococci)

Cellulitis (always cover for staphylococcus and β-hemolytic streptococci since a positive culture is often difficult and may only be obtainable from a blood culture if patient is septic)

Cutaneous necrosis (cover for staphylococcus, β-hemolytic streptococci and if indicated by history for *vibrio vulnificus* infection or if indicated by clinical setting for sepsis and immunocompromise, pseudomonas, candidiasis, or aspergillosis)

Vasculitis (cover for Rocky Mountain spotted fever and meningococcus)

Staphylococcal scalded skin syndrome (cover for staphylococci including methicillin-resistant staphylococci, which may now be community acquired and streptococci)

Atypical mycobacteria (histopathology and culture may be falsely negative, so may have to treat based on clinical impression alone)

Table Principles.2 Topical vs Systemic Therapy for Skin Infections

	Topical Therapy	Systemic Therapy
Pro	1. Less systemic side effects	1. More efficacious, faster
	2. No access site needed	2. Treats concomitant disease in other organs
	3. Gastrointestinal absorption not essential	3. Can monitor blood levels
	4. No gastrointestinal symptoms	
	5. Less chance of sensitization	
	6. Healing benefit of a base as well as an anti-infectious agent	
Con	1. Topical therapy may obscure disease progression	1. Serious allergic reaction more likely
	2. Contact sensitization can occur	2. May need access site
	3. Less efficacious, slower	3. May be much more expensive
	4. Systemic absorption can still result in systemic side effects	4. May not be available
		5. Absorption of oral drugs may be erratic
		6. Drug interactions are an important consideration

Table Principles.3 General Guidelines for Topical Therapy of Skin Infections

1. Ointments' (hydrophobic) bases repel water and tend to hold the product on the skin longer and increase penetration. Ointments also protect the skin better and facilitate re-epitheliazation.

2. If a skin condition is weeping or oozing then an initial period of 2 to 5 days may be needed when the exudate is debrided chemically or surgically or the wound is dried with water, saline, Aveeno (oatmeal), or Domeboro compresses. A cream (hydrophilic base) may be used if more drying is felt to be indicated.

3. A thick adherent eschar may need surgical debridement to allow healing and treatment of the underlying infection.

4. Incision and drainage may be as important or more important (as shown in the recent outbreak of MRSA skin infections) than any topical or even systemic therapy.

5. Restoration of the epidermal barrier (such as in eczema) is necessary to prevent the need for continual therapy.

6. Signs of increased heat, spreading redness, regional lymphadenopathy, fever, and increased tenderness may indicate that systemic therapy needs to be added to topical therapy.

7. Allergic contact dermatitis due most commonly to antibiotics, antifungals, antiyeast, preservatives, and adhesives in tape and other surgical dressings needs to be considered in the differential diagnosis of any worsening skin infection. Clues to this include itching, blistering, and sudden increased redness without fever or regional lymphadenopathy. Unless accurately diagnosed, the condition will continue to worsen.

8. Systemic absorption of the drug is always a consideration. This is especially a concern when the epidermal barrier is compromised, in intertriginous areas where absorption is increased, large areas are treated, and in infants where the body surface area is increased, when large areas compared to the body mass.

Table Principles.4 Topical Therapy for Skin Infections

Antibacterial	Bacitracin
	Neosporin cream and ointment contains polymyxin B, Neomycin, bacitracin; neomycin allergy 1%
	Polysporin cream and ointment contains polymyxin B and bacitracin; can use if neomycin allergy
	Centany (Bactroban) cream and ointment contains mupirocin, and is effective against MRSA in addition to the same coverage as polysporin and neosporin. Resistance by some staphylococci is reported
	Silver-containing compounds used in chronic ulcers, burn patients, and patients with toxic epidermal necrolysis
	0.5 % silver nitrate solution poured over dressing
	Silvadene Cream (cannot use if sulfa allergy is present)
	Aquacel Ag Hydrofiber
	Acticoat Absorbent Fiber
	Silvercel
	Contreet Foam
	Polymem Silver Foam
	Urgotal S. Ag
	Silvasorb Hydrogel
	Iodine-containing products
	Betadine solution, surgical scrub, hand cleanser, and ointment
	Tincture of iodine
	Lugol's solution
	Altabax (retapamulin) ointment
	Gentamicin cream and ointment

Antibacterial	Bacitracin
Antifungal	Imidazoles effective against yeast and dermatophytes
	Micatin (Monistat) cream contains miconazole
	Lotrimin cream contains clotrimazole
	Lotrisone lotion contains clotrimazole and betamethasone
	Spectazole cream contains intraconazole
	Oxistat cream contains oxiconazole
	Nizoril cream, shampoo, lotion contains ketoconazole
	Ertaczo contains sertaconazole
	Ciclopirox effective against yeast and dermatophytes
	Loprox gel, lotion and shampoo and Penlac nail lacquer
	Whitfield's ointment (6% salicylic acid, 12% benzoic acid) is also antiyeast and antibacterial
Antiyeast	See above
	Nystatin cream, ointment, oral suspension contains nystatin
	Mycolog II cream and ointment contains nystatin and triamcinolone
Antiviral	Denavir contains penciclovir for herpes simplex
	Zovirax contains acyclovir for herpes simplex
	Aldara contains imiquimod for warts (esp. genital warts), molluscum contagiosum
Antiparasitic	Thiabendazole for cutaneous larva migrans
	Aldara (imiquimod) for leishmaniasis
	Permethrin for lice and scabies
	Malathione for lice
	Gammabenzene hexachloride for lice and scabies but permethrin has largely replaced this medication since it is less toxic
	Results (50% isopropyl myristate) for lice
Nonspecific (helps all infections by changing pH and acting as a drying agent)	Domeboro compresses (dilute in water with packets or tablets)
	Vinegar compresses (mainly for pseudomonas or gram-negative infections) can use equal parts white vinegar and water
	Bleach compresses (mainly recurrent *Staphylococcus aureus* infections) can use 1 tbsp in 1 pint of water or one cup to a full tub of water as a soak

Topical therapy has some general guidelines, which helps when trying to select the correct topical agent (see Table Principles.3)

A formulary for the most commonly used topical agents is listed in Table Principles.4. When dealing with infected ulcers and wounds, chemical or surgical debridement is an important fundamental part of therapy.

Infectious diseases of the skin may be transmitted by insect vectors, and it is important, therefore, to discuss repellants of these pests (Table Principles.5). Prevention of these potentially hazardous envenomations is the best treatment. Bees, wasps, hornets, and yellow jackets are not repelled by insect repellants. They can become secondarily infected with streptococci and staphylococci. There is no proven effective repellant for ticks, and tsetse flies also do not respond to insect repellants. Insect bed netting should have 1.5 mm openings or less for mosquitoes. If coated with permethrin there is more protection. Finer mesh is needed for sandflies.

No discussion of dermatology and infection would be complete without mentioning the importance of cutaneous transmission of infections. Universal precautions in the hospital or outpatient setting are a mandatory part of any attempt to control the spread of disease. Antiseptic liquids that can be applied without water are very easily accessed in both the hospital and outpatient clinics and have become a mainstay of decreasing skin transmission of infectious diseases.

Table Principles.5 Insect Repellants for Mosquitoes and Sandflies

DEET (N,N-diethylmeta-toluamide)	Effective against mosquitoes, especially at higher concentrations above 20%
	Available in a longer-acting formula (Ultrathon-lasts 8 hours)
	20 to 30% used as directed is safe
	Effective when applied to clothes
	May damage some plastics
	Avoid repetitive use to large areas of skin especially in children
Picaridin (KBR 2033)	Available in Europe, Asia, Australia and Latin America for years
	New 7% variant available in United States
	No odor, will not damage plastic
	Not a dermal sensitizer
	Good repellent for mosquitoes flies, no see-ums, fleas
	No toxicity
	According to WHO best repellant for preventing malaria
	Reapply after several hours
Permethrin (Permanone)	Apply to clothing only
	0.5% permethrin spray is applied to clothing and may last up to 6 weeks
	Examples of sprays are Repel and Sawyer
	Permethrin Tick Repellant
	The best way to apply is to spray on clothes outside and let it dry (it is inactivated in 15 minutes on the skin)
	Potent dermal sensitizer
	May help repel and kill ticks,
Oil of Lemon Eucalyptus	Not approved in children under 3 y/o
	Active ingredient should be oil of lemon eucalyptus (PMD) and not the essential or pure oil of lemon eucalyptus
	Repels mosquitoes, flies, gnats
	Safe but odiferous
	Examples are Repel Eucalyptus Oil (6 hour Protection), Cutter Lemon Eucalyptus Spray
Cintronella	As a candle possibly some benefit
	No evidence of topical application benefit
Precipitated Sulfur	Shake powder in socks or shoes
	Effective for most insects, possibly even ticks, but has a "rotten egg" odor
Catnip Oil (nepatalactone)	Probably ineffective
Soybean Oil	Repels, mosquitoes, gnats, no see-ums, ticks
	Safe even in children
	Relatively sweat and waterproof
Vitamin B1	Example is Bite Blocker for Kids
	Don't Bite Me for Kids Patch
	Waterproof and safe
	Mosquitoes, gnats, no see-ums, ticks may be repelled
Composite Repellants	Example is Sawyer Gold Repellant (Contains DEET 17% and MGK 2645)
Callicarpenal (derived from Beauty Berry shrub)	Appears to be safe and effective for mosquitoes, ticks, fireants
	Not yet available for commercial use

Table Principles.6 Skin Diseases Associated with Increased Infection

Eczema	Interruption of epidermal barrier.
	Decrease in immunity especially to staphylococcus.
Psoriasis	Interruption of epidermal barrier. Not as well documented as in eczema.
Burns	Second- or third-degree causes loss of epidermal barrier, especially *Pseudomonas aeruginosa*.
Toxic Epidermal Necrolysis	Loss of epidermal barrier and sepsis is the usual cause of death frequently acquired through the skin.
Epidermolysis Bullosa	Especially in the more severe recessive form of the disease.
Hailey-Hailey Disease	Control of yeast and bacterial infection is an important
(Chronic Benign Familial Pemphigus)	part of therapy. Loss of epidermal barrier in intertriginous macerated areas.
Pemphigus Vulgaris	Loss of epidermal barrier. Sepsis is usual cause of death, often entering through the skin
Wiskott-Aldrich Syndrome	Decreased immunity
Interdigital tinea pedis	Especially in diabetics this can be a nidis for tinea, candida and ultimately staph and strep and can lead to a limb threatening infection. Related to local factors of warmth and wetness and increased susceptibility in a diabetic patient.
Chronic leg ulcers	Decreased circulation either arterial (ischemic ulcers) or venous (stasis ulcers) and no epidermal barrier.
Puncture wounds	Be sure tetanus vaccinations up to date. Copious irrigation.
Animal bites	Augmentin is probable drug of choice.

Table Principles.7 Noninfectious Skin Diseases that Mimic Infection

Disease	Infections Mimicked
Pyoderma gangrenosum	Furuncle or carbuncle early
	Infected ulcer or granulomatous infection late.
Eosinophilic fasciitis	Cellulitis
Sclerosing panniculitis	Cellulitis
Thrombophlebitis	Cellulitis with lymphangitis
Steroid folliculitis	Staphylococcous Folliculitis
Eosinophilic pustular folliculitis	Staphylococcous Folliculitis
Angioedema	Erysipelas
Relapsing polychondritis	Cellulitis
Pityriasis rosea	Secondary syphilis
Acute generalized eruptitve pustular drug eruption	Staphylococcous folliculitis
Pustular psoriasis	Staphylococcous folliculitis
Inflammatory breast cancer	Cellulitis
Subcutaneous emphysema	Cellulitis
Nummular eczema	Impetigo
Contact dermatitis	Cellulitis
Fixed drug eruption	Herpes simplex
Guttate psoriasis	Secondary syphilis
Hidradinitis suppurativa	Carbuncles, furuncles
	Granuloma inguinale
	Abscesses
Dissecting cellulitis of the scalp	Abscesses
Pustular acne	Staphylococcal folliculitis
Cystic acne	Abscesses
Lethal midline granuloma (lymphoma)	Granulomatous infections such as deep fungi or mucormycosis
Stewart-Treves syndrome	Cellulitis
Vasculitis	Cellulitis
Squamous cell cancer	Granulomatous infections such as deep fungi, mycobacteria, mycetoma or leishmaniasis, verrucae
Actinic keratosis	Verrucae
Seborrheic keratosis	Verrucae
Ruptured sebaceous cyst	Abscess
Brown recluse spider bite	Cellulitis, necrotizing fasciitis
Sweet's syndrome	Cellulitis
Well's syndrome	Cellulitis
Lymphoma	Granulomatous infection
	Cellulitis
	Nodular scabies

Disease	Infections Mimicked
Dermatitis herpetiformis	Scabies
Herald patch of Pityriasis rosea	Tinea corporis
Granuloma annulare	Tinea corporis
Insect bites	Hot tub folliculitis (Pseudomonas)
Verrucous carcinoma	Verrucae
Oral lichen planus	Candidiasis (Thrush)
Psoriasis of the nails	Onychomycosis
Bowen's disease in the groin	Tinea cruris (especially if unilateral)
Extramammary Paget's in the groin	Tinea cruris (especially if unilateral)
Dyshidrotic eczema	Vesicular tinea pedis
Pilonidal cyst	Abscess
Morbilliform drug reaction	Viral exanthem
Panniculitis	Cellulitis
Parasitophobia	Scabies
Fiberglass dermatitis	Scabies
Psoriasis	Crusted or Norwegian scabies
Factitial dermatitis	Almost any infection in which culture and histopathology are repeatedly negative for organisms and especially if the course is atypical

In the general population, infection is more apt to be acquired through skin that has had epidermal barrier damage. The opportunity to treat these infections early is apt to make the overall burden of disease much less. The commonest examples of these are listed in Table Principles.6.

Just as infections can mimic a multitude of noninfectious skin conditions, noninfectious skin conditions can also mimic infection. Some of those most common of these pseudoinfections of the skin are listed in the following Table Principles.7.

SUGGESTED READINGS

Elliott DC, et al. Necrotizing soft tissue infections. Risk factors for mortality and strategies for management. *Ann Surg.* 1996;224(5):672–683.

Liu YM et al. Microbiology and factors affecting mortality in necrotizing fasciitis. *J Microbiol Immunol Infect* (2005);38(6):430–435.

Misago N, et al. Necrotizing Fasciitis due to group A streptococci: a clinicopathological study of six patients. *J Dermatol.* 1996;23(12):876–882.

Vulgia JD, et al. Necrotizing fasciitis 24 cases in children with varicella. *Renal Fail,* 1995;17(4):438–447.

PART I: COMMON INFECTIONS

1 | COMMON BACTERIAL INFECTIONS

Tammie Ferringer

INTRODUCTION

Uncomplicated skin and skin structure infections (uSSSIs) are frequent causes of office visits. The most common bacterial uSS-SIs include impetigo, ecthyma, folliculitis, furuncles, carbuncles, abscesses, erysipelas, and cellulitis.

Folliculitis

Follicular pustules, often with a rim of erythema, characterize folliculitis (Fig. 1.1). Bacterial is one cause, but physical and chemical irritations are also etiologic factors. Predisposing factors include shaving, occlusion, oily topicals, staphylococcal carriage, and friction. Children and young adults are most commonly affected, but folliculitis can occur at any age. Areas of involvement include the face, scalp, beard, axillae, buttocks, and legs.

Hot-tub folliculitis is a variant associated with the use of contaminated hot tubs, whirlpools, and heated swimming pools. This characteristically pruritic folliculitis commonly develops on the trunk 1 to 4 days after exposure.

Furuncles/Carbuncles/Abscesses

Folliculitis, furuncles, and carbuncles represent a continuum of follicular infection. Furuncles or "boils" (Fig. 1.2) are similar to folliculitis, however, the suppurative infiltrate extends beyond the follicle into the dermis and subcutaneous fat. These lesions are fluctuant and tender but typically do not have systemic symptoms. These nodules eventually rupture and discharge pus. The most commonly involved areas are those prone to friction, including the breasts, axillae, buttocks, and thighs. A carbuncle

is a confluence of furuncles with multiple sinus tracts. The posterior neck is a typical location. Occasionally these more complex lesions are associated with fever, malaise, and lymphadenopathy. Chronic staphylococcal carriage, diabetes, and obesity are predisposing factors. Similar to furuncles and carbuncles, abscesses are tender, fluctuant nodules (Fig. 1.3) with surrounding erythema. Abscesses are usually not associated with a follicle.

Cellulitis

Cellulitis is also a nonfollicular infection but typically lacks the purulence of abscesses. Spreading erythema, edema, and warmth

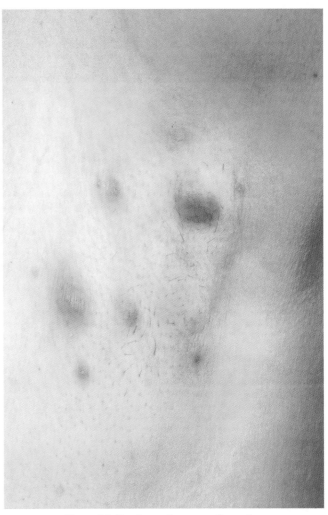

Figure 1.2. Tender erythematous furuncles.

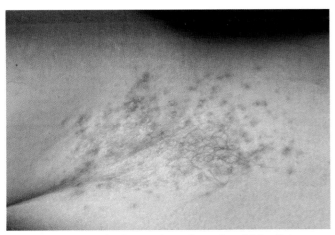

Figure 1.1. Follicular papules and pustules of folliculitis.

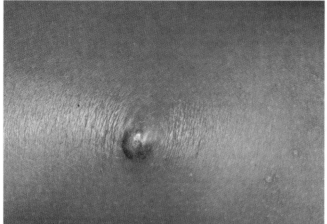

Figure 1.3. Fluctuant nodule consistent with abscess.

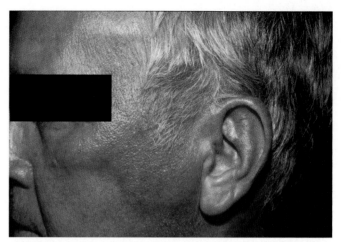

Figure 1.5. Sharply defined erythematous raised border of erysipelas.

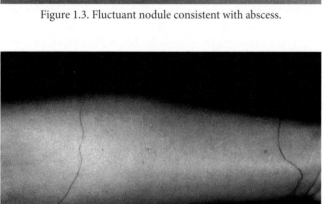

Figure 1.4. Erythema of cellulitis.

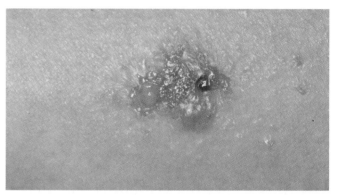

Figure 1.6. Vesicles, pustules, and honey colored crust of impetigo.

characterize cellulitis (Fig. 1.4). The infection involves the deep dermis and subcutaneous tissue and may be associated with mild systemic symptoms including fever and chills. The body area involved varies with age. For children the head and neck are most commonly affected, while in adults the lower extremities are more commonly affected. The breach in skin integrity, which serves as the portal of entry for infection, can be clinically subtle. An underlying dermatosis, macerated interdigital tinea, trauma, surgical incisions, and foreign bodies can all allow entry. Chronic lymphedema, venous insufficiency, diabetes, alcoholism, malignancy, IV drug abuse, and immunosuppression are predisposing factors.

Erysipelas

Erysipelas is a superficial variant of cellulitis that reveals erythema, warmth, tenderness, and peripheral extension. Unlike cellulitis, there is a sharply defined, raised border (Fig. 1.5), and blisters, pustules, and focal hemorrhagic necrosis may be identified. Regional adenopathy, occasionally lymphangitis, and systemic symptoms are often present. The face and legs are the most common sites involved.

Impetigo

Impetigo is a contagious, superficial skin infection. Vesicles and pustules develop on an erythematous base and evolve into the characteristic honey colored crusts (Fig. 1.6). The central face and extremities are the most common areas involved. Skin trauma and a diminished cutaneous barrier from preexisting dermatoses, like eczema, can predispose to impetigo. Other predisposing factors include warm, humid environments and staphylococcal colonization. Although it can affect patients of any age, impetigo is the most common skin infection in pediatric patients. Fewer than one-third of cases of impetigo are of the bullous form. This variety occurs mostly in infants and on normal skin. Bullae larger than 5 mm can be seen.

Ecthyma

Ecthyma is a deeper version of impetigo. The lower extremities are most often affected. This disease is characterized by thick, adherent crusts over ulcers (Fig. 1.7) with an indurated border that often heals with scars.

HISTORY

Penicillin was introduced in the early 1940s as a treatment for infections caused by gram-positive cocci, such as *Staphylococcus aureus*. Shortly after, antibiotic resistance became increasingly obvious. Currently, the majority of staphylococci are resistant to penicillins due to the production of β-lactamase. Surprisingly, over the years, *Streptococcus pyogenes* has still remained susceptible.

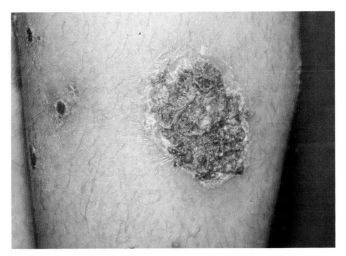

Figure 1.7. Thick adherent crust over ulceration that characterizes ecthyma.

Table 1.1: Bacterial Infections and Associated Organisms

Infection	Organism
Folliculitis	*Staphylococcus aureus* *Pseudomonas aeruginosa* (Hot-tub folliculitis)
Furuncles/Carbuncles	*S. aureus*
Abscess	Polymicrobial reflecting regional flora *S. aureus* alone in one-quarter
Erysipelas	*Streptococcus pyogenes*
Cellulitis	*S. aureus* *Streptococcus pyogenes*
Ecthyma	*St. pyogenes* *S. aureus*
Impetigo	*S. aureus* *St. pyogenes*

Table 1.2: Characteristics of CA-MRSA and HA-MRSA

Characteristic	CA-MRSA	HA-MRSA
Risk factors	Day care attendees, athletes, prisoners, soldiers, IV drug users, homosexual men, homeless, Native Americans, Alaska natives, Pacific Islanders	Nursing home residents, hemodialysis patients, prolonged hospitalization, indwelling catheters
Resistance	β-lactam resistance	Multidrug resistance
Infection	Folliculits, furuncles, and abscesses	Pneumonia, catheter-related urinary or bloodstream infection, postoperative infection

CA-MRSA, community-acquired methicillin-resistant *Staphylococcus aureus*; HA-MRSA, hospital-acquired methicillin-resistant *Staphylococcus aureus*.

Methicillin was introduced in 1959 to overcome the problem of resistance, but this was rapidly followed by identification of methicillin-resistant *Staphylococcus aureus* (MRSA). Since then, hospital-associated MRSA (HA-MRSA) has steadily increased. More recently, community-acquired MRSA (CA-MRSA) came to national attention after reports of outbreaks in prisons and athletic teams in 2002. To this day there continues to be an alarming increase in the incidence of CA-MRSA.

EPIDEMIOLOGY

S. aureus and Group A β-hemolytic streptococci (*Streptococcus pyogenes)* are the organisms most commonly associated with uSSSIs. Table 1.1 lists the most common causes of the uncomplicated bacterial skin infections.

S. aureus is the most common cause of bacterial folliculitis. However, under certain conditions other organisms may be the cause. For example, hot-tub folliculitis is caused by *Pseudomonas aeruginosa*, and patients receiving chronic oral antibiotics for acne may develop gram-negative folliculitis, most commonly due to *Klebsiella pneumoniae* and Enterobacteriaceae.

Like folliculitis, the most common cause of furuncles and carbuncles is *S. aureus*. Abscesses, on the other hand, are often polymicrobial and reflect the regional skin flora. However, *S. aureus* is identified alone in about one-fourth of cases.

Erysipelas is caused almost exclusively by *Streptococcus pyogenes*. In most immunocompetent adults, cellulitis is due to *S. aureus* and *St. pyogenes*. Certain circumstances are also associated with other infectious etiologies. Gram-negative bacilli may be causative in neutropenic patients. Cat and dog bites are typically due to *Pasteurella* species or *Capnocytophaga*. Periorbital cellulitis in unimmunized children is due to *Haemophilus influenza*. Etiologic bacteria may reflect the regional skin flora. For example, infection of the ear or toe webs may involve gram-negative organisms while infection adjacent to the gastrointestinal or respiratory tract may include anaerobes.

Streptococcus pyogenes, sometimes with secondary *S. aureus* infection, is the cause of ecthyma. The majority of cases of impetigo are caused by *S. aureus* and less commonly *St. pyogenes*.

S aureus, phage group II type 71, is the predominant causative organism of bullous impetigo. The bulla is due to staphylococcal toxins that cause acantholysis of the granular layer similar to what takes place in staphylococcal scalded skin syndrome.

In addition to possible bacteremia, the primary cutaneous site of infection can rarely be associated with other significant consequences. Some strains of streptococci have the ability to cause acute glomerulonephritis and some produce toxins associated with streptococcal toxic shock syndrome. Treatment of the cutaneous infection does not seem to alter the risk of glomerulonephritis but treatment can decrease spread of the nephrotoxic strain. Toxins produced by some strains of *S. aureus* can result in staphylococcal scalded skin syndrome or staphylococcal toxic shock syndrome.

Methicillin-sensitive *S. aureus* (MSSA) is the most common form of *S. aureus* identified in association with superficial skin infections. However, MRSA has become increasingly frequent. There are two forms of MRSA, health care associated (HA-MRSA) and community acquired (CA-MRSA) (Table 1.2). Antibiotic resistance is a concern with HA-MRSA while CA-MRSA remains sensitive to antibiotics including trimethoprim–sulfamethoxazole and tetracycline. CA-MRSA has increasingly been identified in association with furuncles and abscesses. CA-MRSA typically affects the young and healthy, especially those living in crowded conditions or in close physical contact, and in certain ethnic groups. Those most commonly affected include athletes, military personnel, injection drug users, homosexual men, the homeless, children in day care, prisoners, Pacific islanders, Alaskan natives, and Native Americans.

The CA-MRSA and HA-MRSA isolates are distinct both epidemiologically and genetically, but there is increasing cross-over in clinical presentation. Therefore, it is best to refer to these strains as "community-type strains" and "health care–type strains."

DIAGNOSIS

USSSIs are typically diagnosed by clinical presentation and treated empirically. Tissue culture, needle aspiration, and blood culture have a poor yield in cellulitis and erysipelas. If bullae or an abscess is present, culture of these areas is more likely to be positive.

The diagnosis of impetigo and ecthyma can be confirmed with culture and Gram stain of the exudate below the crust. Culture of the purulent material associated with folliculitis, furuncles, carbuncles, and abscesses is useful to help tailor the antibiotic therapy.

THERAPY

In some uSSSIs, conservative treatment alone is sufficient but in other cases oral antibiotics are necessary. Rarely, resistant cases and complicated skin infections require intravenous antibiotics.

Folliculitis typically resolves spontaneously; however, topical clindamycin, mupirocin, or benzoyl peroxide can accelerate the healing. Disposal of razors and treatment of predisposing factors is required to prevent reinfection. In the case of hot-tub folliculitis, resolution occurs in 1 to 2 weeks with or without treatment. In the case of persistent infection, oral ciprofloxacin is the treatment of choice. The contaminated water source should be identified and corrected to prevent further outbreaks.

In the case of furuncles, carbuncles, and abscesses, pain is relieved with drainage, which can be promoted with moist heat or surgically via incision and drainage. Drainage alone is often sufficient; however, drainage with systemic antibiotics is recommended when there is surrounding cellulitis, deep extension, systemic symptoms, gas-containing lesions, lesions on the central face, and in patients with serious comorbidities such as immunosuppression. Culture at the time of drainage is recommended to allow susceptibility testing to guide the choice of alternative antibiotics in the event of a poor response to empiric therapy.

Treatment of localized impetigo includes topical mupirocin with debridement of the infectious crust. However, mupirocin resistance limits use. Retapamulin ointment was recently approved by the FDA for treatment of impetigo. In nonresponsive or extensive cases of impetigo and in ecthyma, systemic antibiotics are required.

Erysipelas and cellulitis in immunocompetent patients is treated with oral antibiotics. When possible, elevation of the affected area is recommended. If infection is recurrent,

Table 1.3: Organism-Directed Therapy

Organism	Treatment	Alternatives
Staphylococcus aureus (MSSA)	Penicillinase-resistant penicillin	Penicillin/β-lactamase inhibitor, cephalosporins, clindamycin, fluoroquinolones
S. aureus (MRSA)	Trimethoprim-sulfamethoxazole, tetracyclines, fluoroquinolones, clindamycin	Vancomycin, linezolid, daptomycin, quinopristin/dalfopristin, tigecycline, newer generation carbapenems, and teicoplanin
St. pyogenes	Penicillin	Erythromycin, cephalosporins, clarithromycin, azithromycin, clindamycin

MRSA, methicillin-resistant *Staphylococcus aureus*

predisposing factors such as lymphedema or tinea pedis should be addressed.

When oral antibiotics are necessary, the initial choice of empiric oral antibiotics should take into account the most likely pathogen (including the local prevalence of MRSA) (Table 1.3), regional drug susceptibilities of these pathogens, as well as patient allergy, and severity of the infection. Purulent lesions, especially in recognized risk groups, suggest possible CA-MRSA, and empiric therapy should be based on this assumption. Therapy is later tailored by culture results for those who fail to improve on empiric therapy.

Although penicillin is sufficient for treatment of erysipelas that is almost exclusively caused by *St. pyogenes*, most uSSSIs require coverage of *S. aureus*. Therefore, empiric treatment of minor skin and soft tissue infections includes penicillinase-resistant penicillins, penicillin/β-lactamase inhibitor (amoxicillin-clavulanic acid), cephalosporins, clindamycin, macrolides, or fluoroquinolones.

CA-MRSA should be suspected in certain risk groups and those not responding to standard therapy for MSSA. Most cutaneous infections with CA-MRSA are purulent; therefore, drainage is the most important intervention but oral antibiotics may be required. Susceptibility is constantly evolving and varies by geographic region but in general, drugs active against CA-MRSA include trimethoprim–sulfamethoxazole and tetracyclines. Tetracyclines should be avoided in children below 8 years of age and during pregnancy. The fluoroquinolones are alternatives but resistance is emerging. Rifampin can be used in conjunction with other antibiotics but not alone because of rapid development of resistance. Clindamycin has been used successfully; however, inducible resistance can emerge during therapy. Erythromycin–clindamycin double-disc diffusion testing is required to check for inducible resistance prior to use of clindamycin.

Vancomycin is reserved for severe systemic infections with multiresistant MRSA strains. Newer agents for MRSA include linezolid, daptomycin, quinopristin–dalfopristin, tigecycline, newer generation carbapenems, and teicoplanin. Many of these drugs require intravenous administration and are usually reserved for treatment of HA-MRSA, which is typically resistant to multiple antibiotics. Susceptibility patterns are constantly evolving, and unfortunately, MRSA strains with resistance to some of these newer antibiotics have already been identified.

Signs of more serious infection include pain out of proportion to clinical findings, extensive necrosis, violaceous to necrotic bullae, anesthesia, rapid progression, or crepitus. If these findings or systemic toxicity (hypotension, tachycardia) is identified, blood culture, complete blood count with differential, hospitalization, and surgical and/or infectious disease consultation should be considered.

Cutaneous and nasal *S. aureus* colonization serves as a reservoir for reinfection. Based on 2001–2002 National Health and Nutrition Examination Survey (NHANES) data, reported by Graham et al., the prevalence of colonization of *S. aureus* and MRSA in the noninstitutionalized US population was 31.6% and 0.84%, respectively. These numbers are on the rise, and in 2003 CA-MRSA colonization was identified in 1.3% of all adults and in 2.5% of all children.

Conditions predisposing to *S. aureus* colonization include intravenous drug use, diabetes, hemodialysis, and skin disorders that impair the cutaneous barrier such as atopic dermatitis. CA-MRSA is associated with crowded conditions and close physical contact.

Unlike treatment of infection, lasting eradication of colonization is difficult to achieve. Attempts at elimination of colonization, in the absence of personal or close contact infection, are not recommended. Various decolonization strategies have been reported but convincing evidence is lacking and has resulted in antibiotic resistance and adverse events from systemic therapy. However, for those with recurrent infection, eradication is an important part of treatment.

Oral antibiotics achieve poor levels on the skin surface requiring topical agents such as chlorhexidine, triclosan, benzoyl peroxide wash, or Dakin's solution to address skin colonization. However, triclosan resistance has been identified in MSSA and MRSA isolates.

Topical mupirocin twice a day for the first 5 days each month is often used to treat nasal carriage but resistance is emerging. Intranasal fusidic acid is an alternative but resistance has similarly been reported. Few systemic antibiotics attain adequate levels in nasal secretions; however, oral clindamycin and rifampin have been used. Failure is not uncommon. Use of rifampin in combination with other antimicrobials may decrease resistance.

Other measures are important in preventing reinfection in the presence of colonization. Laundering of clothing, towels, and linens, in addition to keeping separate towels and washcloths, is required. Predisposing conditions such as eczema should be treated. Just as hand washing in hospitals reduces spread of infection, decontamination of fomites, such as athletic equipment, is helpful in community-acquired outbreaks.

PITFALLS AND MYTHS

Folliculitis is not always due to a bacterial infection. Other causes include an acneiform process, a fungal, or a viral infection. Culture of associated pustules may be required for confirmation. Similarly, not all abscesses are infectious and culture and/or biopsy can help differentiate from ruptured cysts and hidradenitits suppurativa.

Erysipelas may resemble contact dermatitis, angioedema, or the butterfly rash of lupus; however, fever and pain are not typical of the later disorders. Ear involvement can be confused with relapsing polychondritis. However, the noncartilaginous earlobe is characteristically spared in relapsing polychondritis.

Lower extremity cellulitis may be confused with stasis dermatitis, panniculitis (especially lipodermatosclerosis), deep venous thrombosis, and superficial thrombophlebitis. Cellulitis is rarely bilateral, unlike stasis dermatitis. However, both conditions can coexist, as stasis dermatitis predisposes to cellulitis. If a palpable cord is not present, duplex ultrasound may be required to identify superficial thrombophlebitis or deep venous thrombosis. Panniculitis is typically associated with induration and may require biopsy for confirmation.

Impetigo may be confused with perioral dermatitis, seborrheic dermatitis, allergic contact dermatitis, herpes simplex, and tinea. Primary dermatoses can acquire secondary impetiginization because of the impaired cutaneous barrier. Culture confirms the presence of impetigo or secondary impetiginization.

One myth associated with bacterial infections is the assumption that all bacterial colonization should be treated, when in reality, lasting eradication of colonization can be difficult to attain and is not necessary in the absence of infection.

Another misconception is that MRSA strains are more virulent and require parenteral therapy. However, the spectrum of disease with MRSA is similar to that of MSSA and particularly in the case of CA-MRSA, remains susceptible to several antibiotics. Intravenous treatment is only required in severe systemic or refractory infections.

SUGGESTED READINGS

Bamberger DM, Boyd SE. Management of *Staphylococcus aureus* infections. *Am Fam Physician* 2005;72(12):2474–2481.

Barton LL, Friedman AD. Impetigo: a reassessment of etiology and therapy. *Pediatr Dermatol* 1987;4(3):185–188.

Berger RS, Seifert MR. Whirlpool folliculitis: a review of its cause, treatment, and prevention. *Cutis* 1990;45(2):97–98.

Centers for Disease Control and Prevention (CDC). Outbreaks of community-associated methicillin-resistant *Staphylococcus aureus* skin infections – Los Angeles County, California, 2002–2003. *MMWR Morb Mortal Wkly Rep* 2003;52(5):88.

Cunha BA. Methicillin-resistant *Staphylococcus aureus*: clinical manifestations and antimicrobial therapy. *Clin Microbiol Infect* 2005;11 Suppl 4:33–42.

Edlich RF, Winters KL, Britt LD, Long WB 3rd. Bacterial diseases of the skin. *J Long Term Eff Med Implants* 2005;15(5):499–510.

Elston DM. Community-acquired methicillin-resistant *Staphylococcus aureus*. *J Am Acad Dermatol* 2007;56(1):1–16; quiz 17–20.

Falagas ME, Bliziotis IA, Fragoulis KN. Oral rifampin for eradication of *Staphylococcus aureus* carriage from healthy and sick populations: a systematic review of the evidence from comparative trials. *Am J Infect Control* 2007;35(2):106–114.

Graham PL 3rd, Lin SX, Larson EL. A U.S. population-based survey of *Staphylococcus aureus* colonization. *Ann Intern Med* 2006 7;144(5):318–325.

Halem M, Trent J, Green J, Kerdel F. Community-acquired methicillin resistant *Staphylococcus aureus* skin infection. *Semin Cutan Med Surg* 2006;25(2):68–71.

Kielhofner MA, Brown B, Dall L. Influence of underlying disease process on the utility of cellulitis needle aspirates. *Arch Intern Med* 1988;148(11):2451–2452.

Kowalski TJ, Berbari EF, Osmon DR. Epidemiology, treatment, and prevention of community-acquired methicillin-resistant *Staphylococcus aureus* infections. *Mayo Clin Proc* 2005;80(9): 1201–1207.

Lee MC, Rios AM, Aten MF, Mejias A, Cavuoti D, McCracken GH Jr, Hardy RD. Management and outcome of children with skin and soft tissue abscesses caused by community-acquired methicillin-resistant *Staphylococcus aureus*. *Pediatr Infect Dis J* 2004;23(2):123–127.

Loeb M, Main C, Walker-Dilks C, Eady A. Antimicrobial drugs for treating methicillin-resistant *Staphylococcus aureus* colonization. *Cochrane Database Syst Rev* 2003;(4):CD003340.

Pankuch GA, Lin G, Hoellman DB, Good CE, Jacobs MR, Appelbaum PC. Activity of retapamulin against *Streptococcus pyogenes* and *Staphylococcus aureus* evaluated by agar dilution, microdilution, E-test, and disk diffusion methodologies. *Antimicrob Agents Chemother* 2006;50(5):1727–1730.

Rayner C, Munckhof WJ. Antibiotics currently used in the treatment of infections caused by *Staphylococcus aureus*. *Intern Med J* 2005;35 Suppl 2:S3–16.

Roberts S, Chambers S. Diagnosis and management of *Staphylococcus aureus* infections of the skin and soft tissue. *Intern Med J* 2005;35 Suppl 2:S97–105.

Stevens DL, Bisno AL, Chambers HF, Everett ED, Dellinger P, Goldstein EJ, Gorbach SL, Hirschmann JV, Kaplan EL, Montoya JG, Wade JC; Infectious Diseases Society of America. Practice guidelines for the diagnosis and management of skin and soft-tissue infections. *Clin Infect Dis* 200515;41(10):1373–1406.

Yang A, Kerdel FA. Infectious disease update: new anti-microbials. *Semin Cutan Med Surg* 2006;25(2):94–99.

COMMON VIRAL INFECTIONS

Alejandra Varela, Anne Marie Tremaine, Aron Gewirtzman, Anita Satyaprakash, Natalia Mendoza, Parisa Ravanfar, and Stephen K. Tyring

HISTORY

Viral diseases may produce mucocutaneous manifestations either as a result of viral replication in the epidermis or secondary to viral replication elsewhere in the body. Most primary epidermal viral infections result from three groups of viruses: human papillomaviruses (HPV), herpesviruses, and poxviruses. Secondary lesions are produced by virus families such as retroviruses, paramyxoviruses, togaviruses, parvoviruses, and picornaviruses.

DNA VIRUSES

1. Poxviruses: replicate in the cytoplasm
   a. Molluscipox: molluscum
   b. Orthopox: vaccinia, smallpox, cowpox
   c. Parapox: Orf, milker's nodules
2. Papillomaviruses: replicate in the nucleus
3. Herpesviruses: replicate in the nucleus
4. Hepadnavirus: replicate in the nucleus
5. Adenoviruses: replicate in the nucleus

POX VIRUSES

Molluscipox (Molluscum Contagiosum)

There are two main subtypes of molluscipox: Molluscum Contagiosum virus (MCV) I and MCV II. Both can be seen in genital and nongenital areas. MCV I is more prevalent than MCV II except in HIV infection. Incubation of the virus ranges from 1 week to months.

Molluscum bodies have large numbers of maturing virons. These virions are sealed off by collagen and lipid-rich sac-like structures that protect the virus from host defenses. Free virus cores can be found in all layers of the epidermis. Histologically, viral particles in infected keratinocytes and eosinophils can be observed. These are known as *Henderson–Paterson bodies* (molluscum bodies).

Clinical Manifestations

This virus is found mainly in the pediatric age-group and is characterized by dome-shaped umbilicated papules. Children often acquire the virus by close contact. The virus can also be transmitted sexually, resulting in genital papules. In immunocompromised patients, especially patients with HIV infection, thousands of papules can be present.

Treatment

Curettage, liquid nitrogen, cantharidin, lactic acid, CO_2, imiquimod, and trichloroacetic acid can be used. Cidofovir is used in immunocompromised patients.

Orthopox

1. Smallpox
2. Vaccinia
3. Monkeypox
4. Cowpox

Smallpox

Smallpox is caused by the variola virus. Variola minor is also known as *alastrim*. Progressive vaccinia can be related to immunosuppression, malignancy, radiation therapy, or AIDS infection. Histologically, smallpox demonstrates balloon and reticular degeneration with hemorrhagic inclusion bodies and polymorphonuclear cells.

Clinical Manifestations

Incubation lasts for 12 to 13 days. Fever, malaise, backache, and exanthema appear after 2 to 4 days. The lesions evolve from macules to papules to vesicles to pustules. There are four clinical types of smallpox: ordinary, modified (by previous vaccination), flat, and hemorrhagic. The latter two have the highest mortality rate, they are 30% fatal.

The lesions are discrete, firm, deep-seated papules that are vesiculated and umbilicated. Crusts will form later. All lesions are in the same stage. Corneal ulceration, laryngeal lesions, encephalitis, and hemorrhage are all possible complications. Variola major can also cause fatal complications such as death secondary to pulmonary edema or heart failure. Patients with immunosuppression, malignancy, radiation therapy, or AIDS are at higher risk for progressive vaccinia.

Treatment

No antiviral treatment exists for smallpox. Cidofovir has been suggested to combat the infection.

Vaccination

The smallpox vaccine provides a high level of immunity for 3 to 5 years, with decreasing immunity thereafter. The vaccine, however, has risks associated with its administration. Postvaccination encephalitis and progressive vaccinia can occur.

Vaccinia

Vaccinia is a laboratory virus used to vaccinate against smallpox and monkeypox. The infection occurs primarily in laboratory workers.

Clinical Manifestations

Papules appear in 2 to 3 days, followed by an umbilicated Jennerian vesicle. A scab ensues and results in a pitted scar. The formation of a pustule at day 7 confirms successful vaccination.

Generalized vaccinia can occur secondary to viremia. It typically occurs 6 to 9 days after vaccination. Eczema vaccinatum can develop, and this occurs more commonly in immunocompromised patients or patients with a nonintact skin barrier.

Treatment

The suggested treatment is Cidofovir.

Monkeypox

This virus occasionally infects humans, predominantly residents of western and central Africa. Populations at risk can receive protection from vaccination with the vaccinia virus.

Cowpox

Cowpox historically infected cows, but is more commonly found in cats. The animals are generally infected at sites of injury – especially at the teats. The virus can infect humans and is transmitted by touch from animals to humans.

Clinical Manifestations

Symptoms of infection of cowpox are localized, pustular lesions generally found on the hands. Lymphadenopathy and fever may also occur.

Parapox

1. Orf
2. Paravaccinia (milker's nodules)

Orf (Ecthyma Contagiosum, Scabby Mouth)

This virus is endemic among sheep, goats, and oxen. Transmission occurs from animals or fomites (especially barn doors and troughs). Sheep farmers and veterinarians are mainly affected. Lesions heal in approximately a month.

The virus is large and ovoid and measures 250×160 nm with surface tubules. It is resistant to drying and lipid solvents, such as ether and chloroform. Incubation period is 4 to 7 days.

Histologically, vacuolization of cells in the upper third of the stratum spinosum is observed with multilocular vesicles, acanthosis, and eosinophilic inclusion bodies in the cytoplasm and nucleus of infected cells. A mixed infiltrate with loss of epidermis over the central part of the lesion is also seen. During the acute stage of this infection, necrosis with massive infiltration of mononuclear cells can be seen.

Clinical Manifestations

Typically nodules are seen around the mouth and nose of animals. Patients present with lymphadenopathy, malaise, fever, and painful lesions (usually on the fingers).

Over a 36-day period, the lesions advance through six clinical stages. Each stage lasts for 6 days.

1. Papular stage: lesions are red and elevated.
2. Target stage: nodule with a red center, white ring, and red halo.
3. Acute stage: weeping surface.
4. Regenerative stage: thin, dry crust with black dots.
5. Papillomatous stage: small papillomas over the surface of the lesion.
6. Regressive stage: thick crusts heal with scarring.

Diagnosis

History and physical examination, confirmed by cell culture, fluorescent antibody, complement fixation, electron microscopy, or histology.

Treatment

Infection spontaneously remits. Direct local care should be aimed at avoiding secondary infection.

Milker's Nodules (Paravaccinia)

Paravaccinia, or milker's nodules, are endemic to cattle. Human disease is contracted through direct transmission (handling of infected cow teats) or through fomites. The virus is 150×300 nm and brick shaped. Histologically, the lesions are similar to those of orf.

Clinical Manifestations

A solitary nodule develops on the finger, which increases slowly in size over a period of 1 to 2 weeks. The nodules are painless and bluish red in color. The lesions typically heal without scarring and patients are often afebrile.

Diagnosis

History and physical examination, confirmed by cell culture, fluorescent antibody, complement fixation, electron microscopy, or histology.

Treatment

Most lesions spontaneously heal within 5 to 7 weeks. Direct local care is aimed at avoiding secondary infection.

HUMAN PAPILLOMAVIRUS

Three categories are used to clinically describe human papillomavirus (HPV):

1. Anogenital/mucosal
2. Nongenital cutaneous
3. Epidermodysplasia verruciformis (EV)

Diseases and Associated HPV Subtypes

Nongenital Cutaneous Diseases (See Table 2.1)

HPV infects the stratified squamous epithelium. The various HPV strains display predilections for specific body sites. They can infect and cause both cutaneous and mucosal disease. HPV gains access

Table 2.1: Nongenital Cutaneous Diseases

Disease	HPV Type
Common warts (verrucae vulgaris)	1, 2, 4, 26, 27, 29, 41, 57, 65
Plantar warts (myrmecia)	1, 2, 4, 63
Flat warts (verrucae plana)	3, 10, 27, 28, 38, 41, 49
Butcher's warts (common warts of people who handle meat, poultry, and fish)	7
Mosaic warts	2, 27, 57
Subungual squamous cell carcinoma	16
Epidermodysplasia verruciformis (benign)	2, 3, 10, 12, 15, 19, 36, 46, 47, 50
Epidermodysplasia verruciformis (malignant or benign)	5, 8, 9, 10, 14, 17, 20, 21, 22, 23, 24, 25, 37, 38

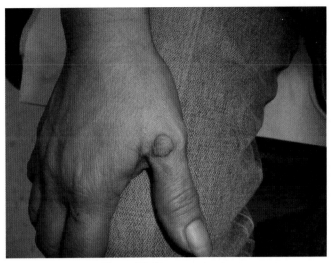

Figure 2.1. Verruca vulgaris.

to keratinocytes, and thus establishes an infection. The viral gene expression influences the proliferation and maturation of the keratinocyte, which results in the growth of a benign tumor. The virus is transmitted by person to person contact. HPV infection is often self-limited and a large portion of the world's population has at some point been infected with the virus.

PALMOPLANTAR WARTS

HPV-1 is the most common type responsible for palmoplantar warts. The lesions may be located anywhere on the palms and/or soles, especially on the fingertips and tips of the toes. Palmoplantar warts may have a number of clinical presentations. They start as minute punctate depressions that coalesce into large, thin, endophytic confluent plaques called mosaic warts. If they coalesce as thick confluent plaques, they are known as myrmecia warts. The borders are sharply demarcated, with a surrounding border of thick callus.

Histologically, the warts display acanthosis, papillomatosis and hyperkeratosis. Myrmecia warts show prominent cytoplasmic, eosinophilic inclusion bodies surrounding the vacuolated nuclei of koilocytes.

Treatment

Available treatments include salicylic acid, 20% trichloroacetic acid, cryotherapy, CO_2 laser, cantharidin, bleomycin, and combination therapy using electrodessication, cryodestruction or surgery and imiquimod.

COMMON WARTS (VERRUCA VULGARIS)

HPV-2 is the most common HPV type associated with common warts, followed by HPV-4, -26, -27, -65, -78. The clinical manifestations include single or grouped scaly, rough papules or nodules especially on the hands (see Fig. 2.1). A close examination would reveal "black dots" which are thrombosed capillaries within the warts. Common warts are very frequent in children and young adults. The lesions tend to koebnerize.

Histologically, common warts are characterized by marked acanthosis associated with hyperkeratosis, elongated rete ridges, prominent koilocytes and stacks of parakeratotic cells and basophilic keratohyaline granules. Dilatation and thrombosed capillaries are evident at the dermis.

Treatment

Treatment includes salicylic acid, 50% trichloroacetic acid, cantharidin, cryotherapy with liquid nitrogen, electrodessication, and combination therapy with cryotherapy or surgery and imiquimod.

FLAT WARTS (VERRUCAE PLANA)

Flat warts are most often caused by HPV-3 and HPV-10, and less frequently by HPV-27, -28, and -49. Flat warts are characterized by grouped, minimally raised, flat-topped, skin colored papules measuring 2–4 mm in diameter. They occur most commonly on the face, hands, beard area, and legs of women. The lesions tend to occur along a line of cutaneous trauma. The koebner phenomenon is also seen with these lesions.

Histologically, flat warts show hyperkeratosis and acanthosis. No papillomatosis is seen. Koilocytes are prominent and the stratum corneum has a "basket-weave" appearance.

Treatment

Treatment involves retinoic acid 0.05% applied daily, which causes desquamation. Mild irritation may occur.

Epidermodysplasia verruciformis

Epidermodysplasia is a very rare genetic chronic disease with autosomal recessive inheritance. It manifests in childhood and is characterized by a unique susceptibility to cutaneous infection by a group of phylogenetically related human papillomavirus (HPV) types, including HPV-5, -8, -9, -12, -14, -15, -17, -19, -25, -36, -38, -47 and -50. Mutations in the EVER1 and EVER2 genes (epidermodysplasia verruciformis susceptibility locus 1 (EV1)) on chromosome 17q25, which encode for membrane proteins in the endoplasmic reticulum, are responsible for the condition.

Clinical manifestations of epidermodysplasia include polymorphic lesions, pityriasis versicolor-like macules, flat wart-like papules and red brown plaques that can undergo malignant transformation. Actinic keratoses start early in life, typically around 30 years of age and 50% will develop squamous cell or bowenoid carcinomas, mainly on sun-exposed areas, in the fourth or fifth decade of life. The HPV types associated with malignant transformation are HPV-5, HPV-8, as well as HPV-14d.

Diagnosis of this disease is clinical and is usually confirmed by biopsy. The histology demonstrates stratum corneum with a basket weave appearance, uneven keratohyaline granules, large,

Table 2.2: Anogenital Disease

Disease	HPV Type
Condyloma acuminata	6, 11, 30, 42, 43, 44, 45, 51, 52, 54
Bowenoid papulosis	16, 18, 34, 39, 42, 45
Bowen disease	16, 18, 31, 34
Giant condylomata	6, 11

coarse granules in the epidermis, koilocytes, and gray cytoplasm. Dysplasia and actinic keratoses may be evident.

Treatment

There is no effective treatment for this condition. For localized malignancies, surgery is the best treatment option; however, for the persistent nonmalignant lesions, surgery is impractical due to the extensive nature of the disease. Counseling is the most important preventive measure; patients with epidermodysplasia must protect the skin from exposure to ultraviolet radiation.

Other therapies, such as long-term oral isotretinoin, have been used to decrease the number of benign lesions, and slow the appearance of premalignant and malignant lesions. Retinoids have an endogenous antiproliferative effect through their control of epithelial cell differentiation. Imiquimod has also been used and has been shown to be effective on the face and body. Additionally, it is a good adjuvant for systemic interferon therapy.

BUTCHER'S WARTS

Butcher's warts are seen in people who frequently handle raw meat. Their morphology is similar to that of common warts, with a higher prevalence of hyperproliferative cauliflower-like lesions. Most commonly, they are seen on the hands.

Histologically, Butcher's warts demonstrate verrucae, prominent acanthosis, papillomatosis, hyperkeratosis, parakeratosis, and elongated rete ridges. Dermal vessels are prominent, as are koilocytotic cells.

Treatment

Treatment includes salicylic acid, 50% trichloroacetic acid, cantharidin, cryotherapy with liquid nitrogen, electrodessication, and combination therapy with cryotherapy or surgery and imiquimod.

Anogenital Disease (See Table 2.2)

BOWENOID PAPULOSIS

Bowenoid papulosis is a focal epidermal hyperplasia and dysplasia induced by HPV infection. Most commonly, it is caused by HPV-16, HPV-18, and HPV-33. It occurs in young, sexually active adults and manifests as papules/plaques on the genitalia.

Histologically, the lesions are characterized by full thickness dysplasia with dysplastic keratinocytes. A circumscribed epidermal proliferation composed of pleomorphic cells with clumped nuclei and abnormal mitoses can be observed.

Treatment

Treatment includes cryotherapy, laser excision, topical retinoids, 5-fluorouracil 5% solution, and imiquimod 5% cream.

CONDYLOMA ACUMINATUM

Condyloma acuminatum (genital warts) are typically caused by HPV-6 and HPV-11. Less commonly, HPV-16, -18, -21, -22,

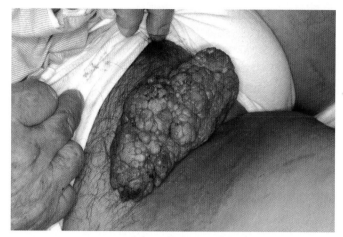

Figure 2.2. Condyloma acuminatum.

and -55 cause the infection. Genital warts are spread through sexual contact. An estimated 500,000 to 1 million new cases of genital condyloma are diagnosed each year.

Histologically, parakeratosis is observed in the mucosa. Papillomatosis, acanthosis, elongated rete ridges, koilocytes, and occasional mitotic figures are also characteristic of the lesions.

Clinical manifestations

Most patients seek care when they notice lumps on the vulva, labia, vaginal introitus, perianal area, or periclitoral area. The lesions are exophytic and cauliflower-like and are found near moist surfaces (see Fig. 2.2). These lesions are generally not painful, but can be associated with pruritus and bleeding.

Cervical cancer can develop from infection with HPV. About 70% of cervical cancers are thought to develop from infection with HPV-16 and HPV-18.

Treatment

Treatment includes trichloroacetic acid, cantharidin, cryotherapy with liquid nitrogen, electrodessication, and combination therapy with cryotherapy or surgery and imiquimod.

Preventative Therapies

Gardasil® is a recombinant quadrivalent vaccine prepared from the highly purified virus-like particles of the major capsid protein of HPV-6, -11, -16, and -18. It is indicated in girls and women ages 9 to 26 years for the prevention of cervical cancer and condyloma acuminatum.

VERRUCOUS CARCINOMA

HPV infection is thought to cause or facilitate the development of verrucous carcinoma. Verrucous carcinoma (VC) presents as a verrucous, exophytic, or endophytic mass that typically develops at sites of chronic irritation or inflammation. The tumor enlarges slowly and may penetrate deeply into the skin, fascia, or bone.

The different types of VC based on the site of occurrence are the following:

Epithelioma cuniculatum: Also known as palmoplantar VC, epithelioma cuniculatum commonly involves the skin overlying the first metatarsal. It manifests as a plaque on the sole of

Table 2.3: Nongenital Mucosal Disease

Disease	HPV Type
Oral focal epithelial hyperplasia (Heck's disease)	13, 32
Oral carcinoma	16, 18
Oral leukoplakia	16, 18

the foot with ulceration. It commonly drains a foul-smelling discharge and can cause pain, bleeding, and difficulty walking. Palmoplantar VC is associated with HPV-2 and HPV-16.

Giant condyloma of Buschke and Lowenstein: This slow-growing, locally destructive verrucous lesion typically occurs on the glans penis (mainly in uncircumcised men), but may appear elsewhere in the anogenital region. HPV-6 and HPV-11 have been linked to these tumors.

Oral florid papillomatosis: The early lesions of oral VC appear as white, translucent patches on an erythematous base. They may develop in areas of leukoplakia, lichen planus, chronic lupus erythematous, cheilitis, or candidiasis. More fully developed lesions may coalesce and extend over large areas of the oral mucosa. Ulceration, fistulation, and local invasion into bones and soft tissue can occur.

Treatment

Treatment includes cryosurgery, curretage and electrodessication, excision with conventional margins, Mohs surgery, and radiation therapy.

Nongenital Mucosal Disease (See Table 2.3)

ORAL FOCAL HYPERPLASIA (HECK DISEASE)

Oral focal hyperplasia is characterized by focal epithelial hyperplasia of the lower labial mucosa. Multiple, flat-topped or dome-shaped pink-white papules are observed ranging from 1 to 5 mm. Some lesions coalesce to form plaques.

Histologically, the lesions demonstrate a hyperplastic mucosa with a thin parakeratotic stratum corneum. Acanthosis, blunting, and anastamosis of rete ridges are commonly observed. The epidermal cells demonstrate pallor as a result of intracellular edema.

Treatments for HPV

Treatments for the multiple presentations of HPV have been discussed in the above sections. For a comprehensive review of HPV therapies, see Table 2.4.

HUMAN HERPES VIRUSES (SEE TABLE 2.5)

Human Herpesvirus 1: Herpes Simplex Virus 1

Herpes simplex 1 (HSV-1) virus belongs to the family Herpesviridae. Humans are the only natural reservoir and there are no vectors associated with transmission. In the US, eighty percent of adults are infected with HSV-1. Worldwide, 85% of adults are infected. Ninety percent of HSV-1 infections are orofacial and 10% are genital. Infection is transmitted by close personal contact.

Viral properties

HSV-1 is neurovirulent. It has the capacity to invade and replicate in the nervous system. Latency is another property of this viral infection. The virus is established and maintained as a latent infection in the nerve cell ganglia. The trigeminal ganglia are most commonly involved in HSV-1 infection. Reactivation of the virus is induced by a variety of stimuli: fever, trauma, emotional stress, sunlight, and menstruation.

The primary infection is subclinical 90% of the time and manifests as gingivostomatitis 10% of time. Forty percent of clinically apparent infections recur three to four times per year.

Clinical Manifestations

GINGIVAL STOMATITIS

Gingival stomatitis has an abrupt onset. It occurs in children aged 6 months to 5 years who present with high fever (102°F to 104°F), anorexia, and listlessness. Gingivitis is the most striking feature of clinical presentation. Vesicular lesions develop on the oral mucosa, tongue, and lips. These lesions later rupture and coalesce, leaving ulcerated plaques. Regional lymphadenopathy, acute herpetic pharyngotonsillitis, pharyngitis, and tonsillitis can also occur. The acute disease lasts for 5 to 7 days and viral shedding may continue for up to 3 weeks.

HERPES LABIALIS

Herpes labialis is the most common manifestation of recurrent HSV-1. A prodrome of pain, burning, and tingling often occurs at the site of infection. Erythematous papules rapidly develop into tiny, thin-walled intraepidermal vesicles that become pustular and ulcerate (see Fig. 2.3). Maximum viral shedding occurs in the first 24 hours of acute illness, but may last for 5 days.

Diagnosis

Histologically, acantholysis, intraepidermal vesicles, balloon and reticular degeneration, intranuclear eosinophilic inclusion bodies, and multinucleated keratinocytes are observed.

LABORATORY CONFIRMATORY STUDIES:

- Viral culture.
- Polymerase chain reaction (PCR) techniques are useful in diagnosis.
- Immunofluorescent staining of tissue culture cells or of smear cells can quickly identify HSV and can distinguish between types 1 and 2.
- Antibody testing.
- Tzanck smear demonstrating multinucleated giant cells.

Treatment

See HSV-2 below.

Human Herpesvirus 2: Herpes Simplex Virus 2

Herpes simplex 2 (HSV-2) is the cause of 70% of primary genital herpes cases (see Fig. 2.4). Greater than 95% of recurrent genital herpes infections are caused by HSV-2. The infection is asymptomatic in approximately 75% of patients. Women are 45% more likely to have the infection than men. Ninety percent of asymptomatic females and males actively shed the virus at some

Table 2.4: Treatments for HPV

Treatment Category	Specific Treatment	Benefits and Drawbacks and Uses
Topical agents	**Salicylic acid**	Over the Counter Removes Surface keratin Cure rates from 70%–80% are reported
	Cantharidin	Dried extract of blister beetle Causes epidermal necrosis and blistering Treatment may require weekly repetition
	Dinitro-chlorobenzene (DNCB)	Powerful sensitizing agent Induces an allergic contact dermatitis Causes local inflammation and an immune response Cure rates from 65%–90% Reported mutagen
	Dibutyl squaric acid	Contact sensitizer Unlike DNCB, it is not a mutagen and therefore may be a safer alternative
	Trichloroacetic acid	Caustic compound Causes immediate superficial tissue necrosis Concentration up to 80% May require weekly applications
	Podophyllotoxin	Derived from the roots of the Indian podophyllum plant Binds to tubulin and prevents microtubule assembly Genital warts: apply twice daily for three consecutive days per week for up to 4 weeks
	Fluorouracil (5FU)	Used primarily to treat actinic keratosis Antimetabolite: fluorinated pyrimidine Active form inhibits DNA synthesis by inhibiting the normal production of thymidine Effective in treating warts but very inflammatory and tetratogenic
	Imiquimod 5% cream	Topical cream approved for treating genital warts; used for other HPV infections Anogenital warts: treat at night, three times per week Common warts: treat nightly under occlusion Palmoplantar warts: treat nightly under occlusion, alternate with a keratinolytic Potent stimulator of proinflammatory cytokine release Works best as part of combination therapy for nonanogenital warts
	Cidofovir	Nucleotide analogue of deoxycytidine monophosphate Used for refractory condyloma acuminata Cidofovir gel must be applied once or twice daily Must be compounded and it is expensive
	Tretinoin	Disrupts epidermal growth and differentiation, thereby reducing the bulk of the wart
Systemic agents	**Cimetidine**	Type 2 histamine receptor antagonist Immunomodulatory effects Results have varied Oral, 25 to 40 ng/kg three times daily for three months
Intralesional injections	**Bleomycin**	Cytotoxic polypeptide that inhibits DNA synthesis in cells and viruses Side effects of bleomycin include pain with injection, local urticaria, Raynaud phenomenon, and possible tissue necrosis If used periungually, bleomycin may cause nail dystrophy or loss
	Interferon-α	Naturally occurring cytokine with antiviral, anticancer, and immunomodulatory effects Intralesional administration is more effective than systemic administration and is associated with mild flu-like symptoms Treatments may be required for several weeks to months before beneficial results are seen Useful for warts that are resistant to standard treatments
Surgical care	**Cryosurgery**	Liquid nitrogen (–196°C) is the most effective method
	Lasers	Carbon dioxide lasers Procedure can be painful and leave scarring Risk of nosocomial infection also exists in health care workers because HPV can be isolated in the plume
	Electrodesiccation and curettage	May be more effective than cryosurgery Painful More likely to scar HPV can be isolated from the plume
	Surgical Excision	Avoid using except in extremely large lesions because of the risks of scarring and recurrence

Table 2.5: Human Herpes Viruses

Herpes Type	Associated Diseases
HHV-1	Herpes simplex 1 (HSV-1): herpes labialis > herpes genitalis
HHV-2	Herpes simplex 2 (HSV-2): herpes genitalis > herpes labialis
HHV-3	Varicella-zoster virus (VZV): chickenpox/ herpes zoster
HHV-4	Epstein-Barr virus (EBV): mononucleosis, Gianotti–Crosti, Burkitt's lymphoma, oral hairy leukoplakia
HHV-5	Cytomegalovirus (CMV): retinitis in AIDS patients
HHV-6	Roseola infantum (exanthema subitum)
HHV-7	Possibly pityriasis rosea
HHV-8	Kaposi's sarcoma

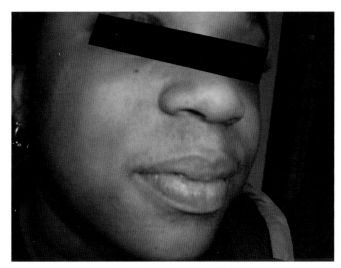

Figure 2.3. Herpes labialis.

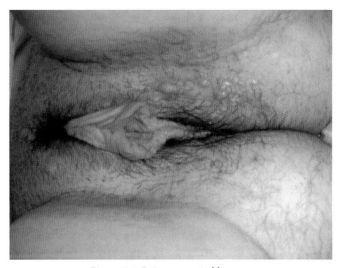

Figure 2.4. Primary genital herpes.

point in time. Eighty percent of transmission occurs secondary to asymptomatic shedding.

Viral properties
Like HSV-1, HSV-2 is also neurovirulent. It has the capacity to invade and replicate in the nervous system. Latency is another property of this infection. The virus is established and maintained as a latent infection in the nerve cell ganglia. Reactivation of the virus is induced by a variety of stimuli, such as fever, trauma, emotional stress, sunlight, and menstruation.

Clinical Manifestations
The infection is spread by sexual contact. The incubation period is 3 to 7 days. Viral shedding lasts for about 12 days. Primary HSV systematic complaints occur in greater than 70% of cases. These include fever, dysuria, malaise, and lymphadenopathy.

Treatment
Acyclovir:
- First episode: 200 mg five times daily or 400 mg three times a day for 10 days.
- Recurrent outbreaks: 200 mg PO five times daily or 400 mg three times a day for 5 days.
- Chronic suppressive therapy: 400 mg twice daily or 200 mg three to five times daily

Valacyclovir:
- First episode: 1 gram twice daily for 10 days
- Recurrent outbreaks: 500 mg twice daily for 3 days or 2 grams twice daily for 1 day
- Chronic suppressive therapy: 500 mg to 1 gram daily

Famciclovir:
- First episode: 250 mg three times daily for 10 days
- Single-day therapy: 1000 mg twice daily for 1 day or 1500 mg once for herpes labialis
- Recurrent outbreaks: 125 mg twice daily for 5 days or 1500 mg once for herpes labialis
- Chronic suppressive therapy: 250 mg twice daily

Herpes Simplex Virus in Immunosuppressed Patients

In patients with HIV, 95% are co-infected with HSV-1, HSV-2, or both. Fifty-two percent of HIV infections among people who have HSV-2 can be associated with infection with the herpes virus. Recurrent HSV episodes may last as long as 30 days, much longer when compared to immunocompetent hosts. Some

Table 2.6: Various Herpes Presentations

Disease	Presentation
Herpetic whitlow	– HSV of the fingers of the hand occurs near the cuticle or at other sites associated with trauma – HSV-2 causes the infection more often than HSV-1
Herpes gladiatorum	– Caused by direct skin to skin contact among wrestlers – Manifests as scattered cutaneous HSV-1 lesions (>HSV-2)
Herpetic keratoconjunctivitis	– Recurrent erosions of the conjunctiva and cornea that can lead to blindness
Lumbosacral herpes simplex virus	– Infection is typically asymptomatic
Herpes associated EM	– Consistent with delayed type hypersensitivity reactions – Targetoid lesions are not always limited to palms and soles
Eczema herpeticum	– Widespread HSV infection in patients with skin disorders such as atopic dermatitis, Darier's disease, pemphigus, or Sezary syndrome
HSV encephalitis	– Most common cause of sporadic encephalitis – Sudden onset of fever, headache, confusion, and temporal lobe signs – 70% mortality if not treated
Ramsay Hunt	– Usually caused by VZV or HSV-1 – Infection of the facial nerve – Symptoms on the affected side typically include facial weakness and a painful herpes-type skin eruption on the pinna of the ear – Frequently, vestibulocochlear disturbances – Recovery of facial movement occurs in about 50% of treated patients

manifestations of HSV in immunosuppressed hosts include the following:

Chronic ulcerative HSV: These are persistent ulcers and erosions that begin on the face or in the perineal area.

Generalized acute mucocutaneous HSV: Characterized by dissemination and fever after localized vesicular eruption.

Systemic HSV: Follows oral or genital lesions. Areas of necrosis are found in the liver, adrenals, and pancreas.

Treatment
In patients with HIV, 5% to 8% are resistant to acyclovir. Acyclovir-resistant HSV in HIV patients can be treated with 1% cidofovir (compounded) or foscarnet. Foscarnet reversibly inhibits viral DNA polymerase and does not require thymidine kinase. Side effects of foscarnet include penile ulcers and nephrotoxicity.

Various Herpes Presentations (See Table 2.6)

Congential Herpes Simplex Virus

Congential herpes simplex virus occurs in 1/3,500 births. The majority of these cases (up to 90%) are caused by perinatal transmission, in which the newborn contracts herpes while passing through the birth canal during delivery. In rare cases (5%–8%), herpes can be acquired in utero. Postnatal transmission is uncommon. Risk of transmission is 50% if the mother has a primary infection and 3% to 5% if the mother had recurrent disease. Birth canal transmission can manifest as lesions on the scalp and face, encephalitis, hepatoadrenal necrosis, pneumonia, and even death.

If lesions appear on an infant during the first 10 days of life, mortality is 20%. If transmission occurs during the first 8 weeks of pregnancy, severe defects can result. Without treatment, the mortality rate of the disease is 65% in transplacental disease, 80% if the patient is infected with HSV-2, and 10% if the patient is infected with HSV-1.

Treatment
In infected females who are pregnant, treatment should be administered from week 36 until delivery. Options include valacyclovir 1 g daily, famciclovir 250 mg twice daily, or acyclovir 400 mg three times daily (due to increased metabolism in pregnant women).

Human herpes virus 3: Varicella-zoster Virus

Varicella-zoster virus manifests clinically as chickenpox and herpes zoster.

CHICKENPOX
Chickenpox is transmitted to others from the skin and respiratory tract. The incubation period is about 2 weeks. Low-grade fever precedes skin manifestations by 1 to 2 days. Lesions begin on the face and appear as "dewdrops on a rose petal" (see Fig. 2.5). They progress to the scalp and trunk while relatively sparing the extremities. The characteristic lesion begins as a red macule that evolves through various stages: papule to vesicle to pustule and finally, to a pruritic crust. Varicella's hallmark is the simultaneous presence of different stages of the rash.

VZV remains dormant in the sensory nerve roots after primary infection.

In utero infections:

CONGENITAL VARICELLA SYNDROME
Congenital varicella syndrome occurs in 2% of children born to women who develop varicella during the first trimester of pregnancy. This syndrome manifests as intrauterine growth retardation, microcephaly, cortical atrophy, limb hypoplasia, microphthalmia, cataracts, chorioretinitis, and cutaneous scarring.

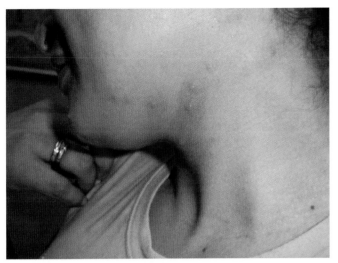

Figure 2.5. Primary VZV.

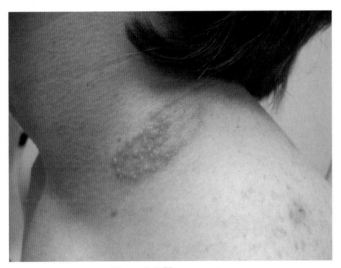

Figure 2.6. Herpes zoster.

INFANTILE ZOSTER

Infantile zoster manifests within the first year of life. The cause is maternal varicella infection after the 20th week of pregnancy. Infantile zoster typically involves the thoracic dermatomes.

NEONATAL VARICELLA

Neonatal varicella can be a serious illness, depending on the timing of maternal infection and delivery of the newborn. If the mother develops varicella within 5 days before and up to 2 days after delivery, the infant is exposed to the secondary viremia of the mother. Mortality is 30% if prophylaxis or treatment with varicella-zoster immune globulin and/or acyclovir is not administered. Onset of varicella more than 5 days antepartum provides the mother sufficient time to develop and pass on protective antibodies to the fetus.

Treatment

CHILDREN

Children with varicella can be treated with acyclovir 20 mg/kg given orally four times daily for 5 to 7 days. Healthy children may not need acyclovir; however, it allows them to return to school more quickly and reduces morbidity. Symptomatic care is the mainstay of treatment. Be cautious to avoid aspirin to prevent Reye's syndrome.

ADULTS

Adults who develop varicella are most effectively treated if one of the following medications is started within the first 24 to 72 hours after the development of vesicles:

Acyclovir: 800 mg five times daily for 7 days
Valacyclovir: 1 g three times daily for 7 days
Famciclovir: 500 mg three times daily for 7 days

Prophylaxis

VARICELLA VACCINE

Give two doses 4 to 8 weeks apart for all children older than 12 months. Seroconversion typically occurs in 78% of adults and adolescents after the first dose and in 99% after the second dose.

HERPES ZOSTER (SHINGLES)

Owing to the reactivation of latent VZV in the sensory ganglion, there is a 20% incidence of herpes zoster in those who have been infected. There is a 66% incidence in patients who are older than 50 years of age.

The rash is preceded by a prodrome that is characterized by fever, malaise, headache, and localized pain in the involved dermatome. It manifests in a unilateral dermatomal distribution with erythema, vesicles, pustules, and crusting (see Fig. 2.6). The rash is contagious until all of the lesions develop crusts. Potential complications of herpes zoster are found in Table 2.7.

Diagnosis

Nonspecific tests:
- Tzanck smear: multinucleated giant cells, nuclear molding
- Histology: intraepidermal vesicle, ballooning degeneration, reticular degeneration, inclusion bodies, margination of chromatin, vascular involvement

Specific tests:
- Viral culture
- PCR

Treatment of herpes zoster

Acyclovir: 800 mg five times daily for 7 days or
Valacyclovir: 1 g three times daily for 7 days or
Famciclovir: 500 mg three times daily for 7 days
Pain and pruritus: analgesics, oral antipruritics, calamine lotion, cool compresses

Treatment of postherpetic neuralgia

- Non-narcotic or narcotic analgesic
- Capsaicin cream
- Topical lidocaine gel or patch
- Tricyclic antidepressants: amitryptiline, maprotiline, or desipramine
- Anticonvulsants: carbamazepine, gabapentin, pregabalin
- Sympathetic nerve blockade
- Steroids: methylprednisolone
- Transcutaneous electrical stimulation
- Acupuncture

Table 2.7: Complications of herpes zoster

Disease	Presentation and Associated Symptoms
Hutchinson's sign	– Zoster on the tip of nose – Could result in herpetic keratitis
Zoster sine herpete	– Segmental pain without lesions
Ophthalmic zoster	– Ocular disease occurs in 20%–70% of patients who develop ophthalmic zoster – Cicatricial lid retraction, ptosis, keratitis, scleritis, uveitis, secondary glaucoma, oculomotor palsies, chorioretinitis, optic neuritis, panophthalmitis
CNS zoster	– Has asymptomatic cerebrospinal fluid changes
Primary varicella pneumonia	– Has a higher incidence in adults and immunocompromised patients
Bacterial super infections	– Usually due to *Staphylococcus aureus*
Acute cerebellar ataxia	– Unsteady gait 11 to 20 days following rash
Guillian-Barré syndrome	– Acute idiopathic polyneuritis
Meningoencephalitis	– Encephalitis with headache, fever, photophobia, nausea, vomiting, and nerve palsies
Motor paralysis	– Extension from sensory ganglion to anterior horn – Occurs within the first 2–3 weeks
Ramsay Hunt	– Facial palsy secondary to herpes-zoster infection of facial (VII) and auditory (VIII) nerves – Affects external ear, tympanic membrane – Causes tinnitus, vertigo, deafness, otalgia, and loss of taste
Postherpetic neuralgia	– Defined as pain greater than one month after vesicles – Occurs in 10%–15% of patients – Resolves in 50% of patients by 3 months, 75% by 1 year – Occurs in 60% of patients over the age of 60

Prophylaxis
VARICELLA-ZOSTER VACCINE

This vaccine is given to increase the immunity in patients who have a history of primary VZV in order to prevent zoster. It is recommended in individuals 60 years of age and older.

Human Herpes Virus 4: Epstein-Barr Virus

This double-stranded DNA virus infects mainly B lymphocytes. After acute infection occurs, EBV persists throughout the patient's lifetime as a latent infection.

Clinical Manifestations (See Table 2.8)

Table 2.8: Clinical Manifestations of EBV

Disease	Presentation and Associated Symptoms
Mononucleosis	– Triad: fever, sore throat, lymphadenopathy – Maculopapular rash present in 3%–15% of patients – 80% of patients develop a rash if they are treated with amoxicillin or ampicillin Treatment: – Supportive care – Antipyretics, analgesics, topical steroids for cutaneous manifestations – Prednisone for complications such as hemolytic anemia, thrombocytopenia, or lymphadenopathy that compromises the airway
Oral hairy leukoplakia	– Usually associated with HIV patients – Secondary nonmalignant hyperplasia of epithelial cells – Accentuated vertical folds laterally on the tongue – Mucosa appears white and thick: does not scrape off – Pathology: papillomatosis – Treatment: acyclovir 400 mg five times daily
Kikuchi's syndrome	– Hyperimmune reaction to an infectious agent causing regional lymph node enlargement
Mucocutaneous lymphoma	– B-cell lymphoma
Burkitt's lymphoma	– High grade B-cell lymphoma – EBV genome can be detected in tumor cells
Nasopharyngeal carcinoma	– Malignant tumor of the squamous epithelium of the nasopharynx – Patients have high levels of antibodies to EBV antigens
Gianotti–Crosti (infantile papular acrodermatitis)	– Symmetric lichenoid papules that spare the trunk – Also associated with hepatitis B, adenovirus, and CMV

Diagnosis of EBV
In patients with EBV, leukocytosis, lymphocytosis, and elevated liver function tests may be observed. Other laboratory tests that can be used in diagnosing EBV include the heterophile antibody test, the monospot test, and EBV serology.

Treatment

Most EBV infections are self-limited and the treatment is symptomatic care.

Human Herpes Virus 5: Cytomegalovirus

Human herpes virus 5, or cytomegalovirus (CMV), is an enveloped dsDNA virus in which a latent infection occurs in the host after infection, and may reactivate during a period of immunosuppression.

The primary infection is usually asymptomatic. Maculopapular rashes and ulcers may develop, as well fever. Enlargement of the lymph nodes and spleen is also observed.

Complications of CMV include CMV pneumonia (in 19% of cases), mononucleosis-like syndrome after treatment with ampicillin or amoxicillin, Guillain-Barré syndrome, and Gianotti–Crosti syndrome. Bone marrow transplant patients that develop CMV have an 85% mortality rate secondary to CMV pneumonia. Patients who have received a solid organ transplant and develop CMV have a four times fold increase in mortality.

Congenital CMV

CMV is the most common congenital infection. Current estimates suggest that 30,000 to 40,000 infants are born with congenital CMV every year in the United States alone. The likelihood of congenital infection and the extent of disease in the newborn depend on maternal immune status. If primary maternal infection occurs during pregnancy, the average rate of transmission is 40%. Most of these infants have cytomegalic inclusion disease at birth. If primary infection occurs during the first trimester, intrauterine growth retardation, retinitis, and optic nerve malformations can manifest. If primary infection occurs after the first trimester, hepatitis, pneumonia, purpura, and disseminated intravascular coagulation (DIC) may occur. With recurrent maternal disease, the risk of transmission to the fetus is lower, ranging from 0.5% to 1.5%. Most of these infants appear normal at birth, but may have subtle growth retardation as compared to noninfected infants.

HIV and CMV

Retinitis is the most common symptom.

Diagnosis

Vasculitis is apparent histologically. "Owl's eyes" inclusions or basophilic intranuclear inclusions are observed. Laboratory studies include viral culture and shell vial assay.

Treatment

Medical care consists of good nutritional support, vigorous supportive care for end-organ syndromes, and specific antiviral therapy. Ganciclovir is the drug of choice for CMV disease. Foscarnet treats CMV that is resistant to ganciclovir. Cidofovir is used for refractory CMV retinitis. Valganciclovir and fomivirsen may also be used to treat CMV disease.

Human Herpes Virus 6: Roseola Infantum

This enveloped DNA virus is spread mainly by oropharyngeal secretions. It is the most common childhood exanthem.

Clinical Manifestations

Typically, the infection occurs in children aged 6 months to 2 years. The incubation period is 5 to 15 days. The virus is spread during the febrile and viremic phase of the illness. Generally, patients present in no apparent distress despite the abrupt onset of high fever (102.2°F –105.8°F). Other clinical signs of infection include a bulging anterior fontanelle, tonsillar and pharyngeal inflammation, tympanic injection, and lymph node enlargement. Fever drops on the fourth day, coinciding with the onset of a rash with characteristic 2 to 5 mm pink macules that begins on the trunk and may spread to the neck and upper and lower extremities. Seizures may occur during the febrile phase of the illness. Other complications include upper respiratory infection, adenopathy, intussusception, thrombocytic purpura, and mononucleosis.

HIV and HHV-6

HHV-6 has a tropism for CD4+ cells. It increases upregulation of CD4 expression, which is needed by the gp120 unit of HIV to infect cells.

Bone marrow transplant patients and HHV-6

Idiopathic bone marrow suppression occurs secondary to HHV-6 infection.

Diagnosis

Diagnosis is based on serology.

Treatment

Symptomatic care is the treatment of choice. Some case reports describe foscarnet and ganciclovir to be successful, but dosages are not known.

Human Herpes Virus 7

HHV-7 has significant homology with HHV-6. No clinical disease has been definitely linked to HHV-7, although the literature describes a questionable relationship to pityriasis rosea. Eighty-five percent of adults are seropositive for HHV-7, and most infections occur during the first 5 years of life. It is transmitted through the saliva.

Diagnosis

HHV-7 is diagnosed through serology.

Treatment

Treatment is symptomatic.

Human Herpes Virus 8: Kaposi's Sarcoma

Kaposi's sarcoma (KS) is a spindle cell tumor thought to be derived from endothelial cell lineage. The condition carries a variable course that ranges from minimal mucocutaneous disease to extensive organ involvement (see Table 2.9).

Histologically, typical findings include proliferations of spindle cells, prominent slit-like vascular spaces, and extravasated red blood cells.

Clinical Manifestations

Lesions can include the skin, oral mucosa, lymph nodes, and visceral organs. Most patients present with cutaneous disease only.

CUTANEOUS LESIONS

Cutaneous lesions can occur at any location, but are most commonly concentrated on the lower extremities and in the head

Table 2.9: Clinical Courses of Kaposi's Sarcoma (KS)

Type of KS	Clinical Course
Epidemic AIDS-related KS	– Occurs in patients with advanced HIV infection – Most common presentation of KS – Visceral involvement is common – Most clinically aggressive form of KS
Immunocompromised KS	– Occurs in patients receiving immunosuppressive therapy, namely organ transplantation patients – Visceral involvement is common – Develops about 30 months following transplantation
Classic KS	– Typically occurs in elderly men of Mediterranean and Eastern European descent – Carries a protracted and indolent course – Common complications: venous stasis and lymphedema – Visceral involvement is uncommon
Endemic African KS	– Occurs in HIV-seronegative persons in Africa – May carry an indolent or aggressive course

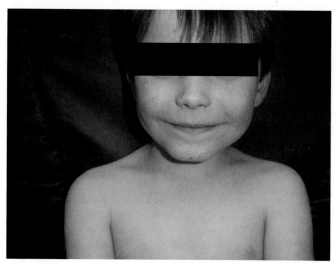

Figure 2.7. Parvo B19.

and neck regions. Nearly all lesions are palpable and nonpruritic. They range in size from several millimeters to several centimeters in diameter. The lesions may be macular, papular, nodular, or plaque-like with colors varying from brown to pink to red or violaceous. In dark-skinned individuals, KS lesions can be difficult to distinguish. The lesions may be discrete or confluent, and characteristically, they appear in a linear, symmetric distribution, following Langer lines.

Tumor-associated lymphedema may occur, especially in cases with facial or lower extremity involvement. This is thought to be secondary to the obstruction of lymph channels.

Diagnosis
A punch biopsy of the skin or an endoscopic, pleural, or transbronchial biopsy is necessary to establish a definitive histologic diagnosis.

Treatment
Treatment includes antiretroviral therapy, excision of solitary KS lesions, radiation, topical retinoids, intralesional vinblastine, interferon α, and chemotherapy.

Herpes Virus B: Herpes Simiae

Herpes virus B is transmitted to humans through primates of the *Macaca* species from a bite, scratch, or open wound. The infection is neurotropic, remaining latent in the ganglia. In humans, initial local erythema occurs with vesicular eruption at the site of

injury. Herpes simiae has a high mortality rate, as death occurs secondary to encephalitis.

Treatment
Treatment is with nucleoside analogues, namely intravenous acyclovir.

PARVOVIRUSES

Parvovirus B19: "Slapped Cheeks," Fifth Disease, Erythema Infectiosum

Parvovirus B19 is the only member of the Parvoviridae family known to cause disease in humans. This single-stranded DNA virus has a tropism for rapidly dividing erythrocyte precursors. Worldwide, B19 infection is very common. Seropositivity rates are 5% to 10% among young children in the United States, and increases to 50% by age 15 and 60% by age 30.

Clinical Manifestations
Twenty percent of B19 infections are asymptomatic. Common symptoms include a mild prodromal illness of fever, malaise, headache, myalgias, nausea, and rhinorrhea. This occurs about 2 days before the onset of a rash. A bright red rash appears on the cheeks; thus the characteristic "slapped cheek" appearance (see Fig. 2.7). This is often followed by a diffuse erythematous eruption with a lacy marble-like appearance that shows up on the trunk and lower extremities. The eruption can last 5 to 9 days and can recur for weeks to months with triggers such as sunlight, exercise, temperature change, bathing, and emotional stress. Arthralgias or arthritis occur in 10% of children.

Alternatively, parvovirus B19 infection can manifest with a purpuric rash, erythema multiforme, or pruritus of the soles and feet. The infection may also cause a papular-pruritic "gloves and socks" syndrome that manifests as an erythematous exanthem of the hands and feet with a distinct margin at the wrist and ankle joints. Pain and edema also occur.

Complications (See Table 2.10)

Table 2.10: Complications of Parvovirus B19

Complication	Presentation
Aplastic crisis	– Occurs in patients with hemoglobinopathies, hemolytic anemias, decreased duration of erythrocyte survival
Chronic anemia	– Occurs in immunocompromised patients
Symmetric postinfectious arthritis	– Affects small joints of hands and feet – More common in women – May persist for weeks to years – May mimic rheumatoid arthritis
Hydrops fetalis	– Occurs when maternal infection occurs before 20 weeks of gestations

Diagnosis
Parvovirus serology (IgM and IgG) can be determined. A complete blood count may demonstrate a low reticulocyte count.

Treatment
Treatment is symptomatic. Red blood cell transfusions may be necessary for aplastic anemia.

HEPADNAVIRUSES

Hepatitis B

Hepatitis B is a disease of the liver caused by the hepatitis B virus. This partially double-stranded circular DNA virus encodes four overlapping reading frames that are as follows:

– S for the surface or envelope gene encoding the pre-S1, pre-S2, and S protein
– C for the core gene, encoding the core nucleocapsid protein and the E antigen
– X for the X gene encoding the X protein
– P for the polymerase gene, which encodes a large protein promoting priming, RNA-dependent and DNA-dependent polymerase and RNase H activities.

The infection is transmitted through exposure to bodily fluids containing the virus. This includes sexual contact, perinatal exposure, blood transfusions, and the reuse of contaminated needles and syringes. Incubation lasts for approximately 75 days.

Clinical Manifestations
PRODROMAL OR PREICTERIC PHASE
An illness similar to serum sickness develops. In 20% to 30% of patients, arthropathy, proteinuria, and hematuria also develop.

ICTERIC PHASE
Jaundice occurs about 10 days after the appearance of constitutional symptoms and can last for 1 to 3 months. Nausea, vomiting, and pruritus are also associated with this phase.

SKIN MANIFESTATIONS
Urticaria and vasculitis may occur secondary to perivascular depositions of immune globulin complexes.

Associated conditions

Transient hypocomplementemia associated with urticaria

Polyarteritis nodosa

Globulinemia

Erythema nodosum

Lichen planus

Leukocytoclastic vasculitis

Gianotti–Crosti

Diagnosis
For active hepatitis B: high levels of the enzymes ALT and AST; HBsAg and HBeAg identified in the serum; HBcAb
For chronic inactive hepatitis: HBsAg, HBcAb of IgG type, and HBeAb identified in the serum
For chronic active hepatitis B: Mild to moderate elevation of the aminotransferases

Treatment
Interferon-α, lamivudine, adefovir dipivoxil, and telbivudine. Prophylaxis is recommended with the hepatitis B vaccine.

RNA VIRUSES

For a brief overview of the RNA viruses, see Table 2.11.

Picornaviruses

Enteroviruses

HAND, FOOT, AND MOUTH DISEASE
This illness is caused by Coxsackie A16 virus and Enterovirus 71 as well as other viruses. The infection is spread by oral–oral transmission, as well as oral–fecal transmission and is highly contagious.

Histologically, intraepidermal blisters, neutrophils, monocytes, necrotic roofs, and intracellular edema are apparent. An edematous dermis as well as intracytoplasmic particles in a crystalline array are also observed.

Clinical Manifestations
Incubation is 3 to 6 days, which is followed by a prodromal exanthem of fever, malaise, and abdominal pain. Oral ulcerative lesions develop on the hard palate, tongue, and buccal mucosa. Two to 10 lesions develop over 5 to 10 days, and these lesions are characterized by vesicles on an erythematous base. Cutaneous lesions develop as well on the hands, feet, and buttocks. A few hundred lesions can develop, more commonly on the hands than on the feet. The lesions are characterized by erythematous macules with a gray center that run parallel to skin lines.

Diagnosis
Diagnosis is made through cell culture and PCR of blood, stool, pharyngeal secretions, and vesicles.

Table 2.11: RNA Viruses

RNA Virus Family	Characteristics
Picornaviruses	– Nonenveloped virions
	– Size ranges from 20 to 25 nm
	– Capsids composed of four different proteins
	– Genome is single-stranded RNA
	– Size ranges from 7500–8500 nucleotides
	• Rhinoviruses
	• Hepatovirus: Hepatitis A virus
	• Enteroviruses
	• Poliovirus
	• Enterovirus
	• Coxsackievirus
	• Echovirus
Togaviruses	– Enveloped
	– ssRNA
	– Rubella
Flaviviruses	– Enveloped
	– ssRNA
	– Hepatitis C
	– Yellow fever
	– Dengue
	– West Nile virus
Retroviruses	– ssRNA
	– Enveloped
	– Contain reverse transcriptase
	– HIV
Paramyxoviruses	– Spherical
	– Enveloped
	– ssRNA
	– Measles
Arenaviruses	– Lassa fever
	– Argentine hemorrhagic fever
Bunyaviruses	– ssRNA – Enveloped
	– Helical symmetry
	– Sandfly fever virus
	– Hantaan virus

Treatment

The infection resolves spontaneously after about 1 week. Treatment is symptomatic care.

HERPANGINA

This infection is spread via the fecal–oral route. It is caused by coxsackievirus A 1–10, 16, and 22; by echovirus 6, 9, 11, 16, 17, 22, and 25; and by enterovirus 71.

Clinical Manifestations

The incubation period is 7 to 14 days with a sudden onset of fever, headache, and back/extremity pain. Lesions occur on mucous membranes, namely, the soft palate, tonsillar pillars, fauces, and uvula. The lesions are gray/white and papulovesicular with surrounding erythema. They range from 1 to 2 mm.

Treatment

Self-limited.

Hepatitis A virus

Hepatitis A

Hepatitis A belongs to the picornaviruses. It is transmitted through fecal–oral contact and has an incubation period of 2 to 7 weeks. Worldwide, there are more than 1.4 million cases of Hepatitis A annually. Fourteen percent of hepatitis cases manifest as transient, discrete, maculopapular, urticarial, or petechial rashes. Rarely, persistent hepatitis A develops into a globulinemia with a cutaneous vasculitis.

Treatment

Supportive care since the infection is mild and self-limited. A combination vaccine for the prevention of hepatitis A and hepatitis B is recommended for persons at risk for infection.

Paramyxoviruses

Rubeola/Measles

Rubeola, or measles, belongs to the family Paramyxoviridae. It is a single-stranded RNA virus that initially infects the respiratory epithelium and is transmitted through respiratory droplets. Measles is responsible for more than 50 million infections and 1 million deaths worldwide annually. It has been called the greatest killer of children in history. The highest incidence of morbidity and mortality is observed in developing countries, but disease still occurs in the United States and other industrialized nations.

Clinical Manifestations

There are four phases to measles infection: incubation, prodrome, enanthem, and exanthem. Measles has an incubation period of 7 to 14 days. It is communicable just before the start of the prodromal symptoms until approximately 4 days following the onset of the exanthem. The prodrome develops on day 0 following incubation and consists of the three Cs: cough, coryza, and conjunctivis. Fever and photophobia are also common during this period. The prodromal symptoms increase in severity up to 3 to 4 days before the onset of the morbilliform rash. The enanthem, Koplik spots, precede the exanthem by about 24 hours. Koplik spots are characterized as red spots on the buccal mucosa with a gray-white center. The exanthem itself begins on the fourth or fifth day following the onset of symptoms and is characterized by nonpruritic red papules that begin on the face and behind the ears that then spread to the trunk and extremities. The exanthem lasts for about 5 days.

Complications

Complications of measles infection include encephalitis, purpura secondary to thrombocytopenia, otitis media, subacute sclerosing panencephalitis, and pneumonia secondary to bacterial infection, tuberculosis.

Diagnosis

Diagnosis is obtained through serology and histology.

Treatment

The treatment for measles is vitamin A and supportive care.

Prophylaxis

The measles vaccine provides protective titers and is usually given with the vaccines for mumps and rubella (MMR).

Togaviruses

Rubella: German Measles

This single-stranded RNA virus belongs to the family of togaviruses. It is a mild viral illness that involves the skin, lymph nodes, and occasionally, the joints.

Histologically, a light perivascular infiltrate of lymphocytes with mild endothelial swelling may be observed. If petechiae or purpura are clinically present, extravasation of erythrocytes may be observed.

Clinical Manifestations

The virus incubates for 2 to 3 weeks and infection is spread by nasal droplets. It is known as "3-day measles," and most commonly presents with generalized lymphadenopathy. It involves all nodes, especially the suboccipital, postauricular, and anterior and posterior cervical nodes.

The exanthem begins as discrete macules on the face that is then spread to the neck, trunk, and the extremities. The macules may coalesce on the trunk. The rash lasts for 1 to 3 days, first leaving the face, and it may be followed by desquamation. Occasionally, a nonspecific enanthem, known as *Forchheimer spots*, can be seen over the soft palate and uvula. The enanthem is characterized by pinpoint red macules and petechiae, and typically occurs just before or along with the exanthem.

Polyarthalgia and polyarthritis may occur along with the infection and may persist for longer than 2 weeks. A syndrome of low-grade fever, chronic fatigue, and myalgias rarely occurs and can persist for months or years after the original infection.

Congenital Rubella Syndrome

Congenital rubella syndrome can occur in the fetus of a pregnant woman without immunity to the virus. Fifty percent of pregnancies result in complications if the fetus is infected during the first trimester. Ophthalmologic complications such as cataracts and retinopathy can result. Cardiac complications include patent ductus arteriosus and pulmonary stenosis. Neurological sequelae of sensorineural deafness, meningoencephalitis, and mental retardation with behavior defects can also occur. Another well-known complication of rubella is a "blueberry muffin" appearance of the infant. This is due to dermal extramedullary hematopoiesis as well as thrombocytopenia with purpura and petechiae.

Diagnosis

Diagnosis is obtained from an isolate from the nose, blood urine, or CSF. However, the diagnosis may also be made on a clinical basis. If the diagnosis is in doubt, a rising titer of IgM antibody over a 2-week period indicates a recent infection.

Treatment

No adequate treatment is available for pregnant women exposed to rubella. The disease is typically self-limited, and symptomatic care is the treatment of choice. The main defense against rubella is immunization (i.e. MMR).

Flaviviruses

Hepatitis C

The World Health Organization estimates that there are 170 million individuals worldwide who are infected with hepatitis C. Medical care costs for treatment of HCV infection in the United States are thought to exceed $600 million dollars per year. Hepatitis C is a spherical enveloped, single-stranded RNA virus belonging to the Flaviviridae family. HCV can produce at least 10 million new particles every day. The natural targets of HCV are hepatocytes, and possibly B lymphocytes.

Clinical Manifestations

Hepatitis C is acquired through parenteral transmission, e.g. blood transfusion as well as via drug abuse, tattoos, body piercing and sometimes by sexual intercourse. Incubation period is 6 to 7 weeks.

ACUTE HCV

Thirty percent of patients present with jaundice. Symptoms are indistinguishable from other types of acute viral hepatitis. Fluctuating serum aminotransferase levels are characteristic.

CHRONIC HCV

HCV is the most common cause of chronic viral hepatitis. Cirrhosis occurs in 8% to 46% percent of patients. The following diseases are associated with chronic hepatitis C infection:

– Immune complexes: skin, kidney (glomerulonephritis)
– Sialadenitis
– Autoimmune thrombocytopenic purpura
– Lymphoma: increased antibodies to HCV in patients with non–Hodgkin's B-cell lymphoma
– Mixed cryoglobulinemia
– Porphyria cutanea tarda
– Lichen planus
– Polyarteritis nodosa
– Pruritus

Treatment

Treatment includes pegylated interferon α + ribavirin.

Retroviruses

Human Immunodeficiency Virus

Human immunodeficiency virus (HIV) is a single-stranded RNA retrovirus that causes acquired immunodeficiency syndrome (AIDS). Infection with HIV occurs by the transfer of blood, semen, vaginal fluid, pre-ejaculate, or breast milk, as the virus is shed in these bodily fluids. The majority of transmission occurs through sexual contact.

Human immunodeficiency virus (HIV) is a Lentivirus, a subgroup of retroviruses. This family of viruses is known for persistent viremia, infection of the nervous system, latency, and weak host immune responses. HIV has a high affinity for CD4+ T lymphocytes and monocytes. The virus binds to CD4+ T cells and replicates itself by generating a DNA copy by reverse transcriptase. In this way, the virus becomes integrated into the host DNA, enabling further replication.

Clinical Manifestations:
HIV infection increases the likelihood of a patient to be afflicted by many different diseases; both infectious and non-infectious (Table 2.12). Primary HIV infection occurs approximately one month after HIV exposure and it is characterized by a self-limited collection of symptoms including fever, malaise, headache, weight loss, gastrointestinal complaints, and sometimes a truncal macular eruption.

HIV infected patients have high rates of infectious conditions which often cause cutaneous manifestations in addition to systemic disease. Viruses including herpesviruses (HSV, VZV, CMV, HHV-8), human papilloma virus, and molluscum contagiosum all cause cutaneous manifestations which have been described previously within this chapter. Epstein Barr virus is a herpesvirus which causes oral hairy leukoplakia. (Table 2.8) Patients with oral hairy leukoplakia present with white, stuck on, verrucous plaques on the tongue which are most often asymptomatic.

Staphylococcus is the most common bacterial agent to cause infection in HIV patients. The infection my result in furuncles, carbuncles, abscesses, cellulitis, folliculitis, impetigo, or necrotizing fasciitis. HIV infected patients are also susceptible to both typical and atypical mycobacterium infections. It is possible for this immunocompromised subset of patients to have cutaneous inoculation with TB or to have cutaneous findings associated with systemic infection. Tuberculous chancre and tuberculosis verrucosa cutis are the two diseases seen with cutaneous inoculation. Tuberculous chancre is a painless ulceration at the inoculation site and tuberculosis verrucosa cutis is a hyperkeratotic plaque at the inoculation site. Disseminated *Mycobacterium tuberculosis* infection can lead to multiple cutaneous findings including; scrofuloderma, lupus vulgaris, and a metastatic tuberculous abscess. Bartonella infection may result in bacillary angiomatosis, which is a cutaneous vascular proliferation. It presents with painful, firm, red nodules that appear very similar to Kaposi's sarcoma lesions. *Treponema pallidum* is the infectious pathogen associated with syphilis. Patients with syphilis and HIV co-infection may have a faster progression through the stages of syphilis, which can have a multitude of manifestations including; nontender genital ulceration (chancre) in primary syphilis; symmetric eruption on the palms and soles, and condyloma lata in secondary syphilis; and destructive granulomatous lesions (gummas) in tertiary syphilis.

Fungal infections with Candida, Histoplamosis, Cryptococcus, and Coccidioidomycosis are common in HIV patients. Infections with Histoplamosis, Cryptococcus, and Coccidioidomycosis can lead to diffuse rashes with varied appearances. Candida, the most common fungal pathogen, causes oral thrush, which presents with white plaques on the tongue and buccal mucosa that can easily be scraped off. Intertriginous eruptions can also occur with candida infection. Histoplamosis infections may lead to mucocutaneous ulcerations or diffuse erythematous eruptions on the body which can be macular, papular, pustular, or psoriasiform. Disseminated skin involvement is rarely seen in HIV patients with systemic Cryptococcus infections and can present with erythematous

Table 2.12: Clinical Manifestations of HIV

Body System	Clinical Manifestation
Constitutional	– Fever – Weight loss – Night sweats – Fatigue/malaise – Lymphadenopathy
Head, ears, eyes, nose, throat	– Oral/esophageal candidiasis – Oral hairy leukoplakia – Blurry vision – Floaters
Central Nervous System	– Confusion – Dementia – Focal deficits – Meningismus – Progressive multifocal leukoencephalopathy – CNS lymphoma

Skin	– Maculopapular rash
	– Primary HIV infection
	– Xerosis
	– Pruritic papular eruption
	– Atopic dermatitis
	– Seborrheic dermatitis
	– Eosinophilic folliculitis
	– Psoriasis
	– Drug rash
	– Photosensitivity
	– Infectious
	  • Bacterial:
	    ▫ Staphylococcus
	    ▫ Bartonella (Bacillary angiomatosis)
	    ▫ Mycobacterium
	      ■ M. tuberculosis
	      ■ Atypical mycobacterium
	    ▫ Treponema (Syphilis)
	  • Viral:
	    ▫ Herpesviruses:
	      ■ Herpes simplex
	      ■ Varicella zoster
	      ■ Cytomegalovirus
	      ■ Epstein-Barr (Oral hairy leukoplakia)
	      ■ HHV-8 (Kaposi's sarcoma)
	    ▫ Human papillomavirus (Condyloma acuminata)
	    ▫ Molluscum contagiosum
	  • Parasitic
	    ▫ Sarcoptes (Scabies)
	  • Fungal
	    ▫ Candida
	    ▫ Dermatophytes
	    ▫ Cryptococcosis
	    ▫ Histoplasmosis
	– Coccidioides

Gastrointestinal	– Nausea – Vomiting – Chronic diarrhea
Genitourinary	– Nephropathy – Cervical cancer
Hematologic	– Burkitt's lymphoma – Diffuse large B-cell lymphoma

papules, nodules, pustules, granulomatous, or verrucous lesions. Patients may also develop ulcerative lesions of the oral mucosa and tongue. Reactivation of pulmonary Coccidioidmycosis can lead to disseminated cutaneous eruptions. These patients may have papules, plaques, nodules, and pustules that overtime coalesce and ulcerate.

Sarcoptes scabiei mite infestation is common in immunocomprimised patients. The female mite burrows under the superficial epidermis leaving distinct linear burrows in the digital webs. In addition, patients have extremely pruritic papular lesions in the axilla, groin, and digital webs. Norwegian scabies consists of hyperkeratotic, scaling, plaques on the scalp, face, back, buttocks, nails, and feet.

There are also several non-infectious dermatologic manifestations of HIV. These skin conditions are common in the general population but when the disease occurs in HIV infected patients it is much more severe and often unresponsive to treatment. Xerotic skin conditions such as acquired ichthyosis (thick fish-like scales) and atopic dermatitis (erythematous scaling plaques) are often much more severe and unresponsive to treatment in HIV infected patients. In general, this patient population has a higher incidence of xerosis; non-erythematous, dry, scaling, cracking skin. Psoriasis, characterized by indurated annular, erythematous plaques with silvery scale, is also more difficult to treat in HIV patients. Explosive episodes of psoriasis may occur with primary HIV infection. Seborrheic dermatitis, consisting of greasy, yellow papules and plaques on the face and scalp, is also more prominent in this patient population. HIV patients may also have involvement of less common areas of the body including the groin, chest, back, and axilla. In addition, HIV infected patients are more prone to photosensitivity reactions compared to the general population.

Pruritic papular eruption (PPE) may occur very early in the course of HIV infection and is characterized by pruritic, hyperpigmented papules on the extremities and trunk that are often chronic in nature. The pruritic lesions do not often respond to anti-pruritic medications.

Eosinophilic folliculitis is an uncommon disease that occurs late in the course of HIV infection and is characterized by pruritic, perifollicular papules and sterile pustules on the trunk. Similar to PPE, anti-pruritic therapy if often unsuccessful.

Adverse drug reactions from HARRT and the antimicrobial therapy used to treat opportunistic infections is frequently seen in the HIV patient population. Zidovudine, a nucleoside reverse transcriptase inhibitor, has been associated with nail dyschromia, brown or blue longitudinal bands that spread down from the proximal nail plate; skin hyperpigmentation, non-specific macular rashes, and urticaria. Nevirapine and delavirapine, non-nucleoside reverse transcriptase inhibitors, may cause transient, pruritic maculopapular eruptions. Protease inhibitors have also been associated with maculopapular eruptions. Trimethoprim-sulfamethoxazole, often used to treat *Pneumocystis carinii* infection, is associated with a wide spectrum of adverse reactions including morbilliform eruptions to Stevens-Johnson syndrome or toxic epidermal necrolysis. Foscarnet, used to treat acyclovir-resistant HSV infections, can cause genital ulcerations from the high concentration of the drug in the urine.

Diagnosis

Human immunodeficiency virus (HIV) is diagnosed by ELISA, Western blot assay, and viral load measured by PCR.

Treatment

Three older, well-established classes of medications exist for the treatment of HIV; three newer classes are also now available. Treatment generally consists of a combination of two or three different medications, as HIV may rapidly develop resistance to single-drug regimens. Patients may undergo testing at various stages of treatment to determine the sensitivities of their virus. All treatments listed below are oral and the adult dosing for treatment-naïve patients, unless otherwise specified.

Nucleoside Reverse Transcriptase Inhibitors (NRTIs):

– Zidovudine: 200 mg TID
– Lamivudine: 150 mg BID
– Stavudine: 40 mg BID
– Didanosine: 20 mg BID
– Zalcitabine: 0.75 mg TID
– Abacavir: 300 mg BID
– Emtricitabine: 200 mg BID
– Tenofovir: 300 mg QD

Several medications are available that are a combination of two or more NRTIs:

– Combivir: zidovudine 300 mg + lamivudine 150 mg, BID
– Trizivir: zidovudine 300 mg + abacavir 300 mg + lamivudine 150 mg, BID
– Epzicom: abacavir 600 mg + lamivudine 300 mg, QD

Non-nucleoside Reverse Transcriptase Inhibitors (NNRTIs):

– Nevirapine: 200 mg for 14 days and then 200 mg BID
– Delavirdine: 400 mg TID in 3 oz of water
– Efavirenz: 600 mg at bedtime
– Etravirine: 200 mg BID

Protease Inhibitors:

– Saquinavir: 1200 mg TID
– Ritonavir: 600 mg BID
– Indinavir: 800 mg every 8 hours
– Lopinavir: 400 mg BID (marketed only in combination with ritonavir 100 mg) or 800 mg QD (marketed only in combination with ritonavir 200 mg)
– Nelfinavir: 750 mg TID
– Amprenavir: 1200 mg BID
– Fosamprenavir calcium: 700 mg BID
– Atazanavir sulfate: 400 mg QD
– Darunavir: 800 mg QD (must be coadministered with ritonavir 100 mg)
– Tipranavir: 500 mg BID (must be coadministered with ritonavir 200 mg)
– Atazanavir: 300 mg QD (coadministered with ritonavir 100 mg) or 400 mg QD (without ritonavir)

Fusion Inhibitors:
– Enfurvirtide: 90 mg BID (subcutaneous injection)

Entry Inhibitors:
– Maraviroc: 300 mg BID

HIV integrase strand transfer inhibitors:
– Raltegravir: 400 mg BID

Multi-class Combination Products:
– Atripla: efavirenz 600 mg + tenofovir 300 mg + emtricitabine 200 mg, at bedtime

PITFALLS AND MYTHS

There are many popular misconceptions about viral infections of the skin. Some of the most popular and egregious beliefs include that frogs transmit warts, herpes can be transmitted through toilet seats, and if someone has chickenpox they cannot bathe or wash their hair, otherwise wind will enter their body and cause rheumatism in their old age. In addition, many members of the lay public believe that a person must have a lesion of genital herpes in order to transmit the virus to a partner.

These common folktales were cleared up in depth throughout the chapter.

SUGGESTED READING

Tyring S, ed. *Mucocutaneous Manifestations of Viral Diseases*. New York: Marcel Dekker; 2002.

Ahmed AM, Madkan V, Tyring SK. Human papillomaviruses and genital disease. *Dermatol Clin* 2006;24(2):157–165.

Balfour HH Jr, Kelly JM, Suarez CS. Acyclovir treatment of varicella in otherwise healthy children. *J Pediatr* 1990;116(4):633–639.

Carrasco D, Vander Straten M, Tyring SK. Treatment of anogenital warts with imiquimod 5% cream followed by surgical excision of residual lesions. *J Am Acad Dermatol* 2002;47(4 Suppl):S212–S216.

Corey L, Wald A, Patel R, et al. Once-daily valacyclovir to reduce the risk of transmission of genital herpes. *N Engl J Med* 2004; 350:11–20.

Fatahzadeh M, Schwartz RA. Human herpes simplex virus infections: epidemiology, pathogenesis, symptomatology, diagnosis, and management. *J Am Acad Dermatol* 2007;57(5):737–763.

Freedberg IM, Eisen AZ, Wolff K, et al. *Fitzpatrick's Dermatology in General Medicine*, 6th Ed. New York: McGraw-Hill; 2003.

Gonzalez L, Gaviria AM, Sanclemente G, et al. Clinical, histopathological and virological findings in patients with focal epithelial hyperplasia from Colombia. *Int J Dermatol* 2005;44:274–279.

Horn TD, Johnson SM, Helm RM, Roberson PK. Intralesional immunotherapy of warts with mumps, Candida, and Trichophyton skin test antigens: a single-blinded, randomized, and controlled trial. *Arch Dermatol* 2005;141(5):589–594

Mertz GJ, Loveless MO, Levin MJ, et al. Oral famciclovir for suppression of recurrent genital herpes simplex virus infection in women. A multicenter, double blind, placebo-controlled trial. *Arch Int Med* 1997;157:343–349.

Nell P, Kohl KS, Graham PL, et al. Progressive vaccinia as an adverse event following exposure to vaccinia virus: Case definition and guidelines of data collection, analysis, and presentation of immunization safety data. *Vaccine* 2007;25(31):5735–5744

Reichman RC, Oakes D, Bonnez W, et al. Treatment of condyloma acuminatum with three different alpha interferon preparations administered parenterally: A double blind, placebo-controlled trial. *J Infect Dis* 1990;162:1270–1276.

Roncalli W, Neto CF, Rady PL, et al. Clinical aspects of epidermodysplasia verruciformis. *J Eur Acad Venereol* 2003;17:394–398.

Tyring S, ed. *Antiviral Agents, Vaccines and Immunotherapies*. New York: Marcel Dekker; 2005.

Tyring SK, Beutner KR, Tucker BA, et al. Antiviral therapy for herpes zoster. *Arch Fam Med* 2000;9:863–869.

Tyring SK, Edwards L, Friedman DJ, et al. Safety and efficacy of 0.5% podofilox gel in the treatment of external genital and/or perianal warts: A double blind, vehicle-controlled study. *Arch Dermatol* 1998;134:33–38.

Scheinfeld N, Lehman DS. An evidence-based review of medical and surgical treatments of genital warts. *Dermatol Online J* 2006;12(3):5.

Lichon V, Khachemoune A. Plantar warts: a focus on treatment modalities. *Dermatol Nurs* 2007;19(4):372–375. Review.

Cox JT. Epidemiology and natural history of HPV. *J Fam Pract* 2006; Suppl:3–9.

Gewirtzman A, Bartlett B, Tyring S. Epidermodysplasia verruciformis and human papilloma virus. *Curr Opin Infect Dis* 2008; 21(2):141–146.

De Oliveira WR, Festa Neto C, Rady PL, Tyring SK. Clinical aspects of epidermodysplasia verruciformis. *J Eur Acad Dermatol Venereol* 2003;17:394–398.

Anadolu R, Oskay T, McGregor JM, et al. Treatment of epidermodysplasia verruciforme with a combination of acitretin and Interferon alfa-2a. *J Am Acad Dermatol* 2001;45:296–299

Baskan EB, Tunali S, Adim SB, Turan A, Toker S. A case of epidermodysplasia verruciformis associated with squamous cell carcinoma and Bowen's disease: a therapeutic challenge. *J Dermatolog Treat* 2006;17(3):179–183

Breman JG, Henderson DA. Diagnosis and management of smallpox. *N Engl J Med* 2002;346(17):1300–8.

Nalca A, Rimoin AW, Bavari S, Whitehouse CA. Reemergence of monkeypox: prevalence, diagnostics, and countermeasures. *Clin Infect Dis* 2005;41(12):1765–1771.

Dohil MA, Lin P, Lee J, Lucky AW, Paller AS, Eichenfield LF. The epidemiology of molluscum contagiosum in children. *J Am Acad Dermatol* 2006;54(1):47–54.

Corey L, Wald A, Patel R, et al. Once-daily valacyclovir to reduce the risk of transmission of genital herpes. *N Engl J Med* 2004; 350(1):11–20.

Wolff K, Johnson R, Suurmond D. *Fitzpatrick's Color Atlas and Synopsis of Clinical Dermatology*. 5th ed. New York: McGraw-Hill Publishing; 2005

Reichman RC, Badger GJ, Mertz GJ, et al. Treatment of recurrent genital herpes simplex infections with oral acyclovir. A controlled trial. *JAMA* 1984;251(16):2103–2107.

Sheffield JS, Hill JB, Hollier LM, et al. Valacyclovir prophylaxis to prevent recurrent herpes at delivery: a randomized clinical trial. *Obstet Gynecol* 2006;108(1):141–147

Tyring SK, Diaz-Mitoma F, Shafran SD, Locke LA, Sacks SL, Young CL. Oral famciclovir for the suppression of recurrent genital herpes: the combined data from two randomized controlled trials. *J Cutan Med Surg* 2003;7(6):449–454.

De Clercq E. Antiviral drugs in current clinical use. *J Clin Virol* 2004;30(2):115–133

Chakrabarty A, Beutner K. Therapy of other viral infections: herpes to hepatitis. *Dermatol Ther* 2004;17(6):465–490

Gnann JW, Jr., Whitley RJ. Clinical practice. Herpes zoster. *N Engl J Med* 2002;347(5):340–346.

Seward JF, Watson BM, Peterson CL, et al. Varicella disease after introduction of varicella vaccine in the United States, 1995–2000. *JAMA* 2002;287(5):606–611

Lesher JL, Jr. Cytomegalovirus infections and the skin. *J Am Acad Dermatol* 1988;18(6):1333–13338.

Zerr DM, Meier AS, Selke SS, et al. A population-based study of primary human herpesvirus 6 infection. *N Engl J Med* 2005; 352(8):768–776.

De Bolle L, Naesens L, De Clercq E. Update on human herpesvirus 6 biology, clinical features, and therapy. *Clin Microbiol Rev* 2005;18(1):217–245.

Parvovirus B19 (erythema infectiosum, fifth disease). Red Book 2006: In: Report of the Committee on Infectious Diseases, 27th edition. Washington, D.C.: American Academy of Pediatrics; 2006

Khetsuriani N, Lamonte-Fowelks A, Oberste S, Pallansch M. Enterovirus surveillance – United States, 1970–2005: Center for Disease Contol and Prevention. *MMWR Surveill Summ* 2006;55(8):1–20.

Measles eradication: Recommendations from a meeting cosponsored by the World Health Organization, the Pan American Health Organization, and CDC: Centers for Disease Control; 1997.

Reef SE, Frey TK, Theall K, et al. The changing epidemiology of rubella in the 1990s: on the verge of elimination and new challenges for control and prevention. *JAMA* 2002;287(4):464–72.

Mendoza N, Diamantis M, Arora A, et al. Mucocutaneous manifestations of Epstein-Barr virus infection. *Am J Clin Dermatol* 2008; 9(5):295–305.

Garman ME, Tyring SK. The cutaneous manifestations of HIV infection. *Dermatol Clin* 2002;20:193–208.

Trent JT, Kirsner RS. Cutaneous manifestations of HIV: A primer. *Adv Skin Wound Care* 2004;17(3):116–129.

Chaker MB, Cockerell CJ. Conconmitant psoriasis, seborrheic dermatitis, and disseminated cutaneous histoplamosis in a patient infected with human immunodeficiency virus. *J Am Acad Dermatol* 1993;29(2 Pt 2):311–313.

Hazelhurst JA, Vismer HF. Histoplamosis presenting with unusual skin lesions in acquired immunodeficiency syndrome. *Br J Dermatol* 1985;113(3):345–8.

Kalter DC, Tschen JA, Klima M. Maculopapular rash in a patient with acquired immunodeficiency syndrome. Disseminated histoplasmosis in acquired acquired immunodeficiency syndrome. *Arch Dermatol* 1985;121(11):1445–1449.

Lindgren AM, Fallon JD, Horan RF. Psoriasiform papules in the acquired immunodeficiency syndrome. Disseminated histoplamosis and AIDS. *Arch Dermatol* 1991;127(5):722–726.

Dimino-Emme L, Gurevitch AW. Cutaneous manifestations of disseminated Cryptococcus. *J Am Acad Dermatol* 1995;32 (5 Pt 2):844–850.

Lynch DP, Naftolin LZ. Oral Cyrptococcus neoformans infection in AIDS. *Oral Surg Med Oral Pathol* 1987;64(4):449–53.

3 | COMMON FUNGAL INFECTIONS

Aditya K. Gupta and Elizabeth A. Cooper

HISTORY

Fungal organisms have a long history of human infection. The "tinea" infections have historically been referred to as "ringworm," because of the presentation of lesions as circular or oval areas of clearing within a red, scaly, elevated "ring." It has only been with the developments in science and medicine in the industrial age that the causal agents were recognized as being microscopic fungi. Taxonomy has only distinguished the dermatophyte organisms most frequently associated with fungal infection (*Trichophyton* sp., *Microsporum* sp. and *Epidermophyton* sp.) since 1934.

In 1958 the first effective oral antifungal agent, griseofulvin, was developed. Following the success of griseofulvin, other oral medications continued to be researched. Ketoconazole was the next major antifungal agent, released in the United States in 1981, followed by fluconazole, terbinafine, and itraconazole within the next decade. These medications are typically classified as azoles (itraconazole, fluconazole, intraconazole, oxiconazole, spectozole, sertaconazole, chlotrimazole, miconazole, bifonazole, sulconazole, ketoconazole) or allylamines (terbinafine, butenafine, naftifine).

Besides the common dermatophyte infections, superficial fungal infections may also result from the *Malassezia* species of yeast. *Malassezia* was first recognized as a pathogen in 1846; however, laboratory culture was unsuccessful until 1927, when the lipid requirement of the species was recognized. Initially only two species under the genus name *Pityrosporum* were described, and only three species were recognized as of 1970. Difficulty in identification was also complicated by the existence of both yeast and mycelial forms, and conversion between forms could not be induced in the laboratory until 1977. Genetic research in the 1990s confirmed that at least seven species of *Malassezia* existed, and more have been discovered since.

Though dermatology and dermatophytosis have a long history, it is only the most recent past that has greatly changed and improved dermatological treatment. The future of these specialties holds great change as biochemistry and genetic research develop and allow for greater understanding of infectious disease. Currently, molecular testing methods are in development and may lead to easier and more accurate fungal identification. Furthermore, molecular research may lead to more targeted treatments that would increase the efficacy of treatment.

EPIDEMIOLOGY

Fungal organisms may infect any location of the body and infections are named on the basis of the area infected. Examples are as follows: tinea corporis/cruris – trunk/face, including arms and legs; tinea capitis – scalp; tinea pedis and manuum – feet and hands; tinea faciei, tinea barbae – face or beard area; tinea unguium, also known as onychomycosis – nails. Three fungal genera cause tinea infections: *Microsporum*, *Trichophyton*, and more rarely, *Epidermophyton*. Species of fungus infecting humans originate from three main sources: other humans (anthropophilic), animals (zoophilic), or less commonly, soil (geophilic). Anthropophilic dermatophytes are the most frequent causes of onychomycosis and other superficial dermatophytoses, and the most frequently seen agents of infection are *Trichophyton rubrum* and *Trichophyton mentagrophytes*. *Trichophyton tonsurans* is currently the most frequent cause of tinea capitis in North America. *Microsporum canis* is a zoophilic organism frequently picked up by humans from contact with animals such as dogs and cats. The major causative species differ geographically and may change in prevalence over time because of population movements from immigration or travel.

The dermatophytes colonize keratinized tissue of the stratum corneum; invasion by anthropophilic species usually results in less inflammation than that of zoophilic or geophilic species. Entry into the stratum corneum may result from trauma to the skin or some other breach of the skin barrier. Excessive sweating and occlusive clothing/footwear aid in providing a warm, moist environment conducive to tinea infection. The presence of health problems such as diabetes and immunocompromised status may also increase the risk of contracting fungal infection.

Autoinoculation can occur, for example, tinea pedis spreading to tinea cruris, tinea capitis to tinea corporis, or onychomycosis to tinea pedis. Infection may also be transmitted between individuals by direct or indirect contact with scales containing fungal arthroconidia from infected individuals, such as those seen in individuals participating in contact sports including wrestling and rugby. Fomites can also play a significant role in transmission. Humans and animals may be asymptomatic pathogen carriers.

Dermatophyte infection in outpatients seen by physicians in the United States was estimated to result in 21.6 million physician office visits between 1990 and 1994. Infection frequencies in subjects with dermatophytoses were as follows: tinea corporis – 27.2%; tinea cruris – 16.9%; tinea pedis – 16.7%; tinea unguium – 15.6%; tinea of hair and beard – 6.9%; and tinea manuum – 1.0%. Tinea pedis is estimated to affect 10% of the world population and occurs most commonly in the web space between the fourth and fifth toes (Figs. 3.1 and 3.2). Onychomycosis has an estimated prevalence of 6.5% to 12.8% in North America, accounting for up to 50% of all nail disease. Tinea pedis is frequently found in association with onychomycosis. Similarly, tinea manuum may accompany tinea

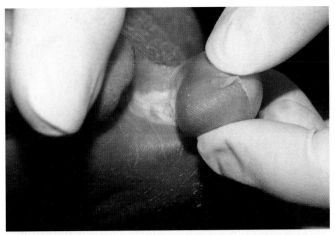

Figure 3.1. Tinea pedis wth interdigital infection.

Figure 3.3. Tinea capitis.

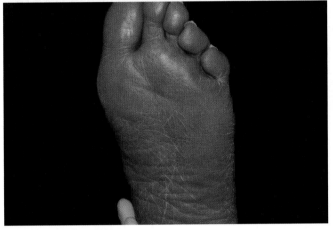

Figure 3.2. Plantar tinea pedis.

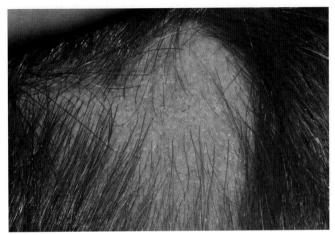

Figure 3.4. Tinea capitis

pedis or onychomycosis, and a two feet-one hand syndrome has been noted to occur.

Tinea capitis shows great variation in epidemiology compared to the other tineas. Unlike the other tineas and onychomycosis, which is associated with increased age, tinea capitis is most prevalent in children between 6 months and before puberty (Fig. 3.3). African-Americans develop tinea capitis at much higher frequencies than the general US population, though this is not the case in the other types of tinea (Fig. 3.4). There also appear to be differences in worldwide distribution of infectious species: In North America, *Trichophyton tonsurans* is the predominant cause of tinea capitis infection; In Western Europe, *Microsporum canis* and *Trichophyton violaceum* are the most common pathogens of tinea capitis; *T. tonsurans* is dominant in the Caribbean and South America; *M. canis*, *Trichophyton mentagrophytes*, and *T. violaceum* dominate in the Middle East. The epidemiology of tinea capitis has shown numerous changes in North America over the past century, with *T. tonsurans* replacing *Microsporum audouinii* as the predominant organism.

Pityriasis versicolor (PV), also known as tinea versicolor, is not strictly speaking a "tinea," as the causative organisms are not dermatophytes, but *Malassezia* yeast. *Malassezia* organisms are a normal part of human commensal skin flora, found particularly in sebaceous skin such as the chest, back, and head. Pityriasis versicolor results when *Malassezia* organisms are converted from the yeast phase to a mycelial phase and are able to infect the stratum corneum, producing the characteristic hypo- or hyperpigmented lesions that can spread into a given area much like a dermatophyte infection (Figs. 3.5 and 3.6). The most common *Malassezia* species contributing to PV lesions are *M. globosa* (50%–60%), *M. sympodialis* (3%–59%), *M. furfur* and *M. slooffiae* (1%–10% each). Pityriasis versicolor (PV) has worldwide distribution, though prevalence is higher in tropical climates compared to temperate climates (30%–40% versus 1%–4%, respectively). PV does not typically affect prepubescent children, but is more frequent in adults where sebaceous gland activity is very high. Equal prevalence between the sexes has been noted. Predisposing factors include high temperature and humidity, malnutrition, the use of oral contraceptives, hyperhidrosis, genetic susceptibility, increased plasma cortisol levels, and immunodeficiency.

DIAGNOSIS

Presentation of tinea infection is typically as annular erythematous plaques with raised leading edges and scaling (central clearing of the lesion may be noticed). Nodules may remain present throughout the lesion (Fig. 3.7). Infection is typically associated

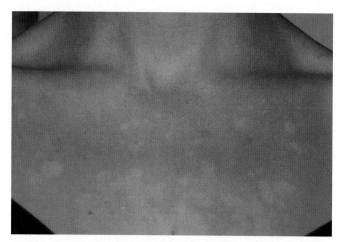

Figure 3.5. Tinea versicolor hypopigmentation.

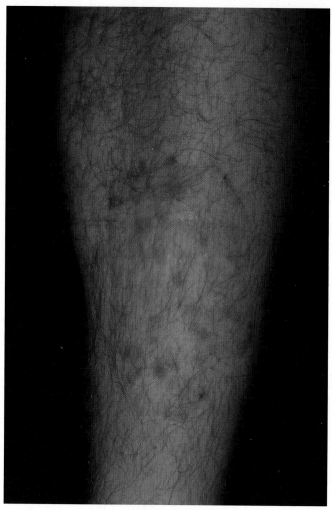

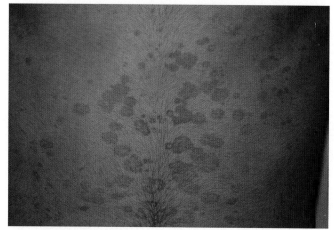

Figure 3.6. Tinea versicolor hyperpigmentation.

Figure 3.7. Tinea corpora of the shin (majocchi granuloma).

with pruritus. Infection may also present as an erythematous papule or series of vesicles. Significant inflammation may result from infection with zoophilic organisms such as *T. verrucosum* or *Microsporum canis* and produce large pustular lesions or a kerion or associated with formation of frank bullae causing tinea corporis bullosa. Infection may also spread down the hair shaft into the dermis producing inflammatory papules and pustules. Typical presentations and variations of the major tinea infections and pityriasis versicolor are listed in Table 3.1.

Definitive diagnosis of tineas requires confirmation of dermatophyte organisms within the affected tissue. For skin infections, scrapings or swabs can be taken from the leading edge of a lesion. Nail clippings and subungual debris can similarly be investigated. Currently, fungal elements are detected using microscopic examination and laboratory fungal culture methods. Potassium hydroxide (KOH) is added to the samples to dissociate hyphae from keratinocytes, and the samples are examined by microscopy. Microscopy can indicate the presence of dermatophytes via the presence of hyphae. However, dermatophyte species cannot be distinguished between each other by microscopy, therefore cultures are required to confirm the causative species.

Microscopic examination of hairs may help differentiate types of tinea capitis infection. Ectothrix infection can be distinguished from endothrix infection by the way that arthroconidia

appear as chains on the surface of the hair shaft or as a mosaic sheath around the hair in ectothrix infections. Inspection under the Wood's light (filtered ultraviolet light with a peak of 365 nm) can aid in diagnosis. Ectothrix infections with *M. audouinii*, *M. canis* and *M. ferrugineum* show bright green fluorescence under the Wood's light. *T. schoenleinii* shows dull green fluorescence. *T. tonsurans*, however, does not fluoresce, and the utility of the Wood's lamp for diagnosis is currently limited in countries where this is the major infecting agent.

As with dermatophyte infections, *Malassezia* organisms should be identified in skin scrapings for definitive diagnosis. They are easily identified by microscopic examination of skin scrapings that reveal fungal hyphae in a typical "spaghetti and meatball" pattern. PV lesions fluoresce yellow/green or gold under the Wood's light. The examination, however, is positive in only one-third of all PV cases, and most likely in cases when the causative organism is *M. furfur*.

THERAPY

Methods of treatment vary widely, depending on the type and extent of infection. However, antifungal medications used will

Table 3.1: Presentation of Common Dermatophyte and Superficial Fungal Infections

Condition	Presentation
Tinea pedis	*Interdigital:* scaling, fissuring, maceration, erosions, hyperhidrosis, pruritus, odor
	Moccasin: fine silvery scales with underlying pink or red skin on soles, heels, sides of feet
	Vesicobullous: inflammatory vesicular or bullous lesions, particularly at in-step
Tinea manuum	Dry, scaly, hyperkeratotic skin particularly of the palmar area, minimal erythema
Tinea corporis	Annular erythematous plaques with raised leading edges and scaling, over glabrous skin of trunk; may be central clearing
Tinea cruris	Annular erythematous plaques with raised leading edges and scaling, over the pubic area, perineal and perianal skin, typically not affecting the scrotum or labia majora
Tinea capitis	*Non-Inflammatory:* erythematous papules around the hair shaft spreading out with fine scaling in noticeable patches and partial or complete alopecia
	Black dot: noticeable black dots where hair breakage at scalp level occurs, scaling with little inflammation (particularly with *T. tonsurans* or *T. violaceum*)
	Inflammatory: kerion with pustules, loose hair, discharge of pus
	Favic: large yellow crusts on the scalp
Onychomycosis	*Distal lateral subungual (DLSO):* infection at the distal end of nail plate; discoloration and thickening of nail plate, onycholysis, subungual debris
	Superficial white (SWO): White spots or patches on the surface of the nail plate
	Proximal subungual (PSO): infection of the proximal nail fold, and extending distally, typically whitish in color
	Endonyx: Milky white discoloration of the nail plate without hyperkeratosis, onycholysis; may show lamellar splitting of the nail plate (typically caused by *T. soudanense* or *T. violaceum*)
Pityriasis versicolor	Well-defined, hyperpigmented or hypopigmented lesions of areas with high concentrations of sebaceous glands such as scalp, chest, back, upper arms and face; showing fine scaling in most cases (caused by *Malassezia* species)

typically be either an azole agent or allylamine (Table 3.2). For most tineas, topical therapy applied directly to the affected areas once or twice daily provides adequate resolution of infection. Topical corticosteroid use is not recommended, as it may lead to suppression of physical signs of infection, with lack of symptoms being wrongly associated with clearance of infection,

leading to treatment relapse. Oral therapy may be considered for patients with larger areas of involvement, where infection presents with unusual severity or persistence, or where oral therapy may be more convenient than daily topical application. Similarly, patients who are immunocompromised may be provided with oral treatment where prompt, thorough resolution of infection is mandatory. Onychomycosis is an exception as topical medications may not penetrate the nail unit adequately, and most cases will require oral rather than topical therapy. Similarly, tinea capitis is most frequently and effectively treated with oral medication, though topical products may be used prophylactically or to prevent relapse of infection.

Cure rates of tinea corporis/cruris/pedis are high, and typically infections resolve with a few weeks of topical therapy. Cure rates for tinea capitis are also high, but longer periods of oral therapy are required (approximately 4–6 weeks of treatment, on average). Cure rates for onychomycosis with oral therapy are not as high as desirable, and reinfection/relapse is common. Oral therapy for onychomycosis is usually given for 12 weeks at a minimum, and extra "booster" therapy may be warranted for cases where improvement is not seen with initial therapy. Also, since diseased nails must be grown out and replaced by new, normal nails, it can take upwards of 9 to 12 months before sufficient efficacy becomes clinically obvious.

Relapse after therapy has been noted with most types of dermatophyte infection. Patients must be encouraged to complete a full treatment cycle, as infection can be present without visible symptoms. Microscopic examination and culture are required to confirm elimination of the pathogen. Infection transmission from symptom-free carriers like family members and pets may need to be controlled with adjunct therapies and techniques. Fomites such as hats and combs must also be treated.

Antifungal Medications

Owing to the numerous types and formulations of topical antifungals, individual discussion of the topical antifungals is not provided here. Antifungals that also provide antibacterial or anti-inflammatory activity are particularly useful, as bacterial superinfection can occur in dermatophytosis, and some dermatophytoses may present with significant inflammation. With topical agents, most adverse events are skin reactions at the application site, which are mild and transient. Safety of therapy is less of a concern for topical medications than oral medications, as serum absorption tends to be minimal with topical dermatophytosis therapy. Current country-specific prescribing information should be consulted prior to prescribing a topical antifungal formulation.

Five main systemic agents are available: terbinafine, itraconazole, fluconazole, griseofulvin, and ketoconazole. Dosing and efficacy vary with indication. The oral antifungal medications may be associated with some potential for severe hepatic toxicity, rare serious skin events such as Stevens-Johnson syndrome, and possible drug-drug interactions due to metabolism through the cytochrome P450 system (Table 3.3). Current country-specific prescribing information for any oral antifungal medication should be consulted prior to providing any medication. Though oral antifungals are typically not approved for use in children, pediatric use has been documented widely in the medical literature. It has typically provided safety profiles similar to those

Table 3.2: Treatment options available for dermatophytoses and pityriasis versicolor.

	Terbinafine	Itraconazole	Fluconazole	Ketoconazole	Griseofulvin	Topicals	
Tinea pedis/ manuum†	*Cream: apply twice daily x 1–4 wks; *1% Solution: apply twice daily for 1 wk; Oral: 250 mg/day 2 wks	**Oral:** 200 mg BID for 1 week	**Oral:** 150 mg once weekly for 2–6 wks	*2% Cream: apply once daily for 6 wks; *Oral: 200–400 mg/day for >4 wks	**Microsize 1** g/day **Ultramicrosize** 660 or 750 mg/day X 4–8 wks	*Ciclopirox 0.77% cream and gel twice daily for 4 wks; Antifungal powder for prevention	*Clotrimazole *Miconazole *Butenafine *Econazole *Naftifine *Oxiconazole
Tinea corporis/cruris	*Cream: apply twice daily x 1–4 wks; *1% Solution: apply twice daily for 1 wk; Oral: 250 mg/day 2–4 wks	**Oral:** 200 mg/day for 1 week	**Oral:** 150–300 mg once weekly for 2–4 wks	*2% Cream: apply once daily for 2 wks; *Oral: 200–400 mg/day for 4 wks	**Microsize 500** mg/day **Ultramicrosize** 330–375 mg/day X 2–4 wks	*Ciclopirox 0.77% cream and gel twice daily for 4 wks	*Clotrimazole *Miconazole *Butenafine *Econazole *Naftifine *Oxiconazole
Tinea capitis	See Table 3.4: Pediatric Dosing	See Table 3.4: Pediatric Dosing	See Table 3.4: Pediatric Dosing	Only effective against *Trichophyton*. 2% shampoo used as adjunct therapy	**See Table 3.4: Pediatric Dosing**	Selenium sulfide shampoo 1% as adjunct therapy	Corticosteroid adjunct therapy for severe inflammatory varieties
Onychomycosis	*Oral: 250 mg/day *Toenail: 12 wks Fingernail: 6 wks*	*Oral: *Continuous therapy: 200 mg/day x 12 wks ‡Pulse therapy: 200 mg BID for 1 week, followed by 3 itraconazole-free weeks *Toenails: 3 pulses *Fingernails only: 2 pulses*	**Oral:** 150 mg once weekly *Toenail:* 9–15 months *Fingernail:* 4–9 months	Oral: 200–400 mg/day x 6 months *Not recommended due to hepatotoxicity risk.*	*Microsize 1 g/day Ultramicrosize 660 or 750mg/day X 4–12 months	*Ciclopirox 8% lacquer once daily x 48 wks	Amorolfine 5% laquer[66] – *Not approved in North America*
Pityriasis versicolor	*1% Solution: apply twice daily for 1 wk; Oral: not effective	Oral: 200 mg/day 5–7 days	2% Shampoo: 5 days; Oral: 300 mg once weekly for 2 wks	*2% Cream: apply once daily for 2 wks; *2% Shampoo: single use; Oral: 200mg/day for 2 weeks, 10 days or 5 days; 400 mg per week for 2 weeks; 400 mg per day for 3 days; 3 doses of 400 mg given every 12 hours.	Not effective	*Ciclopirox 0.77% cream; *Selenium sulfide	*Clotrimazole *Miconazole *Butenafine *Econazole *Oxiconazole

* FDA approved indication

† There are no approved treatments specifically for tinea manuum; treatments shown are for tinea pedis which are effective in the treatment of tinea manuum.

‡ Current standard of care used by US dermatologists where itraconazole is prescribed.

seen in adults. Oral suspensions are available for many of the oral antifungals, providing easier dosing for children.

Oral terbinafine is indicated by the U.S. Food and Drug Administration (FDA) for the treatment of adults with dermatophyte onychomycosis of the toenails and/or fingernails. Terbinafine has been safely used in general population, as well as in children, the elderly, transplant patients, diabetics, and HIV patients. The more common adverse effects with terbinafine use are headache, gastrointestinal symptoms, and dermatologic manifestations (Table 3.3). Less frequently, liver enzyme abnormalities ($\geq$2 times the upper limit of normal), taste disturbances and visual disturbances have been reported. Serum transaminase tests (alanine transaminase, ALT, and aspartate transaminase, AST) are suggested before beginning oral terbinafine to check for preexisting liver dysfunction/disease. Patients should periodically repeat liver function tests while using terbinafine, and be monitored for symptoms of liver dysfunction such as persistent nausea, anorexia, fatigue, vomiting, right upper abdominal pain or jaundice, dark urine, or pale stools. Terbinafine has been reported infrequently to precipitate or exacerbate cutaneous and systemic lupus erythematosus, and should be discontinued in patients showing signs of lupus erythematosus. Furthermore, physicians should consider monitoring complete blood counts in patients with known or suspected immunodeficiency who are administered oral terbinafine for longer than 6 weeks. Terbinafine is metabolized through the CYP2D6 enzymes, and thus may interfere with other CYP2D6 drugs. Other drug interactions are possible, and a current country-specific product monograph should be consulted for complete listing of known drug interactions, warnings and monitoring requirements prior to prescribing. Terbinafine is not recommended for patients with existing liver disease. Terbinafine may be taken in a fasted or fed state without affecting absorption.

Oral itraconazole is indicated by the FDA for the treatment of adults with dermatophyte onychomycosis of the toenails and/or fingernails, and for systemic mycoses such as blastomycosis, histoplasmosis, and aspergillosis. The most commonly reported adverse effects are headache, gastrointestinal disorders, and cutaneous disorders (Table 3.3). Liver function tests should be considered for any subject before dosing and periodically during dosing. Testing is required for any subject with preexisting hepatic function abnormalities or previous experience of liver toxicity with other medications. Abnormal liver function tests were found in 3% of 1845 patients treated with continuous itraconazole compared to 1.9% of 2867 patients treated with pulse itraconazole (200 mg BID for 1 week out of 4 in a month). Itraconazole is metabolized through the CYP3A4 pathway and thus has potential for numerous drug interactions, limiting its use in some patients. Itraconazole is prohibited in patients showing ventricular dysfunction such as current or past congestive heart failure. A current country-specific product monograph should be consulted for complete listing of known drug interactions, warnings, and monitoring requirements before prescribing. Capsules must be taken with a meal or cola beverage to ensure adequate absorption.

Oral fluconazole is indicated by the FDA for the treatment of (1) vaginal candidiasis (vaginal yeast infections due to *Candida* species), (2) oropharyngeal and esophageal candidiasis, and (3) cryptococcal meningitis. Fluconazole may also by used as prophylactic therapy to decrease incidence of candidiasis in patients undergoing bone marrow transplantation who receive cytotoxic chemotherapy or radiation therapy. Fluconazole has shown a favorable adverse effects profile, with the most frequently reported adverse events being nausea (3.7%), headache (1.9%), skin rash (1.8%), vomiting (1.7%), abdominal pain (1.7%), and diarrhea (1.5%) as reported in 4048 clinical trial patients (Table 3.3). When fluconazole and cyclosporine are given concomitantly, careful monitoring of cyclosporine concentration and serum creatinine concentration is recommended. Similarly, blood glucose levels should be closely monitored when using oral hypoglycemics concomitantly with fluconazole, and prothrombin time should be monitored where patients receive coumarin-type anticoagulants concomitantly with fluconazole.

Oral griseofulvin is indicated in the United States for the treatment of tinea infections of the skin, hair, and nails. As with other oral antifungal agents, the use of griseofulvin is not justified for the treatment of tinea infections that would be expected to respond satisfactorily to topical antifungals. Griseofulvin is not effective in the treatment of pityriasis (tinea) versicolor, bacterial infections, candidiasis (moniliasis), or deep mycotic infections. During prolonged griseofulvin therapy, periodic assessment of renal, hepatic and hematopoietic functions should be performed (Table 3.3).

Oral ketoconazole is indicated for the treatment of patients with severe recalcitrant cutaneous dermatophyte infections who have not responded to topical therapy or oral griseofulvin, or who are unable to take griseofulvin, as ketoconazole has been associated with a potential for liver damage (Table 3.3). Patients using oral ketoconazole should be tested for signs of liver dysfunction before initiating therapy. While on therapy, patients should be closely monitored for signs of hepatotoxicity, both clinically and biochemically, using liver function tests including serum AST, ALT, alkaline phosphatase, gamma-glutamyl-transferase and bilirubin (e.g., biweekly during first 2 months of therapy; monthly or bimonthly afterward). Patients should be instructed to report any symptoms of liver dysfunction such as persistent nausea, anorexia, fatigue, vomiting, right upper abdominal pain or jaundice, dark urine, or pale stools.

Tinea Pedis/Manuum

There are no approved treatments specifically for tinea manuum. Treatments for tinea pedis are effectively used to treat tinea manuum. Topical formulations of terbinafine, butenafine, miconazole, econazole, ketoconazole, clotrimazole, and ciclopirox are FDA-approved for tinea pedis/manuum (Table 3.2). Topical formulations may be used for milder, limited presentations. Many topical agents (e.g., miconazole nitrate 1%, ciclopirox olamine 1%, naftifine hydrochloride 1%, sulconazole nitrate 1%) provide antibacterial activity and may be preferred where bacterial superinfection is suspected. Formulations allowing once-daily application rather than twice daily (e.g. naftifine 1% cream, bifonazole 1%, ketoconazole cream 2%) may aid patient compliance and subsequent efficacy.

Chronic infection may warrant the use of oral antifungals, particularly if previous topical regimens have failed. Off-label use of oral itraconazole, terbinafine, or fluconazole may be practical where the tinea involvement is extensive and application of a topical is not feasible. Studies have shown that oral terbinafine and itraconazole may be the most effective treatments, and a higher cure rate has been shown with topical allylamines than

Table 3.3: Summary of Systemic Antifungal Agent Properties

	Terbinafine	Itraconazole	Fluconazole	Griseofulvin	Ketoconazole
Chemistry	Allylamine Available as tablet Inhibits squalene epoxidase = ergosterol deficiency (fungistatic) and accumulation of squalene (fungicidal) Lipophilic; Binds strongly (>99%) and nonspecifically to plasma proteins Extensively metabolized in liver	Triazole Available as capsule, oral solution or IV formulation Inhibits fungal lanosterol 14-α demethylase = ergosterol deficiency (fungistatic) Lipophilic; binds strongly to plasma proteins (>99%) Extensively metabolized in the liver predominantly by CYP3A4	Bis-triazole Available as tablet, oral suspension or IV formulation Inhibits fungal lanosterol 14-α demethylase = ergosterol deficiency (fungistatic) More hydrophilic than other azoles Protein binding of 11% to 12% No significant first-pass hepatic metabolism	Spiro-benzo[b]furan Available as tablet or oral suspension Disruption of fungal cell mitotic spindle, arresting cell division (fungistatic) Concentrated in skin, hair, nails, liver, fat and skeletal muscles; deposited in keratin precursor cells, and bound to new keratin Oxidative demethylation principally in liver	Imidazole Available as tablet Inhibition of cell membrane sterols (e.g., lanosterol); fungistatic at high concentrations 84–99% bound to plasma proteins Partially metabolized in liver
Metabolism	Reported to inhibit CYP2D6 in vitro: use with caution in patients with concomitant 2D6 substrates such as tricyclic antidepressants	Potential for itraconazole metabolism alteration where CYP3A4 is altered by other medications	Potent inhibitor of CYP2C9, and CYP2C19; weaker inhibition of CYP3A group – potential for drug interactions	Induces hepatic enzymes- potential for adverse events, drug interactions	May inhibit synthesis of adrenal steroids, testosterone Potent inhibitor of CYP3A group – possible drug interactions
Contraindications	None	Patients with evidence of ventricular dysfunction such as congestive heart failure (CHF) or a history of CHF; cisapride, midazolam (oral), triazolam, terfenadine, astemizole, pimozide, quinidine, dofetilide, Levacetylmethadol (levamethadyl) HMG CoA-reductase inhibitors: lovastatin, simvastatin, etc; Ergot alkaloids metabolized by CYP3A4: dihydroergotamine, ergometrine (ergonovine), ergotamine, methlerg ometrine(methylergovovine)	Severe liver disease; Use with caution in patients sensitive to other azoles Cisapride Terfenadine	Patients with porphyria or hepatocellular failure	Cisapride Triazolam Terfenadine, Astemizole
Cautions	Monitor CYP2D6-metabolized drug concentration for increases (tricyclic antidepressants, selective serotonin reuptake inhibitors, beta-blockers and monoamine oxidase inhibitors type B) Not recommended for patients with chronic or active liver disease; baseline LFTs for all patients Not recommended for patients with renal impairment (creatinine clearance ≤ 50 mL/min) Discontinue in patients with clinical signs or symptoms of lupus erythematosus Monitor complete blood counts in patients with known or suspected immunodeficiencies (terbinafine used >6 weeks), for decrease in lymphocyte counts, neutrophil counts	Use is strongly discouraged for patients with elevated or abnormal liver enzymes or active liver disease, or who have experienced liver toxicity with other drugs Baseline LFTs for all patients; Discontinue in patients showing signs/symptoms of liver disease Use with caution in patients sensitive to other azoles Advise patients with risk factors for CHF (ischemic and valvular disease, significant pulmonary disease, renal failure or other edematous disorders) to watch for signs and symptoms of CHF Discontinue if signs of neuropathy develop Patients using oral hypoglycemics should closely monitor blood sugar; may need to adjust hypoglycemic dosing Drug (capsules) should be taken after a full meal or with an 240 mL cola beverage	Discontinue in patients showing signs/symptoms of liver disease Use with caution in patients with potential proarrhythmic conditions Monitor patients developing rashes closely for signs of exfoliative skin disorders Patients using oral hypoglycemics should closely monitor blood sugar; may need to adjust hypoglycemic dosing	Use with caution in patients with penicillin sensitivity Female patients should be aware that there is a possibility of decreased oral contraceptive efficacy with griseofulvin use	Close monitoring of hepatic function required; Discontinue in patients showing signs/ symptoms of liver disease Recommended dosage should be followed closely to avoid depression of adrenocortical function and serum testosterone Patients using oral hypoglycemics should closely monitor blood sugar; may need to adjust hypoglycemic dosing

Adverse Events	GI: Diarrhea (5.6%), dyspepsia (4.3%), nausea (2.6%), abdominal pain (2.4%), flatulence (2.2%), taste disturbance (2.8%) Cutaneous: Rash (5.6%), pruritus (2.8%), urticaria (1.1%) CNS: Headache (12.9%) Hepatic/Renal: Liver enzyme abnormalities (≥2× upper limit of normal) (3.3%) Other: Visual disturbance (1.1%) *Rare events based on worldwide experience with terbinafine tablets:* Idiosyncratic and symptomatic hepatic injury and cases of liver failure, some leading to death or liver transplant; serious skin reaction (Stevens-Johnson syndrome, toxic epidermal necrolysis); changes in ocular lens and retina; agranulocytosis; thrombocytopenia, angioedema and allergic reactions (including anaphylaxis); transient decreases in absolute lymphocyte count; cases of severe neutropenia; precipitation and exacerbation of cutaneous and systemic lupus erythematosus; malaise; fatigue; vomiting; arthralgia; myalgia; hair loss	GI: Diarrhea (4%), dyspepsia (4%), abdominal pain (4%), nausea (3%), appetite increase (2%), constipation (2%), gastritis (2%), gastroenteritis (2%) Cutaneous: Rash (4%) CNS: Headache (10%), dizziness (4%), abnormal dreaming (2%) Hepatic/Renal: Liver function abnormality (3%), liver enzyme abnormalities (≥2× upper limit of normal) (4%), urinary tract infection (3%) Other: Rhinitis (9%), upper respiratory tract infection (8%), sinusitis (7%), cystitis (3%), myalgia (3%), asthenia (2%), fever (2%), pain (2%), tremor (2%), herpes zoster (2%), pharyngitis (2%) *Post-marketing experiences (rare):* Rare cases of serious hepatotoxicity including liver failure and death; vomiting; peripheral edema, congestive heart failure, pulmonary edema; peripheral neuropathy; menstrual disorders; reversible increases in hepatic enzymes, hepatitis, liver failure; hypokalemia, hypertriglyceridemia; alopecia; allergic reactions (pruritus, rash, urticaria, angioedema, anaphylaxis); Stevens-Johnson syndrome; anaphylactic, anaphylactoid and allergic reactions; photosensitivity; neutropenia; congenital abnormality including skeletal, genitourinary tract, cardiovascular and ophthalmic malformations as well as chromosomal and multiple malformations (causal relation to itraconazole not established)	GI: Nausea (3.7%), vomiting (1.7%), abdominal pain (1.7%), diarrhea (1.5%) Cutaneous: Skin rash (1.8%) CNS: Headache (1.9%) *Post-marketing experiences (rare):* Rare cases of serious hepatic reactions ranging from mild transient elevations in transaminases to clinical hepatitis, jaundice, cholestasis, and fulminant hepatic failure, including fatalities; rare cases of anaphylaxis (including angioedema, face edema and pruritus); QT prolongation, torsade de pointes; seizures; dizziness; alopecia; exfoliative skin disorders including Stevens-Johnson syndrome and toxic epidermal necrolysis; leucopenia, including neutropenia and agranulocytosis; thrombocytopenia; hypercholesterolemia, hypertriglyceridemia, hypokalemia; dyspepsia, vomiting, and taste perversion	GI: Epigastric distress; nausea, vomiting, excessive thirst; flatulence; diarrhea; oral thrush Cutaneous: Hypersensitivity reactions including rash, and urticaria CNS: Headache, fatigue, dizziness, insomnia *Post-marketing experiences (rare):* Paresthesia of hands and feet; mental confusion; impairment of performance of routine activities and psychotic symptoms with large doses; GI bleeding; angioedema; erythema multiform-like reaction, serum-sickness-like reaction; photosensitivity; lupus erythematosus, lupus-like syndrome or exacerbation of preexisting lupus erythematosus; toxic epidermal necrolysis; proteinuria, nephrosis; hepatotoxicity; menstrual irregularity, amenorrhea; estrogen-like effects in children; transient diminution of hearing; reversible leucopenia; elevated concentrations of porphyrins in feces and erythrocytes; tachycardia, flushing when concomitant with alcohol, and potentiation of alcohol effects	GI: Nausea and/or vomiting (3–10%); 1% or less of patients: Abdominal pain, constipation flatulence, GI bleeding, diarrhea Cutaneous: Pruritus (2%) Less than 1%: Rash, dermatitis, purpura, urticaria CNS: Less than 1%: Headache, dizziness, somnolence, lethargy, asthenia, nervousness, insomnia, abnormal dreaming, photophobia, paresthesia Hepatic/Renal: Transient increases in serum AST(SGOT), ALT (SGPT) and alkaline phosphatase Other: Less than 1%: Arthralgia, fever and chills, dyspnea, tinnitus, impotence, changes in sweat patterns, alopecia, signs of increased intracranial pressure, hemolytic anemia, thrombocytopenia, leucopenia *Post-marketing experiences (rare):* Hepatotoxicity (hepatocellular, cholestatic or mixed pattern), typically reversible, death rarely; Bilateral gynecomastia with breast tenderness in some men; Adrenocortical insufficiency; Transient decrease in serum cholesterol, alterations in serum triglyceride concentrations; Anaphylactic reactions after first dose; Neuropsychiatric disturbances including suicidal tendencies, severe depression; Hypertension in several subjects receiving 400 mg every 6–8 hours for metastatic prostate carcinoma; disulfiram reactions (flushing, rash, peripheral edema, nausea, headache) when ingesting alcohol

Table 3.4: Tinea Capitis Dosing in Children*

Regimen	Duration	Weight (kg)				
		10–20	*21–30*	*31–40*	*41–50*	*50+*
Terbinafine (continuous)	5 mg/kg/d	2–4 weeks	62.5 mg QD	125 mg QD	125 mg QD	250 mg QD	250 mg QD
Itraconazole (continuous)	5 mg/kg/d	2–4 weeks	100 mg QD, every second day	100 mg QD	100 mg QD/BID on alternate days	200 mg QD	200 mg QD
Itraconazole (pulse) ‡	Capsules: 5 mg/kg/d	1 to 3 pulses	100 mg QD, every second day	100 mg QD	100 mg QD/BID on alternate days	200 mg QD	200 mg BID §
	Oral suspension: 3 mg/kg/d	1 to 3 pulses					
Fluconazole (continuous)	Oral suspension: 6 mg/kg/d	20 days					
Fluconazole (pulse) ‖	Oral suspension: 6 mg/kg/d	8–12 weeks					
Griseofulvin† (continuous)	Microsize: 20–25 mg/kg/day	6–12 weeks					
	Ultramicrosize: 10–15 mg/kg/day	6–12 weeks					
Griseofulvin† (continuous)	Oral suspension: # 15–25 mg/kg/d	6–12 weeks					

* Durations of treatment are for *Trichophyton tonsurans* infection. Longer durations for *Microsporum canis* infections may be required
† Currently only griseofulvin is approved by the FDA for use in tinea capitis
‡ Itraconazole pulses are given for 1 week, with 3 weeks "off" before starting the next pulse
§ Itraconazole adult dose 200 mg BID (approved for pulse use in fingernail onychomycosis); No standard has been established in clinical trials for tinea capitis for children >50 kg, and use varies from once-daily as with continuous regimen to twice-daily 200 mg dosing
‖ Fluconazole pulses are 1 day on, 6 days off, before beginning next pulse
Dosing based on Grifulvin V suspension 125 mg/5 mL

with topical azoles. Terbinafine 250 mg/day has been used for tinea pedis with a duration of 2 to 6 weeks. Itraconazole regimens of 100 mg/day for 30 days or 4 weeks, 400 mg daily for 1 week, and 200 mg/day for 2 to 4 weeks have been reported. The dose of fluconazole for tinea pedis most frequently reported is 150 mg once weekly administered for 2 to 6 weeks.

Though oral griseofulvin is approved in the United States for treatment of tinea infections that are not expected to respond satisfactorily to topical antifungals, griseofulvin has lower efficacy than the newer antifungals, poor keratin adherence, and narrow-spectrum activity (dermatophytes only). This may be a limitation when a superimposed bacterial infection is present. Where griseofulvin dosing is used, the suggested dosage for tinea pedis is 660 or 750 mg daily for 4 to 8 weeks. Similarly, use of ketoconazole tablets has been discouraged due to the potential for hepatic side effects. However, ketoconazole dosing of 200 to 400 mg daily for 4 to 8 weeks has been used for the treatment of tinea pedis infection.

Prevention of reinfection is important, and education of the patient on proper foot hygiene is essential. Patients should avoid walking barefoot in communal areas such as bathrooms, showers or swimming areas, and ensure that feet are dried thoroughly after bathing, showering, or swimming. Occlusive footwear should be avoided, or shoes should be alternated every 2 to 3 days, with frequent sock changes to reduce moisture in the foot

environment. Wicking socks decrease moisture as does powder in socks.

Tinea Corporis/Cruris/Faciei

Topical therapies approved by the FDA for treatment of tinea corporis/cruris include terbinafine, butenafine, econazole, miconazole, ketoconazole, clotrimazole, and ciclopirox (Table 3.2). Topical formulations may eradicate smaller areas of infection, but oral therapy may be required where larger areas are involved or where infection is chronic/recurrent.

Off-label use of oral antifungals may be practical when the tinea involvement is extensive and application of a topical is not feasible. Oral itraconazole, terbinafine, and fluconazole have been used successfully in the treatment of tinea corporis/cruris, though none of these agents are currently approved by the FDA for use in these conditions. Terbinafine 250 mg/day has been used for tinea corporis/cruris with a regimen generally lasting 2 to 4 weeks. A continuous itraconazole regimen of 200 mg/day for 1 week is recommended for tinea corporis/cruris. Another regimen of 100 mg/day for 2 weeks has also been reported to be effective. The dose of fluconazole suggested for tinea corporis/cruris is 150 to 300 mg once weekly administered for 2 to 4 weeks. These oral agents are preferred over ketoconazole, due to the potential for hepatic side effects with ketoconazole use, and griseofulvin is not recommended as it does not adequately bind the keratin in the stratum corneum, which reduces its efficacy. When griseofulvin is used for these indications, the suggested dosage is 250 mg twice daily until cure is attained. Similarly, when the decision is made to provide ketoconazole, the suggested dosage is 200 to 400 mg daily for 4 to 8 weeks.

Tinea faciei infections are typically cleared with topical treatment. Topical ciclopirox and terbinafine may provide good anti-inflammatory effects as well as antifungal activity. Miconazole or similar azoles may also be effective. Azoles should be used for 3 to 4 weeks, or at least 1 week after resolution of lesions. Resistant lesions, cases of extensive disease, or more severe cases of infection may require oral therapy.

Tinea Capitis

Unlike most dermatophytoses, topical monotherapy is not recommended for tinea capitis. Oral therapy is required to adequately treat tinea capitis, as the dermatophytes are able to penetrate the infected hair shaft whereas topical therapies cannot. Topical antifungals such as antifungal shampoos (ketoconazole, selenium sulfide, povidone iodine, zinc pyrithione) can be used as adjunct therapy with or without oral antifungals to prevent reinfection or to treat asymptomatic carriers (Table 3.2).

Griseofulvin is the only oral antifungal treatment approved by the FDA. However use of terbinafine, itraconazole and fluconazole for tinea capitis are also reported extensively in the medical literature. The efficacies and safety profiles of terbinafine, itraconazole and fluconazole are similar to those of griseofulvin, and may be used when griseofulvin therapy has failed. Itraconazole, terbinafine, and fluconazole have the advantage of shorter treatment durations when compared to griseofulvin. Dosages are typically given on a weight-based scale, and infections with *Microsporum* may require higher dosing or longer therapy durations than infections with *Trichophyton* (Table 3.4). Oral suspensions are available for griseofulvin, itraconazole, and fluconazole to aid pediatric dosing. Terbinafine and griseofulvin tablets can be crushed, and itraconazole capsules can be opened and added to a fatty food such as peanut butter.

Griseofulvin suggested dosing is 20 to 25 mg/kg/day using the microsize formulation, for 6 to 12 weeks (Table 3.4). Where the ultramicrosize formulation is used, a dose of 10 to 15 mg/kg/day is suggested, as it is more rapidly absorbed than the microsize form. The oral suspension (microsize griseofulvin) contains 125 mg per 5 mL. Treatment should be continued for 2 weeks after the resolution of clinical symptoms. Mycological cure rates are generally high, being in the range of 70% to 100%.

The standard terbinafine dosing regimen for tinea capitis daily dosing is based on weight (less than 20 kg = 62.5 mg; 20–40 kg = 125 mg; greater than 40 kg = 250 mg per day) (Table 3.4). The duration of therapy is generally 4 weeks, though pulse dosing regimens and shorter durations have also been reported to be effective. Higher dosages or longer duration of therapy may be required for *M. canis* infection. Limited studies suggested that doses greater than 4.5 mg/kg/day may increase cure rates in both *Trichophyton* and *Microsporum* infections, with duration of therapy being less important.

Both continuous and pulse regimens of itraconazole have been used to treat tinea capitis. The continuous regimen is 5 mg/kg/day for 4 weeks, and the pulse therapy regimen is 5 mg/kg/day for 1 week a month, given for 2 to 4 months (Table 3.4). When the oral solution is used, dosages are reduced to 3 mg/kg/day, whether used as continuous or pulse therapy.

A limited number of studies have shown that therapy with fluconazole 6 mg/kg/day lasting 2 to 3 weeks can effectively treat tinea capitis (Table 3.4). A comparative study of 5 mg/kg/day for 4 weeks showed similar efficacy to griseofulvin 6 mg/kg/day for 6 weeks. Once weekly therapy with fluconazole for tinea capitis has also been found to be effective.

Transmission of infection from patients and from symptom-free carriers has been a concern for clinicians treating tinea capitis. Adjunct therapies can be provided to the patient and family members to control transmission. Infection frequently may initiate from contact with animals, and treatment of pets may be required. Patients and family members should be counseled to avoid sharing items such as caps, combs and toys. Hats, combs, pillows, blankets, scissors, etc, may be disinfected with bleach. Most clinicians agree that infected children do not need to be kept out of school once treatment is initiated, particularly children in higher grades where little physical contact between students is expected.

Tinea unguium (Onychomycosis)

Onychomycosis is difficult to cure and has a high rate of recurrence. Fingernails may show higher treatment success rates than toenails due to faster rates of outgrowth, and suggested dosing regimens are shorter for fingernail infection than toenail infection. It must also be remembered that nails showing past injury or abnormal growth patterns may never return to "normal" appearance even though the infection may be completely eradicated. Also, due to the high rate of recurrence, long-term follow-up is important, so control of relapse can be undertaken as soon as possible. It is therefore important that patients are informed that most cases of onychomycosis require long-term therapy, with improvements being slow to appear, and in some cases the nail will not return to a normal appearance.

Ciclopirox nail lacquer 8% solution is a topical therapy approved for mild to moderate *Trichophyton rubrum* onychomycosis without lunula involvement (Fig. 3.8). Application is once daily for 48 weeks, and it is suggested that routine nail debridement be provided in conjunction with lacquer applications. The mycological cure rate at week 48 was 33% in the pivotal clinical trials. Its use is not associated with any of the potential adverse effects that might occur with oral antifungals, for example, hepatotoxicity and cutaneous reactions. However, while it is practical to use ciclopirox nail lacquer in situations where three or fewer nails are involved with onychomycosis, an oral antifungal agent should be considered when a greater number of nails are involved, or if the severity of onychomycosis involves greater than 60% of the nail plate area (Fig. 3.9). Amorolfine 5% nail lacquer has not been approved for use in North America, and has proved to be effective therapy in fingernail and toenail onychomycosis without matrix involvement.

Tinea pedis infection is frequently reported in conjunction with onychomycosis infection, and topical agents to control tinea pedis may be given along with onychomycosis treatment for this reason. Topical therapy may also be useful as an adjunctive therapy with oral medications for more severe presentations of infection. Topical monotherapy with allylamines or azoles

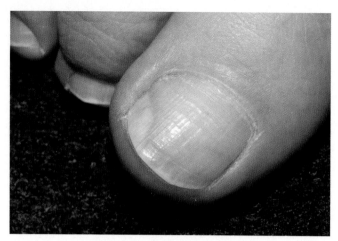

Figure 3.8. Mild onychomycosis.

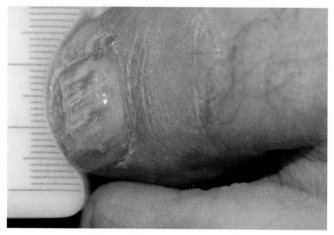

Figure 3.9. Severe onychomycosis.

would not be expected to provide effective therapy in any but the least severe cases of infection. Use of topical azoles or allylamines as prophylactic therapy has rarely been reported. Limited reports with miconazole powder did not show successful prophylaxis of infection.

Terbinafine and itraconazole are the most frequently used oral medications. Though griseofulvin is approved for tinea infection of the nails, its affinity for keratin is low and long-term therapy is required. Efficacy in the treatment of onychomycosis is also low, and the newer azole and allylamine agents have largely replaced griseofulvin for this indication. Ketoconazole is not recommended for therapy of onychomycosis due to the potential for hepatotoxicity (blocking human CYP-dependent demethylation of ergosterol at higher concentrations) and the availability of alternative oral treatments. Fluconazole has shown high efficacy, low relapse rates, and usefulness with yeast co-infection However, there have been few studies on this treatment method.

The FDA-approved oral therapy regimens for onychomycosis are as follows: terbinafine 250 mg/day for 12 weeks (toenails) or 6 weeks (fingernails only); itraconazole 200 mg/day for 12 weeks (toenails with or without fingernail involvement); and itraconazole 200 mg twice daily as pulse therapy (one pulse: 1 week of itraconazole followed by 3 weeks without itraconazole)

using two pulses (fingernails only). Though only a continuous regimen of itraconazole is FDA-approved for toenail onychomycosis, the current itraconazole standard of care of toenail onychomycosis is a pulse regimen (one pulse: 1 week of itraconazole followed by 3 weeks without itraconazole; three pulses given). In countries where fluconazole is approved for the treatment of onychomycosis, the most frequently used schedule is fluconazole 150 to 300 mg once weekly given until the abnormal-appearing nail has grown out (fingernails: 3–6 months; toenails: 9–12 months).

Mycological cure rates (KOH negative and culture negative) for terbinafine use in dermatophyte onychomycosis are estimated at 76% in a meta-analysis of clinical trial data from the medical literature. By comparison, itraconazole mycological cure rates are 59% (continuous therapy) and 63% (pulse therapy). Clinical response rates (infection cleared or showing marked improvement) were as follows: terbinafine – 66%, itraconazole continuous therapy – 70%, and itraconazole pulse therapy – 70%. The complete cure rate (mycological cure and no residual nail area affected) in the terbinafine prescribing information is 38% versus 14% for continuous 12-week itraconazole dosing. For cases of nondermatophyte mold infections, cure rates may be significantly lower, and such cases are known to be difficult to cure.

It has been suggested that oral antifungals with differing mechanisms of action may provide synergistic destruction of nail fungal infection (i.e., terbinafine/itraconazole combination therapy). Use of a topical medication (amorolfine, ciclopirox nail lacquer, etc.) in combination with an oral antifungal may improve the efficacy and cost-benefit rates for severe onychomycosis treatment. These combination methods require further study to determine efficacy, and are not currently accepted treatment methods.

It may also be beneficial to combine oral therapy with routine nail debridement, particularly where the nail is thickened, or where the infection presents as a dermatophytoma, spike or lateral infection. Caution must be taken not to damage the underlying skin during debridement, particularly in subjects who are vulnerable to severe lower limb complications, such as diabetics or individuals with reduced lower limb profusion.

Nail avulsion by surgical or chemical means is one of the traditional options available to manage onychomycosis, as this eliminates most of the fungi and frees the underlying surface for topical antifungal treatment. Avulsion may be full or partial. Avulsion has not been examined in large randomized, controlled trials. There is some potential for permanent nail plate alteration, and it can be painful for the patient.

As with tinea pedis, proper foot and nail hygiene may help prevent reinfection. Patients should avoid walking barefoot in communal areas such as bathrooms, showers or swimming areas, and ensure that feet are dried thoroughly after bathing, showering or swimming. Nails should be kept short and clean. Shoes should fit properly and socks should be made from absorbent material such as cotton.

Pityriasis versicolor

Topical treatment is frequently effective for PV, though systemic therapy may be desirable when infection is widespread, or when short-duration oral therapy is preferable to frequent application of a topical agent. Topical azoles (ketoconazole, fluconazole, bifonazole, clotrimazole, miconazole) have demonstrated efficacy in both cream formulation or shampoos. Terbinafine solution, cream, gel or spray has also been effective. Topical ciclopirox provides both antifungal and anti-inflammatory activity against *Malassezia*. Oral therapy with ketoconazole, itraconazole and fluconazole shows a similarly high efficacy in the medical literature. Oral terbinafine and griseofulvin are not effective for PV. Treatment does not vary with hyperpigmentation versus hypopigmentation. Pigmentation may not return to normal until well after infection is mycologically eradicated, particularly when hypopigmentation is noted.

Ketoconazole and itraconazole may be prescribed prophylactically, as there is a high rate of relapse of PV infection. Rates as high as 60% to 90% in 2 years post-treatment have been reported. Prophylactic doses given are as follows: ketoconazole – single 400 mg dose or 200 mg daily for 3 days once monthly; itraconazole – single 400 mg dose once monthly for 6 months.

PITFALLS AND MYTHS

A primary pitfall for dermatophytosis treatment is not obtaining mycological confirmation of the infectious agent via fungal culture on, particularly for onychomycosis. Onychomycosis is mimicked by many other conditions such as psoriasis or trauma, and proceeding to oral therapy in these cases without identifying an infectious agent is inappropriate. Also, standard oral therapies may be ineffective when the infectious fungi are nondermatophytes. It is not uncommon to require repeat samples to identify a dermatophyte agent in onychomycosis. For nondermatophyte infections, multiple samples are required to confirm their status as the causative agent.

A further pitfall is to assume a negative mycology exam represents a cured infection. Fungal organisms may frequently fail to present on culture. Where clinical signs of infection remain, and particularly where microscopy shows fungal organisms present though culture is negative, there remains a potential for infection relapse. Repeat sampling may be prudent, and follow-up of the clinical condition is warranted.

For most tineas, topical corticosteroid monotherapy is not recommended, as it may lead to suppression of the physical signs of infection, with lack of symptoms sometimes being wrongly associated with clearance of infection, leading to treatment relapse.

It is a myth that children do not get onychomycosis. Though it is much more frequent in elderly patients, and typically develops over years, there are many reports of children presenting with classic dermatophyte onychomycosis infections. Children have also presented with other types of onychomycosis. A suspicion of onychomycosis should not be dismissed due to patient age. Cultures should be obtained to evaluate the presence of fungal organisms.

Onychomycosis represents a challenge for clinicians, in that it is difficult to motivate patients to continue with long periods of follow-up. "Cured" subjects may feel follow-up is a waste of time, while "non-cured" subjects may feel there is no point in continuing to try treatments. As the slow growth of the nails would require years of observation to adequately determine relapse rates, the potential for relapse has not been adequately determined through clinical study. However, reports suggest that the potential for relapse is high. Assessment of cure and relapse is complicated by the high rate of false negative cultures in mycological assessment. Long-term follow-up is necessary to observe the clinical appearance of nails, as a clue to whether relapse is developing when culture remains falsely negative. Follow-up also provides the only non-invasive method to sample greater portions of the nail unit. As the nail grows out and portions that were too deep for sampling earlier now move towards the distal edge, further opportunities for discovering viable fungi are presented. Patient education on the difficulties of treating onychomycosis is essential at the start of treatment, so that expectations are clear, and not set too high.

SUGGESTED READINGS

American Society of Health-System Pharmacists, Inc. Miscellaneous Antifungals – Griseofulvin. In: AHFS Drug Information® 2005. Bethesda, MD, 2005, pp. 535–537.

American Society of Health-System Pharmacists, Inc. Azoles – Ketoconazole. *In:* AHFS Drug Information® 2005. Bethesda, MD, 2005, pp 510–516.

Anaissie EJ, Kontoyiannis DP, Huls C, et al. Safety, plasma concentrations, and efficacy of high-dose fluconazole in invasive mold infections. J Infect Dis 1995;172: 599–602.

Arrese JE, Pierard GE. Treatment failures and relapses in onychomycosis: a stubborn clinical problem. Dermatology 2003;207(3):255–260.

Ashbee RH, Evans EGV. Immunology of diseases associated with Malassezia species. Clin Microbiol Rev 2002;15:21–57.

Baran R, Hay RJ, Haneke E, Tosti A. Review of current antifungal treatment. Onychomycosis: the current approach to diagnosis and therapy. London: Martin Dunitz Ltd.; 1999. p. 44–69.

BERTEK Pharmaceuticals Inc. Mentax®-TC (butenafine HCl) cream, 1%. Prescribing Information. Research Triangle Park, NC, USA. October 2002.

Bonifaz A, Saul A, Mena C et al. Dermatophyte onychomycosis in children under 2 years of age: experience of 16 cases. J Eur Acad Dermatol Venereol 2007;21(1):115–117.

Chan Y, Friedlander SF. New treatments for tinea capitis. Curr Opin Infect Dis 2004;17:97–103.

Crawford F. Athlete's foot. In: Williams H, Bigby M, Diepgen T, Herxheimer A, Naldi L, Rzany B, eds. Evidence based dermatology. London: BMJ Books, 2003:436–440.

Daniel CR, Gupta AK, Daniel MP, Daniel CM. Two feet-one hand syndrome: a retrospective multicenter survey. Int J Dermatol 1997;36:658–660.

Daniel CR, III. Traditional management of onychomycosis. J Am Acad Dermatol 1996;35:S21–S25.

Dastghaib L, Azizzadeh M, Jafari P. Therapeutic options for the treatment of tinea capitis: griseofulvin versus fluconazole. J Dermatolog Treat 2005;16:43–46.

De Doncker P, Gupta AK, Marynissen G, et al: Itraconazole pulse therapy for onychomycosis and dermatomycoses: an overview. J Am Acad Dermatol 1997;37:969–974.

Del Aguila R, Montero Gei F, Robles M, et al: Once-weekly oral doses of fluconazole 150 mg in the treatment of tinea pedis. Clin Exp Dermatol 1992;17:402–406.

Dermik Laboratories (a division of sanofi-aventis). Penlac® Nail Lacquer (ciclopirox) Topical Solution, 8% Prescribing Information. Bridgewater, NJ. July 2006.

Duswald KH, Penk A, Pittrow L: High-dose therapy with fluconazole greater than or equal to 800 mg per day. Mycoses 1997;40:267–277.

Elewski BE. Clinical diagnosis of common scalp disorders. J Investig Dermatol Symp Proc 2005;10:190–193.

Evans EGV. Drug synergies and the potential for combination therapy in onychomycosis. Br J Dermatol 2003;149 (Suppl. 65):11–13.

Faergemann J, Mork NJ, Haglund A, et al: A multicentre (double-blind) comparative study to assess the safety and efficacy of fluconazole and griseofulvin in the treatment of tinea corporis and tinea cruris. Br J Dermatol 1997;136:575–577.

Faergemann J. Management of seborrheic dermatitis and pityriasis versicolor. Am J Clin Dermatol 2000;1:75–80.

Faergemann J. Pityrosporum infections. J Am Acad Dermatol 1994; 31:S18–S20.

Feuilhade de Chauvin M. New diagnostic techniques. J Eur Acad Dermatol Venereol 2005;19(Suppl 1):20–24.

Finch JJ, Warshaw EM. Toenail onychomycosis: current and future treatment options. Dermatolog Ther 2007;20:31–46.

Friedlander SF, Aly R, Krafchik B et al. Terbinafine in the treatment of Trichophyton tinea capitis: a randomized, double-blind, parallel-group, duration-finding study. Pediatrics 2002;109(4):602–607.

GlaxoSmithKline Consumer Healthcare LP. *Oxistat® (oxiconazole nitrate cream) cream 1%; Oxistat® (oxiconazole nitrate lotion) lotion 1%*. Prescribing Information. Pittsburgh, PA, USA. January 2004.

Gomez M, Arenas R, Salazar JJ, et al: Tinea pedis. A multicentre trial to evaluate the efficacy and tolerance of a weekly dose of fluconazole. Dermatologia Revista Mexicana 1996;40:251–255.

The United States Pharmacopeial Convention, Inc. Griseofulvin (Systemic). In: Drug Information for the Health Care Professional, USP DI, ed 24, Taunton MA, 2004, Micromedex: 1493–1496.

Gupta AK, Batra R, Bluhm R, Faergemann J. Pityriasis versicolor. Dermatol Clin 2003;21:413–429.

Gupta AK, Chaudhry M, Elewski B. Tinea corporis, tinea cruris, tinea nigra, and piedra. Dermatol Clin 2003;21:395–400.

Gupta AK, Chow M, Daniel CR, Aly R. Treatments of tinea pedis. Dermatol Clin 2003;21:431–462.

Gupta AK, Cooper EA, Ginter G. Efficacy and safety of itraconazole use in children. Dermatol Clin. 2003;21(3):521–535.

Gupta AK, Cooper EA, Lynde CW. The efficacy and safety of terbinafine in children. Dermatol Clin. 2003;21(3):511–520.

Gupta AK, Cooper EA, Montero-Gei F. The use of fluconazole to treat superficial fungal infections in children. Dermatol Clin. 2003;21(3):537–542.

Gupta AK, Cooper EA, Ryder JE, et al. Optimal management of fungal infections of the skin, hair, and nails. Am J Clin Dermatol 2004;5(4):225–237.

Gupta AK, De Doncker P, Heremans A, et al: Itraconazole for the treatment of tinea pedis: a dose of 400 mg/day given for 1 week is similar in efficacy to 100 or 200 mg/day given for 2 to 4 weeks. J Am Acad Dermatol 1997;36:789–792.

Gupta AK, Dlova N, Taborda P, et al: Once weekly fluconazole is effective in the treatment of tinea capitis: a prospective, multicentre study. Br J Dermatol 2000;142:965–968.

Gupta AK, Jain HC, Lynde CW, et al. Prevalence and epidemiology of onychomycosis in patients visiting physicians' offices: A multicenter Canadian survey of 15,000 patients. J Amer Acad Dermatol 2000;43:244–248.

Gupta AK, Konnikov N, MacDonald P, et al. Prevalence and epidemiology of toenail onychomycosis in diabetic subjects: a multicentre survey. Br J Dermatol 1998;139:665–671.

Gupta AK, Lambert J, Revuz J, Shear N. Update on the safety of itraconazole pulse therapy in onychomycosis and dermatomycoses. Eur J Dermatol 2001; 11(1):6–10.

Gupta AK, Onychomycosis Combination Therapy Study Group. Ciclopirox topical solution, 8% combined with oral terbinafine to treat onychomycosis: a randomized, evaluator-blinded study. J Drugs Dermatol 2005;4(4):481–485.

Gupta AK, Ryder J, Bluhm R. Onychomycosis. In: Williams H, Bigby M, Diepgen T, Herxheimer A, Naldi L, Rzany B, eds. Evidence based dermatology. London: BMJ Books, 2003:441–468.

Gupta AK, Ryder JE, Chow M, Cooper EA. Dermatophytosis: the management of fungal infections. Skinmed 2005;4:305–310.

Gupta AK, Ryder JE, Johnson A.M. Cumulative meta-analysis of systemic antifungal agents for the treatment of onychomycosis. Br J Dermatol 2004;150:537–544.

Gupta AK, Ryder JE, Lynch LE, Tavakkol A. The use of terbinafine in the treatment of onychomycosis in adults and special populations: a review of the evidence. J Drugs Dermatol 2005;4(3):302–308.

Gupta AK, Ryder JE, Skinner AR. Treatment of onychomycosis: pros and cons of antifungal agents. J Cutan Med Surg 2004;8:25–30.

Gupta AK, Ryder JE, Summerbell RC. The diagnosis of non-dermatophyte mold onychomycosis. Int J Dermatol 2003;42:272–273.

Gupta AK, Ryder JE. How to improve cure rates for the management of onychomycosis. Dermatol Clin 2003;21:499–505.

Gupta AK, Ryder JE. The use of oral antifungal agents to treat onychomycosis. Dermatol Clin 2003;21:469–479.

Gupta AK, Scher RK. Management of onychomycosis: a North American perspective. Dermatol Ther 1997;3:58–65.

Gupta AK, Skinner AR. Onychomycosis in children: a brief overview with treatment strategies. Pediatr Dermatol 2004;21(1):74–79.

Gupta AK, Solomon RS, Adam P: Itraconazole oral solution for the treatment of tinea capitis. Br J Dermatol 1998;139:104–106.

Gupta AK, Summerbell RC. Tinea capitis. Med Mycol 2000;38: 255–287.

Gupta AK, Taborda P, Taborda V, et al. Epidemiology and prevalence of onychomycosis in HIV-positive individuals. Int J Dermatol 2000;39:746–753.

Hainer BL Dermatophyte infections. Am Fam Physician 2003;67: 101–108.

Haroon TS, Asghar HA, Aman S, et al: An open, non-comparative study for the evaluation of oral fluconazole in the treatment of tinea corporis. Specialist 1997;13:417–423.

Haroon TS, Hussain I, Aman S, et al: A randomized double-blind comparative study of terbinafine for 1, 2 and 4 weeks in tinea capitis. Br J Dermatol 1996;135:86–88.

Hay RJ, Baran R, Haneke E. Fungal (onychomycosis) and other infections involving the nail apparatus. In: Baran R, Dawber RPR, de Berker DAR, Haneke E, Tosti A, editors. *Baran and Dawber's diseases of the nails and their management*. Osney Mead, Oxford: Blackwell Science Ltd.; 2001; 129–171.

Heikkila H, Stubb S. Long-term results in patients with onychomycosis treated with terbinafine and itraconazole. Br J Dermatol 2002;146:250–3.

Janssen Pharmaceutica Products, L.P. Sporonox® (itraconazole) Capsules Prescribing Information (Ortho-McNeil Inc). Titusville, NJ. June 2006.

King B. Pain at first dressing change after toenail avulsion: the experience of nurses, patients and an observer: 1. J Wound Care 2003;12:5–10.

Kotogyan A, Harmanyeri Y, Tahsin Gunes A, et al: Efficacy and safety of oral fluconazole in the treatment of patients with tinea corporis, cruris or pedis or cutaneous candidiasis. A multicentre, open, non-comparative study. Clin Drug Invest 1996;12:59–66.

Lange M, Roszkiewicz J, Szczerkowska-Dobosz A, et al. Onychomycosis is no longer a rare finding in children. Mycoses 2006;49(1):55–59.

Lecha M, Effendy I, Feuilhade de Chauvin M, Di Chiacchio N, Baran R. Treatment options-development of consensus guidelines. J Eur Acad Dermatol Venereol 2005;19(Suppl 1):25–33.

Lin RL, Szepietowski JC, Schwartz RA. Tinea faciei, an often deceptive facial eruption. Int J Dermatol 2004;43:437–440.

Lipozencic J, Skerlev M, Orofino-Costa R, et al. A randomized, double-blind, parallel-group, duration-finding study of oral terbinafine and open-label, high-dose griseofulvin in children with tinea capitis due to Microsporum species. Br J Dermatol 2002;146:816–823.

Mahoney JM., Bennet J, Olsen B. The diagnosis of onychomycosis. Dermatol Clin 2003;21:463–467.

McNeil Consumer & Specialty Pharmaceuticals. Nizoral® (ketoconazole) 2% shampoo. Prescribing Information. Fort Washington, PA, USA. October 2003.

MEDICIS, The Dermatology Company. Loprox® Gel (ciclopirox) 0.77%. Prescribing Information. Scottsdale, AZ. July 2005.

Merz Pharmaceuticals. Naftin® Naftifine HCl 1% gel/cream. Prescribing Information. Greensboro, NC. May 2007.

Montero Gei F: Fluconazole in the treatment of tinea capitis. Int J Dermatol 1998;37:870–871.

Nandedkar-Thomas MA, Scher RK. An update on disorders of the nails. J Am Acad Dermatol 2005;52:877–887.

Noble SL, Forbes RC, Stamm PL. Diagnosis and management of common tinea infections. Am Fam Physician 1998;58:163–168.

Nolting S, Bräutigam M, Weidinger G: Terbinafine in onychomycosis with involvement by non-dermatophytic fungi. Br J Dermatol 30(Suppl 43):16–21, 1994.

Novartis Pharmaceuticals Corporation. Lamisil® (terbinafine hydrochloride tablets) Prescribing Information. East Hanover, NJ. November 2005.

Olafsson JH, Sigurgeirsson B, Baran R. Combination therapy for onychomycosis. Br J Dermatol 2003;149 (Suppl. 65):15–18.

Padhye AA, Weitzman I. The dermatophytes. In: Collier L, Balows A, Sussman M, Ajello L, Hay RJ, eds. Topley and Wilson's medical mycology. New York, NY: Oxford University Press, 1998:215–236.

Papini M, Difonzo EM, Cilli P, et al: Itraconazole versus fluconazole, a double-blind comparison in tinea corporis. J Mycologie Medicale 1997;7:77–80.

Parent D, Decroix J, Heenen M: Clinical experience with short schedules of itraconazole in the treatment of tinea corporis and/or tinea cruris. Dermatology 1994;189:378–381.

Pfizer Inc. Diflucan® (fluconazole tablets) (fluconazole injection – for intravenous infusion only) (fluconazole for oral suspension) Prescribing Information. New York, NY. August 2004.

Roberts BJ, Friedlander SF. Tinea capitis: a treatment update. Pediatric Annals 2005;34(3):191–200.

Romano C, Papini M, Ghilardi A, Gianni C. Onychomycosis in children: a survey of 46 cases. Mycoses 2005;48(6):430–437.

Savin R. Diagnosis and treatment of tinea versicolor. J Fam Pract 1996;43:127–132.

Scher RK, Baran R. Onychomycosis in clinical practice: factors contributing to recurrence. Br J Dermatol 2003;149 Suppl 65:5–9.

Seebacher C, Brasch J, Abeck D, et al. Onychomycosis. Mycoses 2007;50(4):321–327.

Sigurgeirsson B, Olafsson JH, Steinsson JP, Paul C, Billstein S, Evans EGV. Long-term effectiveness of treatment with terbinafine

versus itraconazole in onychomycosis. Arch Dermatol 2002; 138:353–357.

Smith ES, Fleischer AB, Feldman SR, Williford PM. Characteristics of office-based physician visits for cutaneous fungal infections: an analysis of 1990 to 1994 National Ambulatory Medical Care Survey data. Cutis 2002;69:191–204.

Stary A, Sarnow E: Fluconazole in the treatment of tinea corporis and tinea cruris. Dermatology 1998;196:237–241.

Stevens DA, Diaz M, Negroni R, et al: Safety evaluation of chronic fluconazole therapy. Chemotherapy 1997;43:371–377.

Suchil P, Montero Gei F, Robles M, et al: Once-weekly oral doses of fluconazole 150 mg in the treatment of tinea corporis/cruris and cutaneous candidiasis. Clin Exp Dermatol 1992;17:397–401.

Sunenshine PJ, Schwartz RA, Janniger CK. Tinea versicolor. Int J Dermatol 1998;37:648–655.

TARO Pharmaceuticals Inc. Ciclopirox olamine cream USP, 0.77%. Prescribing Information. Brampton, Ontario, Canada. March 2005.

TARO Pharmaceuticals Inc. Clotrimazole cream USP, 1%. Prescribing Information. Bramalea, Ontario, Canada. June 1996.

TARO Pharmaceuticals Inc. Econazole nitrate cream 1%. Prescribing Information. Brampton, Ontario, Canada. September 2001.

Tosti A, Piraccini BM, Iorizzo M. Management of onychomycosis in children. Dermatol Clin 2003;21:507–509.

Tosti A, Piraccini BM, Lorenzi S, et al. Treatment of nondermatophyte mold and Candida onychomycosis. Dermatol Clin 21:491–497, 2003.

Tosti A, Piraccini BM, Lorenzi S: Onychomycosis caused by non-dermatophyte molds: clinical features and response to treatment of 59 cases. J Am Acad Dermatol 42:217–224, 2000.

Tosti A, Piraccini BM, Stinchi C, Colombo MD. Relapses of onychomycosis after successful treatment with systemic antifungals: a three-year follow-up. Dermatology 1998;197:162–166.

Tosti A, Piraccini BM, Stinchi C, et al: Onychomycosis due to Scopulariopsis brevicaulis: clinical features and response to systemic antifungals. Br J Dermatol 135:799–802, 1996.

Trent JT, Federman D, Kirsner RS. Common viral and fungal skin infections. Ostomy Wound Manage 2001;47:28–34.

The United States Pharmacopeial Convention, Inc. Antifungals, Azole (Systemic). In: Drug Information for the Health Care Professional, USP DI, ed 24, Taunton MA, 2004, Micromedex, pp 315–323.

Warshaw EM, St Clair KR. Prevention of onychomycosis reinfection for patients with complete cure of all 10 toenails: results of a double-blind, placebo-controlled, pilot study of prophylactic miconazole powder 2%. J Am Acad Dermatol. 2005;53(4):717–720.

Yamamoto T, Yokoyama A. Superficial white onychomycosis of the fingernails in a 1-year-old child with hypoxemia. Pediatr Dermatol 2007;24(1):95–96.

PART II: LESS COMMON INFECTIONS

4 | CUTANEOUS TUBERCULOSIS

Bhushan Kumar and Sunil Dogra

HISTORY

Tuberculosis (TB) was a disease familiar to the most ancient civilizations, judging from the inscriptions on Babylonian tablets, which represent the earliest human records. Hippocrates (460–376 BC) was the first to give an intelligent description of this disease as "phthisis," which meant to dry up. Aristotle, a contemporary of Hippocrates, notes that it was a general belief among the Greeks of his day that phthisis was contagious. A similar reference has been made in the Sanskrit works of the Indo-Aryans, namely the Rigveda (1500 BC), Ayurveda (700 BC), and in the Laws of Manu (1000 BC). Galen (AD 131–201) considered the disease an ulceration that should be treated by measures designed to dry the secretion. The Roman acquaintance with TB is reflected in the writings of Pliny the Elder (AD 23–79), while John Bunyan called it "The Captain of the Men of Death," referring to its devastating course and prognosis.

Lupus vulgaris seemed to have been prevalent in Palestine before and during the time of Christ, and was included in the conditions termed *Tsara'ath* in the Old Testament and Gospels. The origin of the Latin word for wolf, "lupus" is unclear, although its usage has been established in the Middle Ages. The great German pathologist, Rudolf Virchow, found that it had appeared in the writings of the Masters of the Salerno School of Medicine (circa 10th century). In 1808, Robert Willan, (1757–1812) the founder of British Dermatology, gave the term lupus to a nodular eruption on the face that progressed to ulceration. In 1887, William Tilbury (1836–1879) used lupus vulgaris specifically for skin TB instead of as a term for any destructive cutaneous condition.

Scrofuloderma was described by the ancient French writers who called it scrofulous gumma. For many centuries, scrofula, along with lupus vulgaris and other nonpulmonary manifestations of TB, was considered curable by the touch of a reigning monarch, hence also known as King's Evil. Rene Laennec's (1781–1826) description of his own prosector's wart in 1826 was the first published case recognizing the association of cutaneous disease with mycobacterial infection. The tuberculous etiology of tuberculosis verrucosa cutis was established jointly by the dermatologist Riehl and the pathologist Paltauf in 1886.

The histopathological characteristics of the disease were described in detail by Carl Rokintansky (1804–1878) and Rudolf Virchow (1821–1902). The credit for describing the giant cells and epithelioid cells in the lupus tissue goes to Forster, who documented these cells in 1855. His findings were later confirmed by Langhans in 1868. Friedlander in 1873 demonstrated the great similarity of the histopathology in lupus vulgaris, scrofuloderma, and TB of other organs. In 1864, Jean Antoine Villemin (1827–1892) established a significant milestone in the history of the evolution of the disease by pronouncing that TB was infectious. Gaspard Laurent Bayle (1774–1816) was the first to discover that TB could affect the entire body and was not confined to the lungs only. In 1865, Jonathan Hutchinson (1828–1913) correlated the incidence of lupus vulgaris with the history of TB in the patient's family. Peters and Brock demonstrated the presence of past or coexisting TB of other organs in relation to cutaneous TB.

Robert Koch (1843–1910) discovered the tubercle bacillus (1882) and confirmed its role in the causation of TB by satisfying the conditions first indicated by Henle and later enunciated and named after Koch, the *Koch's Postulate*. Hutchinson (1888) first used the term "apple-jelly nodule" to describe its peculiar transparency. Scarification, application of caustics, blowing steam through tubes on to the lesion, freezing with carbon dioxide snow, cautery, ultraviolet radiation therapy, X-ray treatment, and vitamin D have all been used in the past, either alone or in combination, to treat lupus vulgaris. Niels Finsen received the Nobel Prize (1903) for his therapeutic results with UV irradiation in lupus vulgaris. One of the major medical advances of the 20th century has been the development of antitubercular therapy.

INTRODUCTION

Tuberculosis (TB), one of the oldest diseases known to mankind, continues to be a significant health problem even as we have entered the 21st century. Worldwide, it remains the leading cause of death by an infectious disease. According to the World Health Organization (WHO), one-third of the world's population is currently infected with the TB bacillus. Approximately 5% to 10% of people who are infected with TB bacilli (but who are not infected with human immunodeficiency virus [HIV]) may manifest disease during their lifetime. People with HIV and TB co-infection are much more likely to develop TB. WHO estimates that the largest number of new TB cases in 2005 occurred in the South-East Asia region, which accounted for 34% of incident cases globally.

Extrapulmonary TB constitutes approximately 10% of all cases of TB and cutaneous TB makes up only 1.5% of all such cases. Although cutaneous TB comprises only a small proportion, when the high prevalence of TB is borne in mind, these numbers become significant. Serious underreporting due to

We are thankful to Dr. BD Radotra for providing us the histopathology photomicrographs and to Drs. JD Wig, V Ramesh, HK Kar, S. Barua, and L Padmavathy for some of the clinical photographs.

diagnostic difficulties and categorization cannot be overlooked. Since 1984, the incidence of extrapulmonary TB has increased at an even faster rate than that of pulmonary TB and is considered a diagnostic criterion in the case definition for AIDS. Because immunocompromised individuals are at increased risk for extra-pulmonary TB, dermatologists are renewing their historic role in the diagnosis of cutaneous lesions of TB.

TB of the skin has a worldwide distribution. While it was more prevalent in regions with a cold and humid climate in the past, it now mostly occurs in tropical regions. Cutaneous TB is still uncommon in industrialized countries despite the rising incidence of extrapulmonary TB in areas with a high prevalence of HIV infection. In developed countries, cutaneous TB has typically been observed in patients with immunosuppression from malnutrition, cancer, prolonged corticosteroid therapy, or immunosuppressive therapy, whereas in developing countries it occurs mostly in the generally healthy patients. In India in the 1950s and 1960s, cutaneous TB affected 2% of all dermatology outpatients and by the 1980s and 1990s, this figure had fallen to 0.15% to 0.1%. This percentage is even less in developed countries. In a recent study from the Philippines, no cases of cutaneous TB were found in 425 patients with pulmonary TB. In another study of 360 patients with TB from Turkey, the incidence of cutaneous infection was found to be 3.5% and the association was much stronger between cutaneous involvement and tuberculous lymphadenitis than with pulmonary infection (44% versus 3%). In a hospital-based study from Tunisia, the estimated incidence of new cases in the dermatology service was 1.2 % per year between 1991 and 2000 compared with 1.4 % between 1981 and 1990. Childhood cases constitute 12.8% to 36.3% of the total patients with cutaneous TB. Childhood TB is a sensitive marker of ongoing transmission of infection within a community and represents a reservoir for future disease.

PATHOGENESIS

Tuberculosis involving the skin is caused by *Mycobacterium tuberculosis, Mycobacterium bovis,* and under certain conditions, the *Bacillus Calmette-Guérin* (BCG), an attenuated strain of *M. bovis.* Mycobacteria are acid-fast bacilli (AFB), weakly gram-positive, nonsporulating, and nonmotile rods. The family Mycobacteriaceae consists of only one genus, *Mycobacteria,* which includes the obligate human pathogens *M. tuberculosis* and the closely related *M. bovis, Mycobacterium africanum,* and *Mycobacterium microti* as well as *Mycobacterium leprae* and a number of facultative pathogenic and nonpathogenic species (the atypical mycobacteria). The AIDS pandemic with its profound and progressive suppression of cellular immune functions has led to a resurgence of TB and to the appearance or recognition of new mycobacterial pathogens.

Even though mycobacterial diseases are widespread and serious, the organisms are neither very virulent nor very infectious. Only approximately 5% to 10% of infections with *M. tuberculosis* actually lead to disease. It is transmitted through inhalation, ingestion, or inoculation. The development of cutaneous TB is dictated by the pathogenicity of the infecting organism, the route of infection (exogenous/endogenous), the patient's prior sensitization to tuberculous protein, and the nature of the patient's cell-mediated immunity (CMI).

The balance between bacterial multiplication and destruction is determined not only by the properties of the invading organisms but also by the immune response of the host to control such an infection. After mycobacteria have invaded the host, they may multiply and lead to progressive disease or their multiplication can be checked or even completely arrested.

Following infection, T lymphocytes interact with mycobacterial antigens displayed on the surface of antigen-presenting cells (APC) and release lymphokines, interleukins (ILs), and interferons. These are then responsible for activation and expression of MHC class II antigens and IL-2 receptors on the T lymphocytes. There is an accumulation of macrophages and resultant granuloma formation at the infection site. Memory T cells generated during initial sensitization remain in circulation and in lymphoid organs for an extended period of time.

Cutaneous TB may evolve either as primary (tuberculous chancre and acute miliary cutaneous TB) or as secondary infection [lupus vulgaris (LV), tuberculosis verrucosa cutis (TBVC), scrofuloderma (SF), and tuberculosis cutis orificialis (TBCO)]. Secondary infection TB manifests in a sensitized host. TB from secondary infection commonly forms a continuous immunopathologic spectrum extending from LV through TBVC, gumma (s), and SF to TBCO, although there is considerable overlap between the clinical presentations. Lupus vulgaris and TBVC represent the "high-immune" pole with active CMI and apparently normal humoral immunity, whereas SF and TBCO represent impaired CMI with a predominantly humoral immune response (Fig. 4.1).

Infection in a sensitized individual by another strain of *M. tuberculosis* results in "reinfection" TB, with LV or TBVC as its cardinal manifestation. Reactivation of the dormant "persister" mycobacteria, consequent to lowered CMl, is responsible for "reactivation" which usually presents as LV or SF but can present as any of the clinical forms indistinguishable from reinfection TB. In reinfection, there is a history of either primary infection or BCG vaccination or both. At times the only evidence of past infection may be pulmonary scarring and calcification visible on X-rays. Subsequently, any event that lowers the CMI may reactivate "persisters." Association of systemic disease with involvement of organs at places distant from cutaneous lesions occurs in all the clinical forms in varying percentages.

In the true clinical setting, this simple categorization may not be entirely true because LV and TBVC may also result from endogenous infection, and SF may result from a continuous smoldering infection in the lymph nodes acquired in infancy. The long-standing infection acts as a microvaccination in the patient. Occurrence of these clinical forms in various combinations seems to fuzz this rather convenient concept based on immunity and resultant histology. Inoculation cutaneous TB after tattooing is quite rare, and is reported mostly from central parts of India, where local customs and rituals result in several tribal women opting for this cheap tattoo ornament. It is likely that the shared tattoo equipment, saliva, or the topical contaminants like soil, cow dung, etc., applied after the procedure might harbor mycobacteria, resulting in cutaneous TB. Simple social custom of nose and ear piercing in developing countries like India are also documented routes of spread of tuberculous infection. Infantile ritual circumcision in the past has been a frequent cause of penile TB when strict sterilized techniques were not practiced. It is still occasionally seen in underdeveloped areas. Sexually transmitted

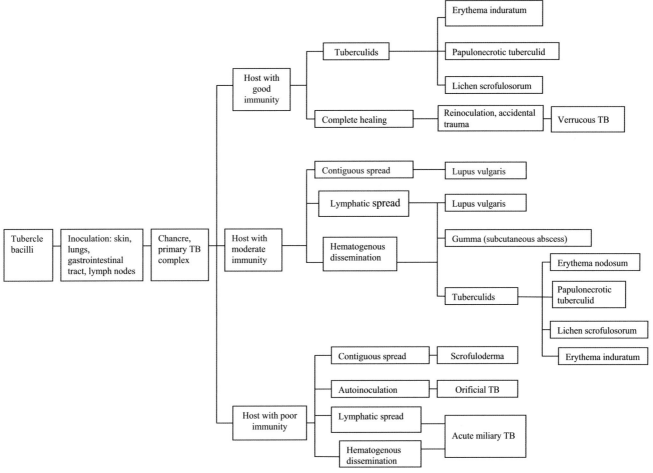

Figure 4.1. Pathogenesis of cutaneous tuberculosis.

primary *Mycobacterium tuberculosis* infection of the penis has been reported in partners of women with endometrial TB. Inoculation TB (accidental) in laboratories handling pathogenic strains of tubercle bacilli has also been reported.

The pathologic deviations observed in different types of cutaneous TB seem to form a spectrum of immunological and histopathological changes extending from scrofuloderma toward LV through TBVC. At one end of this spectrum is scrofuloderma, with a comparatively lower immunity, mild to moderately positive Mantoux test, small to moderate number of lymphocytes in granulomas in the histopathologic sections, and easy demonstrability of bacilli in tissue sections. Lupus vulgaris, on the other hand, forms the opposite pole with a high degree of immunity, moderate to strongly positive Mantoux test, abundant lymphocytes in the granulomas with absent or scant tubercle bacilli, and absence of any immunologic abnormality. TBVC probably occupies an intermediate position showing a moderately positive Mantoux test and ample lymphocytes in granulomas with scant bacilli. It is likely that TBCO occupy a position on the extreme left of the spectrum beyond scrofuloderma.

DIAGNOSIS

Diagnosing cutaneous TB is not always easy if we strictly follow Koch's postulates for any infection. The suggestive clinical picture, careful history of contact with a TB patient or previous tuberculous disease, tuberculin test, and histology contribute to a diagnosis of TB. The definitive diagnosis can only be made by identification of *M. tuberculosis* on the smear and the recovery of organisms on culture, guinea pig inoculation, and their demonstration in the tissue section (Table 4.1).

However, the sensitivity for isolating *M. tuberculosis* on culture is often low and culture in Lowenstein–Jensen medium may take up to 6 to 8 weeks or longer. Smear for demonstration of AFB is particularly helpful in lesions with a high bacillary load such as disseminated miliary TB, scrofuloderma, and gummatous TB lesions. Polymerase chain reaction (PCR) can aid in rapid diagnosis but requires expertise, as it is prone to contamination and false positives. The low yield from PCR and culture may be due to the low number of viable bacilli within the specimen and/or to degradation of DNA material. Combination of dot hybridization with PCR has markedly increased the sensitivity and specificity of PCR in detecting cutaneous TB. Mantoux test with purified protein derivative (PPD) indicates through the skin the cell-mediated hypersensitivity to tuberculin. No definite correlation has been found between Mantoux reactivity and the presence, extent, and type of cutaneous TB. However, it is still a good indicator of the presence of infection if strongly positive, especially in an adult. As the yield from culture and PCR is often low, diagnosis is usually based on clinical features, histological findings, and retrospective review of response to treatment. A successful response to treatment

Table 4.1: Diagnosis of cutaneous tuberculosis

Criteria for the diagnosis of cutaneous tuberculosis

Absolute Criteria

1. Demonstration of AFB in tissue smear/histopathology

2. Positive Culture

3. Positive guinea pig inoculation

4. Positive PCR for *M. tuberculosis*

Relative Criteria

1. Personal or family history of TB and a morphology compatible with cutaneous TB

2. Active, visceral tuberculosis

3. Positive tuberculin-purified protein (PPD) derivative reaction

4. Positive serological tests for detection of antibody to *M. tuberculosis* antigen

5. Compatible histopathology

6. Response to specific antituberculosis therapy

*PCR = polymerase chain reaction

over the course of 6 weeks strongly corroborates a clinical possibility of cutaneous TB, especially in resource-poor settings with lack of sophisticated tests to confirm the diagnosis. However, there may be critics to this therapeutic response diagnostic approach.

Histological interpretation is often difficult in TB. Differences in the histopathological appearances depend on the balance between infection and immunological response. Classical tuberculous histology in the form of tuberculous granuloma is found in not more than two-third of cases. The fully formed granuloma consists of a focus of epithelioid cells containing a variable, but usually sparse number of Langhans' giant cells and a varying amount of caseation necrosis in the center. This is surrounded by a rim of lymphocytes and monocytes. While this tuberculous granuloma is highly characteristic, it is not pathognomonic and is not always found. In the remaining, the histological picture could only be interpreted as chronic inflammation or granulomatous pathology consistent with TB, and the final diagnosis again depends on the clinical picture, other investigations, and therapeutic response. Deep fungal infections, syphilis, leprosy, sarcoidosis, etc. among other diseases can produce an identical picture difficult to distinguish from the characteristic tuberculous histology.

CLASSIFICATION

Numerous attempts have been made to classify cutaneous TB based on clinical morphology, route of entry of organisms, the immune status of the host, and so forth, but none of them is completely satisfactory. The clinical manifestations comprise a considerable number of skin changes, usually subclassified into more or less distinct disease forms. True cutaneous TB skin lesions show a spectrum of morphological presentations that are the outcome of pathological changes characterized by

granulomatous inflammation, variable caseation necrosis, and the presence of *M. tuberculosis* demonstrable by special staining, culture, or polymerase chain reaction. In tuberculids, the pathogenesis is believed to be a hypersensitivity reaction to the presence of *M. tuberculosis* or its antigens. The tuberculids, like true cutaneous TB, also show a spectrum of morphological presentations modified by granulomatous inflammation, variable necrosis, and vasculitis. While mycobacteria have not always been demonstrated from tuberculid lesions, most experts believe *M. tuberculosis* to be an etiologic factor.

New information has allowed further classification of true cutaneous TB based on the route of infection and the immune status of the patient. The system proposed by Tappeiner and Wolff uses this new approach (Table 4.2). Under this system, true cutaneous TB is classified as being acquired either exogenously or endogenously. Exogenous infection occurs following the direct inoculation of the organism into the skin of an individual who is susceptible, either naïve or previously infected or sensitized with BCG. Endogenous infection denotes the occurrence of disease after variable periods of quiescence in treated or untreated tuberculosis patients. This endogenous infection can be in the same site or region or at a distant site/region.

CLINICAL FEATURES

Lupus Vulgaris

Lupus vulgaris is an extremely chronic and progressive form of cutaneous TB occurring in a person with a moderate to high degree of immunity. Lupus vulgaris is the most common form of cutaneous TB reported in studies from Africa and India.

Lupus vulgaris originates from TB elsewhere in the body by hematogenous, lymphatic, or contiguous spread, most often from cervical adenitis or pulmonary TB, sometimes from an old, apparently quiescent primary complex. Rarely, it follows primary inoculation TB or is found at the site of BCG vaccination. The condition is more common in females than in males, and all age groups are equally affected. The lesions are usually solitary or few, but two or more sites may be involved simultaneously. In patients with active pulmonary TB, multiple foci may develop. Though lupus vulgaris can arise at the site of a primary inoculation, around the ostia of an active lesion of scrofuloderma, or at the site of a BCG vaccination, it commonly appears in normal-looking skin. Following a transient impairment of immunity, particularly after measles (thus the term lupus postexanthematicus), multiple disseminated lesions of lupus vulgaris may arise simultaneously in different regions of the body due to hematogenous spread from a latent tuberculous focus. During and following the eruption, a previously positive tuberculin test may become negative but will usually revert to positive as the general condition of the patient improves.

The disease shows a predilection for the face and almost 80% of the lesions are seen over the head and neck. On the face it tends to involve the nose, earlobes, upper lip and frequently extends to the contiguous mucosal surfaces. Next in frequency are the arms and legs. Involvement of the trunk is uncommon. In India the face is affected less often and the buttocks and limbs more frequently. This has been attributed to the prevailing local habit of children playing without clothing and defecating in the

Table 4.2: Classification of Cutaneous Tuberculosis

Exogenous infection	**Nonimmune host**
	• Primary inoculation tuberculosis (primary complex)
	Immune host
	• Tuberculosis verrucosa cutis
	• Inoculation tuberculosis (tattoo, accidental trauma, laboratory personnel)
	• Lupus vulgaris
Endogenous Infection (spread)	• Lupus vulgaris
	• Scrofuloderma
	• Metastatic tuberculous abscess (tuberculous gumma)
	• Acute miliary tuberculosis
	• Orificial tuberculosis (including colostomy opening)
Tuberculids	**True tuberculids**
	• Lichen scrofulosorum
	• Papulonecrotic tuberculid
	Facultative tuberculids
	• Erythema induratum (Bazin)
	• Erythema nodosum

Modified from Tappeiner and Wolff.

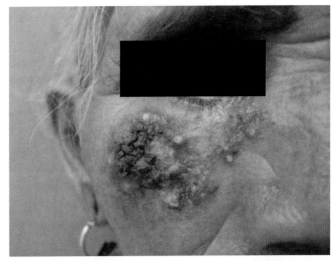
Figure 4.2. Lupus vulgaris over face; note scarring and ectropion.

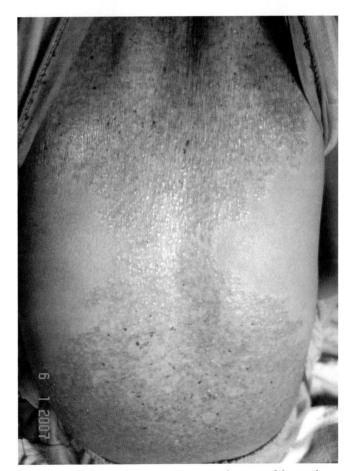
Figure 4.3. Lupus vulgaris – extensive involvement of the trunk.

open and so the possibility of sitting on the dried sputum of patients with TB.

The characteristic lesion is a plaque, composed of nodules of an "apple-jelly" color, which extends irregularly in some areas, while scarring occurs in one edge, causing considerable tissue destruction over many years. In general, lupus vulgaris is asymptomatic. The earliest lesion is a small, reddish-brown, flat plaque of soft consistency, which gives the impression of being embedded in the skin. The lesion gradually becomes darker, slightly raised, more infiltrated and, by slow peripheral extension, gyrate or discoid in shape. Slight scaling may be the only indication of the presence of the lesions. The lesion extends peripherally, leaving behind an atrophic scar, on which new lesions may develop (Figs. 4.2–4.4). Pressing on the lesion with a glass slide may display the characteristic "apple-jelly" color of the nodule/papule, which is often not appreciated in people with darker skin. The hypertrophic form displays soft tumorous nodules, and is rather deeply infiltrating (Fig. 4.5). In the ulcerative form, the underlying tissue becomes necrotic and breaks down (Fig. 4.6 and 4.7). This may result in marked destruction, particularly if auricular or nasal cartilage is involved. The vegetative form consists of papular and nodular forms, and is marked by necrosis and ulceration. Typical lupus vulgaris plaques do not present diagnostic problems. Sometimes they have to be distinguished from lesions of sarcoidosis, lymphocytoma, discoid lupus erythematosus, tertiary syphilis, leprosy, blastomycosis or other deep mycotic infections, lupoid leishmaniasis, and chronic vegetating pyodermas.

In 40% of patients with lupus vulgaris, there is associated tuberculous lymphadenitis, and 10% to 20% have pulmonary TB or TB of the bones and joints or a focus in another system. In many cases,

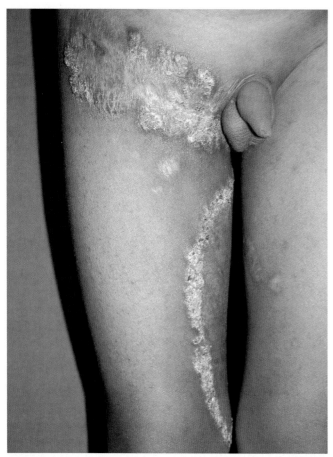

Figure 4.4. Lupus vulgaris – multiple lesions involving the groin and leg showing central scaring.

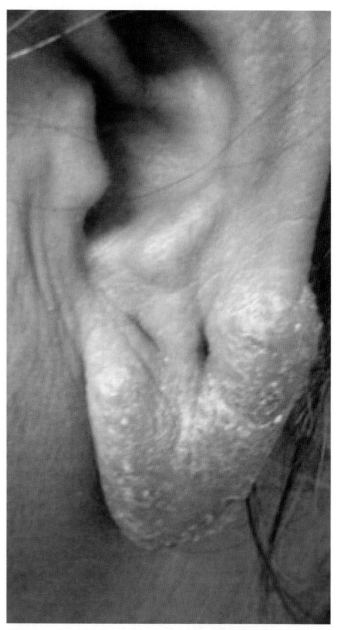

Figure 4.5. Lupus vulgaris (hypertrophic type) involving ear lobule following ear piercing.

lupus vulgaris may be regarded as a symptom of another tuberculous disease running a serious course. The morbidity of lupus vulgaris in patients with pulmonary TB is 4 to 10 times higher than the rest. Its course is chronic and, without treatment, may extend over many years or even decades. Complete healing without therapy is only rarely observed. In developing countries, neglect and lack of awareness about cutaneous TB is responsible for delayed diagnosis and complications in long-standing cases in the form of dissemination of the disease, contractures, myiasis, and even malignant transformation (Fig. 4.8).

Scrofuloderma

Scrofuloderma results from the involvement and breakdown of the skin overlying a tuberculous focus, usually a lymph gland, but sometimes an infected bone, joint, subcutaneous gumma, tuberculous pleural abscess, infected epididymis, or even a lacrimal gland. It occurs most commonly over a lymph node, particularly the cervical lymph nodes. In India, scrofuloderma is a common presentation in children unlike in Europe where adults are more often afflicted.

In developing countries, consumption of unpasteurized milk containing *M. bovis* is a common source of infection causing scrofuloderma, especially in the cervical region. Bluish red skin overlying the infected gland or tuberculous focus (cold abscess) breaks down to form undermined ulcers with a floor of granulating tissue (Fig. 4.9). Numerous fistulae may intercommunicate beneath ridges of the necrosed/necrosing skin. The resulting ulcers and sinuses may drain watery, purulent, or caseous material (Fig. 4.10). Progression and scarring produce irregular adherent masses, densely fibrous in places and fluctuant or discharging in others. After healing, characteristic puckered scarring marks the site of the infection (Fig. 4.11 and 4.12).

M. avium-intracellulare lymphadenitis and the more benign *Mycobacterium scrofulaceum* infection have to be excluded by bacterial cultures. If there is an underlying tuberculous lymphadenitis or bone and joint disease, the diagnosis usually presents no difficulty. Syphilitic gummas, deep fungal infections, particularly sporotrichosis, actinomycosis, severe forms of acne conglobata, and hidradenitis suppurativa may have to be excluded. Scrofuloderma may heal spontaneously, but this can take years.

Tuberculosis Verrucosa Cutis (Warty Tuberculosis)

This is the verrucous form of reinfection TB that localizes at the skin sites prone to trauma of a previously infected patient who usually has a moderate or high degree of immunity. Lesions arise in many ways: by accidental infection from an extraneous source – physicians, pathologists and postmortem attendants are traditionally at risk (thus, "anatomist's wart," "prosector's wart," "verruca necrogenica"); autoinoculation in a patient with active TB; and in children and young adults already infected/BCG vaccinated, who have some degree of immunity.

The lesion starts as a small, symptomless, indurated, warty papule with a slight inflammatory areola. By gradual extension a verrucous plaque is formed. Irregular extension at the edges leads to a serpiginous outline (Fig. 4.13). The center may involute leaving an atrophic scar, or the whole lesion can form a massive, infiltrated papillomatous excrescence. It may be purplish, red, or brown in color with firm consistency but there may be areas of relative softening. Pus and keratinous material may sometimes be expressed from these soft areas or from fissures. Lymphadenitis is rare and may be due to secondary pyococcal infection. This form of TB needs to be differentiated clinically from common warts, keratoses, blastomycosis, chromoblastomycosis, actinomycosis, leishmaniasis, tertiary syphilis, hypertrophic lichen planus, and

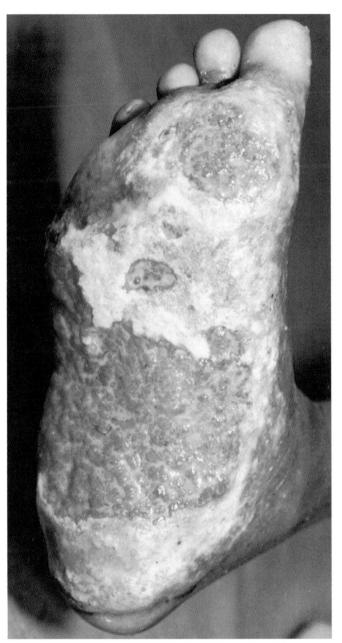

Figure 4.6. Lupus vulgaris (ulcerative type) over foot.

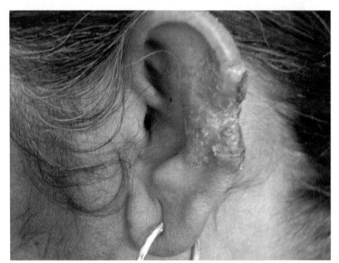

Figure 4.7. Lupus vulgaris showing mutilation of the ear.

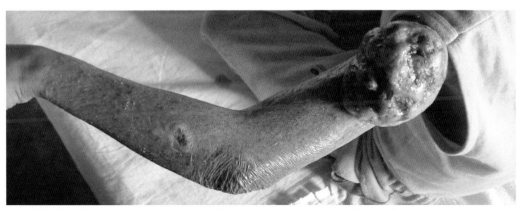

Figure 4.8. Squamous cell carcinoma developing over lupus vulgaris.

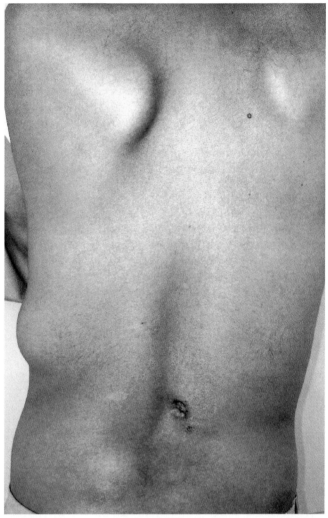

Figure 4.9. Cold abscess over trunk (left flank); note healed sinus over midback.

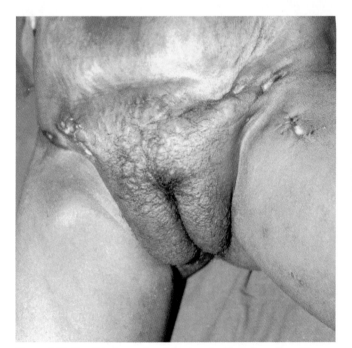

Figure 4.10. Scrofuloderma involving inguinal lymph nodes with vulval edema.

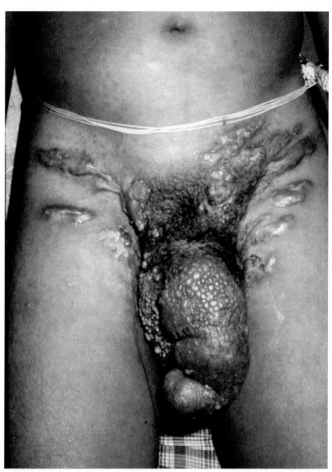

Figure 4.11. Scrofuloderma – chronic scarring resulting in genital lymphedema.

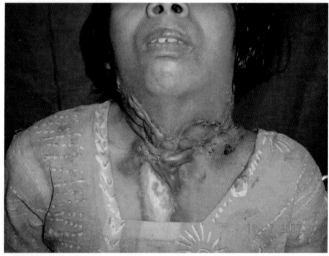

Figure 4.12. Scrofuloderma – extensive scarring, keloid formation and webbing of the neck.

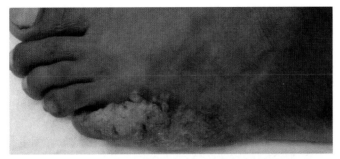

Figure 4.13. Tuberculosis verrucosa cutis over foot.

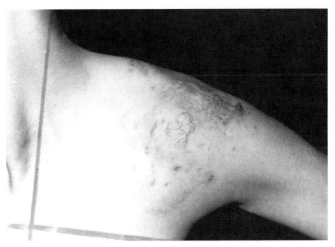

Figure 4.14. BCG vaccine-induced lupus vulgaris.

squamous cell carcinoma. Extension is usually extremely slow and lesions may remain virtually inactive for months or years. Spontaneous remission has been reported.

Primary Inoculation Tuberculosis (Tuberculous Chancre)

A tuberculous chancre is the result of the inoculation of *M. tuberculosis* into the skin of an individual without natural or artificially acquired immunity to this organism. The tuberculous chancre and the affected regional lymph nodes constitute the tuberculous primary complex of the skin. The skin lesion appears 2 to 4 weeks after inoculation as a small papule, scab, or wound with little tendency to heal. A painless ulcer develop that may be quite insignificant or may enlarge to attain a diameter of over 5 cm. It is shallow with a granular or hemorrhagic base studded with miliary abscesses or covered by necrotic tissue. The ragged edges are undermined and of a reddish-blue hue. As the lesions grow older, they become more indurated, with thick adherent crusts. A slowly progressing, painless regional lymphadenopathy develops 3 to 8 weeks after the infection and may rarely be the only clinical symptom. After weeks or months, cold abscesses may develop that perforate to the surface of the skin and form sinuses. Body temperature may be slightly raised. Occasionally, lymph node enlargement, abscess formation, and suppurations may take a more acute course.

Wounds inoculated with tubercle bacilli may heal temporarily but break down later, giving rise to granulating ulcers. Mucosal infections result in painless ulcers or fungating granulomas. Inoculation TB of the finger may present as painless paronychia. Inoculations of mycobacteria in puncture wounds have resulted in subcutaneous abscesses. Clinical differential diagnoses include tularemia, sporotrichosis, cat-scratch fever, and *M. marinum* infections.

Without anti-TB medications, the primary lesion heals with scarring after several months, and may occasionally evolve into tuberculosis verrucosa cutis or lupus vulgaris. Scrofuloderma may evolve if regional lymph nodes break down and cause contiguous extension into the overlying skin. The incidence of post-BCG cutaneous TB caused by the *Bacillus Calmette Guerin* is extremely low in comparison to the great number of vaccinations performed. Usually the BCG reactions run a milder course than "spontaneous" TB of the skin, and they occur more often after revaccination. Specific lesions following BCG vaccination include: inoculation site lupus vulgaris (Fig. 4.14), regional adenitis (which can sometimes be severe), scrofuloderma, and generalized tuberculid-like eruptions. In addition, there is the occasional occurrence of generalized adenitis, osteitis, and tuberculous foci in distant organs.

Acute Disseminated Miliary Tuberculosis

Disseminated miliary tuberculosis (Tuberculosis cutis miliaris acuta generalisata) of the skin, once a rare form of TB that occurred mainly in infants in the prechemotherapy era, has now reemerged among patients infected with HIV. It is an uncommon form of TB secondary to hematogenous dissemination of tubercle bacilli (classically from a pulmonary or meningeal source) to multiple organs including the skin. It has also been described in a few patients with immune dysfunction secondary to malignancy, chemotherapy, or other immunosuppression; post organ transplant or after treatment of autoimmune disease; and in some healthy individuals. The initial presentation of this condition is as a widespread erythematous papular rash. Tiny central vesicles then develop, and these rupture or dry up a few days later, forming a crust. Healing occurs within 1 to 4 weeks, as a depressed scar, with a brownish halo. Lesions may appear anywhere on the body, and usually number between 20 and 50.

Diagnosis is sometimes only made by the biopsy of a skin lesion showing AFB. The eruption occurs in individuals already gravely ill, which requires a high index of suspicion for diagnosis in the early stage. A multitude of maculopapular and purpuric rashes must be excluded, but the diagnosis is usually substantiated by the evidence of acute miliary disease of the internal organs. In the untreated or in those with delayed diagnosis, the prognosis is poor, but a favorable outcome after treatment is possible. With the increased prevalence of HIV disease and the accelerated transmission of TB among patients with HIV, more cases of this once-rare condition are likely to be encountered.

Orificial Tuberculosis

Tuberculous infection of the mucosa or the skin adjoining orifices in a patient with advanced internal TB is now very rare. It occurs particularly in those with pulmonary, intestinal, or urogenital disease from where tuberculous bacilli are regularly shed. In orificial TB of the mouth, the tongue, and particularly the tip and the lateral margins, are most frequently affected, but the soft and hard palate are also common sites of involvement. The lesions are usually mildly symptomatic but can be very painful. In cases with intestinal TB, lesions develop on and around the anus, and active genitourinary disease may lead to involvement of vulva and glans penis. A small yellowish or reddish nodule appears on the mucosa and breaks down to form a circular or irregular ulcer with a typical punched-out appearance, undermined edges, and soft consistency. Its floor is covered by pseudomembranous material and often exhibits multiple areas of yellowish slough and granulation tissue. The surrounding mucosa is swollen, edematous, and inflamed. Lesions may be single or multiple and range from being almost asymptomatic to being extremely painful.

Orificial TB is a symptom of advanced internal disease with a most unfavorable prognosis. Individuals developing orificial TB run a downhill course, and as the internal condition progresses, the orificial lesions enlarge and spread. Chronic ulcers of the mouth in patients with pulmonary TB should arouse suspicion. Large numbers of acid-fast organisms can be detected in smears, and culture confirms the diagnosis. Syphilitic lesions, aphthous ulcers, and carcinoma have to be excluded.

Tuberculous Gumma

This form of TB is the result of hematogenous dissemination from a primary focus during periods of bacillemia and lowered resistance. It usually occurs in undernourished children or in patients who are severely immunosuppressed. Nontender and fluctuant subcutaneous abscesses may arise as single or multiple lesions on the trunk, extremities, or head. The underlying abscesses often invade the overlying skin and it breaks down, forming ulcerative lesions and sinuses indistinguishable from scrofuloderma. The extremities are more often affected than the trunk. Secondary lesions may occur rarely along the draining lymphatics. This condition may occur with progressive organ TB but may also occur without any identifiable underlying tuberculous source. Acid-fast stains usually reveal copious amounts of mycobacteria. Clinical conditions like panniculitis, deep fungal infections, syphilitic gumma, and hidradenitis suppurativa have to be excluded by histopathology and culture.

Tuberculids

The term *tuberculid* is applied to any of a group of eruptions, which arise in response to an internal focus of TB as evidenced by strong PPD reactivity and response of lesions to antituberculous therapy (ATT). The lesions are usually symmetrical and disseminated. Such tuberculids may be thought of as belonging to either one of the two groups: the true tuberculids and the facultative tuberculids. The "true tuberculids" are papulonecrotic tuberculid and lichen scrofulosorum, and are deemed such because *M. tuberculosis* is considered to be the only etiological agent. The "facultative" tuberculids are erythema induratum of Bazin and erythema nodosum.

Papulonecrotic tuberculids

The eruption consists of recurring lesions of symmetrical, hard, dusky-red papules. These soften, ulcerate, and heal with pigmented, mostly atrophic scars, over the course of a few weeks (Figs. 4.15, 4.16a and 4.16b). Presence of active lesions adjacent to areas of scarring is considered a diagnostic aid to papulonecrotic tuberculid. The lesions are generally asymptomatic and

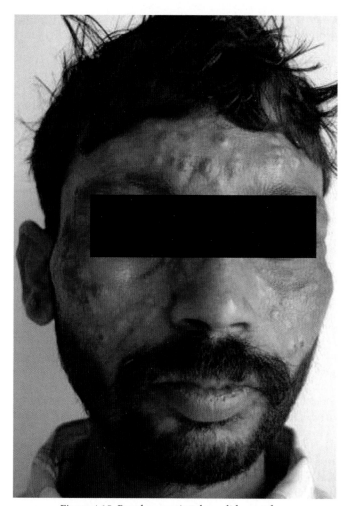

Figure 4.15. Papulonecrotic tuberculids over face.

new crops of lesions may continue over months or years. The legs, knees, elbows, hands, and feet are the sites of predilection, but ears, face, buttocks, and glans penis alone may sometimes be affected. Young adults are predominantly affected, but papulonecrotic tuberculid has also been seen in infants and young children. As a rule, tubercle bacilli are not seen on tissue examination and cannot be cultured, but in many cases mycobacterial DNA has been detected by PCR. Patients usually have strongly positive Mantoux (tuberculin) test and many have clinical manifestations of TB. Clinical conditions like vasculitis, pityriasis lichenoides et varioliformis acuta (PLEVA), and secondary syphilis should be excluded by histopathology. The lesions respond satisfactorily to ATT. The rarity of the condition today and the frequent absence of an obvious focus of TB may deceive the unwary. Biopsy and tuberculin testing should be carried out in all doubtful cases. A therapeutic test is usually decisive.

Lichen scrofulosorum

Lichen scrofulosorum (LS) was first described by Hebra in 1868. It has been considered a rare immunological manifestation of cutaneous TB. Much of the current information is based on case reports and small case series. It is mostly observed in children, though it can also be seen in adolescents and adults. LS is most frequently associated with concurrent tuberculous

a

b

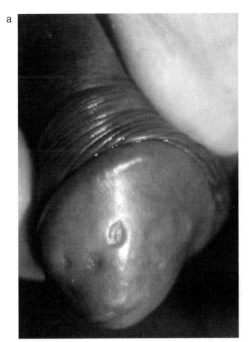
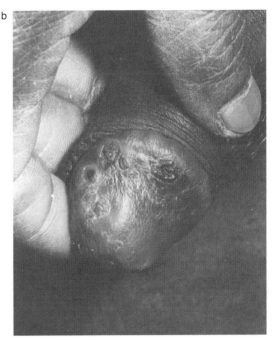

Figure 4.16. (a & b). Papulonecrotic tuberculids over glans penis.

involvement of lymph nodes, bone, or other organs and exhibits an excellent response to ATT. In a series of 39 cases from India, 72% of the patients had an associated tubercular focus elsewhere in the body. Patients presenting primarily with LS should be thoroughly screened for a possible occult tubercular focus. High incidence of a positive Mantoux test also suggests the presence of a high degree of tissue hypersensitivity in these patients. It has also been reported following BCG immunotherapy.

The disease is characterized by eruptions on the trunk of grouped, closely set, minute lichenoid papules, which are often perifollicular. These lesions consist of yellow to reddish-brown papules, 0.5 to 3 mm in diameter, sometimes slightly scaly and occasionally capped by a minute pustule. They develop in groups or discoid patches, and involute slowly over a period of months, without scarring (Fig. 4.17). As these lesions are subtle and asymptomatic, neither the patient nor the physician may give it enough importance and thus may miss the diagnosis. A high index of suspicion and awareness about this entity is needed for diagnosis. Conditions like lichen planus, lichen nitidus, lichenoid secondary syphilis, and micropapular forms of sarcoidosis, which resemble LS morphologically, should be excluded.

Erythema Induratum of Bazin

Originally described by Ernest Bazin in 1861, erythema induratum of Bazin is the tuberculid with an overwhelming female preponderance. It is characterized by indurated, often ulcerated erythrocyanotic nodules that arise on the calves, especially the posterolateral aspect, of those with heavy legs. The nodules may at first regress during warm weather but eventually persist and even ulcerate. The ulcers are ragged, irregular, and shallow, with a bluish edge. Resolution is slow, even with adequate therapy, since the underlying circulatory dysfunction

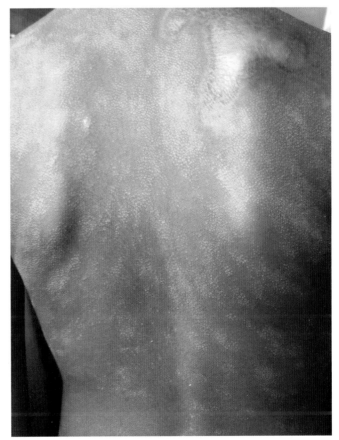

Figure 4.17. Lichen scrofulosorum over trunk; note scar of treated lupus vulgaris over upperback.

is not readily amenable to treatment. Past or active foci of TB are usually present and the tuberculin test is positive. The term *erythema induratum* should perhaps be reserved for cases with

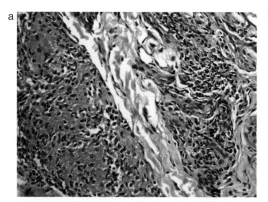
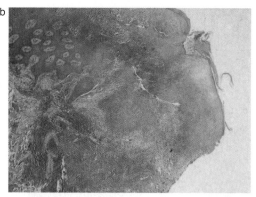

Figure 4.18. Lupus vulgaris (a) epidermal hyperplasia with granulomas in the upper dermis (H&E ×40). Lupus vulgaris (b) higher magnification of the granulomas (H&E ×200).

a proven tuberculous origin though an identical clinical picture can occur without this association. The peripheral T lymphocytes of patients with erythema induratum show an exaggerated response to PPD.

Erythema Nodosum

Erythema nodosum (EN) is the most frequent cause of acute panniculitis characterized clinically by erythematous tender nodules distributed bilaterally over the lower extremities and histologically by septal inflammation. EN is associated with a variety of disease processes and results from inflammatory reactions that may be triggered by a multitude of antigenic stimuli including viral, bacterial, and mycobacterial antigens. In developing countries, where TB is still a major public health problem, it is a predominant cause of EN. It preferentially affects women and can occur at any age, with a peak incidence between the second and third decades of life. The individual lesions are 1 to 5 cm in size, tender, do not ulcerate, and spontaneously involute within a few weeks.

EN has been associated mostly with primary TB. However, there are reports of its association with secondary or reactivation extrapulmonary TB as well. EN was considered to be a favorable finding as it ensured early diagnosis and prompt institution of appropriate therapy. Since majority of patients with EN show a strong tuberculin test, these inflammatory nodules are considered to represent a morphologic expression of hypersensitivity to hematogenous tuberculous antigen. In patients having recurrent/persistent EN, without any other identifiable cause and a strongly positive tuberculin reaction, ATT is indicated even in the absence of other specific signs of infection in an endemic area.

HISTOPATHOLOGY

The microscopic picture of the infectious granuloma due to *Mycobacterium tuberculosis* ranges from well demarcated tuberculous granulomas to a diffuse inflammatory infiltrate with loose granulomas or even nonspecific inflammation. The most prominent histologic feature in lupus vulgaris is the formation of typical tubercles, usually in the upper part of dermis with epithelioid and Langhans giant cells. Secondary changes may be superimposed: epidermal thinning and atrophy or acanthosis with

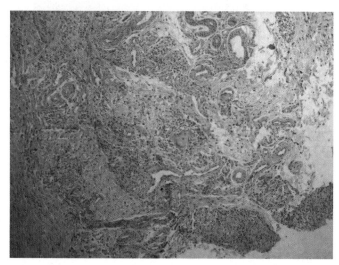

Figure 4.19. TBVC – epithelioid cell granulomas close to the adnexal structures with a multinucleate giant cell (H&E ×200).

excessive hyperkeratosis or even pseudoepitheliomatous hyperplasia (Fig. 4.18a and 4.18b). Old lesions are composed chiefly of epithelioid cells and it may at times be impossible to distinguish it from sarcoidal infiltrates. Lymphocytes are scattered throughout the lesion. The early histopathologic changes in tuberculous chancre are those of acute neutrophilic inflammation with necrosis. Numerous bacilli are present. After 3 to 6 weeks, the infiltrate becomes more granulomatous and caseation appears, coinciding with the disappearance of the bacilli. In tuberculosis verrucosa cutis (Fig. 4.19), there is a striking pseudoepitheliomatous hyperplasia, hyperkeratosis, acanthosis, and papillomatosis with the dermis showing varying amounts of chronic inflammation and at times superficial abscess formation. The intense, mixed infiltrate may show only sparse tuberculous foci. Occasionally the epidermis may show marked hyperkeratosis and the dermis may show a varying amount of chronic inflammation. Serial sections may be required to identify a granuloma. Scrofuloderma reveals massive necrosis and abscess formation in the center of the lesion on histopathology. However, the periphery of the abscesses or the margins of the sinuses contain tuberculoid granulomas and true tubercles, and *M. tuberculosis* can be more easily found (Fig. 4.20). Eosinophils may be present in sizeable

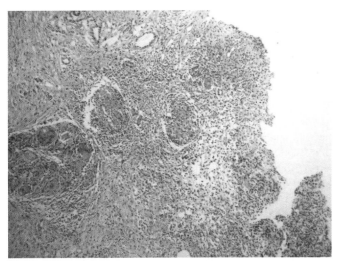

Figure 4.20. Scrofuloderma – multiple epithelioid cell granulomas in the deep dermis with Langhans type of giant cells (H&E ×100).

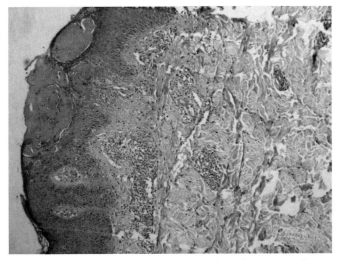

Figure 4.21. Papulonecrotic tuberculid – epidermal necrosis with vasculitis and dense infiltrate in the upper dermis (H&E ×100).

numbers. Rarely biopsy may be nondiagnostic showing only granulation tissue. As in scrofuloderma, massive necrosis and abscess formation are found in tuberculous gumma. Acid-fast stains usually reveal copious amounts of mycobacteria. In orificial TB, there is a heavy nonspecific inflammatory infiltrate and necrosis, but tubercles with caseation may be found only deep in the dermis and mycobacteria are easily demonstrable. Lesions of miliary TB initially reveal necrosis and nonspecific inflammatory infiltrate and small abscesses occasionally with signs of vasculitis.

Mycobacteria are present both in and around blood vessels. In later stages (if the patient develops immunity), lymphocytic cuffing of the vessels and even classical tubercles may be observed. Among tuberculids, the most characteristic feature on histopathology in papulonecrotic tuberculid is a wedge-shaped necrosis of the upper dermis extending into the epidermis, and there may be a leukocytoclastic or lymphocytic vasculitis or granulomatous infiltrate present (Fig. 4.21). In lichen scrofulosorum, superficial tuberculoid granulomas consisting primarily of epithelioid cells are found usually distributed around hair follicles. Necrosis is infrequent. Mycobacteria are not demonstrable in the sections or on culture. Histopathological features in erythema induratum are usually nonspecific like those of a nodular vasculitis with areas of tuberculoid granulomas, fat necrosis, and foreign-body giant cell reactions. Erythema nodosum is a septal panniculitis of the subcutis characterized by a widening of septa with inflammatory infiltrate and inflammation around the vessels, but with no evidence of vasculitis (Fig. 4.22a and 4.22b). In the early stages, there is edema and widening of septa with an inflammatory infiltrate comprised of lymphocytes and histiocytes. In late stages, granuloma formation with giant cells may be seen.

SYSTEMIC INVOLVEMENT

Systemic organ involvement, which is quite common in all forms of cutaneous TB, has not received the attention it deserves. This may precisely be the reason for the very widely differing protocols recommended for the treatment of cutaneous TB. Understanding and accepting the significance of endogenous spread of the disease would automatically imply the presence

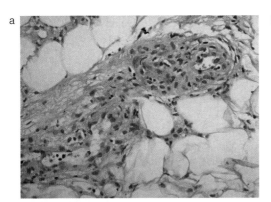

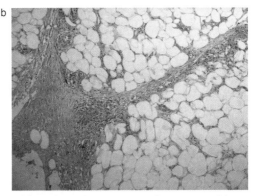

Figure 4.22. Erythema nodosum (a) subcutaneous tissue showing thickening and dense inflammation of the septae (H&E ×100). Erythema nodosum (b) entrapped blood vessels with perivascular infiltrate (H&E ×200).

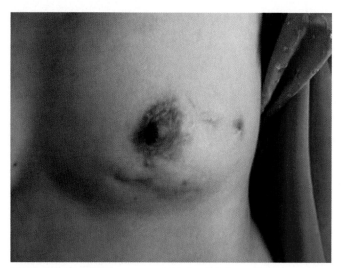

Figure 4.23. Scrofuloderma – multiple healed sinuses involving breast

of an active focus of infection somewhere inside (which may or may not be identifiable with the presently available diagnostic tools) and the obvious necessity to treat it adequately. Needless to state that complete treatment of the patients with cutaneous TB and the focus of infection inside is imperative. Although for adequate treatment the concept of making all efforts to locate the focus somewhere in the body is sound, there are only two studies available, which have investigated for a focus of infection and reported its presence in 18.8% to 22.1% of patients. The infective focus was found in all variants of the disease but it was more often seen in patients with scrofuloderma and tubercular gummas. All body organs, namely, lungs, abdomen, and bones, hosted a focus and rarely even the CNS and heart were found to be affected. The identification of the focus gains further significance because the recommended regime of 6 months of antitubercular therapy may not be sufficient for TB of the CNS, heart or bone. It would be worthwhile recommending that in all patients with cutaneous TB, all possible efforts should be made to identify a focus with relevant investigations for ensuring complete treatment.

TUBERCULOSIS OF THE BREAST

Tuberculosis is rarely localized to the breast. It may be an isolated disease or may be a part of the disseminated disease spread hematogenously or by contiguity or through lymphatics (Fig. 4.23). Coincidental TB of the faucial tonsils of the suckling infant is suggested as one of the modes of infection. The lesions occur as an ulcerated plaque or a nodule present unilaterally. Though the controversy between the entity of granulomatous mastitis and true TB of the breast is probably only of semantics, the patient would be better off if treated for a tubercular etiology. On histology, tuberculoid granulomas with fat necrosis are seen. Despite a strongly positive Mantoux test, AFBs are not present. However, the basic principles of diagnosis, that is, a suggestive history, compatible clinical picture, strongly positive Mantoux test, presence of TB elsewhere, and poor response to treatment for conditions mimicking granulomatous pathology should help in confirming the diagnosis.

HIV AND CUTANEOUS TUBERCULOSIS

Mycobacterium tuberculosis is a common pathogen in persons infected with HIV. The risk of active TB in people infected with HIV and *M. tuberculosis* is 3% to 8% per year, with a lifetime risk of 50% or more. As many as 50% of AIDS patients may be infected with AFB at some stage of their disease. The prevalence of TB in AIDS patients may be 100 times that in the general population. Several studies have documented a high prevalence of extrapulmonary disease in HIV-seropositive patients with TB. However, the skin has remained a relatively unusual site of dissemination. Specific skin lesions of TB in HIV-infected patients are rare, probably because of the shorter life expectancy of most HIV-infected patients after reactivation of TB, which allows insufficient time for TB of the skin or mucous membranes to develop fully.

Fatal cases can occur in tuberculosis presenting in the skin. This is especially true with the advent of multidrug resistant tuberculosis and the increasing occurrence of tuberculosis in AIDS patients. In most cases, these poor prognostic types are the multibacillary forms of infection such as miliary TB. Other types of cutaneous TB reported in HIV-infected patients are tuberculous gumma, tuberculids, cold abscess, and orificial TB.

Cutaneous miliary TB in the setting of HIV infection as well as other forms of immunosuppression is typically characterized histologically by a lack of granulomatous response and a high bacillary load – analogous to lepromatous leprosy. HIV/TB with low CD4 counts shows less pronounced cellular immune response to PPD than to *M tuberculosis*. A negative PPD test, therefore, does not rule out the diagnosis of TB in patients with HIV and a low CD4 count.

BCG PROPHYLAXIS

In developing countries, where morbidity and mortality due to TB are much greater, disease prevention is most desirable. BCG vaccination against TB, which is relatively safe, inexpensive, and easy to use in the field, has been used for many years. BCG vaccine was developed from *M. bovis* in 1908 and first used in 1921. BCG vaccination does not prevent all tuberculous infections. It has been used extensively to prevent the more serious forms of disease caused by *M. tuberculosis*, such as meningoencephalitis and miliary TB. There is very extensive worldwide experience with BCG, and it is generally considered a very safe vaccine with very rare side effects. The standard dose is 0.1 mL for children and adults, and 0.05 mL for infants up to 12 months of age. Currently the intradermal route is preferred. Subcutaneous injection is considered second line, but is also acceptable. Approximately 3 to 4 weeks after vaccination, a 5 to 15 mm erythematous, inflamed, and infiltrated papule appears. Frequently, a central crust develops, which then falls off, leaving an ulcer that usually heals by the 13th week following vaccination. This crusted ulcer then evolves into a small, flat scar.

Currently used strains, maintained by many laboratories, are by no means identical, and this fact may in part explain the very different protection rates ranging from 0% to 80% found in the 10 major trials of BCG vaccination conducted since the 1930s. The protective effect of BCG in children is likely to last for at least 15 years. It is most effective in preventing meningitis and miliary disease. Protection from cutaneous TB may be provided by the BCG vaccine. This is demonstrated by the fact that patients with disseminated disease (any systemic organ involvement or the presence of generalized lymphadenopathy, multiple sites) are less likely to have been BCG vaccinated than those with localized disease. One study showed more unvaccinated individuals in a group with disseminated types of cutaneous TB (80.3%) than those with localized cutaneous TB (65.5%). A different problem concerns BCG vaccination for TB or leprosy in children in countries with a high prevalence of AIDS, since attenuated BCG organisms may become pathogenic, leading to active disease in children infected with HIV.

TREATMENT

Historically, scarification, application of caustics, blowing steam through tubes onto the lesion, freezing with carbon dioxide snow, cautery, ultraviolet radiation therapy, X-ray treatment, and vitamin D have all been used in the past, either alone or in combination, to treat cutaneous TB. Volk (1924) highly recommended roentgen therapy, heliotherapy, and tuberculin for treating scrofuloderma. Presently, except for an additional use of cryotherapy and electrocautery for destroying small lupus nodules within scarred areas, all the other means of treatment are obsolete. One of the major medical advances of the 20th century has been the development of antitubercular therapy. As in TB of other organs, chemotherapy is the treatment of choice for cutaneous TB.

Essentially, the treatment of TB of the skin is the same as that of TB in general. Attention to the patient as a whole is an essential part of the proper management of any tuberculous lesion. This involves a careful search for an underlying focus of disease. The public health aspect should be taken into consideration when following these patients. Don't forget that improvement in general nutrition can be an important therapeutic intervention. The optimal treatment for cutaneous TB consists of a multiple drug regimen for a duration that is long enough to kill all viable organisms, thus preventing the emergence of resistant strains and recurrences. Since most patients with cutaneous TB have systemic disease involvement as well, the treatment of TB of the skin is the same as that of TB in general. It is inferred that anti-TB regimens used for pulmonary TB are adequate for treating cutaneous TB. The Centers for Disease Control and Prevention recommends chemotherapy that is split into two phases. The initial intensive phase, which consists of daily isoniazid, rifampin, pyrazinamide, and either ethambutol or streptomycin for 8 weeks, is directed at rapidly destroying large numbers of viable organisms. The maintenance or continuation phase, which consists of isoniazid and rifampin given daily, three times weekly or twice weekly for 16 weeks, is aimed at eliminating the remaining, persistent organisms. Isoniazid, rifampicin, pyrazinamide and ethambutol may be as efficacious when given three times weekly as when given daily. Fully intermittent regimens (directly observed therapy, DOTS) were used in the two largest TB programs (India and China) with a high level of effectiveness under program conditions.

Patients with cutaneous TB usually have no demonstrable AFBs and should be monitored clinically. In all cases of cutaneous TB, there is always a good response observed rather early to anti-TB treatment. This response is reassuring since there have been only isolated case reports of multidrug-resistant cutaneous TB. However, the rise in the advent of multidrug resistant bacilli and the presence of the infection in HIV-positive individuals can pose serious management problems. HIV-infected patients who strictly adhere to standard treatment regimens do not have an increased risk of treatment failure or relapse. Drug interactions, especially between protease inhibitors or non-nucleoside reverse-transcriptase inhibitors and rifampin, may result in either toxic blood levels of rifampicin or non-therapeutic blood levels of various other antiretroviral agents. Intermittent treatment regimens should not be used in HIV-infected patients with CD4+ cell counts less than 100 cells/μL so as to avoid an unacceptable rate of treatment failure or relapse.

Surgical excision is sometimes necessary as an adjunct to chemotherapy, especially in the management of scrofuloderma and localized lesions of TB verrucosa cutis and lupus vulgaris. In some cases of LV corrective plastic surgery may be indicated depending on the degree of mutilation and skin deformity. In conjunction with ATT, steroids may also have a place in therapy in a few instances, especially in cases of tuberculids and erythema nodosum.

The treatment of cutaneous TB in most cases is the same as for pulmonary TB, as lesions in the skin often represent hematogenously or lymphatically dispersed disease from the internal foci of infection. Along with the increase in the number of patients who have both AIDS and TB, developing countries are more likely to face the problem of cutaneous TB including its diagnosis, treatment, and even drug resistance in the future.

PITFALLS AND MYTHS

Cutaneous TB has not received due importance in the developed world where it has become a rarity seen only in immigrants and HIV-infected individuals. The classification system, though useful in understanding the clinical spectrum, does not always help in ascertaining the endogenous or exogenous mode of spread of the disease. Morphology of any chronic skin lesion(s) like TB can mimic any other infections or even malignancy depending upon the course of the disease, presence of signs of acute inflammation, discharging sinuses, and mutilations caused by the disease. Spread of the tubercular process by contiguity, through lymphatics and via involvement of regional lymph nodes enlarges the list of diseases that need to be considered and/or excluded in the differential (Table 4.3). The difficulty can be more serious in the presence of a developing malignancy as can happen in a long-standing inflammation and ulceration of the skin due to any cause.

Diagnosis of cutaneous TB may require more than pure clinical skills in areas where it is less frequently seen and in HIV-positive patients in whom the course of the disease is altered and atypical lesions are seen. Demonstration of a classical tubercular granuloma on histopathology is diagnostic but caseation necrosis is usually sparse or absent. The infiltrate can be nonspecific in up to one-third of the patients. Demonstration of AFB in Ziehl-Neelsen–stained tissue smears, histopathological sections, or their recovery in culture is disappointing in most instances. The diagnostic value of a positive Mantoux test is ambiguous if

Table 4.3: Common conditions that mimic cutaneous tuberculosis

1. Sarcoidosis

2. Tuberculoid leprosy

3. Deep fungal infections

4. Leishmaniasis

5. Syphilis (tertiary stage)

6. Lymphocytoma cutis

7. Discoid lupus erythematosus

8. Blastomycosis like pyoderma

9. Squamous cell carcinoma

10. Verrucous carcinoma

11. Hypertrophic lichen planus

12. Atypical mycobacterial infections

the patient has had BCG vaccination or exposure to the other environmental mycobacteria. A strongly positive test is significant but the sensitivity decreases with advancing age, early treatment, and conditions that reduce delayed hypersensitivity. Other than these factors and technical errors (e.g., subdermal injection of tuberculin), about 5% of patients do not react to ordinary strength of tuberculin for reasons unknown. Other sophisticated tools like PCR and detection of mycobacterial DNA are either not easily available or are also not always reliable.

Lupus vulgaris is the most common variant of cutaneous TB, accounting for nearly 59% of secondary skin TB cases in India with an average prevalence of 0.37% among general dermatology patients. It has become so rare in developed countries that "Lupus," unqualified, means lupus erythematosus and not lupus vulgaris.

Typical lupus vulgaris plaques do not present diagnostic problems; however, they have to be distinguished from lesions of sarcoidosis, lymphocytoma cutis, discoid lupus erythematosus, tertiary syphilis, leprosy, blastomycosis or other deep mycotic infections, lupoid leishmaniasis, and chronic vegetating pyodermas. Criteria helpful in the diagnosis are the softness of the lesions, a brownish-red color, and a slow evolution of disease. The apple-jelly nodules revealed by diascopy are highly characteristic, but not pathognomonic. Other diseases with similar lupoid infiltrates that look like apple-jelly nodules include lupoid leishmaniasis, sarcoidosis, lupoid rosacea, pseudolymphoma of the skin, and chronic granulomatous disease. In lupus vulgaris, a blunt probe easily breaks through the overlying epidermis into the nodule because of the caseous necrosis present in the lesions. The nodules of leprosy are firmer and signs of nerve involvement are present. The nodules of sarcoidosis resemble grains of sand rather than "apple-jelly." This applies to the feel on probing rather than to the color, which is instead often grayish. Biopsy with special stains for organisms and culture are important diagnostic procedures to differentiate from other lupoid or infiltrative conditions. Leprosy and sarcoidosis, however, are still the chief causes for difficulty in differentiating from cutaneous TB.

Tuberculoid leprosy is differentiated by its neural and perineural granulomatous inflammation. Scattered, noncaseating, compact epithelioid cell granulomas sparsely surrounded by lymphocytes are characteristic of sarcoidosis.

Tertiary syphilis shows more pronounced vascular changes and a plasma cell infiltrate. Demonstration of causative organisms in histologic sections or cultures will be diagnostic in leishmaniasis and deep mycoses. Lupus vulgaris may resemble psoriasis but is more infiltrated, is of a longer duration, and usually has only a single to few lesions present. Bowen's disease can closely resemble cutaneous TB clinically but its chronicity, specific location, and characteristic histology help to differentiate it.

Tuberculosis verrucosa cutis (TBVC) usually affects the hands and feet and is more scaly and verrucous than lupus vulgaris. Early lesions resemble warts or keratoses. Blastomycosis, chromomycosis, and actinomycosis may simulate exuberant forms, and crusted lesions may resemble leishmaniasis. Negative fungal cultures and the presence of tuberculous foci on histology are diagnostic aids. Chronic vegetating pyoderma and hyperkeratotic lesions due to other, atypical mycobacteria may be difficult to exclude. Hypertrophic lichen planus is pruritic and more disseminated and mucosae may be involved. Tertiary syphilis is generally more aggressive in course unlike indolent TBVC and has diagnostic serology.

Primary inoculation TB may simulate primary syphilis, tularemia, cat-scratch disease, sporotrichosis, and other ulceroglandular infectious diseases. Dark-field microscopy can confirm syphilis. The clinical setting, culture from the lesion, and specific serology are most useful for distinguishing these conditions. Any ulcer with little or no tendency to heal and unilateral regional lymphadenopathy in a child and even an adult should always arouse suspicion. Acid-fast organisms can be demonstrated in histologic sections or in smears obtained from the primary ulcer. They can also be seen by draining lymph nodes by fine needle aspiration cytology (FNAC) in the initial stages of the disease but may be difficult to find in older lesions. Diagnosis is verified by mycobacterial culture. Reaction to intradermal PPD is negative initially but becomes positive during the course of the disease.

Miliary TB needs to be differentiated from Letterer-Siwe syndrome, pityriasis lichenoides et varioliformis acuta (PLEVA), secondary syphilis, and drug reactions. In syphilis, serology and biopsy are definitive.

Scrofuloderma: *M. avium-intracellulare* lymphadenitis and the more benign *M. scrofulaceum* infection have to be excluded by bacterial cultures. If there is an underlying tuberculous lymphadenitis or bone and joint disease, the diagnosis usually presents no difficulty. Syphilitic gummas, deep fungal infections, particularly sporotrichosis, actinomycosis, severe forms of acne conglobata, and hidradenitis suppurativa can masquerade this condition. A confirmation of the clinical diagnosis is achieved by bacterial culture and supportive histology.

TB gumma: All forms of panniculitis, deep fungal infections, syphilitic gumma, and hidradenitis suppurativa pose a diagnostic challenge. A confirmation of the clinical diagnosis is obtained by histopathology, aspiration cytology, and bacterial culture.

TB orificialis: Painful ulcers of the mouth in patients with pulmonary TB should arouse suspicion. Similar ulcers can occur in the perianal region. Large numbers of acid-fast organisms can be detected in smears, and bacterial culture confirms the diagnosis. Syphilitic lesions and aphthous ulcers have to be excluded.

Lichen scrofulosorum: Lichen planus, lichen nitidus, lichenoid secondary syphilis, and micropapular forms of sarcoidosis should be differentiated. Histology and syphilis serology always help.

Papulonecrotic tuberculid: The exclusion of PLEVA may present difficulties. Eruptions in leukocytoclastic necrotizing vasculitis also have to be distinguished. Prurigo and secondary syphilis can easily be excluded. The clinical appearance, indolent lesions with resultant scarring, and histology confirm the diagnosis.

Erythema nodosum: Apart from TB, which is the commonest cause in developing countries, it is often associated with a variety of disease processes, drugs, and infections. Strongly reactive Mantoux test helps differentiate it from other etiologies.

We feel that a high index of clinical suspicion is of foremost importance in the diagnosis of cutaneous TB. This is particularly true for areas where the disease is seen rarely. It remains a disease of great importance as it can be treated effectively. Considering all this, it can be suggested that in areas where TB of the skin is not common, and in the immune compromised patient, a high degree of suspicion should be supplemented with laboratory help in the form of histopathology, smear and culture for mycobacterium tuberculosis. Mantoux test (strongly positive test is very helpful), PCR, mycobacterial antigen detection, looking for evidence of TB elsewhere in the body, and past and family history of TB are other helpful factors. A therapeutic trial with ATT for not less than 4 weeks may be indicated if tests are nonconfirmatory and disease is highly suspected.

SUGGESTED READINGS

Arora SK, Kumar B, Sehgal S. Development of a polymerase chain reaction dot-blotting system for detecting cutaneous tuberculosis. Br J Dermatol 2000; 142:72–76.

Barbagallo J, Tager P, Ingleton R, Hirsch RJ, Weinberg JM. Cutaneous tuberculosis: diagnosis and treatment. Am J Clin Dermatol 2002; 3:319–328.

Chong LY, Lo KK. Cutaneous tuberculosis in Hong Kong: a 10-year retrospective study. Int J Dermatol 1995; 34:26–29.

Jacinto SS, de Leon PL, Mendoza C. Cutaneous tuberculosis and other skin diseases in hospitalized, treated pulmonary tuberculosis patients in the Philippines. Cutis 2003; 72:373–376.

Kivanc-Altunay I, Baysal Z, Ekmekci TR, Koslu A. Incidence of cutaneous tuberculosis in patients with organ tuberculosis. Int J Dermatol 2003; 42:197–200.

Kumar B, Muralidhar S. Cutaneous tuberculosis: a twenty-year prospective study. Int J Tuberc Lung Dis. 1999; 3:494–500.

Kumar B, Rai R, Kaur I, et al. Childhood cutaneous tuberculosis: a study over 25 years from northern India. Int J Dermatol 2001; 40:26–32.

Ramam M, Tejasvi T, Manchanda Y, Sharma S, Mittal R. What is the appropriate duration of a therapeutic trial in cutaneous tuberculosis? Further observations. Indian J Dermatol Venereol Leprol 2007; 73: 243–246.

Sehgal V. Cutaneous tuberculosis. Dermatol Clin 1994; 12:645–653.

Tappeiner G, Wolff K. Tuberculosis and other mycobacterial infections. In: Fitzpatrick TB, Eisen AZ, Wolff K, et al., editors. Dermatology in General Medicine. 5th edition. New York: McGraw Hill, 2004: 2274–2292.

5 | LEPROSY

Arturo P. Saavedra and Samuel L. Moschella

INTRODUCTION

Leprosy, or Hansen's disease, is caused by the acid-fast, rod-like *Mycobaterium leprae*. Although effective treatment did not become available until the 1940s, the organism was discovered by Gerhard Henrik Armauer Hansen in 1873 and became the first bacterium known to cause disease in man. Since then, the dramatic, chronic, and debilitating consequences of the disease have been stigmatizing to those affected. Worldwide, it is still the most common cause of peripheral neuropathies, and is superseded in developed countries only by diabetes and alcoholism. Social containment and isolation are not just historical remnants, as those currently treated continue to face social challenges not only in the Third World but also in developed societies.

HISTORY

Hansen's disease has been reported as early as 1400 BC. Evidence of bone disease has been found in Egyptian mummies. During the 13th century, it became widespread in Europe, but it is still endemic in Portugal, Spain, Greece, and Italy.

Despite this fact, the early diagnosis and prevention of leprosy continues to escape health-care providers. In India, the *Vedas* included instructions for the prevention of leprosy, yet today we have been unable to identify cases early before neurologic and dermatologic sequelae ensue. Leprosy is still the main cause of peripheral neuropathies worldwide. As education programs become more prevalent and basic science evolves (the entire genome of *Lepra* is now sequenced), we hope that historical trends in incidence and disease progression will also change.

EPIDEMIOLOGY, MICROBIOLOGY, AND TRANSMISSION

According to estimates by the World Health Organization (WHO), the global registered number of cases of leprosy in 2006 approximated 219,826. Although this figure suggests a general decrease in prevalence of disease, incidence has been stable (if not increasing) and several countries such as India, Brazil, and some central African countries still struggle to contain spread of disease. In Brazil, 38,410 new cases were detected in 2005 and prevalence was estimated to be approximately 1.5%. In the United States, the disease is uncommon, but the greatest number of cases have been found in Louisiana, Hawaii, and Texas. Immigration patterns from endemic communities account for a large number of these cases. Much of the progress achieved so far has been secondary to the use of multidrug therapy (MDT) as well as the development of programs aimed at eradicating disease (defined as a prevalence of less than one case of leprosy per 10,000 members in a population). However, given the difficulties with early detection, compliance with prolonged therapy, and management of permanent disabilities, leprosy continues to be a public health problem and many believe that complete eradication is still far into the future, if at all obtainable. Some have estimated that even after a complete course of antibiotics aimed to be curative, up to one-third of patients will remain with cutaneous and neurologic disabilities. These data suggest that care of the patient with Hansen's disease will transcend "cure" and the health-care system must be prepared to meet these needs.

Mycobacterium leprae is an obligate intracellular, gram-positive, acid-fast bacterium that is tropic for macrophages, smooth muscle, and nerve tissue. The organism can survive singly or be found in aggregates (globi) in infected tissues. It replicates slowly with a generation time of 13 days and a calculated incubation period of 3 to 5 years. Its genome has now been entirely sequenced and because of its limited number of genes, interest in *Mycobacterium leprae* has increased as a model system in which to study obligate intracellular parasitism, infection of neurons, and modulation of the immune response by parasitism. Though armadillos are the most notable animal reservoir for the organism in the United States, the organism has also been recovered from chimpanzees and the Mangabey monkey. Though it cannot be cultured, the mycobacterium may be grown in the footpad of mice, which has been of particular importance in determining drug resistance profiles.

The exact mechanisms of transmission are unknown. Close human contact with prolonged exposure and high-titer inoculums are required for transmission. Nonetheless, conjugal transmission of leprosy is under 8%. In addition, socioeconomic factors such as poor hygiene, sanitation, close living quarters, and poor nutrition appear to be risk factors. The disease is observed twice as often in men as it is in women. The average onset of disease is between 20 and 30 years of age, and childhood cases of Hansen's disease are rarely reported in the absence of another case in the same home.

Leprosy is acquired through close physical contact, particularly from patients with lepromatous disease. Once on therapy, patients are not infectious. Respiratory and nasal secretions are most contagious and account for most transmitted cases; much less commonly, the organism is acquired from the surface of the skin. The route of entry is the respiratory tract and there is no evidence of sexual transmission. Direct inoculation at sites of cutaneous trauma has been reported. Although animal reservoirs are not likely an important source of transmission, the nine-banded armadillo can develop a fully disseminated *M. Leprae* infection. Through intravenous inoculation, they have been the source of in vivo propagation of *M. Leprae* for more than 30 years (Fig. 5.1). Though low levels of vitamins A and E and minerals like calcium and magnesium are seen in leprosy, diet is not believed to be a risk factor in acquiring the infection.

PATHOGENICITY AND IMMUNOLOGY

Perhaps the most fascinating aspect of the disease is that its clinical expression, pathology, and response to treatment are determined by the immune response of the affected patient to mycobacterial antigens. Because bacterial isolates do not vary widely in virulence, it is unlikely that these clinical differences are due to infection with different strains of *M. Leprae*. Patients with high cellular immunity, low mycobacterial load, and well-developed granulomatous responses on pathology are classified on the "tuberculoid" end of the spectrum. Patients with low cellular immunity against the organism, high mycobacterial loads and humoral immunity, and poorly formed granulomas with infiltrates of foamy cells are categorized as having "lepromatous" leprosy. The majority of patients however, exhibit less "polarized" responses. Those near the tuberculoid end are termed borderline tuberculoid (BT), those near the lepromatous end are labeled borderline lepromatous (BL) and those who exhibit mixed features are termed mid-borderline leprosy (BB). An uncharacteristic clinical and histologic lesion is usually the first expression of leprosy and is classified as indeterminate leprosy (the WHO's single paucibacillary lesion of leprosy).

Interestingly, 95% of people are not susceptible to infection. In addition, the disease is only rarely found in children, and when present, there is usually an index case in the home. Whether these observations are related to the mycobacterium's long replication time or to the immune milieu of childhood is currently unknown. Interestingly, there are racial differences in acquiring infection. For instance, Caucasians have a much higher rate of acquiring lepromatous leprosy, followed by Asians, Indians, and African-Americans in that order.

Two major mechanisms of resistance to infection have been postulated. Innate resistance mediated by monocytes provides the first layer of protection. Specifically, the promoter region of PARK2, which has been associated with early-onset Parkinson's disease, has been linked to susceptibility to infection by *Mycobacterium leprae*. The acquired arm of the immune response, mediated by T lymphocytes and dendritic cells, serves as a second layer of protection against infection that may also modulate the expression of disease. HLA-DR2 and DR3, chromosome 10p13, and the transporter associated with antigen processing, (TAP)-2, have been linked to increased risk of acquiring tuberculoid-type leprosy. On the other hand, HLA-DQ1 has been associated with lepromatous leprosy. Tumor necrosis factor A gene (TNF-A), toll-like receptor (TLR)-2, as well as certain polymorphisms of the vitamin D receptor gene, have also been associated with an increased risk for infection. Finally, cytokines such as interleukin IL-12 and IL-18 are linked to resistance to infection and accordingly are found in high levels in patients with polar tuberculoid (TT) disease.

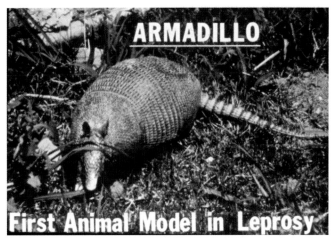

Figure 5.1. The nine-banded armadillo can develop disseminated infection with *Mycobaterium Leprae* and has become a vector in which to replicate the organism for research purposes.

It is unclear whether the number and activity of lymphocytes and dendritic cells determine the phenotype of and susceptibility to infection. For instance, fewer Langerhans cells are detected in skin biopsies of both normal and lesional skin of patients with lepromatous leprosy (LL). On the other hand, the number of Langerhans cells is higher in patients with TT. In general, tuberculoid lesions are associated with higher levels of Th1 type of cytokines like IL-2, TNF-α. and IFN-γ, whereas lepromatous lesions show a Th2-like response and exhibit higher levels of IL-4 and IFN-γ. Coincident with these findings, Th1-like cytokines are associated with activation of TLR-1 and TLR-2, whereas Th2-like cytokines appear to prevent activation of these toll-like receptors.

Overall, impairment in cellular immunity is important for acquiring the infection. Anergic responses and defects in cellular immunity appear to be lasting, and evidence suggests that such defects persist in spite of therapy. Though patients with LL are anergic to these antigens, this does not imply that they are immunocompromised. As explained by Scollard et. al., these patients are not at increased risk of other opportunistic infections or of developing cancer. Interestingly, co-infection with leprosy does not increase transmissibility or risk of infection with human immunodeficiency virus (HIV), as is the case with tuberculosis, herpes, and leishmaniasis. Co-infection with leprosy does not lead to progression or clinical deterioration in HIV/AIDS (acquired immunodeficiency syndrome).

CLINICAL FINDINGS AND CLASSIFICATION CRITERIA

Consistent with its optimal growth temperatures of 27° C to 30° C, *Mycobacterium lepra* tends to infect cooler areas of the body such as the ears and the nose. The skin, peripheral nerves, the testes, and the anterior chamber of the eye are generally the most commonly affected sites. In addition, the upper respiratory tract, lymph nodes, and rarely the viscera (particularly the liver and spleen) may be affected. Though peripheral sensory nerves are most commonly affected, autonomic and motor nerves may also become damaged. Usually, temperature sensation is affected first, followed by light touch, pain, and pressure. In fact, skin lesions need not be present to make a diagnosis of leprosy. In the absence of skin lesions, the differential diagnosis elicited in cases that turn out to be "neuritic" leprosy includes primary amyloidosis, progressive hypertrophic familial neuropathy, carpal tunnel syndrome, diabetic neuropathy and congenital indifference to pain. In neuritic leprosy, the ulnar nerve is most commonly affected and upper motor neuron signs are never elicited. Furthermore, proximal muscles are not involved, the central nervous system is spared, reflexes are intact, and coordination examination is within normal limits. Biopsy is required for diagnosis but electromyography may also be helpful.

Ridley–Jopling Classification

On the basis of the immunologic criteria discussed earlier, clinical classification of leprosy was devised by Ridley and Jopling in 1966. On the basis of the immunological response of the host to the organism, the disease was categorized into five presentations: polar tuberculoid (TT), borderline tuberculoid (BT), borderline (BB), borderline lepromatous (BL) and lepromatous leprosy (LL).

Patients with strong immunity to the organism are diagnosed with polar tuberculoid (TT) leprosy. As a result, only one or a few lesions are noted on cutaneous examination. These lesions can be well-demarcated macules, patches, or plaques with superficial scaling. Fine erythema and hypopigmentation may be detected (Fig. 5.2). Hypopigmentation is thought to result from a decrease in the total number of melanocytes in infected skin. A local xerotic surface accompanies the primary lesion. The morphology may approximate an oval, but geometric configurations of discrete papules in annular or circinate arrays have also been reported. The primary lesion may be confused for tinea corporis, psoriasis, gyrate erythema, granuloma annulare, necrobiosis lipoidica, lupus vulgaris, and tuberculosis verrucosa cutis. The skin may show hair loss and central atrophy at sites noted to be anesthetic. Peripheral nerve enlargement can be palpated on examination, usually in only one or two trunks, depending on the site of infection. Lesions of tuberculoid leprosy may heal spontaneously.

Borderline tuberculoid (BT) leprosy presents with a greater number of lesions, which may be hypopigmented, but may also show erythema and other brownish dyspigmentation patterns (Fig. 5.3). Macules, patches, and plaques with scale constitute the primary lesion, but in addition, smaller "satellite" lesions may be noted in the periphery of a larger lesion. Annular disease is also common and may be misdiagnosed as granuloma annulare, erythema multiforme, lupus vulgaris, and tinea circinata. The disease has often been confused with mycosis fungoides, B-cell lymphoma, lichen planus, and pityriasis alba. Close inspection of the primary lesion may show local hair loss, xerosis, and thick granular margins. Papulonodular lesions and infiltrative plaques may also develop, with a rough surface and anesthesia. There are a larger number of asymmetric lesions and the central portions may show atrophy. There is peripheral nerve involvement and lesions need not be anesthetic to make the diagnosis (Fig. 5.4). Screening for peripheral neuropathy is best accomplished with the use of microfilaments as is currently performed for diabetic neuropathy. Lesions that resolve spontaneously or during therapy

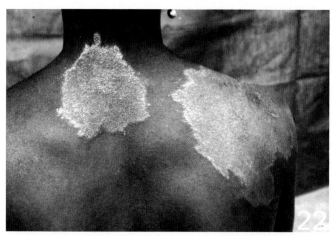

Figure 5.2. Female patient with polar tuberculoid (TT) disease. Note that lesions are well demarcated and show focal areas of hypopigmentation and scaling.

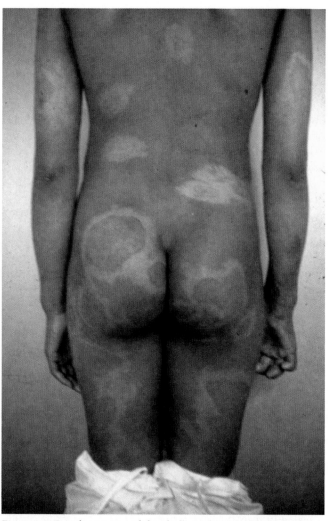

Figure 5.3. Female patient with borderline tuberculoid (BT) disease. Note the arcuate but asymmetrical hypopigmented lesions which are greater in number when compared to patients with polar tuberculoid (TT) disease. In addition, there is a claw hand deformity in the right upper extremity. The patient had evidence of both sensory and motor deficits on neurologic exam.

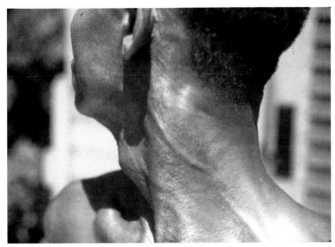

Figure 5.4. This patient with borderline tuberculoid (BT) disease exhibits auricular nerve enlargement, easily seen and palpated on exam.

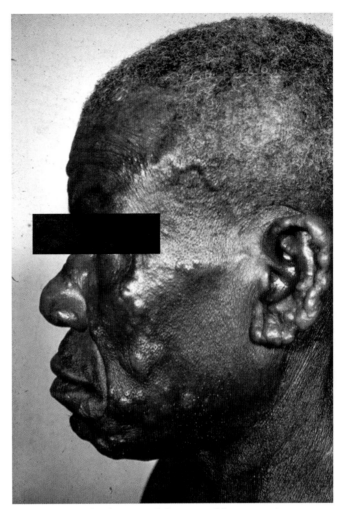

Figure 5.5. Nodules that cause deformities of the nose and ears, as well as madarosis, can be appreciated in this patient with advanced lepromatous leprosy (LL).

may show central clearing within a background of browny erythema. The differential diagnosis may be similar to that listed for TT, but annular syphilides, sarcoidosis, and leishmaniasis must be added.

Patients with borderline disease (BB) exhibit more extensive disease. Many lesions are noted, mostly patches and plaques with sharp demarcation and edges that slope into surrounding skin. Plaques tend to be erythematous and are arranged as infiltrated bands with central areas of anesthesia. "Punched-out" lesions may be seen. In general, the inner margins of the primary lesion are easier to discriminate than the outer margin. Disease is asymmetric and peripheral nerve involvement is more widespread. Neuritis in these cases can be more severe than in other types of leprosy, as multiple trunks may be damaged asymmetrically very early in the course of the disease. In general, loss of sweating precedes sensory nerve damage. As a result, some have advocated the use of sweat function tests in patients with uncertain neurologic exams. Pilocarpine nitrate and acetylcholine tests are sometimes used in the diagnosis of leprosy and in the evaluation of impending sensory nerve damage.

Those patients with lower immunity to the organism tend to express more disseminated and symmetrical cutaneous and neural disease. Those with borderline lepromatous (BL) disease present with several plaques resembling those seen in borderline disease (BB). Macules, patches, papules, and plaques with a smooth, shiny erythematous surface are commonly seen. Erythema and hypopigmentation are common. Primary lesions are more irregularly shaped and bilaterally distributed. Annular lesions can be seen. Though lesions are infiltrated, they are poorly demarcated and borders are hard to discriminate and may be slightly anesthetic. The neurologic exam can appear to be within normal limits. Occasionally, tinea versicolor, vitiligo, psoriasis, secondary syphilis, contact dermatitis, pityriasis rosea, onchocerciasis, and scleroderma may figure into the differential diagnosis.

Lepromatous (LL) leprosy presents the other "polar" end of the disease spectrum, when compared to tuberculous (TT) leprosy, and is the most infectious form of the disease. The patient presents with symmetrically distributed macules, papules, plaques, and nodules that show hypopigmentation, erythema,

and a browny dyschromia commonly compared to copper. Nodules are not subcutaneous and as a result, the skin cannot be moved over them. This may be an important maneuver in establishing a diagnosis. Punched-out papules may be seen and smaller macules and papules may coalesce into infiltrated plaques. Rare forms of "digitate" morphology have also been reported. The disease tends to spare the axilla, groin, and perineum. General xerosis and acquired icthyosis may ensue. The face may become generally infiltrated, causing leonine-like faces, with a shiny, smooth texture. Madarosis, or loss of hair in the lateral aspect of the eyebrows, is commonly seen. Complete loss of eyelashes has also been reported. The nasal mucosa may become inflamed and ulcerated and the septum may perforate. Saddle nose deformities can also result. Recurrent epistaxis is not an infrequent sign of the disease. In advanced stages, disease may become nodular, especially in cooler parts of the body and may cause deformities of the nose, ears, eyelids, joints, and trunk (Fig. 5.5). The conjunctiva, cornea, and iris are involved and cataract-like opacities develop. In earlier stages, corneal insensitivity may be a treatable and reversible finding. The viscera may also become involved, particularly the reticuloendothelial system. However, glomerulonephritis and secondary amyloid

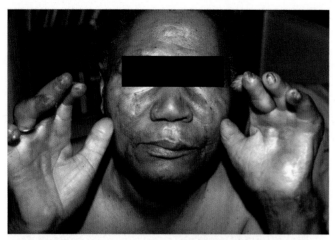

Figure 5.6. Note ulcerations in the fingertips, claw hand deformities, madarosis, and left-sided facial palsy in this patient with lepromatous leprosy (LL). This patient had both median and ulnar neuropathies with both motor and sensory deficits.

Table 5.1: Comparison between Paucibacillary and Multibacillary Disease

Category of Disease	Paucibacillary	Multibacillary
Bacillary Index	2 or less	Greater than 2
Number of lesions	5 or less	Greater than 5
Patients affected	TT, BT	BB, BL, LL

TT, polar tuberculoid disease; BT, borderline tuberculoid disease; BB, borderline leprosy; BL, borderline lepromatous disease; LL, lepromatous leprosy.

have also been reported. At this stage, the differential diagnosis may include neurofibromatosis, multiple lipomatosis, leukemia cutis, disseminated fungal and parasitic disease such as anergic cutaneous leishmaniasis and Kala-Azar, as well as disseminated xanthomatosis. Usually, there is no sensory nerve involvement in early stages but symmetric peripheral neuropathies can ensue in untreated patients. Classic stocking and glove anesthesia develops first but as long nerves become progressively involved, sensory levels may be detected on examination. The facial nerve is very commonly involved. Muscle atrophy may ensue with time; claw deformities in hands and feet, foot drop, and the so-called "papal" hand may also develop (Fig. 5.6).

The term "indeterminate" disease (single paucibacillary lesion) may be used for those patients presenting with one or few macules that are hypopigmented and/or mildly erythematous, generally on exposed skin surfaces. There is no anesthesia, but some lesions may show hypoesthesia and hypohidrosis. Peripheral nerve enlargement is usually not detected. Pathologic examination reveals a mixed inflammatory infiltrate involving the neurovascular bundle. This stage is often considered the very earliest stage of the disease and, most commonly, it leads to spontaneous resolution.

Histoid leprosy is a special case that deserves mention. Patients present with multiple papules, nodules, and plaques interspaced by relatively uninvolved skin. The surface of these plaques is smooth and shiny, and is sometimes described as pearly. They may occur at different stages, particularly in disseminated disease, and have been reported to occur near the eye, in intertrigenous areas, and near fossae of the extremities. The lesions vary in color from pink to yellow to brown to violaceous and often exhibit secondary changes such as an excoriated surface. Most patients are thought to be in the lepromatous disease spectrum, who prematurely interrupted treatment, are drug-resistant (particularly to dapsone), or who are relapsing.

WHO Classification

In addition to using clinical criteria established by the Ridley and Jopling classification, the WHO introduced the concept

of skin-slit smears as a simplified way of categorizing disease. A smear is examined under oil for the total number of acid-fast bacilli recovered. A bacillary index represents a logarithmic count of organisms seen. For instance, a bacillary index of 2 represents 1 to 10 organisms per high-power field. The WHO initially classified those patients with a bacillary index of less than 2 or fewer than five clinical lesions as "paucibacillary" disease. Whereas those patients with an index greater than 2 and at least six clinical lesions were classified as having multibacillary disease (Table 5.1). In general, patients with TT and BT tend to be paucibacillary, whereas those with BB, BL, and LL disease fulfill the criteria for multibacillary disease. However, to prevent undertreatment, any patient with a positive smear or organisms on biopsy is currently is said to have "multibacillary" disease, regardless of the index. Generally, the terms paucibacillary and multibacillary are more helpful in designing a therapeutic regimen than in establishing clinical classification and prognosis (see section on treatment). However, patients with multibacillary disease are known to be about 5 to 10 times more infective than patients with paucibacillary disease.

HYPERSENSITIVITY REACTIONS

Leprosy is a disease that presents with two "clinical faces." The first one is a result of a host response to the infective organism. The other is a hypersensitivity reaction to antigens of the viable or dead bacillus, the so-called "reactions." The nature of the reaction depends on the cell-immune status of the patient. Those patients with BT and BB disease who have a relatively intact cell-mediated immunity clinically express a reversal reaction (Type I). In contrast, those patients with LL and BL are anergic or almost anergic to *M. Leprae* and respond with immune-complex disease and clinically with erythema nodosum leprosum (Type II reaction). These reactions occur in 30% to 50% of all patients with leprosy as a result of stress, medical illness, pregnancy, injury, surgery, concurrent infection, vaccination, and multiple drug therapy. Unfortunately, no laboratory tests are available to specifically diagnose these reactions or to predict who among those infected will develop them.

Type I reactions are more common in patients with borderline states, particularly borderline lepromatous leprosy (BL), and occur during the first 6 to 18 months of treatment but have been reported up to 7 years after initiating therapy.

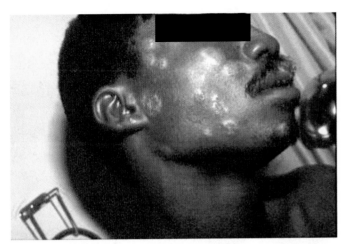

Figure 5.7. In this patient with BL disease, a reversal Type 1 reaction is exhibited by painful erythematous, edematous, nodular, and infiltrated nodules. These nodules appeared acutely.

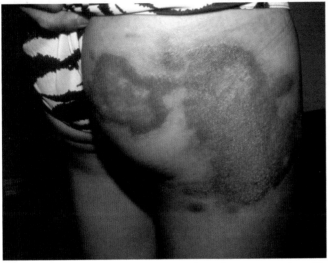

Figure 5.8. Type 1 reaction in a patient with BL disease, presenting with a new, large erythematous plaque in the setting of general malaise.

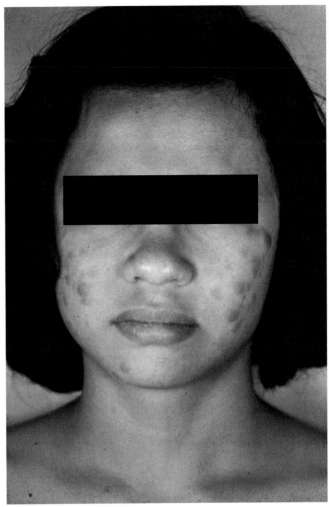

Figure 5.9. This patient was treated unsuccessfully with tetracycline for acne vulgaris in the setting of diffuse lepromatous leprosy. Note that the acute and fleeting nature of the lesions, as well as the erythematous and deep nodular morphology, suggests the correct diagnosis of ENL.

Reversal reactions are rarely observed in patients with TT. Type I reactions belong to the Type IV, cell-mediated, allergic-type delayed hypersensitivity reactions and appear after an acute shift toward high cellular immunity. Cytokines such as IL-1, IL-2, IL-12, IFN-γ, and TNF-α are upregulated, suggesting a predominant Th1-like response. Most commonly, this type of reaction occurs as the patient shifts to a higher degree of cellular immunity, termed *upgrading*. Patients are acutely ill but disease may also develop over days or weeks. Patients present with edema of the hands, feet, and face as well as tenderness along nerves and joints. The ulnar, median, facial, greater auricular, common peroneal, and posterior tibial nerves are most commonly affected. Abscesses have been reported to develop along nerves. Patients may acutely develop foot drops, facial palsy, and claw hands. Eye involvement may present as lagopthalmus with complicating exposure keratitis. The skin lesions become more erythematous and infiltrated and may ulcerate (termed *Lazarine leprosy*). Patients can develop new lesions in the setting of a Type I reaction. If untreated, lesions typically resolve after 3 to 4 months (Figs. 5.7 and 5.8). Systemic lupus erythematosus and drug reactions often figure into the clinical differential diagnosis.

Type II reactions, termed *Erythema nodosum leprosum* (ENL), are characterized by the acute onset of cutaneous and subcutaneous erythematous nodular lesions that bear no relationship to other lesions that the patient had before this attack (Fig. 5.9). Some may be very deep seated, may suppurate, and ulcerate (erythema induratum leprosum). A varicelliform vesicular and necrotic papular eruption that favors the upper extremities and face has also been described. Generally, this reaction is a subtype of Type II humoral lepromatous hypersensitivity reactions and is more common in borderline cases and in LL disease. Its incidence appears to decrease with increasing age and with decreasing inoculums during primary infection. Rarely, ENL may be the presenting sign of leprosy, and in these cases, findings consistent with primary infection may not be seen on physical examination. IFN-γ, TNF-α, and IL-12 are found in high levels in the serum of affected patients. In fact, injection of IFN-γ into a lesion in leprosy has reportedly lead to the development of ENL. This immune-complex deposition disease leads to a strong polyclonal antibody response that may be associated with general edema, nerve tenderness, bone and joint pain, and fever and chills. Neuritic night pain has also been reported. The associated neuritis can result in an acute paralysis. In addition, epistaxis, orchitis, proteinuria, and consequent glomerulonephritis can develop. Stress reactions like those associated with Type I lepra reactions can also lead to ENL. An important feature of ENL is that it most commonly occurs late in the treatment course. Mild cases of ENL may spontaneously remit; however, severe cases can be progressive and more apt to recur. Death rarely occurs from renal insufficiency.

An uncommon third type of reaction is Lucio's phenomenon, which is usually restricted to Central and South America and immigrants from those areas. It is usually associated with high mortality rates. It occurs in a subtype of lepromatous leprosy called *primary diffuse lepromatous leprosy*, the so-called "la lepra bonita." The face is diffusely infiltrated (pseudomyxedematous facies). Madarosis, anhidrosis, and infiltration of the nasal mucosa with persistent epistaxis and destruction of nasal cartilage are seen. Diffuse body hair loss is also seen but orchitis and iritis are not observed. Unlike in ENL, systemic symptoms such as fever, malaise, chills, joint pain, and nerve tenderness are rare but anemia and cryoglobulinemia may be observed. Visceral findings such as hepatosplenomegaly and lymphadenopathy occur. The eruption of Lucio's phenomenon is characterized by the presence of symmetrical black stellate necrotic lesions of the extremities (erythema necrotisans). The lesions may resemble the cutaneous flame figures seen in coagulopathic states (Fig. 5.10).

LABORATORY TESTS

Work up of leprosy is somewhat different than other infectious diseases because the mycobacterium cannot be cultured. As a result, clinicopathologic correlation is of utmost importance. At this time, the role of laboratory tests is adjunctive. Cultures are taken to exclude other organisms rather than to recover the mycobacterium. PCR tests are used mostly in experimental analysis, and no true serologic tests exists for routine diagnosis. However, because the diagnosis can be stigmatizing and requires long periods of treatment with medications that may not be innocuous, it is important to highlight those tests that may be useful in establishing the diagnosis or in affecting treatment. In this section, we will review the clinical utility of skin-slit smears, the lepromin test, polymerase chain reaction tests, as well as other investigational assays.

As stated earlier, skin scrapings were initially introduced to aid in the classification of disease into either paucibacillary or multibacillary disease. Currently, the role of skin scrapings is limited as it does not provide high sensitivity or specificity. Skin smears are only positive in 10% to 50% of cases and are most helpful when taken from multibacillary patients or from those with recurrence or clinical relapse. It is more reliable when used by experienced clinicians and is most helpful in determining drug therapy rather than in making the diagnosis. On the other hand, a positive index may be obtained in BB, BL, and LL

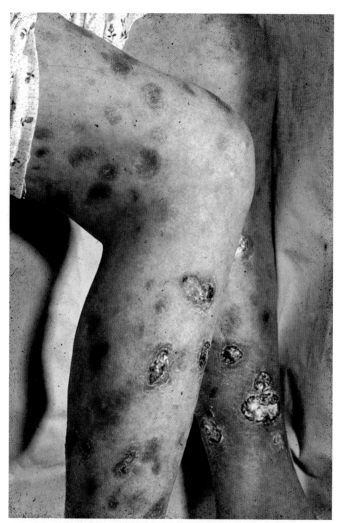

Figure 5.10. **A** patient with Lucio's phenomenon, who portrays stellate scarring and ulceration, commonly confused with cutaneous manifestations of hypercoagulation syndromes.

disease. The lack of specificity results from the fact that other cutaneous mycobacterial infections may have a positive skin-slit test.

Though it is not approved by the U.S. Federal Drug Administration in the United States, the lepromin (Mitsuda) test has been used worldwide. The test lacks both specificity and sensitivity. It is not diagnostic of leprosy and it is not required to make a diagnosis. A suspension of whole autoclaved leprosy bacilli is injected intradermally and the induration response is measured 4 weeks later, ideally with the aid of a pathologist to establish the presence of a granulomatous reaction pattern on histopathologic evaluation. The lepromin test is negative in BB, BL, and LL disease. It is most helpful in patients with a strong cellular immunity to the organism. Therefore, a strong reaction is observed in TT disease. The intensity of reaction decreases along the spectrum (i.e. patients with BT may show a weakly positive result). Results are highly variable in indeterminate leprosy. Though a positive result may be caused by prior exposure to the mycobacterium, it reflects the presence of cell-mediated immunity and the ability of patients to eliminate mycobacterial loads.

Enzyme-linked immunosorbent assays have been developed to test for antibodies against phenolic glycolipid 1 (PGL-1). PGL-1 is the main lipid component of the outer leaflet of the mycobacterial cell wall that affords the test its specificity. It is also responsible for binding laminin 2 and thereby infecting Schwann cells. Because patients with paucibacillary disease have strong cellular immunity against the organism but have poor humoral responses, anti-PGL-1 testing is rarely positive in these patients. However, even when present, humoral responses to mycobacterial antigens are not robust, stable, or detectable. Like other tests discussed in this section, PGL-1 ELISA lacks specificity and sensitivity and is a better marker for the presence of multibacillary disease rather than a way of making the diagnosis. The test has been used mostly in epidemiological studies and at this time is mostly of interest to the research community. Similar lipoarabinomannan tests, fluorescent antibody absorption tests (FTA-ABS), and radioimmunoassay techniques are also available but used less frequently than PGL-1 ELISA.

Mycobacterium leprae cannot be cultured, but it may be grown in the footpad of the mice to establish sensitivities to antibiotics. PCR tests that may become increasingly useful in this regard have been developed. In addition to mutation analysis, PCR techniques have added greatly to our ability to detect drug-resistant strains. For instance, missense mutations in *rpoB* are associated with resistance to rifampin. Using this technique, in which microorganisms are detected on Fite-stained sections, mycobacterial DNA can be isolated from skin samples in patients before therapy when the diagnosis is still questionable. PCR tests are not indicated in patients in whom no microorganisms could be identified on stains or in patients who are improving with therapy. Because PCR techniques can detect DNA from both viable and nonviable organisms, it should not be solely used to make a diagnosis of active infection at this time. Novel techniques that expand 16S rRNA sequences (which are quickly degraded once the mycobacterium is not viable) may circumvent this problem. Though positive PCR results can also be obtained from other sites such as nasal mucosa, blood, nerve, and ocular tissue, their use remains limited to research laboratories of centers that specialize in the care of patients with Hansen's disease.

Importantly, no serologic studies are available that identify carriers or that facilitate segregation of patients who are likely to fail treatment or endure relapse. In addition, though co-infection with HIV and *Mycobacterium leprae* does not lead to progression of either disease, those with leprosy may have a false negative HIV ELISA test because the mycobacterium may generate antibodies that cross-react with HIV screening assays. In addition, patients with LL and BL may have false-positive VDRL and FTA-ABS. Given the extent of hyperglobulinemias, false-positive antinuclear antibodies and rheumatoid factor can also be reported.

PATHOLOGY

In general, histopathologic evaluation benefits from a deep biopsy obtained from the advancing border of a lesion suspicious for leprosy. The atrophic center should not be biopsied. Because the disease exhibits a spectrum of clinical and histopathologic findings, the most important aspects to evaluate include (1) the extent of granulomatous inflammation, (2) the presence or absence of mycobacteria (which usually requires special stains such as the modified Fite stain due to the fact that this organism is less acid fast than other mycobacteria), and (3) the location of granulomas and organisms, whether present diffusely in the dermis or clustered around (and invading) peripheral nerves. As an obligate intracellular pathogen, *M. Leprae* is found in macrophages when it affects the skin and in Schwann cells when it affects nerve tissue. The extent to which each of the above three criteria is noted on histopathologic sections helps categorize the disease along the spectrum suggested by Ridley and Jopling.

Tuberculoid leprosy is characterized by epithelioid granuloma formation, often surrounding nerves and appendages that may become completely replaced. Dense foci of lymphocytes may be noted surrounding granulomas as well. Occasionally, the granulomas may extend superficially to abut the epidermis. Microorganisms are rarely encountered on Fite-stained sections, and when observed, they are found near nerves, which may exhibit caseation. Unlike in lepromatous disease where damage to the nerve is caused initially by disrupting the perineurium, in tuberculous disease infiltration of the nerve by microorganisms is generally the rule. When T-cell subtypes are analyzed, CD4+ cells are found throughout the lesion whereas CD8+ cells are only present at the periphery of lesions in TT. They are found at a ratio of 1.9:1 (normal ratio is about 2:1). On the other hand, in lesions of lepromatous leprosy, the CD4+/CD8+ ratio is 0.6:1 and CD8+ cells are distributed throughout the entire lesion. Of note, Langerhans cells are not uncommonly seen and infiltrates and lesional skin can be positive for CD1 and langerin. This finding should not detract the pathologist from making a diagnosis of leprosy in favor of Langerhans cell histiocytosis. The level of CD1+ expression is much higher in TT lesions than in LL lesions.

The histopathology of lepromatous leprosy is on the other end of the spectrum. A diffuse infiltrate of sheets of foamy histiocytes and a clear Grenz zone are observed. Abundant microorganisms are seen singly or in large collections called *globi*. Virchow cells (Lepra cells) may be seen, which are classically described as large macrophages with foamy, fatty changes, containing globi. Lymphocytes can be scant and plasma cells are notable. Microorganisms cause neural destruction by either disrupting the perineurium, by their high concentration in Schwann cells, or by eliciting inflammation and fibrosis.

Patients with borderline disease show histopathology that is between those seen in tuberculoid and lepromatous disease. True BB disease is rarely diagnosed histopathologically as most patients will shift into BT or BL and the biopsy must be interpreted in correlation with clinical findings. In BT, a Grenz zone is commonly seen within a loosely-formed granuloma surrounded by lymphocytes. Nerves and the adnexa may be involved but they are usually not replaced by the inflammatory response. Acid-fast bacteria can be found. As the disease trends toward BB, epithelioid granulomas are not commonly rimmed by lymphocytes. Langerhans cells are less common than in BT and acid-fast bacilli are found in greater numbers. Finally, in BL disease, a diffuse granulomatous response is seen, in which foamy histiocytes predominate. Lymphocytes are commonly admixed within the lesion and a well-formed Grenz zone is observed. Perineural infiltration is common and microorganisms are readily observed on Fite-stained sections.

The findings of indeterminate leprosy include a mild mononuclear cell infiltrate around nerves, vessels, and appendages. When organisms can be demonstrated on Fite stain, a diagnosis is easier to make. Without this finding, histopathologic examination can be nonspecific.

In histoid leprosy, a nodular infiltrate of epithelioid and spindled histiocytes is seen surrounded by an atrophic epidermis. A Grenz zone is observed and microorganisms are readily identifiable, singly or in globi.

Lucio's phenomenon may show necrotizing vasculopathy associated with a high level of infected endothelial cells. Leukocytoclastic vasculitis, thrombosis, and resultant epidermal hemorrhagic infarction are seen in.

Pathology in Type I reactions is nonspecific but may show perivascular and perineural lymphocytic infiltration. Type 2 reactions show marked edema and a neutrophilic dermal infiltrate, often aggregating in microabscesses and surrounding the vasculature and adnexa. The subcutaneous tissue is often involved. Endothelial cell swelling and edema may be observed. Microorganisms can be identified on stains but they are usually degenerated.

Neuritic leprosy (no evidence of cutaneous disease) is best diagnosed by biopsy. In the absence of cutaneous disease, a high index of clinical suspicion is required to make the diagnosis. Histopathological examination shows epithelioid granuloma formation with bacilli present inside nerves in higher concentrations than in other areas. This pathology most closely resembles the findings in cutaneous TT and BT.

TREATMENT AND THERAPY

Classification of disease as paucibacillary or multibacillary is most helpful in establishing treatment protocols for patients. In general, multidrug treatment is encouraged to prevent resistance to dapsone. Rifampin is generally employed in all treatment regimens because of its potent bactericidal action against the mycobacterium. The treating clinician should remember that to treat the disease effectively, attention only to drug therapy is not sufficient. The cost of therapy and availability of medications is important to consider, particularly in resource-poor settings. More importantly, encouraging adherence to long periods of therapy is perhaps the most important role of the treating clinician. In those with deformities, physical therapy and a systemic approach to the disease is essential. Finally, all patients, their friends and family, must be educated about the infection, its course, and potential social ramifications of the disease. Patients often require support systems from social workers and clinicians as they face discriminatory policies.

According to WHO guidelines, paucibacillary disease may be treated with rifampin 600 mg every month for 6 months in addition to dapsone 100 mg daily for 6 months. In the United States, the Public Health Service (PHS) recommends that treatment with both drugs be for an entire year. Patients should be followed up every 6 months for the first 5 years after treatment is finished. Though still under clinical investigation, a single paucibacillary lesion may be treated with one dose of ROM

Table 5.2: Alternative Agents for Use in Leprosy

Rifabutin
Rifapentine*
Moxifloxacin*
Ofloxacin
Perfloxacin
Sparfloxacin
Levofloxacin
Minocycline
Ansamycins
Clarithromycin
Telithromycin

* Represent the most active bactericidal agents

therapy (rifampin 600 mg, ofloxacin 400 mg, and minocycline 100 mg).

Patients with multibacillary disease should be treated with rifampin 600 mg and clofazimine 300 mg every month in addition to dapsone 100 mg and clofazimine 50 mg every day for 12 months. Unlike the WHO, PHS recommends dapsone 100 mg daily, rifampin 600 mg daily, and clofazimine 50 mg daily for 2 years. Follow-up every 6 months for a period of 10 years following completion of treatment is encouraged. Table 5.2 shows alternative drugs with activity against *Mycobacterium leprae* for those patients who are allergic to commonly used medications or otherwise present contraindications to their use. In addition, important side effects to medications are listed in Table 5.3. Prompt therapy is important in limiting infectivity and spread of the organism.

Therapy of household contacts and prophylaxis is controversial, but currently, it is not recommended. Dapsone prophylaxis may lead to resistance or delay in onset of disease, rather than to prevention. Regular clinical follow-up of household contacts is encouraged.

Treatment of reversal reactions usually requires some level of immunosuppression. Mild type I reactions may be treated with nonsteroidal anti-inflammatory medications (NSAIDs). Severe cases, those that present with neuritis, potential involvement of the facial nerve, or those that do not respond to conservative therapy, require oral steroids. Dosing should begin at 1 mg/kg and gradually titrated or tapered as permitted by symptoms. Though neuritis may respond quickly if it is caused by compression or edema, once there is nerve trunk damage, symptoms may take much longer to improve. Similarly, mild cases of ENL may be treated with NSAIDs, colchicine, pentoxyfilline, and antimalarials. However, unless contraindicated, standard therapy is with thalidomide at doses ranging from 100 to 400 mg/day. Some patients may respond to an increase in dosage of clofazimine whereas nonresponders may benefit from oral steroids. The presence of neuritis usually also requires treatment with systemic steroids. Ocular disease is treated with topical steroids and atropine. Opthalmic

Table 5.3: Commonly Used Drugs in Hansen's Disease: Important Side Effects

Drug	Side Effects	Screening Labs
Dapsone	Hemolytic anemia (mild and dose dependent); Agranulocytosis (rare) Hypersensitivity Reaction	CBC (every 6 months); G6PD (before starting)
Clofazimine	Red/grey discoloration, particularly in lesional skin; Diarrhea, abdominal pain, intestinal obstruction at higher doses	Review of systems, abdominal exam
Rifampin	Transaminitis (address if higher than 2.5× normal), thrombocytopenia, drug interactions (steroids, anticoagulants, oral contraceptives)	CBC and platelets, electrolytes, and liver function tests (every 3 months)
Floroquinolones	Rash, visual disturbance, vasculitis, hematuria, cartilage erosion	
Minocycline	Pigmentation, vestibulitis, transaminitis, lupus-like syndrome	CBC, LFTs
Clarithromycin	Headache, rash, gastrointestinal upset, increased PT time and BUN	CBC, electrolytes, coagulation tests
Thalidomide	Teratogenicity and neurotoxicity	CBC and differential, physical exam, pregnancy test

CBC, complete blood count; LFT, liver function test.

evaluation and referral is strongly suggested. Alternative therapeutic agents that may be helpful in treating ENL are presented in Table 5.4.

Lucio's phenomenon is best treated with systemic corticosteroids. Unlike ENL it is not responsive to thalidomide. It carries a high mortality rate and morbidities eventually require wound care akin to that of a burn victim with admission to intensive care units.

As mentioned earlier, it is not uncommon for leprosy to present during pregnancy or early puerperium. Hypersensitivity reactions, Type I and Type II, relapses, and downgrading of the disease are more prevalent during pregnancy, especially during the third trimester, lactation, and the puerperium. The infection can be treated with dapsone and clofazimine, as well as a monthly dose of rifampin. Reversal reactions may be treated with clofazimine and steroids, but thalidomide is always contraindicated in pregnancy.

Though various vaccines have been developed, their efficacy is poor, particularly among certain populations. Given the relative utility of MDT, less attention has been focused on improving currently available vaccines. Nonetheless, given their immunologic benefits, particularly in improving bacterial clearance and inducing a fall in bacillary index among MDT nonresponders, research on potential vaccines should be pursued particularly for use in countries such as Brazil and India, where prevalence continues to be high. Among the vaccines currently investigated in the field are BCG, mycobacterium ICRC, and mycobacterium W. A vaccine that protects not only against tuberculosis but also against leprosy could be the answer to the problem of vaccination.

Importantly, the care of the patient with leprosy must be multidisciplinary. Given the sequelae of the disease, neurologists, orthopedic surgeons, otorhinolaryngologists, podiatrists, occupational therapists, rehabilitation specialists, and social workers

Table 5.4: Alternative Agents in the Treatment of ENL

Colchicine

Pentoxifylline

Cyclosporine A

Aziathioprine

Mycophenolate mofetil

Methotrexate

Cyclophosphamide

Etanercept

Adalimumab

Infliximab

Intravenous IgG

Plasmapheresis

ENL, Erythema nodosum leprosum; IgG, immunoglobulin G.

are invaluable adjuncts to the dermatologist, infectious disease specialist, or the primary practitioner caring for those who are actively treated or who battle the various disabilities created by the disease. Even if deformities are not readily visible, care must be taken to monitor areas such as the feet, hands, and eyes, where the incidence of insensitivity is high (Fig. 5.11). Cutaneous ulcers and eye disease may develop as a result of decreased protection from physical and thermal trauma. Importantly, there is a documented increase in the development of squamous cell carcinoma in chronic foot ulcers. Neuropathy may be responsive in up to 60% of patients. Early consultation and referral should be

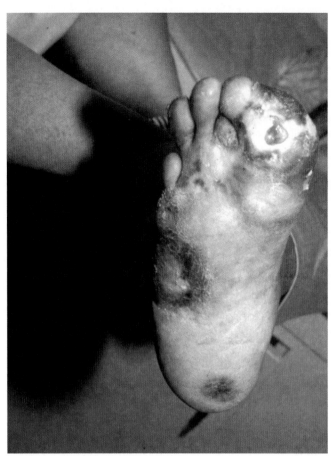

Figure 5.11. This patient with advanced lepromatous leprosy (LL) has developed foot ulcers at sites of pressure due to developed neuropathies and insensitivity. An increase in the incidence of squamous cell carcinomas has been documented in these ulcers. At this stage, neurologic changes are often irreversible and require careful follow-up by the clinical team.

Table 5.5: Clinical "Masquerades" in the Diagnosis of Leprosy

A.	Infectious
	Tinea versicolor
	Tuberculosis verrucosa cutis
	Annular syphilis
	Leishmaniasis
	Deep fungal infection
B.	Inflammatory Disease
	Psoriasis
	Gyrate erythema
	Granuloma annulare
	Necrobiosis lipoidica
	Pityriasis alba
	Lichen planus
	Sarcoid
	Contact dermatitis
	Leukoderma
	Postinflammatory hypopigmentation
C.	Malignancy
	Mycosis fungoides
	B-cell lymphoma
	Leukemia cutis
D.	Metabolic Diseases
	Xanthomatosis
E.	Connective Tissue and Autoimmune Disease
	Lupus
	Vitiligo
	Scleroderma/morphea

obtained by those who are not able to perform sensory testing, surveillance, and follow-up treatment.

PITFALLS AND MYTHS

Patients with Hansen's disease have been subject to great social stigma since the beginning of times. In fact, skin disease described in early literature and the Bible likely represents papulosquamous diseases rather than leprosy. Yet, to this date, despite increasing information about susceptibility of hosts, infectivity, and efficacy of antimicrobial therapy, many patients suffer from social disparity. Employment discrimination is illegal in the United States, yet many patients fear social isolation and inability to secure and maintain employment. In addition, because a high index of suspicion must be kept to make the diagnosis, either clinically or pathologically, many patients escape the health-care system, misdiagnosed or untreated. As detailed in Table 5.5, because the differential diagnosis may be vast, the diagnosis is important to consider, particularly in those patients from endemic areas.

Because antibody tests and PCR studies are mostly experimental, tests such as the Mitsuda reaction lack specificity, and skin smears require a well-trained examiner for adequate utility; laboratory tests are often not helpful in making the diagnosis. Pathologic examination is paramount, and may also pose challenges when the diagnosis is not considered early. Particularly in cases of paucibacillary disease, it is necessary to carefully examine cutaneous nerves, as only few mycobacteria may be evident even when the index of suspicion is very high. Often, organisms may not be observed, or only fragments of organisms may be seen, and they are easily confused with nonspecific binding of Fite reactants. Methenamine silver stains may be helpful in identifying fragmented portions of the bacilli. Empiric therapy or repeat biopsy may be indicated in these cases.

Unlike other infectious diseases, the incidence, course, and prognosis of leprosy do not appear to be affected by co-infection with HIV. Reactivation disease in the setting of immune reconstitution syndrome in the early treatment of HIV does not appear to be a concern as has been reported in other disorders like herpetic disease, tuberculosis, leishmaniasis, or sarcoidosis.

Remember most of the leprosy patients are from "third-world countries" and have comorbidities, which can be potentially fatal if activated by immunosuppressive drugs such as corticosteroids given for reactions and neuritis. Consequently, it behooves the attending physician to do a PPD, a hepatitis B surface antigen test, and an immunoassay for strongyloidiasis.

Leprosy is a reportable disease. Early treatment drastically reduces infectivity and some believe that after the first dose of antibiotics, transmission is virtually eliminated. Vertical transmission is below 8% and conjugal transmission also appears to be in that range. Because early therapy also prevents the devastating sequelae of the disease, referral to centers that specialize in the care of Hansen's disease is recommended. Particularly in multibacillary disease and in the setting of reversal reactions, treatment prevents neurologic and cutaneous disability.

CONCLUSIONS

Whether or not the disease is eradicated in the future, Hansen's disease continues to affect people across the world. Regardless of microbiologic cure, treatment of disabilities will continue to be a public health concern. Because clinical signs of infection can be subtle, a high index of suspicion must be maintained in those that present with either neural, cutaneous disease, or both. As the most common cause of peripheral neuropathies in developing countries, Hansen's disease should continue to be on the agenda of every country, as an increase in availability and affordability of transportation have facilitated immigration patterns. Importance should not only be placed on treatment and prevention but also on establishing educational programs that can mitigate the social difficulties that people with this disease often face. The battle in reducing incidence will necessitate new policies in primary health care, which should promote early detection, adequate treatment, as well as disability prevention, management, and further research.

SUGGESTED READINGS

Anderson H, Stryjewska B, Boyanton B, et al. Hansen disease in the United States in the 21st century: A review of the literature. Arch Path Lab Med 2007;131:982–986.

Britton W, Lockwood D. Leprosy. Lancet 2004;363:1209–1219.

Haimanot R, Melaku, Z. Leprosy. Curr Op Neurol 2000;13:317–322.

www.who.int/lep/leprosy/en/index.html

Jacobs M, George S, Pulimood S, et al. Short-term follow-up of patients with multibacillary leprosy and HIV infection. Int J Lepr Other Mycobater Dis 1996;64:392–395.

Mallick SN. Integration of leprosy control with primary health care. Lepr Rev 2003;74:148–153.

McKee P, Calonje E, Granter, S. Pathology of the Skin, 3rd edition. Elsevier, London, 2005.

Moschella S. Leprosy: epidemiology and present and possible future therapeutic approaches. Drugs Fut 2006;31:961–7.

Moschella SL. An update on the diagnosis and treatment of Leprosy. J Am Acad Dermatol 2004;51:417–426.

Oskam L, Slim E, Buhrer-Sekula S. Serology: Recent developments strengths, limitations, and prospects: A state of the art overview. Lepr Rev 2004;75:192–193.

Ramos e Silva M, De Castro M. Mycobacterial Infections. In: Dermatology, 1st edition. Mosby, London, 2003.

Ridley DS. Skin biopsy in leprosy: Histological interpretation and clinical application. Documenta Geigy, Basle, 1977.

Sabin TD, Swift TR, Jacobson RR. Leprosy. In: Dyck PJ, Thomas PK, eds. Peripheral neuropathy. Philadelphia: Saunders, 1993;1354–1379.

Sasaki S, Takeshita F, Okuda K, et al., Mycobacterium leprae and leprosy: a compendium. Microbiol Immunol 2001;45:729–736.

Schurr E, Alcais A, Singh M, et al. Mycobacterial infections: PARK2 and PACRG associations in leprosy. Tiss Antig 2007;69:231–233.

Scollard DM, Adams LB, Gillis TP et al. The continuing challenges of Leprosy. Clin Microbiol Rev 2006;19:338–381.

Utianoski AP, Lockwood, DN. Leprosy: current diagnostic and treatment approaches. Curr Opin Infect Dis 2003;16:421–427.

Yawalkar SJ. Leprosy for medical practitioners and paramedical workers, 5th edition, CIBA-GEIGY, Basle, 1992.

6 | ATYPICAL MYCOBACTERIA

Francesca Prignano, Caterina Fabroni, and Torello Lotti

HISTORY

The nontuberculous mycobacteria are species different from *Mycobacterium tuberculosis*. In the past these organisms were referred to as "atypical" (as they were thought to be unusual M. tuberculosis strains), as "anonymous," as "tuberculoid," or as "opportunistic," but actually they are widely known as *environmental mycobacteria* because their peculiar ability to exist in the environment.

Their existence has been known since the nineteenth century, but their role as human pathogens was not seriously considered until the middle of the twentieth century when a new mycobacterial skin disease called *swimming pool* or *fish tank granulomas,* due to *Mycobacterium marinum*, was described by Linell and Norden and Runyon published his classification of the mycobacteria.

Environmental mycobacteria (Table 6.1) are acid-fast mycobacteria, have a wide distribution, and can be found in up to 90% of biofilms (the slim layer present at the water–solid interfaces) taken from piped water systems. They are extremely hardy and thrive in even the most hostile environments; some species such as the *Mycobacterium chelonae* or *Mycobacterium abscessus* group resist the activity of disinfectants and biocides such as organomercurials, chlorine, and alkaline gluteraldehyde. Pseudo-outbreaks of mycobacteriosis related to contaminated surgical instruments have been described all over the world. Mycobacteria, therefore, can easily affect the skin; in some cases, especially in immunosuppressed patients, they are able to spread toward the pulmonary or lymphoglandular system and even reproduce a systemic illness. They are characterized by a low pathogenicity, and for mycobacteria to infect, the tissue has to be damaged or there must be an immunocompromised host. Clinically, skin lesions are characterized by nodules or plaques, which at the very beginning remain localized at the inoculation site, or the infection can spread along the lymphatic vessels toward lymph nodes to reproduce the so-called sporotrichoid syndrome. Histopathology can be helpful in diagnosis, but the real diagnostic tools are the isolation of the bacteria on a selective media and the PCR technique (if the first proves not to be sufficient).

CLASSIFICATION

For the more than 30 species of nontubercular mycobacteria, the most available classification criteria is by Runyon, based on the growth rate, colony morphology on the Loewenstein–Jensen

We wish to thank Prof. Elisa M. Difonzo for providing the pictures used in this chapter.

medium and on the ability to form a pigment spontaneously or after photoexposition (Table 6.1).

Group 1 includes slowly growing photochromogens such as *M. marinum* and *Mycobacterium kansasii*. Group 2 includes slowly growing mycobacteria that produce pigment either in the presence or in absence of light and therefore are called *scotochromogens*. This group includes *Mycobacterium scrofulaceum*, *Mycobacterium szulgai*, and *Mycobacterium gordonae*. Group 3 includes the nonchromogens, which are always slow growing; examples are intracellular *Mycobacterium avium*, *Mycobacterium malmoense*, and *Mycobacterium xenopi*. Group 4 includes rapidly growing nonchromogens such as *Mycobacterium fortuitum*, *Mycobacterium chelonae*, and *Mycobacterium abscessus*, which are also the most pathogenic for human beings. The identification of the different species has been performed in recent years with molecular methods such as genetic sequencing and PCR-based techniques. In the case of slow-growing mycobacteria, PCR is used through the direct sequencing of the gene codifying the 16S of ribosomal RNA. In the case of rapidly growing mycobacteria, identification of species is possible through PCR-restriction fragment length polymorphism analysis of the heat shock protein 65 (hsp65) gene.

Mycobacterium marinum

Mycobacterium marinum was originally reported after its discovery on saltwater fish in the Philadelphia Aquarium in 1926. The first human skin infection was reported in 1951 and occurred in contaminated swimming pools. *M. marinum* is usually found on plants, in soil, and on fish in household aquariums, and in fresh and saltwater worldwide. Its optimal growth temperature is 30°C to 32°C, and it will not grow if the temperature is ≥37°C.

Mycobacterium marinum causes infections that are typically localized to the skin. Infection only occasionally involves deeper structures, like the joints and tendons. Disseminated infections are extremely rare and, if they occur, they occur in immunocompromised individuals only.

Mycobacterium kansasii

This organism is found in fresh water, particularly in temperate regions. It is primarily a pulmonary pathogen and causes a tuberculosis-like illness with a predilection for middle-aged or elderly men with chronic obstructive pulmonary disorder. Cutaneous manifestations vary widely and include erythematous granulomatous plaques, verrucous plaques, and verrucous nodules with sporotrichoid spread.

Table 6.1: Mycobacteria classification

Group	Growth Rate	Pigment Growth	Organism
I	Slow 2–3 weeks	**Photochromogen**	*Mycobacterium kansasii, Mycobacterium marinum, Mycobacterium simiae*
II	Slow 2–3 weeks	**Scotochromogen**	*Mycobacterium scrofulaceum, Mycobacterium szulgai, Mycobacterium gordonae*
III	Slow 2–3 weeks	**Nonphotochromogen**	*Mycobacterium malmoense, Mycobacterium xenopi, Mycobacterium avium–intracellulare*
IV	Rapid 3–5 days	**Nonchromogen**	*Mycobacterium fortuitum, Mycobacterium chelonae, Mycobacterium abscessus*

Taken from Runyon, et al (1959).

Mycobacterium scrofulaceum

This form is widely distributed but most prevalent in the southeastern United States, where it has been isolated from soil, tap water, raw milk, and pooled oysters. *M. scrofulaceum* may cause pulmonary disease but primarily causes local lymphadenitis in childhood, which can result in fistula formation.

Mycobacterium avium Complex

Mycobacterium avium complex includes *Mycobacterium avium* and *Mycobacterium intracellulare* and is ubiquitous in nature. Both mycobacteria survive in soil, water, house dust, vegetables, eggs, and milk. In immunocompromised hosts, these mycobacteria cause widespread, disseminated disease involving the liver, spleen, gastrointestinal tract, lymph nodes, bone marrow, and skin. Skin is typically involved in the setting of disseminated infection. Sporadically, primary cutaneous infections occur after traumatic inoculation or in association with a contaminated water source.

Mycobacterium fortuitum Complex

Mycobacterium fortuitum complex includes three species (isolated in recent years with biomolecular techniques): *Mycobacterium fortuitum*, *Mycobacterium peregrinum* type 1, and *Mycobacterium peregrinum* type 2.

Mycobacterium fortuitum is the most important member of the rapidly growing mycobacteria. The organism is found in water, dust, soil, marine life, and other animals. The sources of infection are contaminated surgical instruments or medical solutions, and the infection is a possible complication of surgery and aesthetic procedures. Clinically *Mycobacterium fortuitum* complex infection can result in cutaneous or extracutaneous manifestations, including endocarditis, osteomyelitis, mediastinitis, meningitis, keratitis, and disseminated infection. Skin infections

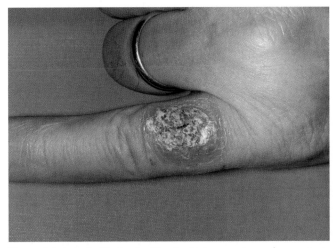

Figure 6.1. A typical lesion by *Mycobacterium marinum* shows a typical erythematous plaque with squamous, crusty elements at the center of the lesion. Courtesy of Prof. M. Elisa Difonzo.

are the most frequent, and the lesions appear after an incubation period of approximately 4 to 6 weeks and are usually painful, erythematous nodules at the site of an inoculation. Cellulitis, furunculosis, ulcers, draining sinus tracts, and abscesses can also form. Cases of infections have been described after intramuscular injections, biopsy, mesotherapy, and pedicure.

Mycobacterium chelonae–Mycobacterium abscessus Complex

This group includes *M. chelonae*, *M. abscessus*, and *Mycobacterium immunogenum*. They are widespread in soil and in water. These organisms are frequently implicated in pulmonary and systemic disease, but they can also localize to the skin as primary involvement or spread to the skin after systemic dissemination.

CLINICAL PRESENTATION

All mycobacteria are characterized by low pathogenicity, and they can only contaminate affected or traumatized skin. The most common occasions and locations for infection are fishing, swimming pools, and aquariums. For quick-growing mycobacteria, medical and aesthetic procedures are the most common predisposing factors. The incubation period varies from 2 weeks to 9 months. A small reddish papule normally appears at the inoculation site. Slowly, the lesion grows and similar lesions can grow and spread through the lymphatic vessels. In accordance with the clinical evolution, it is possible to distinguish three different clinical patterns:

1. A unique lesion at the inoculation site (Fig. 6.1)
2. Multiple lesions with a sporotrichoid morphology (Fig. 6.2)
3. Deeper infections with involvement of subcutaneous structures

The outcome of the lesions is strictly linked to the characteristics of the infecting mycobacterium and to the immunological condition of the host. Cutaneous mycobacteriosis should be

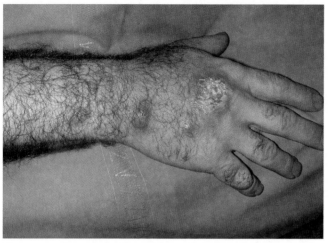

Figure 6.2. Sporotrichoid syndrome. Courtesy of Prof. M. Elisa Difonzo.

Table 6.2: Differential Diagnosis

Diagnosis	Discriminative Criteria
Cutaneous leishmaniasis	Demonstration of amastigotes in Giemsa-stained smears from infected skin by direct microscopy
Subcutaneous mycoses (Majocchi's granuloma)	Positive direct microscopic examination and cultures for Trichophyton rubrum
Cutaneous sporotrichosis	Positive direct microscopic examination for Sporothrix schenckii
Skin tuberculosis	Positive cultures and/or positive PCR for *Mycobacterium tuberculosis*

considered in the differential diagnosis of any granulomatous/nodular dermatosis (see Table 6.2).

DIAGNOSIS

There are three tools to perform a correct diagnosis:

1. The most important is a culture performed on a selective medium, usually Loewenstein–Jensen agar (Fig. 6.3).
2. Histopathology.
3. Biomolecular techniques, if available.

No single diagnostic criteria by itself is highly specific or sensitive or both. Application of the three together is the best way to make a definitive diagnosis.

THERAPY

The variability of clinical presentations and the complexity of laboratory techniques often leads to a delay in the diagnosis of cutaneous mycobacteriosis. The lack of an antimicrobial susceptibility profile causes most cases to be treated empirically, with

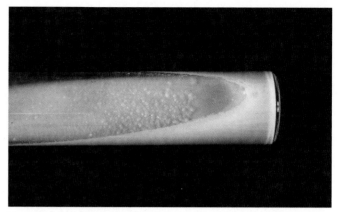

Figure 6.3. A colony of *Mycobacterium marinum* with the classic milky color. Courtesy of Prof. M. Elisa Difonzo.

the possibility of therapeutic failure. In addition, many mycobacteria display both in vitro and in vivo drug resistance to antimicrobial agents. Combination treatment is preferred to avoid the emergence of resistant strains and/or relapse of the disease. The most often used drugs are tetracycline, antitubercular drugs, macrolides, quinolones, and trimethoprim–sulfamethoxazole. *M. marinum* strains are most often susceptible to quinolones and doxycycline, clarithromycin, and erythromycin and are resistant to pyrazinamide and isoniazid.

The treatment of infections due to rapidly growing mycobacteria may be difficult because of multiresistant strains, and surgery may be the best treatment option.

PITFALLS AND MYTHS

Cutaneous mycobacteriosis is a challenge for the dermatologist because the diagnosis requires a high index of suspicion and, contrary to popular belief, immunocompetent subjects, apparently without risk factors, are frequently affected.

This circumstance is linked to the difficulty of detecting in the personal history of the patient a dangerous activity or event that happened weeks or months before the appearance of skin lesions and to the clinical presentation of skin lesions. *M. scrofulaceum* lymphadenitis, for example, may be indistinguishable from *M. tuberculosis* infection (scrofuloderma), or a *M. marinum* granulomatous nodular lesion with central ulceration has to be considered in the differential diagnosis along with other granulomatous skin infections.

The risk factors linked to these infections are changing. In the past century a large number of swimming and bathing related infections were described. Now, the incidence of these outbreaks has been drastically reduced because of the improvement in the construction and maintenance of these facilities. The most important chance of infection is mainly related to hobbies and to medical procedures.

A recent study stressed the capability of environmental mycobacteria to grow as aggregated "sessile" communities attached to living and nonliving surfaces (including medical devices), forming a *biofilm*. A biofilm develops when the attached cells excrete polymers that facilitate adhesion, matrix formation, and alteration of the organism's phenotype with respect to growth rate and gene transcription. The physical and genetic profiles of microorganisms within the protected biofilm community are deeply different from their existence as unprotected independent cells. The hallmark of biofilm-related infections is the dramatic resistance to antimicrobials and host defenses.

SUGGESTED READINGS

Ang P, Rattana-Apiromyakij N, Goh CL. Retrospective study of Mycobacterium marinum skin infections. Int J Dermatol 2000; 39:343–347.

Aziz SA, Faber WR, Kolk AHJ. Atypical cutaneous mycobacteriosis diagnosed by polymerase chain reaction. Br J Dermatol 2004; 151:719–720.

Bartralot R, Pujol RM, Garcia-Patos V et al. Cutaneous infections due to nontuberculous mycobacteria: histopathologic review of 28 cases. Comparative study between lesions observed in immunosuppressed patient and normal host. J Cutan Pathol 2000; 27:124–129.

Breathnach A, Levell N, Munro C. Cutaneous *Mycobacterium kansasii* infection: case report and review. Clin Infect Dis 1995; 20:812–817.

Cassetty CT, Sanchez M. *Mycobacterium marinum* infection. Dermatol Online J 2004;10:21.

Cummins DL, Del Acerba D, Tausk A. *Mycobacterium marinum* different response to second-generation tetracyclines. Int J Dermatol 2005;44:518–520.

Devallois A, Goh KS, Rastogi N. Rapid identification of Mycobacteria to species level by PCR-restriction fragment length polymorphism analysis of the hsp65 gene and proposition of an algorithm to differentiate 34 mycobacterial species. J Clin Microbiol 1997;35:2969–2973.

Grange JM. The Mycobacteria. In: Topley and Wilson's Principles of Bacteriology, Virology and Immunity. 8th edition, Vol. 2, Parker MT, Duerden BI, eds. London: Eduard Arnold, 1990; 73–101.

Han XY, Tarrand JJ, Infante R. Clinical significance and epidemiological analyses of *Mycobacterium avium* and *Mycobacterium intracellulare* among patient with AIDS. J Clin Microbiol 2005 Sep;43:4407–4412.

Hautmann G, Lotti T. Atypical mycobacterial infections of the skin. Dermatol Clin 1994;4(12):657–668.

Hautmann G, Lotti T. Atypical mycobacterial infections: a difficult and emerging group of infectious dermatoses. Int J Dermatol 1993;32:499.

Hautmann G, Lotti T. Diseases caused by *Mycobacterium scrofulaceum*. Clin Dermatol. 1995 13;3:277–280.

Jenkins PA. Mycobacteria in the environment. J Appl Bacteriol Symp 1991;70:137S-141S.

Jogi R, Tyring SK. Therapy of nontuberculous mycobacterial infections. Dermatol Ther 2004;17:491–498.

Muthusami JC, Vyas FL, Mukundan U, Jesudason MV, Govil S, Jesudason SR. Mycobacterium fortuitum: An iatrogenic cause of soft tissue infection in surgery. ANZ J Surg 2004;74:662–666.

Palenque E. Skin disease and nontuberculous atypical mycobacteria. Int J Dermatol 2000; 39:659–666.

Pesce RR, Fejka S, Colodny SM. *Mycobacterium fortuitum* presenting as an asymptomatic enlarging pulmonary nodule. Am J Med 1991;91:310–312.

Philalay JS, Palermo CO, Hauge KA et al. Genes required for intrinsic multidrug resistance in *Mycobacterium avium*. Antimicrob Agents Chemother 2004;48:3412–3418.

Runyon EH. Anonymous mycobacteria in pulmonary disease. Med Clin North Am 1959;45:273–290.

Sungkanuparph S, Sathapatayavongs B, Pracharktam R. Infections with rapidly growing mycobacteria: report of 20 cases. Int J Infect Dis 2003;7:198–205.

ARTHROPOD-BORNE INFECTION

Dirk M. Elston

INTRODUCTION

Arthropod-borne diseases remain a major cause of death and morbidity throughout the world. Malaria alone kills thousands of people every year. Dengue, trypanosomiasis, leishmaniasis, viral encephalitis, and viral hemorrhagic fevers are important public health threats. Modern technology affords us some protection from arthropod-borne disease. Window screens and an indoor life-style results in lower rates of infection in developed countries. During a recent outbreak of dengue fever along the US–Mexican border, the incidence of disease was much lower in Laredo, Texas, than in Nuevo Laredo, Mexico, even though the vector, *Aedes aegypti*, was more abundant on the Texas side of the border. This demonstrates the magnitude of the effect of screens and indoor living, even when vector-control measures have failed.

In areas where disease activity is endemic rather than episodic, state health departments administer aggressive mosquito control programs. Considerable manpower and equipment are contributed by military reserve units, and recent conflicts have demonstrated that war disrupts vector control efforts at home as well as in the zone of conflict. Disruption of the public health infrastructure in Iraq and Afghanistan as well as the failure to deliver repellent to our troops contributed to the much publicized cases of leishmaniasis among American troops in Iraq.

Mosquito-borne outbreaks of West Nile fever in the United States have also gained national attention. Rocky Mountain spotted fever and equine encephalitis remain the most lethal vector-borne diseases in North America, but many other illnesses are commonly transmitted by mosquitoes, flies, ticks, and fleas. Mosquitoes transmit West Nile fever, St. Louis encephalitis, and equine encephalitis. Even malaria has resurfaced as an endemic infection within the United States. Ticks transmit Lyme disease (Fig. 7.1), Rocky Mountain spotted fever, babesiosis, ehrlichiosis, Colorado tick fever, relapsing fever, and tularemia. In the West, fleas transmit plague and endemic typhus. In the East, house mouse mites transmit rickettsial pox. Sandflies (Fig. 7.2) in Texas carry leishmaniasis (Fig. 7.3).

The world is full of bugs. Even if we lived sealed inside our homes, pets, bats, birds, and rodents carry disease vectors into the house. Among the homeless, ectoparasite infestation contributes to a high prevalence of infection with *Bartonella quintana*. It is important to note that the vector may influence the expression of disease. *Bartonella* organisms transmitted by a louse produce endocarditis, while the same organism causes cat scratch disease or bacillary angiomatosis when transmitted by a flea.

While some diseases have a single vector, others have multiple possible vectors. Tick bites and handling of infected animals are the usual mode of transmission for tularemia, but deerfly bites and bites by horseflies are also responsible for transmission.

HISTORY

Vector-borne diseases are at least as old as mankind. Credible evidence of bartonellosis has been found in a 4000-year-old human tooth. Important elements of patient history include

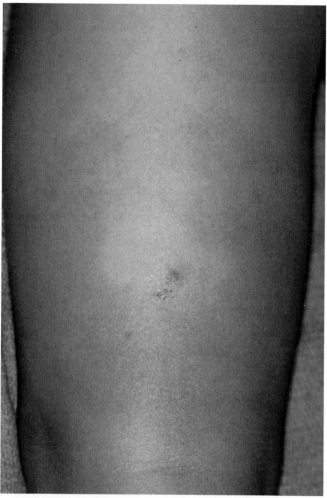

Figure 7.1. Erythema chronicum migrans of Lyme disease.

Images were produced while the author was a full-time federal employee. They are in the public domain.

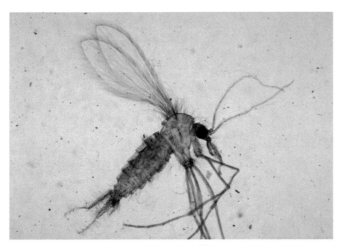

Figure 7.2. Sandfly.

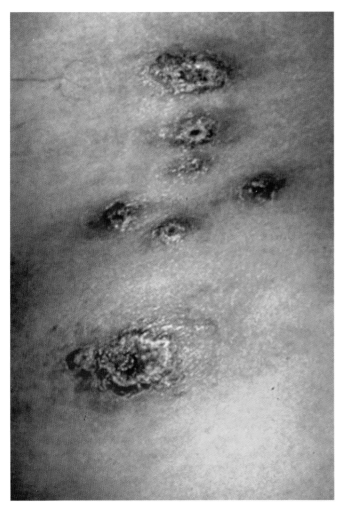

Figure 7.3. Leishmaniasis.

Table 7.1: Tick-Borne Diseases and Associated Vectors

Disease	Vector
Malaria	Anopheline mosquitoes
Dengue	*Aedes* mosquitoes
Yellow fever	*Aedes* mosquitoes
Arboviridae	*Culex* mosquitoes
Bartonellosis	Fleas, lice, sandflies
Leishmaniasis	Sandflies
American trypanosomiasis (Fig. 7.4)	Triatome bugs (Fig. 7.5)
African trypanosomiasis	Tsetse flies
Rocky Mountain Spotted Fever	*Dermacentor variabilis Dermacentor andersoni* (Fig. 7.6) *Amblyomma americanum*
Human monocytic ehrlichiosis	*Amblyomma americanum* (Fig. 7.7)
Human anaplasmosis	*Ixodes scapularis* (Fig. 7.8)
Lyme disease	*Ixodes scapularis*
Babesiosis	*Ixodes scapularis*
Tularemia	*Amblyomma americanum Dermacentor andersoni Dermacentor variabilis Chrysops* deerflies Horseflies
Tick-borne Relapsing Fever	*Ornithodoros* genus (soft tick)
Tick paralysis	*Dermacentor andersoni* (wood tick) *Dermacentor variabilis* (dog tick)
Plague	*Xenopsylla cheopis* (Fig. 7.9) and *Pulex irritans* (Fig. 7.10)
Typhus	*Pediculus humanus*
Endemic typhus	*Ctenocephalides felis* (Fig. 7.11) and *Xenopsylla cheopis*

travel and the use of repellents and prophylactic antibiotics. Travelers who follow the Centers for Disease Control and Prevention (CDC) guidelines for malaria prophylaxis are far less likely to become infected. Of the 891 reported cases of malaria among US travelers abroad in 2001, only 180 had followed the recommended prophylaxis regimen. It is also important to note if repellents, protective clothing, and mosquito netting were used as recommended. The degree of engorgement of a removed tick or the duration of attachment can be used to estimate the risk of disease transmission.

EPIDEMIOLOGY

Epidemiology of vector-borne illness varies geographically as well as by season. CDC websites provide detailed risks in various areas of the country and the world. Table 7.1 lists some important arthropod-borne diseases and their major vectors.

DIAGNOSIS

The type of exposure, vector, and disease prevalence may be as important in establishing a presumptive diagnosis as the subsequent signs and symptoms of disease. Periodic fevers suggest malaria. Headache is common to a wide variety of tick and

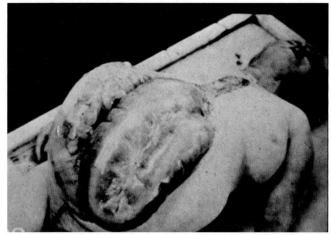

Figure 7.4. Chagas disease, toxic megacolon.
Image courtesy of Walter Reed Army Medical Center teaching file.

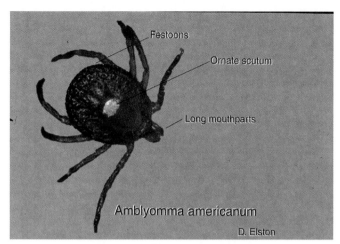

Figure 7.7. *Amblyomma americanum.*

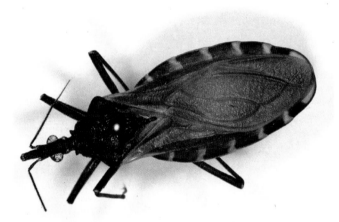

Figure 7.5. Triatome bug.

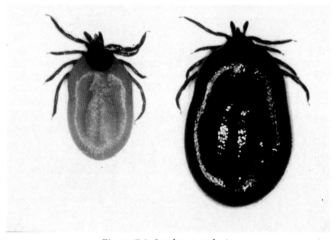

Figure 7.8. *Ixodes scapularis.*

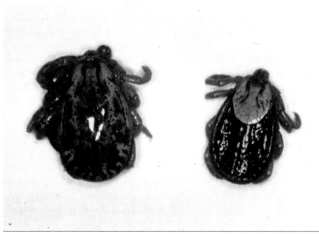

Figure 7.6. *Dermacentor andersoni.*

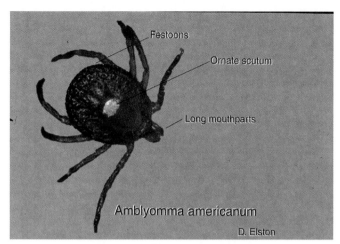

Figure 7.9. *Xenopsylla cheopis.*

mosquito-borne diseases. In endemic areas, fever and headache after a tick bite suggest a diagnosis of Rocky Mountain spotted fever until proved otherwise. Empiric therapy is appropriate in this setting, and it is never appropriate to withhold therapy until a diagnosis is established by laboratory studies.

THERAPY

Once disease has occurred, treatment depends on the disease as well as the age of the patient and severity of illness. The CDC and the Infectious Disease Society of America (IDSA) list recommendations for a wide array of arthropod-borne diseases. Most

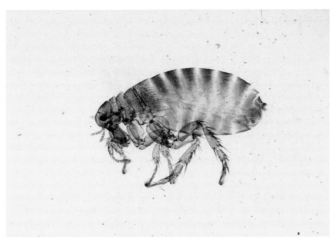

Figure 7.10. *Pulex irritans.*

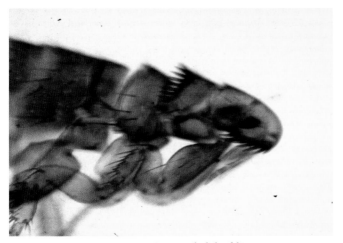

Figure 7.11. *Ctenocephalides felis.*

tick-borne illnesses are best treated with doxycycline. Notable exceptions include tularemia, where streptomycin remains the drug of choice, and babesiosis, where drugs such as atovaquone, azithromycin, clindamycin, and quinine are used. The reader is advised to consult the guidelines listed for full details.

The best intervention is prevention. Use of mosquito netting, repellents, and malaria prophylaxis are the mainstays of primary prevention. Prevention of mosquito and sandfly bites focuses on the use of protective clothing and chemical repellents, as these flying arthropods do not need to crawl over clothing to reach exposed skin. Efforts to reduce the numbers of flies and mosquitoes are important in areas with endemic disease. Anopheline mosquitoes that carry malaria bite mostly at night; therefore, those who must be outside after dark are at greatest risk. Pyrethroid-impregnated mosquito netting has been shown to be helpful. As noted earlier, all travelers to malaria-endemic areas should take the CDC-recommended chemoprophylactic regimen. The *Aedes* mosquitoes that carry dengue bite during the day. In areas where the disease is endemic, repellents and protective clothing should be worn whenever there is a risk of exposure. Public health measures, such as control of standing water, stocking ponds with fish, turtles, and frogs to consume mosquito larvae, and area sprays play an important role in overall management. Mosquito traps such as the Mosquito Magnet are effective for small areas such as a backyard. Several such traps

are now marketed. In general, the propane-powered units are more versatile and provide better results.

DEET (*N,N*-diethyl-3-methylbenzamide, previously called *N,N*-diethyl-m-toluamide) remains the gold standard against which other repellents are measured. Extended release products are preferred. Picaridin is a newer repellent effective against a broad range of mosquitoes.

Secondary prevention of Lyme disease and rickettsial diseases is possible in highly endemic areas with the use of prophylactic doxycycline. However, it should be noted that treatment is only highly effective when appropriately high doses are started early in the course of clinical disease, so prophylaxis may not always be in the best interest of the patient. My practice is to provide the prescription, but instruct the patient not to fill it unless signs or symptoms occur. For rickettsial disease, this would include fever and headache (regardless of the absence of rash). For Lyme disease, an expanding red ring (erythema migrans) or arthritis would be reasons for treatment.

PITFALLS AND MYTHS

Myth 1: Skin-so-soft is a highly effective repellent. Some years ago, Skin-so-soft bath oil achieved cult status as a repellent. It does exert a short-lived repellent effect on some mosquitoes, and insect wings easily become plastered down to the thick oily film. It has not, however, performed well in comparison to traditional repellents such as DEET in controlled trials.

Myth 2: DEET is dangerous in children. Although there are rare reports of anaphylaxis, toxic encephalopathy, and bullous dermatitis in both children and adults, DEET products have a well-established overall safety record. The Academy of Pediatrics currently recommends sustained release formulations and notes that there is no evidence of any advantage to concentrations higher than 30%.

There are two critical points to remember. Rocky Mountain spotted fever has a high mortality rate if antibiotic treatment is delayed. In endemic areas, empiric treatment should be started in any patient who presents with fever and a headache, regardless of the history of tick bite and regardless of the absence of rash. The second point is that prevention is the best form of management. Appropriate use of protective clothing, repellents, mosquito nets, and chemoprophylaxis can reduce the burden of arthropod-borne disease.

SUGGESTED READINGS

Brown M, Hebert AA. Insect repellents: An overview. J Am Acad Dermatol 1997;36:243–249.

Carnevale P. Protection of travelers against biting arthropod vectors. Bull Soc Pathol Exotique 1998;91:474–485.

Coosemans M, Van Gompel A. The principal arthropod vectors of disease. What are the risks of travelers' to be bitten? To be infected? Bull Soc Pathol Exotique 1998;91:467–473.

Fradin MS. Mosquitoes and mosquito repellents: a clinician's guide. Ann Intern Med. 1998;128:931–940.

Kline DL. Comparison of two American biophysics mosquito traps: the professional and a new counterflow geometry trap. J Am Mosq Control Assoc. 1999;15(3):276–282.

8 | DEEP FUNGAL INFECTIONS

Evandro Ararigbóia Rivitti and Paulo Ricardo Criado

INTRODUCTION

Fungal diseases affect a considerable number of people worldwide and can cause significant morbidity and mortality. The number of cases has multiplied with the increase in world travel and immunosuppression. Generally speaking, fungal infections can be classified as either superficial or deep. Superficial fungal infections, including dermatophytes, have an affinity for keratin and, therefore, are typically limited to either the epidermis or adnexal structures. Deep fungal infections affect deeper structures, including internal organs.

Cutaneous manifestations of deep fungal infections occur from primary infection of the skin or from cutaneous dissemination due to a systemic infection.

Deep fungal skin infections are chronic diseases, caused by various groups of fungi. The clinical spectrum of these infections can be classified into (i) subcutaneous mycoses and (ii) systemic mycoses.

Subcutaneous mycoses are due to a large and diverse group of fungus that produce disease when traumatically introduced into the skin and subcutaneous tissue. Sporotrichosis, mycetoma, chromomycosis, and lobomycosis are the most common subcutaneous mycoses.

Systemic mycoses are caused by "true" fungal pathogens and opportunistic fungi. The "true" fungal pathogens are agents of histoplasmosis, blastomycosis, coccidioidomycosis, and paracoccidioidomycosis. The opportunistic deep mycoses comprise a spectrum of diseases, including zygomycosis, cryptococcosis, aspergillosis, phaeohyphomycosis, and hyalohyphomycosis.

Dermatologists from all over the world should be able to recognize and diagnose deep mycoses. Many of the deep mycoses, such as sporotrichosis, commonly occur in the United States, and others can infect travelers from endemic areas.

In Table 8.1, we summarize the current nomenclature for most fungi reviewed in this chapter.

HISTORY

Tropical medicine was born with Sir Patrick Manson (1984–1922), the famous Scottish parasitologist who worked for 24 years in China. While there, he studied superficial mycoses, malaria, and filariasis. In 1908 Lutz (a Brazilian scientist) described the paracoccidioidomycosis, and Splendore (in 1912) classified the agent in the Zymonema genus. In 1928, Almeida and Lacaz, in Brazil, suggested the name *Paracoccidioides* and finally the agent then became known around the world as *Paracoccidioides brasiliensis,* the fungus of the South American blastomycosis. In 1914 the German physician Max Rudolph, while living in Brazil, described the first six cases of chromomycosis and isolated the fungus in four patients.

Systemic tropical mycoses have been emerging since the beginning of the deep fungal infections epidemic. The incidence of these infections is probably even underestimated since most cases occur in populations with poor access to medical care and in regions where modern diagnostic methods are unavailable. This scenario is especially applied in third-world countries, which are localized to tropical areas of the planet. In these areas access to modern therapy for acquired immune deficiency syndrome (AIDS) (HAART regime) is difficult because of the elevated financial costs associated. In developed countries, especially in North America, Europe, and a few countries in Asia, AIDS is sometimes observed in returning travelers, aid workers, immigrants, and often in organ-transplanted patients who have been using immunosuppressive therapy. The differential diagnosis of imported systemic tropical mycoses may be especially difficult for uninformed physicians.

In several countries, medical mycology is not taught adequately to medical students (in graduation and in residency programs). Consequently, there is little awareness of the importance of fungal infections, especially in tropical countries, where these diseases often show up in medical practice. In addition sometimes the personal concern with aesthetic dermatology is favored among medical students and dermatology residents.

Table 8.1: Current Nomenclature of the Fungi and Diseases Frequently Involved in Deep Fungal Infections

Fungi Molds	Infection
Black fungi	Chromoblastomycosis Mycetoma Pheohyphomycosis
Non-Black Fungi	Aspergillosis Hyalohyphomycosis Mycetoma
Dimorphic Fungi	Blastomycosis Coccidioidomycosis Histoplasmosis
Yeasts	Candidiasis Cryptococcosis
Fungi whose classification is uncertain	Lobomycosis Rhinosporidiosis

Table 8.2: General Classification of Mycetoma

Actinomycetoma (Bacterium)

- Endogenous Actinomycosis: caused by anaerobic actinomycetes: *Actinomyces israelli, Actinomyces viscous, Actinomyces odontolyticus, Arachinia propionica*

- Exogenous Actinomycosis (Nocardiosis): caused by aerobic actinomycetes: Genus: *Actinomadura, Nocardia and Streptomyces*

Eumycetomas (Fungi)

- Maduromycosis: exogenous origin due to several aerobic fungi: *Petrellidium, Acremonium, Madurella, Leptosphera and others*

SUBCUTANEOUS MYCOSIS

Subcutaneous mycoses consist of a heterogeneous group of infections caused by a broad spectrum of taxonomically diverse fungi. Fungi gain entrance into the subcutaneous tissue usually following traumatic implantation, where they remain in localized microenvironmental niches and are often associated with abscess formation. These mycoses include pheohyphomycosis, hyalohyphomycosis, chromoblastomycosis, and mycetoma. Subcutaneous mycoses tend to remain localized and rarely result in systemic infections.

Mycetoma

Mycetoma is a chronic granulomatous infection that is caused by either a fungus (eumycetoma) or by a bacterium (actinomycetoma). Classification of mycetomas is shown in Table 8.2.

Although mycetoma is not endemic in the United States, the continual entry of immigrants from areas where the disease is endemic creates a need for increased awareness and studies regarding the clinical presentation and treatment of this disease. Mycetoma is more common in individuals who have more frequent and direct contact with the field environment, such as farmers, herdsmen, and other field laborers.

The disease is endemic in tropical and subtropical areas. The majority of cases occur in the "mycetoma belt," which stretches between the latitudes of 15° south and 30° north. Within this belt are countries such as Sudan, Somalia, Senegal, India, Yemen, Mexico, Venezuela, Colombia, Brazil, and Argentina. Geographic areas in the *mycetoma belt* are characterized by short rainy seasons that last for 4 to 6 months with fairly consistent daily temperatures (30°C–37°C) and relative humidities of 60% to 80%. These rainy seasons are followed by dry seasons of 6 to 8 months with variable daytime temperatures (45°C–60°C) and relative humidities of 12% to 18%.

Mycetoma is not contagious and typically remains localized, involving cutaneous and subcutaneous tissue, fascia, and bone. All subcutaneous mycoses are caused by fungi or bacteria that enter the skin via an incisive injury, often a thorn prick or splinter. The incubation period for the disease is variable.

Mycetomas are characterized by abscesses that contain grains, or large aggregates of fungi or actinomycete filaments (Fig. 8.1). They enclose cells with modified internal and cell wall structures and a hard extracellular matrix. Without therapy, this disease may lead to severe local tissue destruction, requiring surgical amputation. Actinomycetomas can spread more rapidly.

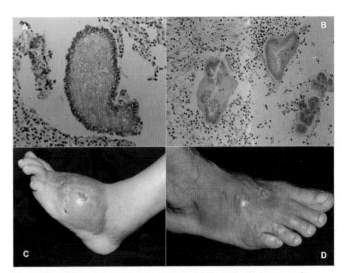

Figure 8.1. Mycetoma. A: eumycetoma (skin with aggregates of brown fungi of *Madurella grisea*, constituted by molds with numerous clamidospores – HE, OM 200x); B: actinomycetoma (skin with grains of *Actinomadura madurae* – HE 100x); C: eumycetoma in foot; D: actinomycetoma in foot.

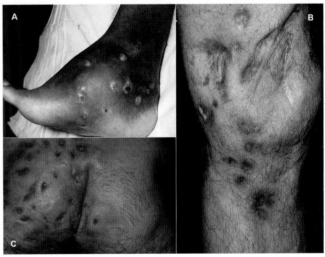

Figure 8.2. Mycetoma: clinical aspects. A: enlargement of the foot and nodules with draining sinuses; B: involvement of the lower limb; C: involvement of the buttocks.

Mycetomas start as small, firm, painless subcutaneous plaques or nodules, usually on the foot or leg (Fig. 8.2), but are also found on the arms, chest wall, and scalp. The most common etiological agents of mycetoma worldwide are eumycetes, particularly *Madurella mycetomatis* (Fig. 8.3), which causes >70% of the cases in certain regions of Central Africa, including Sudan. The infection involves the skin and the subcutaneous tissues as well as bone. In Central America and Mexico, mycetomas are more commonly caused by the actinomycetes *Nocardia brasiliensis, Streptomyces somaliensis, Actinomadura madurae*, and *A. peletierii*. Scalp mycetomas are rare but can be caused by *Streptomyces somaliensis*. Mycetomas as a result of *Nocardia* are often found on the chest wall and can invade the lung. In most cases, mycetomas can spread locally, but they rarely disseminate.

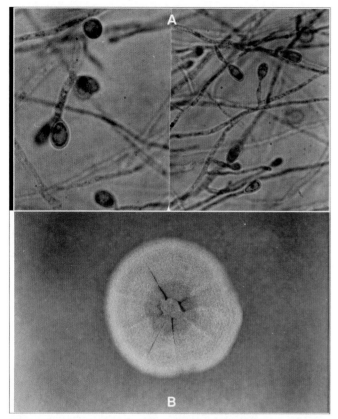

Figure 8.3. Mycetoma and etiologic agents. A: *Pseudallescheria boydii* microcultive (septated fungal hyphae with piriform conidia); B: *Madurella mycetomatis* macroculture (potato agar at room temperature).

Eumycotic mycetoma is a localized chronic infection and is caused by true fungi. The most important fungi are of the genera *Acremonium*, *Exophiala*, *Pseudallescheria*, *Madurella*, *Pyrenochaeta*, and *Leptosphaeria*. In the United States, mycetoma is most commonly caused by the fungus *Pseudallescheria boydii* (Fig. 8.3). The disease starts as painless, cutaneous papules or nodules that increase in size and spread to the connective tissue.

Eumycotic mycetoma is characterized by tumefaction, draining sinuses, and the presence of grain (organized, interwoven mycelial aggregates) formation, usually appearing on the foot. Mycetoma is typically unilateral, and most often (~70%–80%) the foot is the primary site of infection, followed by the hands (~12%), legs, and knee joints.

Ultimate diagnosis is made by visualization of grains, which can be collected by opening up pustules and expressing the contents or by deep surgical incision. After that the grains are fixed in a solution of 20% potassium hydroxide, they can be seen on a glass slide. Usually, fungal hyphae may be seen, and the characteristic colors (black, white, yellow, red or mixed colors) of the grains are useful in differentiating between the various agents that cause mycetomas.

Eumycetes that usually have *white grains* are *Acremonium falciforme*, *Acremonium kiliense*, *Acremonium recifei*, *Cylindrocarpon cyanescens*, *Cylindrocarpon destructans*, *Pseudallescheria boydii*, *Fusarium oxysporum*, *Fusarium solani*, *Fusarium moniliforme*, *Neotestudina rosatii*, *Polycytella hominis*, and *Aspergillus*

nidulans. *Black grains* are found in following eumycetes: *Plenodomus avrami*, *Corynespora cassiicola*, *Curvularia geniculata*, *Curvularia lunata*, *Leptosphaeria senegalensis*, *Leptosphaeria thompkinsii*, *Madurella grisea*, *Pseudochaetosphaeronema larense*, *Pyrenochaeta mackinnoni*, *Pyrenochaeta romeroi*, *Madurella mycetomatis*, *Exophiala jeanselmei*, *Phialophora verrucosa*. *Aspergillius flavus* shows *green grains*.

MRI can exhibit the extent of involvement. Periosteal thickening, bone lytic lesions, and increased bone density can be seen on radiographic films.

Management of actinomycetomas can be started with streptomycin (14 mg/kg daily) intramuscularly for 4 weeks. After this initial four weeks of therapy, dapsone (1.5mg/kg twice daily) should then be added to the treatment regiment on alternate days with streptomycin. If this regimen fails, dapsone should be replaced by trimethoprin/sulfamethoxazole (14mg/kg twice daily) or rifampicin (15–20mg/kg daily).

Surgery is often performed as a first-line therapy for eumycetes. To be effective, the surgery must be done before the infection has extended to the underlying bone and must be followed by systemic antifungals. Care must be taken throughout any surgical procedure to avoid contamination and further infection, with emphasis placed on maintaining the integrity of the capsule. Aggressive wide excision or amputation should be performed for early localized lesions. Less aggresive surgery should be performed for extensive disease with bone involvement. Following completion of surgery, treatment of the wound with iodine is recommended to eliminate any residual fungi.

Medical treatment of eumycetomas is initiated with ketoconazole (400–800 mg daily) or itraconazole (400 mg daily). Cure rates with ketoconazole seem to be dose dependent, with some patients needing treatment for months or years. Use of itraconazole has been associated with good clinical response with a low recurrence rate. Liver function tests should be monitored. The following findings are needed for a presumptive cure: disappearance of the subcutaneous mass with healing of the sinuses and the appearance of normal skin, three consecutive negative immunoelectrophoresis tests one month apart, restoration of the normal radiological appearance of bone with remodeling, absence of hyperreflective echoes and cavities upon ultrasonic examination, and absence of grains on fine needle aspiration.

Chromomycosis

The synonyms for this disease include chromoblastomycosis, cladosporiosis, Fonseca's disease, Pedroso and Lane's mycosis, and phaeosporotrichosis. First described by Pedroso and Gomes in 1920, in Sao Paulo, as "a verrucous dermatitis of infectious origin" (Fig. 8.4), the disease was later named *chromoblastomycosis* by Moore and Almeida in 1935. These fungi produce sclerotic bodies that mostly partition by separation along the septa, and show brownish spherical formations called *fumagoid bodies*.

Chromomycosis is a chronic, often debilitating, suppurative, and granulomatous mycosis of the skin and subcutaneous tissues established after inoculative trauma. Chromomycosis occurs worldwide, but is prevalent in many tropical and subtropical countries, like Brazil, and probably occurs when spores are implanted from soil or decaying vegetation after minor trauma.

This mycosis is caused by several species of dematiaceus hyphomycetes: *Fonsecaea pedrosoi* (Fig. 8.5), *Phialophora verrucosa, Cladophialophora carrionii, Fonsecaea compacta, Rhinocladiella aquaspersa,* and *Wangiella dermatitidis.*

The host defense mechanism in chromomycosis in some studies demonstrates a predominantly cellular immune response, with the activation of the macrophages involved in fungus phagocytosis. Although phagocytosis occurs, death of fungal cells is rarely observed. The ability of *Fonsecaea pedrosoi* to produce secreted or wall-associated melanin-like components protects the organism against destruction by host immune cells.

After inoculation there is an adherence by the fungus to epithelial cells. The fungus then differentiates into sclerotic forms (sclerotic bodies, muriform cell, Medlar body). Phaeoid (dark-colored) hyphae may also be observed in infected tissues. *Sclerotic bodies* are dark-brown (melanin produced in the cell wall), spherical or polyhedral, thick-walled structures which have horizontal and vertical septa inside. They may be found singly, in clusters, or within giant cells.

Clinically, chromomycosis is chronic with the development of nodules, verrucous, cauliflower-like lesions, tumors, plaques, and scar lesions (Fig. 8.6a & b). Differentiation requires microscopic examination.

The lower limbs are most frequently affected, and upper limb disease occurs in only 15% of cases (Fig. 8.4). The condition usually remains confined to the skin and subcutaneous layer, although lymphatic spread can occur and rare cases of cerebral involvement have been reported. General health state is not affected. There is a characteristic odor of secondary fusospiral organisms. Long-standing cases can also be complicated by lymphedema and, occasionally, squamous cell carcinoma.

Pseudoepitheliomatous hyperplasia, intraepidermal abscesses, and suppurative and granulomatous inflammatory infiltrates into the dermis are often found. Spherical, dark, or brown bodies (muriform cell and Medlar bodies) are sometimes present in the dermis in giant cells.

The major differences between genera are the microscopic features.

- *Fonsecaea* type: Conidia are one-celled and arise on swollen dentils that are located at the tips of the conidiophores. These primary conidia function as sympodial conidiogenous cells, becoming irregularly swollen at their apices. These in turn give rise to one-celled, pale brown, secondary conidia

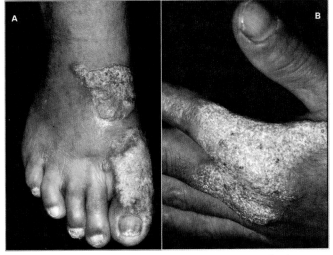

Figure 8.4. Chromomycosis. A: verrucous dermatitis on the foot; B: verrucous dermatitis on the hand.

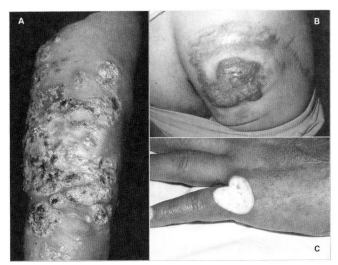

Figure 8.6. Chromomycosis. Polymorphous skin manifestations. A: nodules, verrucous cauliflower-like lesions, and tumors; B: plaques and scar lesions; C: a lesion in treatment with liquid nitrogen.

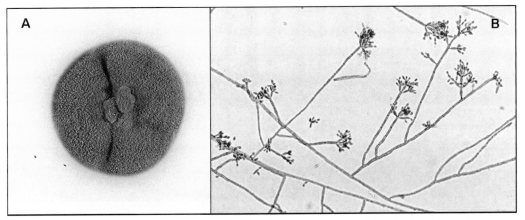

Figure 8.5. Chromomycosis. *Fonsecaea pedrosoi* cultive. A: macrocultive in potato agar for 21 days at room temperature; B: microcultive showing *Fonsecaea* type of conidiogenesis (OM 400x).

on swollen dentils. The secondary conidia often produce tertiary series of conidia like those formed by the primary conidia, resulting in a complex conidial head. Long chains of conidia are not formed in this type of conidiogenesis.

- *Cladosporium* type: Conidiophores give rise to primary shield-shaped conidia, which then generate long, branching chains of oval, dematiaceous conidia. The conidia have visible dark hila, which are actually the attachment scars. This type of conidiogenesis is primarily observed for the strains belonging to the genus *Cladosporium*, but may also be observed in strains of *Fonsecaea*.
- *Phialophora* type: In this type of conidiogenesis, conidia are located at the apices of the phialides, which are vase-shaped and have collarettes. This type of conidiogenesis is primarily observed for the strains belonging to the genus *Phialophora*, but may also very rarely be observed in strains of *Fonsecaea*.
- *Rhinocladiella* type: Conidiophores are sympodial and have dentils, which bear one-celled, pale brown conidia. The conidia may be located at the tips and along the sides of conidiophores. Formation of secondary conidia is very rare. This type of conidiogenesis is primarily observed for the strains belonging to the genus *Rhinocladiella*, but may also be observed in strains of *Fonsecaea*.

The clinical differential diagnosis of the verrucous lesions of chromomycosis should include verrucous leishmaniasis, verrucous tuberculosis, sporotrichosis, and verrucous carcinoma.

Treatment

For small and localized chromomycosis lesions, extensive excision is the treatment of choice. Other therapies are carbon dioxide laser, cryotherapy, and heat therapy. Cryotherapy is performed with two freezing cycles lasting 30 to 60 seconds (Fig. 8.6c).

A number of systemic therapies have been used, including ketoconazole, itraconazole, amphotericin, flucytosine, fluconazole, thiabendazole, saperconazole, terbinafine, and potassium iodide. However, chromomycosis is often resistant to treatment, especially when the causative organism is *Fonsecaea pedrosoi*. In this setting, itraconazole is used at a dose of 200 mg/day associated with flucytosine at a dose of 150 mg/kg/day for several months. Extensive disease requires treatment with intravenous amphoterecin B, 25 mg on alternate days (see infusion technique in Paracoccidioidomycosis) as well as flucytosine at a dose of 150 mg/kg/day, over 2 to 3 months.

Damian *et al.* reported the use of regional chemotherapy using the isolated limb infusion (ILI) technique, with melphalan and actinomycin D. Apart from cytotoxicity-induced desquamation and necrosis, the ILI procedure also produces hyperthermia of the skin and subcutis, which could contribute to its effectiveness against thermosensitive fungi. Melphalan and actinomycin D are also likely to have direct cytotoxic effects on the causative fungus, similar to what is observed in vitro and in vivo with 5-fluorouracil therapy.

Sporotrichosis

Sporotrichosis is a subacute or chronic subcutaneous mycosis caused by the thermally dimorphic organism *Sporothrix*

schenckii. It is found throughout the world as a saprophytic organism, particularly in temperate and tropical areas. This mycosis develops mainly through (i) penetration of the fungus into the dermis after wounds or an abrasion of the skin from infected materials such as hay, thorns, wood, splinters, barbed wire, gardening tools, flowers, pottery, or contact with cattle and feed; (ii) inhalation of spores through the respiratory tract; or (iii) insect stings or animals bites. Sporotrichosis is the most common subcutaneous mycosis in Latin America.

Most cases of sporotrichosis involve primarily the skin and neighboring lymphatic channels. Dissemination to other organs and tissues such as bones and joints occurs in immunocompromised patients (i.e., patients with diabetes, alcoholism, AIDS, or on corticosteroid therapy).

In most cases, the disease localizes to the upper limbs or the face. It is exceedingly rare in the trunk (Fig. 8.7).

The clinical spectrum of the sporotrichoses is divided into the following forms: Cutaneous and Extracutaneous forms. The Cutaneous form is classified into:

- Cutaneous lymphatic form (75%, Fig. 8.8C): This common presentation usually shows papulonodular lesions, and sometimes ulcerative lesions. It occurs at the site of inoculation (sporotrichoid chancre). Following this, the disease causes a lymphangitis cord of nodules or gummatous lesions that can ulcerate in the configuration of a rosary. Often there is no regional lymphadenopathy. In adults the initial lesion is most common on the extremities and in children on the face.
- Cutaneous localized forms (20%)
  1. Papulonodular form (Fig. 8.8a & b): There are papulosquamous lesions, crusts, nodular lesions and originating plaques that resemble acne or furuncles. There are no observed signs of lymphangitis.
  2. Ulcerative form: single or multiple ulcers, irregular borders, and variable extension (Fig. 8.9). Sometimes in the periphery of the lesions there are gummas.

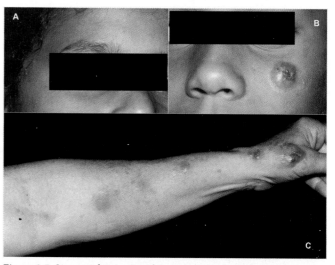

Figure 8.7. Sporotrichosis. A and B: Cutaneous localized form on children's faces (Papulo-nodular form); C: cutaneous-lymphatic form (papulo-nodular, ulcerative lesions and lymphangitis).

3. Verrucous form: Generally a single verrucous plaque, with variable form and extension, showing a central scar. There are no signs of lymphangitis. Under examination, the lesions show a purulent discharge. This form is classified under the clinical spectrum of *cutaneous verrucous syndrome* (leishmaniasis, sporotrichosis, chromomycosis, and tuberculosis).

- Cutaneous disseminated form: Rare, characterized by nodules or gummas dispersed on extensive areas of the body, which can ulcerate. It is observed in patients with human immunodeficiency virus (HIV).

Extracutaneous forms: In rare cases of sporotrichosis there are lesions in bones, lungs, testis, oronasal mucosa, larynx, and pharynx. Usually, this form is due to ingestion, inhalation, or is associated with cutaneous disseminated disease.

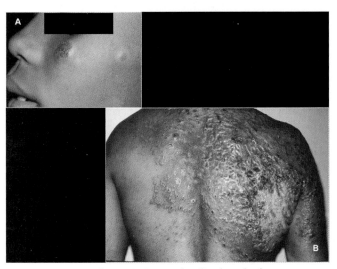

Figure 8.8. Sporotrichosis. A: Disease localized on the face; B: Extensive lesions on trunk.

Diagnosis

- Mycological studies:
  1. Direct examination: In KOH preparations this fungus cannot be recognized. Gram stain can demonstrate gram-positive oval or cigar corpuscles. The better diagnostic technique is fluorescent antibodies, which must be incubated at 37° C for 12 hours.
  2. Culture: The gold standard for diagnosing sporotrichosis is fungal culture (Fig. 8.10). The pus or scrapings are cultured on Sabouraud dextrose agar and a medium containing cycloheximide. At 30°C growth is usually present in 3 to 5 days. Microscopically, thin branching hyphae with pyriform conidia can be seen. This is the mycelia form. *S schenckii* is a dimorphic fungus, growing as yeast at 37°C and mycelium at room temperature. The mold-to-yeast form conversion is necessary since other fungi are morphologically similar. Transferring the fungus to brain heart infusion agar and incubating at 37°C in 5% to 10 % CO_2 produces mold-to-yeast form conversion. In culture, *S schenckii* appears as a white, smooth, or verrucous colony with aerial mycelium, which subsequently turns brown, and then black.
- Histopathological examination: This can be falsely negative. It can show a granuloma with a central suppurative reaction and secondary histiocytic epithelioid and plasmocytoid reaction in the periphery of the lesion. In hematoxylin-eosin (H&E) stain, "asteroid bodies" can be observed, which represent fungal elements surrounded by eosinophilic material.
- Intradermal tests: Intradermal skin tests using sporotrichin as the antigen are useful in epidemiological studies and as an auxiliary method for detecting atypical forms of the disease. They can yield false-positive and false-negative results.
- Serology: It is possible to use immunodiffusion (ID) and immunoelectrophoresis tests in the diagnosis of sporotrichosis

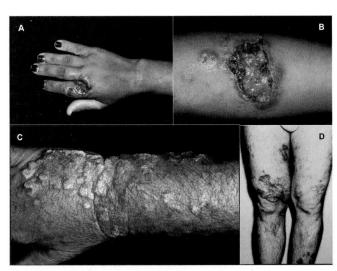

Figure 8.9. Sporotrichosis. A and B: Ulcerative lesions; C: verrucous form; D: scars of extensive involvement of the lower limb.

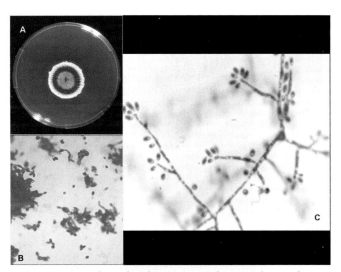

Figure 8.10. *Sporothrix schenckii*. A: macrocultive in Sabouraud dextrose agar at room temperature (white, smooth or verrucous colony with aerial mycelium); B: microscopic features of the yeast form at 37°C; C: mycelium with conidia on marguerite collection (microcultive at room temperature).

using a fungal culture filtrate employing sera from patients with the disseminated cutaneous form. These methods are mainly used in cases of extracutaneous sporotrichosis or atypical forms This permits the selection of an adequate treatment regimen. ELISA test shows 90% sensitivity and 86% overall efficacy when tested against sera obtained from patients with the lymphocutaneous, fixed cutaneous, disseminated cutaneous or multiple and extracutaneous forms of sporotrichosis.

Treatment

Potassium iodide (KI) was the first drug successfully used in the treatment of sporotrichosis and is used for localized cutaneous forms. It is formulated as a saturated solution containing approximately 20 g potassium iodide in 20 mL distilled water. Each 10 drops of this solution contains 0.5g of KI. Treatment is initiated with 5 drops administered twice a day, and the dose is increased by one drop/dose/day until reaching a total of 4 to 6 g/day (40–60 drops, twice a day) (Fig. 8.11). If there is gastric intolerance, intravenous sodium iodide in doses of 1 to 2g/day can be given. KI is not suggested during pregnancy. Adverse effects include nausea, metallic taste, hypothyroidism, iododerma, and iodism. Itraconazole is administered orally at a dose of 100 to 400 mg/day. Terbinafine is not formally indicated for the treatment of sporotrichosis but reports have shown therapeutic success. Treatment with fluconazole is cited in the literature, but this is not a first choice drug. Fluconazole is administered orally at 200 to 400 mg/day and has the advantage of the action on the central nervous system. Amphotericin B is indicated for treatment of moderate to severe clinical forms in immunosuppressed individuals and those who did not respond to other drugs. Amphotericin B is nephrotoxic and cardiotoxic. The drug is administered intravenously, with a maximum daily dose of 50 mg and a total cumulative dose of 500 to 1000 mg. The duration of treatment until clinical cure is 6 to 8 weeks, on average, in immunocompetent patients.

Lobomycosis

Lobomycosis or Jorge Lobo's disease was described in 1931 by Jorge Lobo, in Brazil. Lobo suspected that his patient had a modified form of paracoccidioidomycosis, which he called *keloidal blastomycosis*. A second human case was reported in 1938, after which the disease was termed *Lobo's disease*. Lobomycosis is a chronic granulomatous infection of the skin and subcutaneous tissues caused by the fungus *Lacazia loboi*.

More than 500 human cases have been reported to date, although the disease appears to be confined to remote tropical areas of South and Central America, especially in communities along rivers. Lobomycosis is rarely reported outside of Latin America. It occurs in tropical and subtropical areas. The condition has been described in Bolivia, Brazil, Colombia, Costa Rica, Ecuador, French Guiana, Guyana, Mexico, Panama, Peru, Suriname, and Venezuela. Brazil and Colombia have the most cases and they are found along the Amazon basin, especially among the Caibi Indians.

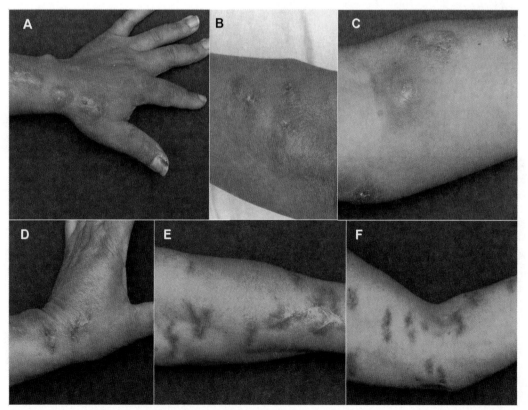

Figure 8.11. Sporotrichosis (cutaneous-lymphatic form) treated with KI. A, B and C: Before the KI treatment. D, E, and F: 60 days after KI treatment.

Attempts to grow *L. loboi* on artificial media have been unsuccessful. Successful inoculation of this fungus has been achieved in a hamster's cheek pouch (*Mesocricetus auratus*). *L. loboi* is a saprophytic fungus in the soil, on vegetables, and in water. It is inoculated in humans by trauma. Aquarium employees and farmers comprise most of the cases. Occupations such as gold mining, fishing, and hunting also put patients at risk.

L. loboi is abundant in tissue under microscopic examination, and shows globoid or elliptic corpuscles of 6 to 12 μm in diameter. Numerous yeast-like, round, thick, and birefringent cell walls are seen (Fig. 8.12, upper left). Chains of yeast cells are typically formed (Fig. 8.12, medium right). This fungus reproduces by gemmulation.

The initial lesion is a superficial or deep papule that can form solitary or multiple plaques or nodular lesions (Fig. 8.12 upper right). It is characterized by the appearance of slowly developing (months, years, or decades), keloid-like (Fig. 8.12, upper left, down left and right), ulcerated, or verrucous nodular or plaque-like cutaneous lesions. These lesions occur usually at the site of local trauma as from a cut, insect bite, animal bite, or ray sting. Lesions tend to occur on exposed, cooler areas of the body, and in particular the lower extremities and ears. The disease is limited to skin and semi-mucosal areas. Other sites reportedly affected include the forehead, face, chest, scapula, lumbosacral spine, buttocks, and scrotum. The patient often complains of pruritus, burning, hypoesthesia, or anesthesia. The disease can

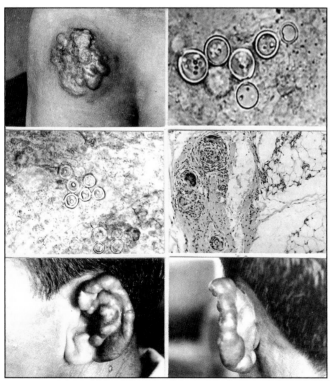

Figure 8.12. Lobomycosis. Upper left: Keloid-like lesion; upper right: numerous yeast-like, round, thick, and birefringent cell walls of *Lacazia loboi;* medium left: chains of yeast cells; down left and down right: clinical aspects of keloid-like lesions on the ear. The genus *Lacazia* was proposed to honor Professor Carlos da Silva Lacaz, eminent mycologist and university lecturer of the Dermatology Department, School of Medicine, Sao Paulo University, Brazil.

be complicated by secondary bacterial infection or carcinomatous degeneration.

The organism rarely spreads to the lymphatics.

Diagnosis

- Histopathological examination shows a granulomatous infiltrate with Langhans cells and numerous parasites, isolated or in chains. The clinical differential diagnosis includes anergic leishmaniasis, leprosy, zygomycosis, sarcoidosis, or benign and malignant neoplasms.

Treatment

Optional treatment of lobomycosis is surgical excision. Full excision of the lesion is required for clinical success. Repeated cryotherapy may also be beneficial. Clofazimine has been effective in some cases of lobomycosis in doses of 100 to 200 mg/day for 12 to 24 months.

Rhinosporidiosis

Epidemiology

Rhinosporidiosis appears as vegetant lesions of the mucosal surfaces. *Rhinosporidium seeberi* has recently been shown to be an aquatic protist. Phylogenetic analysis of rDNA and rRNA from rhinosporidiosis tissue samples suggests that *R. seeberi* is the first known human pathogen from the DRIPs (*Dermocystidium*, the Rosette agent, *Ichthyophonus*, and *Psorospermium*) class of microbes.

Rhinosporidiosis has been documented in both tropical and temperate areas worldwide. The infection is usually found in young males. The mechanism of infection is not known, but some patients have a history of fresh water exposure. It is hypothesized that aquatic animals are natural hosts of *R. seeberi* and humans become infected when they come into contact with these animals and their parasites.

Rhinosporidiosis occurs in the Americas, Europe, Africa, and Asia but is far more common in the tropics. The greatest prevalence is in southern India and Sri Lanka, where the incidence is estimated at 1.4% in the pediatric population. Some arid countries of the Middle East also show a high incidence of the disease. South America is the second most common source of rhinosporidiosis, and the disease is endemic in the northeast part of Brazil, in a transitional environment between the Amazon rain forest and some arid areas where the rainfall is highly irregular, known as *Caatinga*. The incidence of rhinosporidiosis in this particular Brazilian province is similar to the most affected areas of India, suggesting that both dry conditions and aquatic environments are related to the disease.

Rhinosporidiosis occurs in healthy people, and there are no predisposing factors, besides an exposure to fresh water. Most infections occur in the nose (Fig. 8.13A), but they can also occur in the oral mucosa, larynx, conjunctiva, and perianal regions. Ocular infection is more prevalent in women, while nasal and nasopharyngeal infections preferentially affect men. The infection causes the development of painless intranasal papules that evolve into large and hyperplastic polyps studded with flecks. The surface of the polyp is irregular and red with some white dots, like small cysts (Fig. 8.13a) that correspond to the sporangia. Visceral dissemination has been reported but is very uncommon.

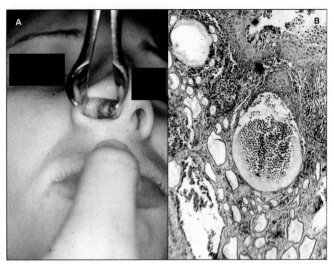

Figure 8.13. Rhinosporidiosis. A: irregular polyp and red surface; B: characteristic thick-walled giant sporangia with multiple spores.

The differential diagnosis must include pyogenic granuloma, coccidioidomycosis, and myospherulosis, which is an iatrogenic condition related to the application of nasal substances.

Diagnosis

*   The diagnosis is based on the histopathologic demonstration of the characteristic thick-walled giant sporangia (Fig. 8.13b). Sporangia can be seen on direct microscopy or on H&E-stained sections and have multiple basophilic spores in a clear material. The submucosa shows chronic inflammation and spherical sporangia in different stages of development and ranging in size from 250 to 300 μm in diameter. When compared with the spherules of *Coccidioides immitis*, the mature sporangia of rhinosporidiosis are larger and do not have a thick outer wall.

Treatment

The best management for rhinosporidiosis is excision because there is no medical treatment known to be effective. To prevent the 20% of cases that recur after surgery, the base of the lesion can be cauterized after excision. Local injection of amphotericin B may be used as an adjunct treatment to surgery to prevent re-infection and spread of the disease.

SYSTEMIC MYCOSIS

Systemic mycoses are those in which the pathogen has disseminated from one organ to another. Frequently, systemic mycoses originate in the lungs, where the pathogens disseminate by the hematogenous route. If a vital organ such as the brain is involved, death may result.

Histoplasmosis

Histoplasmosis is a systemic mycosis caused by *Histoplasma capsulatum*. It mainly affects the lungs where it is generally asymptomatic. *Histoplasma capsulatum* is a saprophyte and

is also found in soil contaminated with chicken feathers or droppings.

Endemic regions are in the western hemisphere, which include southern Mexico and some areas in the southeastern United States. Generally, it is a chronic or acute pulmonary disease. However, depending on the immune status of the host, it can also occur in disseminated form, especially in the setting of HIV.

Cutaneous lesions of histoplasmosis in HIV-infected patients may take on a wide variety of patterns, including hemorrhagic, papular, and ulceronecrotic patterns (Fig. 8.14). The cutaneous and mucocutaneous manifestations of histoplasmosis are frequently a consequence of the progression of a primary infection to disseminated histoplasmosis (DH). Rarely, the infection can appear as a few primary cutaneous lesions with a good prognosis. The acquired immunodeficiency syndrome (AIDS)-related incidence of DH is 0.5% to 2.7% in nonendemic regions, and up to 10% in endemic regions. It is important to point out that many AIDS-related cases present initially as DH.

Diagnosis

*   Mycological studies: on fungal culture, on Sabouraud agar, white colonies grow at 30°C. Tuberculate macroconidia can be visualized on microscopic examination.
*   Histopathological examination: skin biopsies are a simple method to diagnose cutaneous histoplasmosis. Owing to the diverse morphologic presentations of the infecting fungus, it is particularly helpful to use periodic acid–Schiff (PAS) stains. Cultures are still the best confirmatory diagnostic test, but serologic tests are also important, especially when biopsies and culture determinations are negative.
*   Antigen detection: Detection of antigen in bodily fluids offers a valuable approach to rapid diagnosis in patients with progressive disseminated histoplasmosis (PDH) and diffuse pulmonary histoplasmosis. Antigen is found in the urine of over 90% of patients with disseminated histoplasmosis and 80% with diffuse pulmonary disease. False-positive results in other mycoses and nonfungal infections have been rare. Antigen can also be detected in bronchoalveolar lavage (BAL) fluid of patients with pulmonary histoplasmosis and in cerebrospinal fluid (CSF) in those with meningitis.
*   Antibody response (serology): These tests are useful. Antibodies measured by ID or complement fixation (CF) first appear 4 to 8 weeks following exposure and persist for several years. However, patients who are immunocompromised may not mount an antibody response. For example, in patients with disseminated histoplasmosis, antibody levels decline slowly in self-limited disease. Several authors reported that there is no complete recovery from histoplasmosis before a CF titer of 1:8 is reached, despite remission of the cutaneous lesions.
*   Polymerase chain reaction: Several molecular biology laboratories offer PCR for diagnosis of histoplasmosis, but the accuracy of those methods is unclear.

Treatment

Immunocompromised patients with disseminated histoplasmosis generally receive IV amphotericin B at a total cumulative dose of 2 g (0.5 to 1 mg/kg/day for 7 days, then 0.8 mg/kg/day). Frequently, it is necessary to start a concomitant or maintenance treatment,

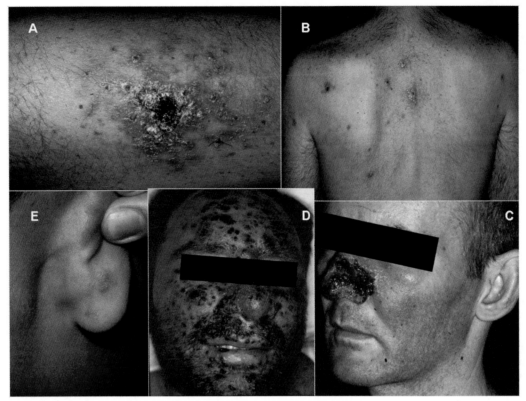

Figure 8.14. Histoplasmosis. A, B, C: hemorrhagic, papular, and ulceronecrotic patterns; D: extensive facial involvement; E: solitary retroauricular sarcoid lesions.

usually with systemic azolic antifungal drugs. Itraconazole 200 to 300 mg/day or fluconazole 100 to 300 mg/day are considered the best options. Most cases in immunocompetent patients without disseminated disease are self-limited and require no treatment.

Blastomycosis (North American Blastomycosis)

Blastomycosis is caused by infection with the dimorphic fungus *Blastomyces dermatitidis*. Like histoplasmosis and coccidioidomycosis, this disease occurs most commonly in defined geographic regions (endemic mycosis). In North America, blastomycosis usually occurs in the southeastern and south central states that border the Mississippi and Ohio Rivers, the mid-western states and Canadian provinces bordering the Great Lakes, and a small area of New York and Canada adjacent to the St. Lawrence River. Within these regions of endemicity, several studies have documented the presence of areas of hyperendemicity where the rate of blastomycosis is unusually high. Point-source outbreaks have been associated with occupational and recreational activities, frequently along streams or rivers, which result in exposure to moist soil enriched with decaying vegetation.

Primary infection initially involves the lungs with hematogenous dissemination to extrapulmonary sites such as the skin even if the pulmonary nidus is not apparent.

The clinical spectrum of blastomycosis is varied, including asymptomatic infection, acute or chronic pneumonia, and disseminated disease. Asymptomatic infection occurs in at least 50% of infected persons. The incubation period is 30 to 45 days.

Acute pulmonary blastomycosis mimics influenza or bacterial pneumonia. Spontaneous cures of symptomatic acute infections do occur. Most patients diagnosed with blastomycosis have an indolent onset of chronic pneumonia indistinguishable from tuberculosis, other fungal infections, and cancer.

In rare cases, cutaneous inoculation with *B. dermatitidis* can cause a syndrome of cutaneous inoculation blastomycosis. Criteria for diagnosis have included skin lesions often with focal lymphadenopathy or lymphangitis, a history of inoculation with material known or likely to contain the organisms, no evidence of systemic involvement (before, during, or after presentation), and recovery of organisms from specimens of skin lesions or lymph nodes by means of culture or direct smear.

Diagnosis

- Definitive diagnosis requires the growth of *B. dermatitidis* from a clinical specimen. Visualization of the characteristic budding yeast form in clinical specimens supports a presumptive diagnosis of blastomycosis and may prompt the initiation of antifungal therapy. Serological tests are generally not helpful for diagnosing blastomycosis.
- Antigen detection: The sensitivity is 93% overall and 89% in disseminated disease. Sensitivity is somewhat higher in urine than in serum, and antigen also can be detected with high sensitivity (~ 80%) in BAL and CSF.
- Serology is not useful.

Treatment

Intravenous amphotericin B, in cumulative doses of >1 g, has been described to result in cure without relapse in 70% to 91%

of cases. Overwhelming pulmonary disease is the most common cause of death. Increased mortality rates have been associated with advanced age, chronic obstructive pulmonary disease, and cancer. Ketoconazole was the first azole shown to be an effective alternative. Ketoconazole must be used at a dosage of ≥400 mg/day. Itraconazole is more readily absorbed, has enhanced antimycotic activity, and is better tolerated. Itraconazole dosage is 200 to 400 mg/day.

Coccidioidomycosis

Paracoccidioidomycosis (South American Blastomycosis)

Paracoccidioidomycosis (Pbmycosis, South American Blastomycosis, formerly termed Lutz-Splendore-Almeida disease) is a chronic, progressive, and insidious systemic mycosis caused by *Paracoccidioides brasiliensis*, a fungus found in the soil of certain areas of Latin America, from Mexico in the north to Argentina in the south, but mainly between latitudes 23° to 34°, altitudes between 150 meters and 2,000 meters, and pluviometric indices between 100 and 400 cm/year (see Chapter 10). Its precise natural history is incompletely understood. In Latin America, Antilleans and Chile are the only countries where this disease is not found. Adolpho Lutz first described the disease in a patient from Sao Paulo, Brazil, and Almeida proposed the name of the species in 1930. Naturally acquired animal infection has been demonstrated only in armadillos (*Dasiypus novemcinctus*). Bats and saguis (small monkeys from the southeastern forest of Brazil) are possible natural reservoirs. Dogs, cattle, and horses also have antibodies against *P. brasiliensis*. It is possible that the normal habitat of the fungus is the soil or the plants that grow in these specific geographic regions, and both animals and men acquire the pathogen by aspiration. The forms of inoculation in several tissues are demonstrated in Table 8.3.

Non-autochthonous cases have been reported outside the endemic areas. All of these patients have either lived in or visited Latin America at least once. Therefore, Pbmycosis can be considered a traveler's disease. Unapparent subclinical infection and minor lung changes are, however, common in affected areas and in Europeans and Americans who lived in these areas.

This disease has long periods of latency. Some non-autochthonous infections develop over 30 or more years after the patient left the endemic region.

The constant movement of people from rural to urban areas and an increase in the average life span will certainly contribute to a higher frequency of this disease. The association of systemic Pbmycosis with pulmonary tuberculosis (Tb) is common.

Table 8.3. Paracoccidioides brasiliensis and Forms of Inoculation in the Host

Organs	Inoculation form
Oro-pharyngeal mucosa	Direct inoculation
Upper respiratory tract and lungs	Inhalation
Bowel mucosa	Ingestion
Skin	Direct inoculation

Pbmycosis is a chronic granulomatous infectious disease. It is fundamentally a pulmonary and lymph node infection but may secondarily disseminate to mucocutaneous sites. Primary infection starts in the lungs after inhalation of fungal propagules, which then transform into the pathogenic yeast form. Active paracoccidioidomycosis is estimated to develop in only 2% of patients.

The *P. brasiliensis* virulence orthologs are placed in groups, based either on their functional or on their structural characteristics. These characteristics include metabolism-, cell wall-, and detoxification-related genes, as well as secreted factors and other determinants.

P. brasiliensis expresses some molecules that account for its ability to evade immunity. P. brasiliensis proteases are potentially associated with the invasion process. However, it is still uncertain whether these proteases help the fungi cause disease. Cell-mediated immune response is the main mechanism of defense against *P. brasiliensis* infection. The protective cell-mediated immune response in Pbmycosis is characterized by the production of cytokines (TNF-α, IL-12 and IFN-γ), which are required for the activation of macrophages. These same macrophages are the main defensive cells against *P. brasiliensis*. In the absence of such cytokines, such as in susceptible hosts, macrophages serve as a protected environment in which the fungi can undergo intracellular replication and disseminate from the lungs to other organs.

P. brasiliensis is a dimorphic fungus, but in humans it presents only in the yeast form and is usually from 2 to 10 μm in diameter, even though cells up to 30 μm or more are also common. The principal characteristic in its parasitic state is the formation of new yeast by evagination of the mother cell wall, which resembles a helm. The image seen in scanning electron microscopy is compared to a "grenade." The fungus is a eukaryote, with one or more nuclei and nucleoli. At 19° to 28°C the fungus develops as a mold and produces slow-growing colonies. The microscopic structures show thin septate hyphae with chlamydospores, which is the same form found in nature.

Chlamydospores are the infectious form of the fungus. In cultures at 37°C, as well as in tissues and exudates, the fungus appears as an oval-to-round yeast cell that reproduces by multiple buddings (Fig. 8.15). The "pilot wheel" cell is characteristic (Fig. 8.15d).

Inhalation is considered the most important route of infection. After inhalation, the chlamydospores transform to the yeast form in the patient's body. The primary site of infection, which is often not apparent, is the lung. A benign and transient pulmonary or oral infection occurs in normal individuals. If the host becomes immunosuppressed, a reactivation occurs in lungs, skin, mucous membranes, lymphatics, or the CNS. It is not contagious from person to person because at body temperature the fungus is in the yeast form.

The clinical manifestations of Pbmycosis are polymorphous. The forms of Pbmycosis are classified into acute/subacute, chronic, and residual or sequel forms.

ACUTE/SUBACUTE FORM (CHILDHOOD/JUVENILE TYPE)

This form represents 3% to 5% of the Pbmycosis cases and predominates in children and adolescents. The patients have involvement of the mononuclear phagocytic system, depressed

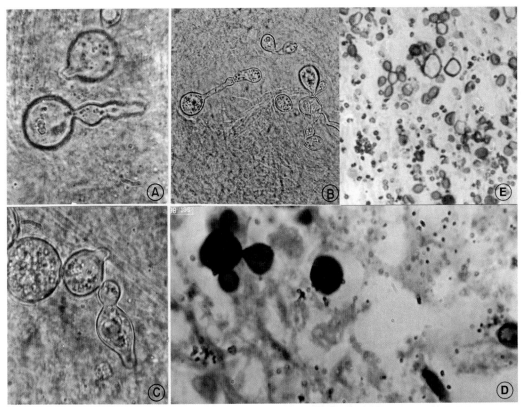

Figure 8.15. *Paracoccidioides brasiliensis*. A, B and C: fungus appears as an oval-to-round yeast cell that reproduces by multiple budding; D: yeast form in tissue with multiple budding and characteristic "pilot wheel" cell (Gomori-Grocott stain); E: mouse testis with numerous *P. brasiliensis* (Gomori-Grocott stain, OM 100x).

cellular immunity, and increased antibodies. Both sexes are equally compromised. This form is characterized by rapid evolution, leaving the patient looking for medical attention 4 to 12 weeks after the onset of infection. Respectively, in order of frequency, the main manifestations include lymphadenopathy, gastrointestinal symptoms, hepatosplenomegaly, osteoarticular involvement, and cutaneous lesions. In the subacute form there is a maintained general state of lymphadenopathy. In the acute form the patient complains of a deteriorated general state, and several internal organs are involved, principally the liver, spleen, and bone marrow, among others.

CHRONIC FORM (ADULT TYPE)
This form comprises at least 90% of the patients and affects patients between 30 to 60 years, usually male patients. The disease progresses slowly, with a silent course for many years. It is subclassified into mild, moderate, and severe forms. The pulmonary symptoms are present in 90% of the patients. This form is called "unifocal" when the Pbmycosis is restricted to one organ. The lungs can be the only organ affected in at least 25% of patients. Frequently, Pbmycosis involves many internal organs simultaneously (multifocal form). The lungs, oral and/or nasal mucosa, and skin are most frequently involved in this form.

Direct inoculation of the parasite in both skin and oral mucous membranes is not common, but can explain some cases of skin and/or mucosal lesions without lung involvement. A common habit in Brazilian rural areas, the use of twigs to clean teeth, is the presumptive cause of these lesions. Conspicuous lesions of Pbmycosis were found in the gingival mucosa of these patients, and fungus was collected from apical teeth granulomas. *P. brasiliensis was* recovered in the amygdales in the absence of clinical lesions (*occult amigdalitis paracoccidioica*). The intestinal mucosa can also be a site of direct inoculation after the accidental ingestion of the fungus. The pulmonary route is the most important one and is the site of inoculation in more than 96% of all patients with Pbmycosis.

One half of the patients develop subsequent oral lesions, often with nasal and pharyngeal ulcers. These ulcerations have a punctate vascular pattern over a granulomatous base, with clinical features of mulberry-like surface, and are known as stomatitis "moriforme" of Aguiar-Pupo (Fig. 8.16). The stomatitis progresses to ulcerovegetant crusts (Fig. 8.17a & b), which compromise large areas of the oral cavity, pharynx, larynx, and nasal cavities. Dysphagia and hoarseness due to laryngeal disease and destruction of vocal cords can ensue. Perioral crusted and granulomatous plaques are common. Gingival involvement may lead to tooth loss. In the end stages, the epiglottis and uvula are also destroyed, the hard palate is perforated, and the lips and tongue may become involved. These oral manifestations are followed by massive bilateral cervical lymph node enlargement. Other lymphoid tissue sites, such as axillary, inguinal, and mesenteric lymph nodes, also can be affected.

The cutaneous lesions of Pbmycosis can vary from crusted papules to ulcers (Fig. 8.17c & d), nodules, plaques, and verrucous lesions. Centrofacial localization is typical of Pbmycosis, and most of the lesions occur through dissemination of the oral and gingival lesions. Most of the skin lesions, however, are the

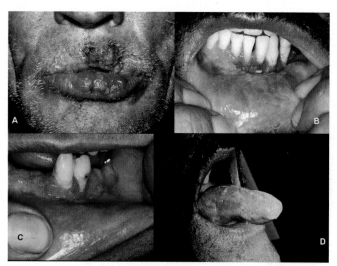

Figure 8.16. Paracoccidioidomycosis. A, B, C and D: mucocutaneous involvement with the classical mulberry-like surface that are known as stomatitis "moriforme" of Aguiar-Pupo. Aguiar-Pupo was an eminent dermatologist, who described this classical mulberry-like mucosal surface in Pbmycosis. Aguiar-Pupo was university lecturer of the Dermatology Department, School of Medicine, Sao Paulo University, Brazil.

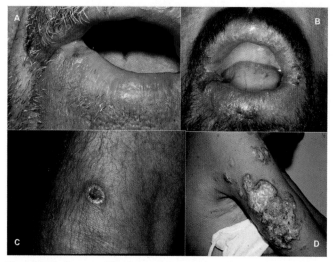

Figure 8.17. Paracoccidioidomycosis. A and B: ulcerovegetant and crusts lesions; C and D: ulcerated lesions.

result of hematogenic dissemination of the fungus from the lungs.

The adrenal glands are affected in 48.2% of Pbmycosis patients submitted to autopsy. Lesions can affect long bones or cranial bones in a symmetric pattern. The bone lesions are characterized by osteolytic radiological images or bone destruction, including articulations. Mesenteric lymph node disease may cause bowel obstruction and symptoms of an acute abdomen. The involvement of the central nervous system includes a spectrum of meningitis, meningoencephalitis, subacute or chronic meningoradiculitis or a combination of any of these. Untreated Pbmycosis can be fatal owing to the possibility of severe pulmonary fibrosis, central nervous system involvement, or adrenal disease.

RESIDUAL OR SEQUEL FORM

This type of disease is from scarring post treatment. Host response fungi cause a chronic granulomatous inflammatory process with resultant fibrosis. There is an elevated level of cytokines such as TNF-α and TGF-β that promote tissue fibrosis, particularly in the lungs. Pulmonary fibrosis occurs in at least 50% of the patients with chronic lung disease and can result in chronic obstructive lung disease.

Patients with Pbmycosis and AIDS generally present in a form similar to that of the more severe acute forms of Pbmycosis. Pbmycosis is seen as an opportunistic infection in patients with AIDS in endemic regions, however, a greater increase in prevalence is expected. It is possible to use trimethoprim–sulfamethoxazole as a prophylaxis for *Pneumocystis carinii* pneumonia. It is also effective against *P. brasiliensis*, which explains in part the scarcity of reported cases of systemic Pbmycosis.

Diagnosis

It is established by visualization of *P. brasiliensis* upon light microscopic examination, isolation of the fungus by culture from biological specimens, and clinical appearance. Material scraped from the mouth can be stained with PAS or placed in 10% potassium hydroxide.

Detection of gp43 glycoprotein and gp70 polysaccharide in serum has been reported as a sensitive and specific method for the diagnosis of paracoccidioidomycosis and for monitoring therapy. The sensitivity and specificity for detection of gp43 and gp70 are estimated at 98% to 100%. Both antigens could also be detected in the CSF, BAL, and urine. Detection of a gp87-kDa antigen has also been reported but would appear to be less useful because of cross-reactions with other fungi and mycobacteria. Polymerase chain reaction with oligonucleotide primers of the gp43 antigen has recently been used to detect *P. brasiliensis* in sputum. However, whether these methods are available for routine clinical use is unknown.

- Serology: Measurement of the antibody response by ID and CF is useful for diagnosis of Pbmycosis. The ID test is more specific than CF but is not quantitative. There are recommendations for quantitative results of ID or other diagnostic tests for Pbmycosis, for better interpretation of the therapeutic response. This is because the antibodies progressively decrease with clinical control of the disease. Serologic cure is probable if the titration of antibodies is negative or the dilution stabilizes at 1:2. Some patients at the time of diagnosis can demonstrate ID titration below 1:4.
- Antigenemia enzyme immunoassay (EIA) methods are more sensitive but less specific than CF, and standardized methods are not yet available for the clinical testing. Clearance of antibodies with therapy or spontaneously can be measured by CF.

Treatment

Sulfas are first choice for the treatment of Pbmycosis. Sulfamethoxazole–trimethoprim (SMZ-TMP) is used in initial doses of 800/160 mg, twice a day for 30 days. Subsequently 400/80 mg (SMZ-TMP) is administrated twice daily for an undetermined time until cicatrization of the lesions, radiological regression of the lung images, and a relevant decrease of serologic titers.

Amphotericin B has elective indication in severe forms of Pbmycosis and in patients with hepatic disease. Amphotericin B is administrated intravenously, drop by drop, into 5% dextrose solution, over 6 hours. In the first infusion, usually it is used in doses of 0.25 mg/kg, and if it is well tolerated, then subsequently it can be increased from 0.5 mg/kg to 1.0 mg/kg/daily or on alternate days. The total cumulative dose depends on the clinical, serological, and radiological progression. Usually, mucocutaneous Pbmycosis is cured with total doses of 30 mg/kg, but in the lymphadenopathy form 60 mg/kg of total dose must be given.

Ketoconazole can be used in a dose of 400 mg/day during 30 days, and then subsequently in a dose of 200 mg/day for 12 to 24 months. Itraconazole is better tolerated and has the same efficacy as ketoconazole. Itraconazole must be used in a dosage of 200–400 mg/day, especially for nervous system lesions.

Zygomycosis

The class *Zygomycetes* is divided into two orders, *Mucorales* and *Entomophthorales*. The term *mucormycosis* is used to describe infections caused by the fungus *Mucorales*. Members of the order *Mucorales* are the etiological agents of the disease traditionally known as "mucormycosis." It is a fulminant disease with high rates of morbidity and mortality that mainly affects immunocompromised patients, especially ketoacidotic diabetic patients. However, species of the order *Entomophthorales* cause "entomophoromycosis" and they are responsible for the chronic subcutaneous disease observed in immunocompetent patients in tropical and subtropical regions.

Mucormycosis

Mucormycosis, the third invasive mycosis in order of importance after candidiasis and aspergillosis, is a disease that may be caused by several species of different genera, which are listed in Table 8.1. Fungi belonging to the order *Mucorales* fall into six families (i.e., Mucoraceae, Cunninghamellaceae, Mortierellaceae, Saksenaceae, Syncephalastraceae and Thamnidaceae). The most important species in order of frequency are *Rhizopus arrhizus (oryzae), Rhizopus microsporus var. Rhizopodiformis, Rhizomucor pusillus, Cunninghmaella bertholletiae, Apophysomyces elegans,* and *Saksenaea vasiformis*.

The incidence of mucormycosis is approximately 1.7 cases per 1000,000 (1.000.000) inhabitants per year, which corresponds to 500 patients per year in the United States. Postmortem evaluation for the presence of agents responsible for mucormycosis shows that mucormycosis is ten- to 50-fold less frequent than candidiasis or aspergillosis. It also reveals that mucormycosis appears in one to five cases per 10,000 autopsies. In patients undergoing allogenic bone marrow transplantation, the incidence may be 2% to 3%.

The main risk factors for the development of mucormycosis are ketoacidosis (diabetic or other), iatrogenic immunosuppression, especially when associated with neutropenia and graft versus host disease in hematological patients, use of corticosteroids or deferoxamine, disruption of mucocutaneous barriers by catheters and other devices, and even exposure to bandages contaminated with these fungi.

Mucorales invade deep tissues via inhalation of airborne spores, percutaneous inoculation, or ingestion. These fungi colonize a high number of patients but do not necessarily cause invasion and disease.

Mucormycosis is very infrequent in immunocompetent patients.

Mucormycosis may occur after traumatic inoculation, especially in those cases where the inoculation is accompanied by contamination with water and soil. Mortality in these circumstances fluctuates between 38% and 80%.

Mucormycosis manifests most commonly, respectively, in the sinuses, lungs, skin, brain, and gastrointestinal tract. After *Aspergillus* and *Candida* infections, *Mucorales* infections are the third most common fungal infections seen in patients with hematologic malignancies.

With the exception of rhinocerebral and cutaneous mucormycosis, the clinical diagnosis of mucormycosis is difficult, and is often made at a late stage of the disease or postmortem.

The number of cases of cutaneous and soft tissue mucormycosis has increased during the last few years. This condition can occur on problem-free skin or follow the rupture of barriers, (i.e., through surgery, trauma, or burns). Sometimes, the infection begins at catheter insertion sites or even after insect bites. It has also been described after the use of contaminated dressings and intramuscular injections.

Most patients with cutaneous mucormycosis have underlying conditions such as diabetes mellitus, solid organ transplants, or leukemia.

There are three clinical patterns of presentation of mucormycosis infection:

(i) Cutaneous infection: This is rare and characterized by the development of erythematous and edematous lesions or papular and nodular lesions, which originate as necrotic vesicobullous or ulcerated lesions (Fig. 8.18). The fungus is an exogenous agent inoculated by trauma or it can be an endogenous agent coming from a visceral focus. The clinical manifestations range from pustules or vesicles to wounds with wide necrotic zones. Mucromycoses are characterized by particularly necrotic skin lesions due to the angiocentric nature of these microorganisms. In their early stages, lesions may be similar to those present in ecthyma gangrenosum. In extensive lesions, a cotton-like growth may be observed over the surface of the tissues, a clinical sign known as "hairy pus." Rapid diagnosis of cutaneous mucormycosis may explain the lower rate of associated mortality.

(ii) Rhinosinus mucormycosis: The acute infection is dramatic. At the onset the sinuses or palate are involved with progressive invasion of the orbit or brain tissues. There is invasion of the nose, orbit, and later, the secondary invasion of the intracranial structures. This form of infection is involved in 33% to 50% of all cases of mucormycosis. The most frequent underlying conditions associated are ketoacidotic diabetes mellitus, and leukemia. Patients that are solid organ or hematopoietic stem cell recipients and patients with HIV infection are also more frequently affected.

(iii) Systemic infection: Fatigue and general symptoms are seen, including weight loss. The infection can disseminate to the lungs or gastrointestinal system, causing organ-specific symptoms.

Tests using cultures of clinical samples have limited sensitivity. Specimens should be cut into small fragments before plating. The presence of wide, nonseptate hyphae in culture or on slides should always be interpreted with care, as they may represent colonization. Histopathological testing does not indicate the genus and species, and should therefore be complemented with culture. Perineural invasion, angioinvasion, and infarction are common histologic findings in *Mucorales* infections. Histological invasion, particularly of vessels, by wide, nonseptate hyphae branched at right angles is diagnostic in the appropriate clinical context.

Treatment

Mucormycosis requires a rapid diagnosis, correction of predisposing factors, surgical resection, debridement, and appropriate antifungal therapy. Some studies have 50% of cases diagnosed postmortem. Predisposing factors that could be addressed include diabetic ketoacidosis, corticosteroids and deferoxamine. Rapid and complete surgery, if possible, is the best treatment for mucormycosis. In fact, partial resection of necrotic tissue is better than none at all, although this is easier in the cutaneous and rhinocerebral forms than in the visceral forms. Pulmonary and disseminated disease in neutropenic patients is impossible to operate on in many cases. Surgery combined with the use of antifungal drugs is always better than antifungal therapy alone. Current data, although indirect, points to high-dose liposomal amphotericin B as the therapy of choice for this condition. Liposomal amphotericin B is better tolerated and has a lower toxicity. Itraconazole, despite its in vitro activity against *Mucorales* and its success in a few clinical cases, is considered an inappropriate therapy choice.

Voriconazole is not active in vitro against *Mucorales* and fails when used in vivo. Posaconazole and ravuconazole have good activity in vitro and, in animal models. Posaconazole has proven to be superior to itraconazole but less effective than amphotericin B deoxycholate. Recent studies indicate that use of posaconazole is effective in clinical failures with amphotericin B and other treatments. Currently, it is the most promising therapeutic alternative to amphotericin B. Some authors consider that further studies should be done to determine the potential role of caspofungin in mucormycosis, as there may be a synergy between caspofungin and amphotericin B lipid complex.

Cytokines such as γ-interferon or granulocyte–macrophage colony-stimulating factor (GM-CSF) have also been used to treat mucormycosis (Table 8.4).

Entomophthoromycosis

For this fungus, the general health state of the patient is not compromised, and it is defined as a chronic disease generally localized tithe subcutaneous tissue or the nasal submucosa.

Usually, the disease consists of two entities, basidiobolomycosis and conidiobolomycosis, which are both capable of inducing chronic subcutaneous granulomatous infections that are histopathologically similar but clinically and mycologically different.

Entomophthorales organisms are aerobic and grow in most culture media after 2 to 5 days of inoculation and at temperatures of 25°C to 37°C whereas *Mucorales* organisms typically show growth at 55°C. Entomophthorales (genera *Conidiobolus*

Table 8.4: Different Genera of Mucormycetes and Species

Family	Genus	Species
Cunninghamellaceae	*Cunninghamella*	*C. bertholletiae*
Mortierellaceae	*Mortierella*	
Saksenaceae	*Saksenaea*	*S. vasiformis*
Syncephalastraceae	*Syncephalastrum*	*S. racemosum*
Mucoraceae	*Absidia*	*A. corymbifera*
	Apophysomyces	*A. elegans*
	Mucor	*M. circinelloides*
		M. hiemalis
		M. racemosus
		M. ramosissimus
		M. rouxianus
	Rhizopus	*R. pusillus*
		R. arrhizus
Thamnidaceae	*Cokeromyces*	*C. recurvatus*

coronatus and *Basidiobolus ranarum*) infect primarily immunocompetent individuals and produce chronic, generally indolent, cutaneous, nasal, or sinus disease.

Basidiobolomycosis is caused by *Basidiobolus ranarum* and is also called subcutaneous phycomycosis, subcutaneous zygomycosis, or entomophthoromycosis basidiobolae. This fungus is usually detected in the intestinal tube of toads, frogs, lizards, and in the insect class.

Conidiobolomycosis is due to *Conidiobolus coronatus* and is also called rhinoentomophthoromycosis, rhinophycomycosis, or rhinophycomycosis entomophthorae. This agent is found in soil, often in the presence of decomposing plant matter.

There are three clinical forms: subcutaneous, centrofacial, and visceral. The agents are soil, saprophytic fungi, organisms found in animal feces, saprophytes or parasites of insects and small animals.

(i) The subcutaneous form of infection is caused by *Basidiobolus haptosporus*, a soil saprophytic fungus. Through cutaneous trauma, the parasite is inoculated in the skin and subcutaneous infection occurs. It can involve the adjacent structures, such as muscles or bones, and disseminate to internal organs by contiguity or hematogenous dissemination. *Basidiobolus ranarum* typically causes a chronic infection of the peripheral or subcutaneous tissue, generally on the arms, trunk, and buttocks. It is usually acquired by traumatic implantation. The disease slowly evolutes after months or years.

(ii) The centrofacial form of infection, named *rhinophycomycosis*, is caused by *Conidiobolus coronatus*. This fungus reaches the nasal mucosa by inhalation or trauma. This form of entomophthoromycosis occurs in adults and rarely in children. The clinical manifestations include nasal obstruction, rhinitis, and epistaxis. On physical examination, there are enanthems of the mucosa, edema, and polypoid or nodular lesions in the nasal cavity. The patients develop cutaneous edema and progressive infiltration in the centrofacial region. The infection progresses to involve the nasopharynx, oropharynx, palate, larynx, and sometimes the blood stream.

(iii) The visceral form is rare, can occur in adults and children, and the symptoms are related to the organ involved. The visceral form is usually caused by *Conidiobolus incongruns* that infects the host via inhalation or trauma.

Because *Entomophthorales* organisms are ubiquitous and may be laboratory contaminants, diagnosis should be verified by histological demonstration of organisms in affected tissues. The fungus is difficult to isolate in culture, with an 85% rate of negative cultures having been reported in several international papers.

Entomophthorales infections are characterized by a mixed granulomatous inflammatory infiltrate with eosinophils, histiocytes, neutrophils, plasma cells, and giant cells. In addition, hyphal elements may be surrounded by a dense eosinophilic sleeve-like material. A polymerase chain reaction (PCR) assay has recently been developed and may be useful in cases in where the diagnosis is suspected but histology and culture findings are negative.

Treatment

Potassium iodide has been the traditional drug employed in the treatment, although several other drugs, such as amphotericin B, cotrimoxazole, ketoconazole, itraconazole, and fluconazole have been successfully tried. A combination of amphotericin B and terbinafine has been reported. Treatment also includes aggressive surgical debridement and control of underlying risk factors. Treatment failures with amphotericin B have been reported, and itraconazole may be preferred as a first-line agent at a dose of 200–400 mg/day.

Cryptococcosis

Cryptococcosis is a fungal infection caused by two varieties of *Cryptococcus neoformans*, with five serotypes. According to some researchers, *C. neoformans* var. *grubii* represents strains of serotype A, var. *neoformans* represents strains of serotypes D and AD, and var. *gattii* represents strains of serotypes B and C. Based on sequential analysis of intergenic rDNA spaces, Diaz *et al.* consider two pathogenic varieties: C. neoformans (serotypes A, D and AD) and *Cryptococcus bacillisporus* (serotypes B and C). The latter corresponds to *C. neoformans* var. *gattii*.

Cryptococcus neoformans is a dimorphic fungus, frequently recovered from pigeon droppings and nesting places, soil, and dust. Immunosuppressed individuals – such as those with HIV (most common risk factor) or malignancies, those receiving immunosuppressive medication after organ transplantation, or those with connective tissue diseases such as systemic lupus erythematosus – are at an increased risk for developing cryptococcosis after exposure. Interestingly, individuals who work with pigeons are not at an increased risk for this disease.

Cryptococcosis is the most common systemic mycotic infection in AIDS patients, affecting 3% to 7% of this population. It occurs in 6% to 13% of patients with AIDS, when their CD4 lymphocyte count is below 200/mm³. Cryptococcosis at other sites follows dissemination from the lungs. Cryptococcal meningitis is the most common condition. Cutaneous involvement and other conditions like endophthalmitis, chorioretinitis

(Fig. 8.19e), conjunctivitis, sinusitis, myocarditis, pericarditis, endocarditis, gastroduodenitis, hepatitis, cholecystitis, peritonitis, renal abscesses, adrenal involvement, arthritis, osteomyelitis, lymphadenitis, and breast masses have also been reported.

When the host is immunocompromised, *C. neoformans* cells try to escape the defenses of the organism by producing sialic acid, capsulated polysaccharides, melanin, mannitol, and phospholipase. In contrast, in immunocompetent hosts, the mechanisms of pathogenicity have not been carefully clarified. In cryptococcosis, melanin seems to interfere with the virulence of the yeast, with great tropism for the central nervous system, which is rich in catecholamines.

Clinically, cryptococcosis manifests as primary cutaneous and disseminated systemic disease (Fig. 8.19). Primary cutaneous cryptococcosis occurs through direct infection from an object contaminated with *Cryptococcus*. This rare presentation manifests as a single lesion at the site of infection; it usually clears without systemic therapy. Cutaneous disease, which affects 10% to 20% of patients, may also appear as a result of disseminated cryptococcosis. The lesions vary greatly in morphology. Cutaneous cryptococcosis in its generalized forms, especially in patients with AIDS, presents with multiple lesions, most of them simulating molluscum contagiosum. Acneiform, nodular or herpetiform lesions, or cellulitis also occur. Cutaneous cryptococcosis is three times more likely to occur in men than in women, possibly because of the protective effects of estrogen.

Disseminated cryptococcosis begins as an infection in the respiratory tract that spreads hematogenously from the primary pulmonary site to the skin, prostate, liver, kidneys, bone, and peritoneum. Disseminated *Cryptococcus* is more common in AIDS and renal transplant patients but may occasionally occur in patients with hematologic malignancies. Cutaneous signs may be the first indication of infection, sometimes preceding the diagnosis of disseminated cryptococcosis by 2 to 8 months. Recognizing cutaneous lesions is important in preventing the severe neurologic sequela of cryptococcosis. Lesions mostly appear on the head and neck, first as painless papules or pustules, then later develop into nodules that ulcerate and ooze purulent material. Vasculitic lesions presenting

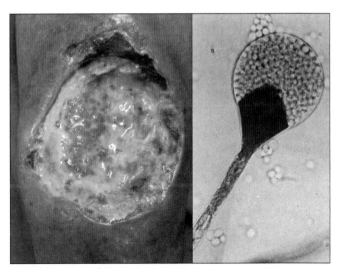

Figure 8.18. Cutaneous mucormycosis. A: ulcerative and destructive lesion on leg; B: Mucor (microcultive).

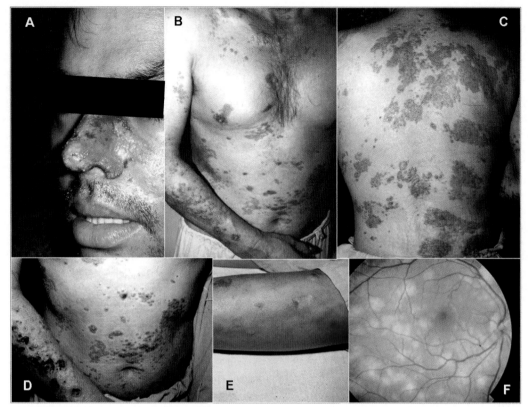

Figure 8.19. Cryptococcosis. A, B, C, D: extensive cutaneous lesions in a immunosuppressed patient; E: chorioretinitis (lesions on retina).

as palpable purpura; eczematous, follicular, or purple papules; nodules; and plaques that resemble Kaposi sarcoma may appear as well. Secondary osteomyelitis may develop; draining sinuses may form as a result of subsequent growth to overlying skin. The mortality of untrearted disseminated cryptococcosis is 70% to 80%.

Diagnosis

- Direct examination and culture: Skin biopsy reveals plenty of budding yeast cells with demarcated capsules of 5 to 10 mm in size by India ink preparation (IIP) and Gram staining. Specimens are inoculated on Sabouraud dextrose agar (SDA) and incubated at 37°C and room temperature (RT). On SDA, creamy flat, shiny, moist mucoid colonies grow with smooth edges. Luxuriant growth on SDA at RT are observed in 2 days.
- Antigen detection: Detection of capsular polysaccharide by latex agglutination (LA) using a variety of U.S. Food and Drug Administration (FDA)-cleared test kits is a most useful method for rapid diagnosis of cryptococcal meningitis, and is positive in about 90% of cases. Antigen also can be detected in serum, especially in patients with AIDS. Antigenemia may be seen in patients with pneumonia but then should undergo prompt evaluation for meningitis or other sites of extrapulmonary dissemination. Antigen may also be detected in BAL in patients with pneumonia. In most studies, specificity is above 95%. Causes for false-positive results include rheumatoid factor, antiidiotype antibodies, infection with cross-reactive organisms (*Trichosporon asahiii, Capnocytophaga*

canimorsus), contaminated agar, use of disinfectants or soaps to wash ring slides, and defective test kits.
- Antibody response: This plays no meaningful role.

Treatment

Most of the recent information regarding treatment of cryptococcosis has been derived from experience in HIV patients. The recommended therapy is a 2-week course of amphoterecin B 0.7 mg/kg/day plus flucytosine 100 mg/kg/day followed by 8 weeks of fluconazole 400 mg/day. Fluconazole at higher doses (400–800 mg/day), alone or in combination with flucytosine, has been used successfully. Although it has been suggested that immunocompromised patients should receive suppressive therapy with low-dose fluconazole (200 mg/day) until recovery of their host defenses, it is uncertain whether this is necessary.

Phaeohyphomycosis

Phaeohyphomycosis encompasses distinct mycotic infections regardless of the site of the lesion, of the pattern of tissue response, or of the taxonomic classification of the etiologic agents. Subcutaneous phaeohyphomycosis (Fig. 8.20a & b), improperly named phaeohyphomycotic cyst, is the most common presentation and also includes cases with dermal involvement. Patients are usually adults, and some of them are immunologically compromised with associated underlying diseases or locally compromised because of the application of topical corticosteroids.

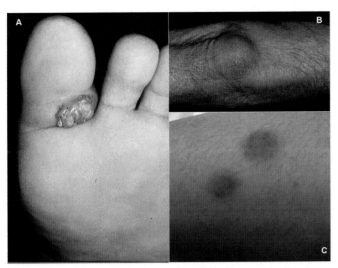

Figure 8.20. Phaeohyphomycosis and Hyalohyphomycosis. A and B: subcutaneous phaeohyphomycosis; C: hyalohyphomycosis due to *Fusarium spp.* Purpuric lesions on the thigh in a patient with severe neutropenia secondary to leukemia.

Isolation and identification of the causative organisms is very important because of variable sensitivity to therapeutic agents.

Because of the increasing number of immunocompromised patients, the number of fungi causing subcutaneous phaeohyphomycosis has been increasing. Among them, members of the genera *Alternaria*, *Bipolaris*, *Curvularia*, *Exophiala*, *Phialophora*, and *Wangiella* are the most common species. Despite the morphological differences among species, the illnesses they produce have common features. Subcutaneous phaeohyphomycosis has occurred with equal frequency in tropical, subtropical, and temperate areas.

Subcutaneous phaeohyphomycosis lesions occur often on exposed body parts and especially on the upper arms. Inoculation of the agent is considered to be caused by wounds made by contaminated plant materials. The spectrum of clinical presentation is broad, ranging from well-localized cysts to aggressive infections that invade surrounding tissue. The most common and typical lesions are subcutaneous cysts or abscesses at the site of trauma, frequently caused by *Exophiala jeanselmei*. The primary lesion occurs as an asymptomatic, small, palpable nodule. The nodule gradually evolves to become an encapsulated, fluctuant abscess with a liquefied center. Occasionally, a granulomatous elevated plaque may also appear. Less frequently, it is manifested as a verrucous nodule or a diffuse extensive infiltration simulating borderline leprosy.

Cutaneous disease may persist for months or years. Immunocompromised patients often present with multiple lesions. Lymph node involvement and dissemination are rare. However, systemic phaeohyphomycosis may occur from the subcutaneous infections in immunocompromised patients.

Hyalohyphomycosis

The great increase in the immunosuppressed patient population has been accompanied by an increasing list of fungal opportunistic infections. The underlying diseases and the intensive immunosuppressive, antineoplastic, antibiotic, and corticosteroid treatments all contribute.

Ajello and McGinnis proposed the name "hyalohyphomycosis" to accommodate mycotic infections in which the etiologic agent's tissue form is septate hyphae with no pigment in the wall and is characterized by hyaline hyphae in tissue.

Hyalohyphomycosis generally occurs in patients with severe underlying systemic disorders such as leukemia, lymphoma, systemic lupus erythematosus, or diabetes mellitus. The skin is one of the most common organs involved, and regional lymph nodes are also often affected. Occasionally, the etiologic fungi invade the blood vessels and evoke fungemia.

Dissemination of hyalohyphomycosis occurs more often than with phaeohyphomycosis. *Acremonium* spp., *Fusarium* spp., *Paecilomyces* spp., *Penicillium* spp., *Scopulariopsis* spp. and *Trichoderma* spp. are known to be common causative organisms, whereas *Pseudallescheria boydii* is less prevalent. Histologically, it may be impossible to differentiate between these organisms based on morphology alone. Definitive identification of the causative organism is needed for effective treatment. In one review of disseminated *Fusarium* infections, for example, the skin was the nidus of infection in 33% of patients. Hematogenous dissemination from primary skin infections generally occurs only in very neutropenic patients and carries a high risk of mortality (Fig. 8.20c). In hyalohyphomycosis, thrombotic phenomenon with local invasion is common, and the majority of organisms show some sensitivity to amphotericin B.

Species of the genus *Fusarium* are usually plant saprophytes and pathogens, known by dermatologists as skin contaminants. Occasionally, however, these organisms may cause disease in man. *Fusarium* species have long been known as rapidly destructive agents in infections of the cornea, burned skin, and subcutaneous lesions following trauma, mainly in immunocompromised patients. The species is almost always *Fusarium solani*.

Treatment

It consists of antifungal medications and surgical debridement. The therapy varies depending on the etiological agent and the clinical state of the patient. *P. boydii* is often resistant to amphotericin B. In most cases, miconazole has shown the best in vitro activity against *P. boydii*. Hyalohyphomycosis caused by *Fusarium spp.* is frequently refractory to antifungal therapy, particularly in granulocytopenic patients, and restoration of host defense is essential in order for treatment to be effective. *Fusarium* dissemination occurs and progresses in spite of amphotericin B therapy. Nowadays, voriconazole associated with amphoterecin B has been successful in these cases.

Voriconazole maintains the general properties of the azoles. However, it has a more pronounced blockage of ergosterol synthesis in the filamentous fungi, for which it acts as a fungicide. It has a more intense in vitro effect than itraconazole on *Aspergillus* species, including *A. terreus*, which is commonly resistant to amphotericin B. It is effective against many species of *Fusarium, Paecilomyces, Alternaria,* and *Bipolaris*, as well as against *Scedosporium apiospermum* and *P. boydii*.

Voriconazole is administered orally or intravenously in a dosage of 6 mg/kg of body weight every 12 hours on the first day and 4 mg/kg of body weight every 12 hours thereafter. Adults receive oral doses of 200 mg (in tablet form) every 12 hours

(100 mg every 12 hours for patients weighing less than 40 kg), which makes it possible to reach a maximum serum concentration of 4 to 6 μg/mL in a state of equilibrium. Absorption does not depend on gastric acidity, and the bioavailability of the oral drug is good. Voriconazole reaches levels inhibitory for fungi in the encephalon and in the cerebrospinal fluid. Because it is metabolized and excreted by the liver, it is necessary to adjust the dosage or avoid its use in cases of hepatic insufficiency. In cases of moderate to severe renal insufficiency, intravenous administration is contraindicated because of the risk of accumulation of the vehicle cyclodextrin.

OTHER OPPORTUNISTIC DEEP CUTANEOUS FUNGAL INFECTIONS

Occasionally, the opportunistic fungi may also cause a variety of other skin lesions such as subcutaneous nodules, abscesses, and folliculitis. There are no pathognomonic features of these skin lesions, and identification of the causative organisms requires tissue biopsy for culture. Primary fungal skin infections may occur at the cutaneous insertion site of intravenous catheters and at the sites of contact with arm boards in pediatric patients.

Most reported cases have involved *Aspergillus* or *Rhizopus* spp. The skin lesion is usually a red plaque, which may be studded with pustules or vesicles. A subsequent eschar often develops within the plaque. Hospitalized neutropenic patients are at a higher risk of primary cutaneous infections by opportunistic fungi (especially *Aspergillus*, *Mucor*, *Rhizopus*, and *Fusarium* spp.). However, these infections are unusual even in this patient population. Damage to the epidermis facilitates local skin infection that may be caused by a number of factors: intravenous catheters directly disrupt the skin, tape and occlusive dressings may cause maceration, prolonged administration of corticosteroids (e.g., for GVHD) may cause cutaneous atrophy and increase the risk of skin infection, and patients with chronic cutaneous GVHD experience a greater number of skin infections (as is seen in other chronic inflammatory dermatoses such as psoriasis and atopic dermatitis).

Because *Aspergillus*, *Fusarium*, and *Rhizopus* spp., etc. are common saprophytes, a positive culture alone is not proof of infection. A skin biopsy specimen that demonstrates tissue invasion is ideal. Repeated cultures that yield only the suspected fungal pathogen are also suggestive. Primary skin infections caused by opportunistic fungi may act as a nidus for fungemia and subsequent multiorgan involvement. These occurrences have been documented in all of the primary skin lesions described earlier (paronychias, infections under adhesive dressings, etc.).

Regionally endemic pathogenic fungi rarely cause primary skin infections in cancer patients; most are caused by *Histoplasma* or *Coccidioides* spp. These skin infections can act as a nidus for dissemination in the neutropenic host. In addition, patients who were immunocompetent at the time of initial skin infection, and who have residual skin lesions, may experience reactivation when immunosuppression occurs.

When treating patients with a combination of two or more antifungal agents, except under certain conditions, care must be taken to avoid the possibility of antagonism between the drugs. The combination of amphotericin B and 5-fluorocytosine presents synergy and is the initial treatment for cryptococcosis and in certain cases of candidiasis and aspergillosis. The same effect occurs with fluconazole and 5-fluorocytosine in cryptococcosis and candidiasis. However, the combination of amphotericin B and azole drugs might result in lower efficacy than that of amphotericin B in isolated use or, simply, in the absence of synergism. In general, the combined use of itraconazole or other azoles and amphotericin B is avoided, and, if possible, the use of amphotericin B in sequence to a therapeutic course of itraconazole or other azoles is also avoided. Terbinafine, echinocandins, and voriconazole are being investigated in sequence with one another and with traditional antifungal agents in infections produced in animals, as well as, experimentally, in patients with severe fungal infections. The results have varied, and it has not yet been possible to clearly make other associations with the synergistic effect on the efficacy of antifungal agents.

In Table 8.5, we summarize the antifungal therapies for adults with disseminated or systemic deep fungal diseases.

PITFALLS AND MYTHS

Mycotic infections are common and their incidence is increasing. Fungal infections are typically diagnosed by culture, serology, or histopathology. They can be difficult to distinguish from other infections, particularly tuberculosis, but there are numerous clinical clues that can help suggest the presence of systemic mycoses. Intradermal tests, serologic tests, and agent isolation can aid in the confirmation of a fungal infection. Diagnosis of deep fungal infections is not straightforward. Definitive diagnosis requires the demonstration of fungi in tissue specimens obtained by biopsy together with a positive culture. Modern molecular techniques are promising, including PCR that is being developed to help with rapid diagnosis of deep fungal infections, since they have higher specificity and sensitivity, particularly with the use of DNA probes.

There are two medical scenarios that represent a challenge to definitive diagnosis on deep fungal infections: (i) the presence of the "verrucous cutaneous syndrome," and/or (ii) the histopathological descriptive diagnosis of pseudoepitheliomatous and granulomatous dermatitis without an identifiable infectious agent.

The verrucous cutaneous syndrome is known by the acronym "LECT," *L*eishmaniasis, *E*sporotricose (Portuguese) (Sporotrichosis, English), *C*hromomycosis, *T*uberculosis, which are infectious diseases that can present like verrucous cutaneous lesions. The specific intradermal tests, cultures of skin fragments obtained by biopsies, and serology studies can help in definitive diagnosis.

The presence of pseudoepitheliomatous hyperplasia (PH) with dermal and/or subcutaneous granuloma is another challenge in the diagnosis of deep fungal disease. PH is a histopathological reaction that is characterized by a downward proliferation of the epidermis, which may suggest a squamous cell carcinoma. These lesions show an epithelial hyperplasia that includes an irregular invasion of the dermis by uneven and jagged epidermal masses. By strict criteria, this process also involves the epithelium of adnexal structures after they undergo squamous metaplasia. PH occurs secondary to a wide range of stimuli, most notably, a chronic inflammatory process (i.e., deep fungal diseases).

Table 8.5: Summary of Treatment Options in Deep Fungal Diseases

Fungal disease/Clinical form	First-Choice Therapy	Alternative Therapy
PARACOCCIDIOIDOMYCOSIS Lungs, oral or laryngeal mucosa	Itra (400 mg/day; 6–18 months*) or SMZ-TMP (2400–480 mg/day or 1600–320 mg/day; 12–24 months*)	Keto (400 mg/day) Fluco (400 mg/day)
Disseminated, severe cases	Amph B-d (total dose 30–60 mg/kg) followed by Itra (400 mg/day; 6–12 months)	Itra, Keto, Fluco
CRYPTOCOCCOSIS Pleuropulmonary localized, in patients without immunosuppression	Fluco (200–400 mg/day; 3–12 months)	Amph B-d (total dose: 20–35 mg/kg)
Disseminated, meningitis or immunosuppression	Amph B-d: 0.7–1.0 mg/kg/day plus 5-FC (100 mg/kg/day: 2 weeks), followed by Fluco (400–800 mg/day; 10 weeks) followed by Fluco (200 mg/day; ≥ 6 months)	Amph B-d (total dose: >35 mg/kg) followed by Fluco (200 mg/day during > 6 months)
COCCIDIOIDOMYCOSIS Pulmonary acute diffuse	Amph B-d (total dose: 20–35 mg/kg)	Itra, Keto, Fluco
Disseminated	Itra (400 mg/day; ≥ 12 months)	
Pulmonary, chronic fibrous-cavitary disease	Itra (400 mg/day; ≥ 12 months)	Keto (400 mg/day); Fluco (400 mg/day); Amph B-d
HISTOPLASMOSIS Pulmonary, acute, severe or prolonged disease	Itra (400 mg/day; 6–12 weeks)	Amph B-d (total dose: 20 mg/kg) followed by Itra (400mg/day; 12 weeks)
Pulmonary chronic; mild disseminated	Itra (400 mg/day; 12–24 months)	Amph B-d (total dose: 20–35 mg/kg) followed by Itra (400 mg/day; 12–24 months)
Disseminated and severe or immunosuppressed patients	Amph B-d (total dose: > 35 mg/kg) followed by Itra (400 mg/day; ≥ 24 months)	Itra (400–600 mg/day)
SPOROTRICHOSIS Cutaneous-lymphatic	Potassium iodide (KI) 4–6 g/day during 2–3 months	Itra (100–400 mg/day)
Pulmonary, disseminated	Amph B-d (total dose 500–1000 mg) or Itra (400 mg/day; 3–6 months)	Itra (400–600 mg/day; 6–12 months)
ZYGO (MURCOMYCOSIS) Pulmonary, invasive, disseminated	Amph B-d (total dose > 35 mg/kg)	Amph B-l
PHAEOHYPHOMYCOSIS pulmonary/systemic (*Bipolaris, Exophiala, Exserohilium, Phialophora, Wangiella ssp, etc*)	Amph B-d (total dose > 35 mg/kg) and / or Vorico 400 mg/day, intravenous	Amph B-l; Itra (400–600 mg/day)
HYALOHYPHOMYCOSIS pulmonary/systemic (*Acremonium, Paecylomices, Scopulariopsis spp*, etc)	Amph B-d (total dose > 35 mg/kg) and / or Vorico 400 mg/day, intravenous	Amph B-l; Itra (400–600 mg/day)
FUSARIOSIS pulmonary/invasive/disseminated	Amph B-d (total dose > 30–35 mg/kg) and / or Vorico 400 mg/day, intravenous	Amph B-l
NEUTROPENIC patients with persistent fever	Amph B-d or Amph B-l	Itra, Fluco, Vorico or Caspo

SMZ-TMP, sulfamethoxazole–trimethoprim; Amph B, amphotericin B desoxycholate – conventional preparation; Amph B-l, amphotericin B in lipid formulations: L-Amph, liposomal / Cd-Amph B, coloidal dispersion/Lc Ampho b, lipid complex; Keto, Ketoconazole; Itra, Itraconazole; Fluco, Fluconazole; Vorico, Voriconazole; Caspo, Caspofungin;* Variable period of treatment, according to case severity.

Neither histopathology pattern is specific of the mycosis because deep fungal infections are able to induce a varied spectrum of inflammatory lesions. So it is very important to evaluate the immunological status of the patient, which in many cases is diminished, because the mycoses are much more frequent in immunodeficient patients. So for an infection to take place, there must exist a series of factors that favor it. Examples of these factors include the immunity of the guest, the virulence, the amount of fungal cells, and the coexistence of other diseases. The first response that the organism produces is a suppurative inflammation by the infiltrates of polymorphonuclear cells. Later, a response of mononuclear cells and, if it evolves, epithelioid macrophage cells and multinuclear giant cells, can give rise to a chronic infection and to fibrosis. Nevertheless, all this can be attenuated if the patient suffers from an immunosuppressive disease or is undergoing immunosuppressive therapy. The most characteristic histopathology finding is the granuloma lesion with multinucleated giant cells, stimulated by the cellular immune response.

The pathologist can observe the fungi with two basic morphologies. The first is with a tubular form or hyphae (multicellular) and the second with an oval form corresponds with the spores or conidia (unicellular). Also, these forms, may or may not be pigmented.

The pathologist can identify and diagnose infections by fungi classified into one of the four groups: dimorphic fungus, classic pathogens, opportunists, and others.

The ubiquitous dematiaceous fungi can be contaminants in cultures, making the determination of clinical significance problematic. A high degree of clinical suspicion as well as correlation with appropriate clinical findings is required when interpreting culture results. Unfortunately, there are no simple serological or antigen tests available to detect these fungi in blood or tissue. PCR is being studied as an aid to the diagnosis of these fungal infections, but as yet is not widely available or reliable. However, studies have begun to examine the potential of identifying species within this diverse group of fungi using PCR of highly conserved regions of ribosomal DNA. The diagnosis of phaeohyphomycosis currently rests on pathological examination of clinical specimens and careful gross and microscopic examination of cultures, requiring the expertise of a mycology reference laboratory. In tissue, they will stain with the Fontana–Masson stain. Longer than normal staining times may be required. This can be helpful in distinguishing these fungi from other species, particularly *Aspergillus*. In addition, hyphae typically appear more fragmented in tissue than seen with *Aspergillus*, with irregular septate hyphae and beaded, yeast-like forms.

Deep fungal infections continue to be an important cause of morbidity and mortality, especially in transplant recipients and other immunosuppressed patients. The insidious nature and atypical manifestations of these infections often delay diagnosis and therapy. In immunosuppressed patients, persistent fever that does not respond to antibacterial therapy should alert the physician to the possibility of fungal infection.

SUGGESTED READINGS

Almeida OP, Jacks Jr. J. Paracoccidioidomycosis of the mouth: an emerging deep mycosis. Crit Rev Oral Biol Med 2003; 14(5):377–382.

Almeida SM. Central nervous system paracoccidioidomycosis: An Overview. Braz J Infect Dis 2005;9(2):126–133.

Artal EM. Diagnóstico histopatológico de las micosis. Rev Iberoam Micol 2004; 21: 1–9.

Bonifaz A, Cansela R, Novales J, de Oca GM, Navarrete G, Romo J. Cutaneous histoplasmosis associated with acquired immunodeficiency syndrome (AIDS). Int J Dermatol 2000;39(1):35–38.

Chapman SW, Bradsher RW Jr, Campbell GD Jr, Pappas PG, Kauffman CA. Practice guidelines for the management of patients with blastomycosis. Infectious Diseases Society of America. Clin Infect Dis 2000;30(4):679–683.

Costa AR, Valente NY, Criado PR, Pires MC, Vasconcellos C. Invasive hyalohyphomycosis due to Fusarium solani in a patient with acute lymphocytic leukemia. Int J Dermatol 2000;39(9):717–718.

Damian DL, Barnetson RC, Thompson JC. Treatment of Refractory Chromomycosis by Isolated Limb Infusion with Melphalan and Actinomycin D. J Cutan Med Surgery 2006;10(1):48–51.

Dharmshale SN, Patil SA, Gohil A, Chowdhary A, Oberoi C. Disseminated crytococcosis with extensive cutaneous involvement in AIDS. Indian J Med Microbiol 2006;24:228–230.

Diaz MR, Boekhout T, Theelen B, Fell JW. Molecular sequence analysis of the intergenic spacer (IGS) associated with rDNA of the two varieties of the pathogenic yeast C. neoformans. System Appl Microbiol 2000;23:535–545.

Elsayed S, Kuhn SM, Barber D, Church DL, Adams S, Kasper R. Human case of lobomycosis. Emerg Infect Dis 2004;10(4):715–718.

Foss NT, Rocha MRO, Lima VTA, Velludo MASL, Roselino AMF. Entomophthoramycosis: therapeutic success by using Amphoteric B and Terbinafine. Dermatology 1996;193:258–260.

Gimenes VM, Criado PR, Martins JE, Almeida SR. Cellular immune response of patients with chromoblastomycosis undergoing antifungal therapy. Mycopathologia 200;162(2):97–101.

Gimenes VMF, de Souza MG, Ferreira KS, Marques SG, Goncalves AG, Santos Dvcl, Silva Cde MP, Almeida SR. Cytokines and lymphocyte proliferation in patients with different clinical forms of chromoblastomycosis. Microbes Infect 2005;7(4):708–713.

Goel R, Wallace ML. Pseudoepitheliomatous hyperplasia secondary to cutaneous aspergillus. Am J Dermatopathol 2001;23(3):224–226.

Gray NA, Baddour LM. Cutaneous inoculation blastomycosis. Clin Infect Dis 2002;34(10):E44–49.

Kimura M, McGinnis MR. Nomenclature for fungus infections Int J Dermatol 1998;37(11):825–828.

Koga T, Matsuda T, Matsumoto T, Furue M. Therapeutic Approaches to Subcutaneous Mycoses. Am J Clin Dermatol 2003;4(8):537–543.

Larone, DH 1995. Medically Important Fungi – A Guide to Identification, 3rd ed. ASM Press, Washington, D.C.

Lopes-Bezerra LM, Schubach A, Costa RO. Sporothrix schenckii and sporotrichosis. An Acad Bras Cienc 2006;78(2):293–308.

Lupi O, Tyring SK, McGinnis MR. Tropical dermatology: fungal tropical diseases. J Am Acad Dermatol 2005;53(6):931–951.

Martinez R. An update on the use of antifungal agents. J Bras Pneumol 2006; 32(5):449–460.

Mays SR, Bogle MA, Bodey GP. Cutaneous fungal infections in the oncology patient: recognition and management. Am J Clin Dermatol 2006;7(1):31–34.

Pincelli TPH, Brandt HCR, Motta AL, Maciel FVR, Criado PR. Fusariosis in an immunocompromised patient: therapeutic success with voriconazole. An Bras Dermatol 2008;83:331–334. Disponível em: http://www.anaisdedermatologia.org.br/artigo_imprimir.php?artigo_id=100887 (text in Portuguese. Abstract in English)

Revankar SG. Dematiaceous fungi. Mycoses 2007; 50: 91–101.

Shikanai-Yasuda MA, Telles Filho FQ, Mendes RP et al. Consenso em Paracoccidioidomicose. Rev. Soc. Bras. Med. Trop. [Online]. 2006, Vol. 39, No. 3 [Cited 2007-02-20], pp. 297–310. Disponível em: http://www.scielo.br/scielo.php?script=sci_arttext&pid=S0037-86822006000300017&lng=pt&nrm=iso> (text in Portuguese).

Wheat LJ. Antigen detection, serology, and molecular diagnosis of invasive mycoses in the immunocompromised host. Transpl Infect Dis 2006;8:128–139.

9 | PARASITOLOGY

Francisco G. Bravo and Salim Mohanna

This chapter will cover most of the organisms that directly or indirectly compromise tissues through human infection. Although in developed countries they are considered exotic diseases just to be diagnosed in travelers, many of them represent a major health problem for developing countries around the world.

HISTORY

Parasites have accompanied mankind since antiquity. Dracunculiasis is described in the Ebers papyrus from 1500 BC, and references to this disease are clearly identified in the Bible. The ancient symbol of medicine, the staff of Asklepios, is believed by some scholars to also represent the treatment of dracunculaisis which involves slowly extracting the worm by winding it around a stick. This treatment is still in use to this day. Tenias were described by the ancient Greeks and are cited by Aristotle in his *History of Animals*.

Protozoa have ancient history in human disease annals. Evidence of *Trypanosoma cruzi* DNA has been found in mummies from Peru and northern Chile dating from 2000 BC to AD 1400. Old world cutaneous leishmaniasis is described on tablets in the library of King Ashurbanipal from the 7th century BC. The famous Arab physician Avicenna already described oriental sore in the 10th century as Balkh sore. New world leishmaniasis, as mucocutaneous disease, is clearly represented in ancient Peruvian pottery from the 5th century. The separation of Old World and New World Leishmaniasis was a contribution of Gaspar Vianna, who in 1911 created a new species, *Leishmania braziliensis*.

PROTOZOA

Globalization has changed patterns of protozoal infection with major implications for world health. The key to the recognition of protozoal infection is knowledge of epidemiological risk factors such as the parasite's geographic distribution and the major modes of clinical presentation.

Leishmaniasis

Leishmaniasis is an infectious process caused by intracellular parasites of the *Leishmania* genera, belonging to the *Trypanosomatidae* family. A particular structure, the kinetoplast, a unique form of mitochondrial DNA, is characteristic of these genera. Up to 21 species have been described as pathogenic for humans. Leishmaniasis is listed among the six most relevant infectious diseases in the world, with 12 million current cases in 88 countries on five different continents. The disease is transmitted from animal reservoirs, such as dogs and rodents, to humans by sandflies of the genera *Phlebothomus* and *Lutzomyia*; humans themselves can also be part of the reservoir. Leishmaniasis can be divided into two broad categories of disease, visceral and cutaneous. Whereas the visceral forms are mainly seen in India, Bangladesh, Sudan, Nepal, and Brazil, 90% of cutaneous cases are seen in Afghanistan, Iran, Saudi Arabia, Syria, Brazil, and Peru. No predilection for race, sex, or age has been demonstrated, although most cases are seen in adult males between the ages of 20 and 40 years.

The *Leishmania* are divided into four groups: *tropica, mexicana, braziliensis (viannia),* and *donovani.* The first three are the cause of cutaneous leishmaniasis whereas *Leishmania donovani* is responsible for the visceral forms. The different forms of cutaneous disease are species specific for certain regions in the world. Cutaneous forms seen in the Middle East are due to *Leishmania tropica*, in Central America they are due to *Leishmania mexicana*, and in South America they are due to *Leishmania braziliensis*, and *Leishmania peruviana*. Different names are given to the disease depending on the geographical location: oriental sore in Asia, chiclero's ulcer in Mexico, uta in the Andes, espundia in the Amazon basin, and pian bois in Northern Brazil. The parasite exists in two different forms, amastigote and promastigote. The amastigote, the form commonly seen in human tissue, is non-flagellated, ovoid in shape, and measures 3 to 5 μm in diameter. Two visible structures can be distinguished on light microscopy, the nucleus and the kinetoplast. The promastigote is the flagellated form seen in the gut of the sandfly. The conversion from promastigote to amastigote takes place as the microorganism, once introduced through the sandfly bite, comes into contact with human macrophages; this transformation is precipitated by low *ph* and lysosomal enzymes.

Regardless of the species involved in the pathogenesis, in most circumstances the classical elementary lesion for purely cutaneous leishmaniasis is an ulcer. It is usually round, with slightly elevated and indurated borders, and with a reddish base. It is commonly located in areas of the body not covered by clothing and therefore, exposed to the sandfly bite, such as the face, neck, and extremities. The lesion itself is painless and tends to regress spontaneously. Some clinical characteristics based on geographic distribution are worthy of mention (Table 9.1).

Old World leishmaniasis is caused by *Leishmania major, Leishmania tropica, Leishmania aethiopica,* and *Leishmania infantum.* Different clinical patterns have been described. The *wet* type is associated with *L. major* and is seen mostly in rural areas of North Africa as well as in Central and West Asia. It is

Table 9.1 Leishmaniasis : Geographic Guide and Clinical Manifestations

Complex	Species	Geographic location	Skin lesion	Internal involvement
Leishmania tropica	L. tropica	OW: Central and west Asia, Western India	Cutaneous ulceration, L. recidivans	
	Leishmania major	OW: North Africa, Central and West Asia	Cutaneous ulceration	
	Leishmania aethiopica	OW: Ethiopia, Kenya	Cutaneous ulceration, limited MCL, DCL	
Leishmania mexicana	L. mexicana	NW: Central America	Cutaneous ulceration	
	Leishmania amazonensis	NW: South America	Cutaneous ulceration, DCL	
	Leishmania pifanoi	NW: Venezuela	Cutaneous ulceration, DCL	
Leishmania (v) braziliensis	L. braziliensis	NW: South and Central America	Cutaneous ulceration, MCL	Can involve upper airways
	Leishmania peruviana	NW : Peru	Cutaneous ulceration, more rare MCL	
	L. panamensis	NW: Central America and Colombia	Cutaneous ulceration	
	Leishmania guyanensis	NW: Central America and Northern Countries of South America	Cutaneous ulceration, more rare MCL	
Leishmania donovani	L. donovani	OW: India, Kenya, East Africa	Post kala-azar	Visceral leishmaniasis
	Leishmania infantum	OW: Mediterranean basin, Central and West Asia	Cutaneous ulceration in adults	Visceral leishmaniasis in children
	Leishmania chagasi	NW: South America	Papules or nodules	Visceral leishmaniasis

OW: Old world; NW: New world; MCL: Mucocutaneous leishmaniasis; DCL: Diffuse cutaneous leishmaniasis

zoonotic, with rodents as the natural reservoir. It has an incubation period of up to 2 months. The lesion is crusty, associated with lymphadenopathy and has a tendency to involute spontaneously in 2 to 6 months. The *dry type*, caused by *L. tropica* and known as *oriental sore*, is seen mostly in Central and West Asia, Western India, Ethiopia, and Kenya. It is urban anthroponotic, and humans and dogs are the main reservoir. The incubation period can be as long as 1 year and takes 8 to 12 months to heal. *L. infantum*, although a cause of visceral disease in children, is associated with cutaneous disease in adults. Another type is associated with *L. aethiopica*. It is seen in Ethiopia and Kenya, and is usually a single facial ulceration, and takes up to 5 years to heal. It is known to cause mucosal involvement by continuity, but never to the extent that is seen with *L. braziliensis* infection. Two forms are remarkable for their chronicity: the lupoid forms seen in the Middle East and caused by *L. tropica* and the diffuse cutaneous form described as lepromatoid or pseudo-lepromatous leishmaniasis caused by *L. aethiopica*.

New World leishmaniasis, the type seen in the Americas, manifests primarily as a skin ulceration. The causal microorganism can belong to two groups: the *mexicana* group and the *braziliensis* (also known as *viannia*) group. Cases produced by the *L. mexicana* group predominate in Mexico and Central America (with a few cases described in the state of Texas). Cases produced by the *L. braziliensis (viannia)* group predominate in South America, from the coastal areas to the highlands of the Andes, the Amazon forest, and other tropical river systems. However, the distribution of both groups seems to overlap, especially in the southern tip of Central America and the northern regions of South America. The clinical variants include purely cutaneous, mucocutaneous, diffuse, and visceral leishmaniasis.

The purely cutaneous forms appear 10 to 90 days following the bite of the vector. The initial papule becomes an ulcer, with raised borders (Fig. 9.1 and 9.2), although sometimes the lesion will be a plaque or nodule, even adopting a sarcoidal appearance. Although single lesions predominate, they can be multiple. They may adopt a sporotrichoid pattern (Fig. 9.3); 10% may have regional lymphadenopathy. Some lesions will have a verrucous appearance, similar to tuberculosis verrucosa (Fig. 9.4). The lesions are distributed in areas exposed to insect bites, including near mucosa. Those locations should be differentiated from true mucocutaneous lesions, which carry a completely different

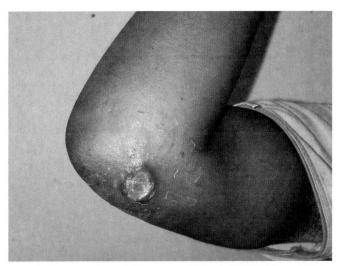

Figure 9.1. Cutaneous leishmaniasis, showing the raised borders.

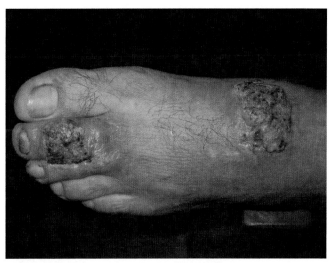

Figure 9.4. Verrucous cutaneous leishmaniasis: can be easily confused with tuberculosis verrucosa.

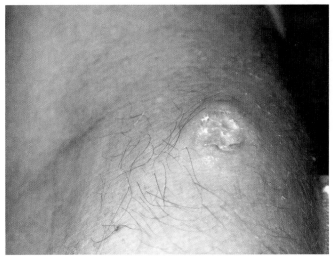

Figure 9.2. Cutaneous leishmaniasis.

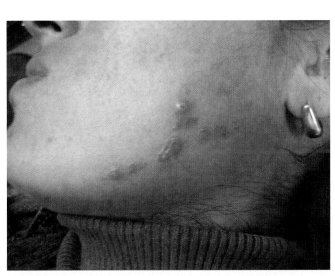

Figure 9.3. Cutaneous leishmaniasis, sporotrichoid pattern.

prognosis. A classical location for the *mexicana complex* is on the ear area, although an identical clinical presentation can be seen in infection by leishmanias of the *braziliensis* complex (Fig. 9.5). Parasites from both groups, *mexicana* and *braziliensis*, will produce purely cutaneous lesions. Most of the lesions produced by the *mexicana* complex will heal spontaneously and never develop mucosal involvement. Some species of the *braziliensis* group, such as *L. (v) peruviana*, will follow the same course, whereas other species such as *L. (v) braziliensis* and *Leishmania (v) panamensis* may carry the possibility of progressing to mucocutaneous involvement.

The variety known as *mucocutaneous leishmaniasis*, which is caused by several species of the *L. braziliensis* complex, is characterized by its ability to produce, after a dormant period (months to years), an ulceration on the mucosa of the nasal septum. This can progress externally causing infiltration of the nose and upper lip or mutilating the whole nose and nasolabial area (Fig. 9.6). It is a consequence of hematogenous dissemination. When the progression is toward the mucosal side, it may destroy the palate, producing a granulomatous infiltration of the pharynx, the larynx, and even the upper respiratory airway. In a patient with the classical presentation of a facial midline destructive lesion involving the nasal pyramid associated with marked edematous infiltration of the upper lip, hoarseness will be a sign of laryngeal involvement.

The diffuse form of leishmaniasis is seen rarely but represents a very particular variant. In the Americas, it is produced by *Leishmania amazonensis* of the *mexicana* group. The patients seem to lack the capability to react against the microorganism, similar to what is seen in the lepromatous pole of leprosy. Multiple microorganisms will be seen inside foamy histiocytes. The clinical expression will consist of multiple large, rarely ulcerated nodules distributed all over the body surface, with nondestructive mucosal involvement.

Visceral disease can be seen in Old World and New World leishmaniasis. It is caused by leishmanias of the *donovani* group, including *L. donovani*, *L. infantum*, and *L. chagasi*. The disease is systemic, with fever and hepatosplenomegaly as the main manifestations. Involvement of the skin can be seen as papular and

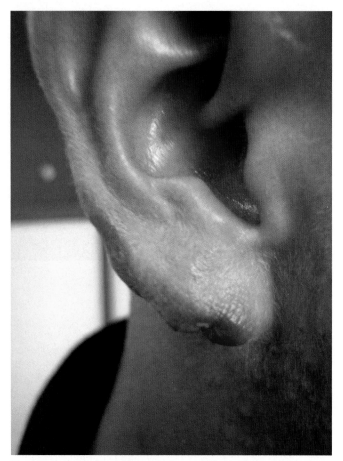

Figure 9.5. Cutaneous leishmaniasis caused by Leishmania peruviana, mimicking chiclero's ulcer.

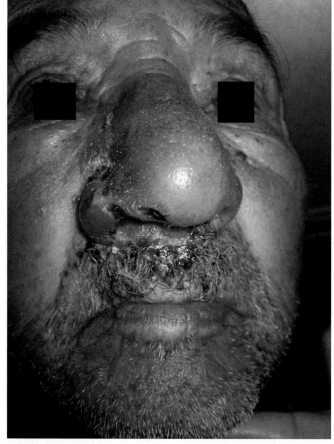

Figure 9.6. Mucocutaneous leishmaniasis.

nodular eruptions. The post kala-azar form is very dramatic as the lesions are quite extensive, ranging from macules to nodules.

In the diagnosis of leishmaniasis it is important to consider the great similarity of lesions produced by different species of leishmanias. Thus, the history of either living or traveling to specific geographic areas will be important to establish a most likely etiological agent. It is quite important to establish the possibility of infection by species with the potential to induce mucocutaneous disease (*L. (v) braziliensis* and *L. (v) panamensis*). This especially applies to patients who acquired the infection in the Amazonic regions of South America, and in a few countries in Central America. It should be kept in mind that none of the methods have 100% sensitivity, and it is better to rely on multiple methods to increase the likeness of a correct diagnosis. Direct examination, either by smear, or microaspiration is often used. Staining techniques include Giemsa, H&E, Romnowsky, and specific immunostaining. Skin biopsy is quite reliable if multiple organisms are seen (such as in early cases), but not so helpful when parasites are scarce, especially in old, granulomatous lesions. Where amastigotes can be confused with other structures, the visualization of the kinetocore seems to be quite specific. Culturing requires specific medium, such as NNM. The sensitivity is 40% in mucocutaneous disease but quite high in visceral disease. Isolation in laboratory animals is cumbersome but it is an alternative for difficult cases. Intradermal reactions, such as the Montenegro test are useful, although it requires some interpretation. Its positivity has diagnostic relevance in

patients not living in endemic areas, but it is not that reliable in the local residents. Serology testing will include immunofluorescent techniques, direct agglutination, ELISA, latex agglutination, and immunoblotting. The most modern methodology is based on molecular biology. PCR techniques are considered quite sensitive and quite specific. The gene targets include 18S-rRNA, small subunit rRNA, miniexon gene repeat, β-tubulin gene, transcriber spacer regions, and microsatellite DNA of the kinetoplast. PCR testing can detect as little as half a parasite, and should be the method of choice when available; unfortunately, that is not the case for most endemic rural areas. In such areas, sometimes the clinical criterion is enough for a therapeutic trial. In travelers who are not residents of endemic areas, the diagnosis should require visualization or isolation of the microorganism or molecular evidence of infection.

Decision for treatment should be based on the precise definition of the species involved, when identification is possible. Old World leishmaniasis may get by with no treatment. Treatment, when indicated, is based on use of antimonial preparations, either injected around the lesion, or systemic administration by the IM or IV route. *L. major* and *L. tropica* usually respond to a 10-day course. For Old World leishmaniasis, methods such as cryotherapy with liquid nitrogen, oral fluconazole, and topical paramomycin are also valid alternatives. One should keep in mind that spontaneous resolution is quite likely in many cases. For American leishmaniasis, either cutaneous or mucocutaneous, treatment is always recommended. The choices include available antimonial preparations, such as *N*-methyl-glucamine and sodium stibogluconate. A dose of 10 to 20 mg per kilogram should be given daily, IM or IV. The treatment should extend to 10 days for patients with cutaneous leishmaniasis with a low risk of developing mucocutaneous disease (such as *L. mexicana*) and for 20 days for those exposed in high-risk areas for developing mucocutaneous disease (*L. braziliensis* group). Active mucocutaneous disease should receive up to 28 days of therapy or receive an alternative therapy such as amphotericin-B or pentamidine. The treatment with antimonials is not free of complications, such as cardiac and renal toxicity. Liposomal amphotericin-B is a costly, but rather effective treatment for mucocutaneous disease. Oral miltefosine has shown high cure rates in areas where *L.* (v) *panamensis* is common (Colombia and Guatemala), but not as effective with infections due to *L.* (v) *braziliensis* and *L. mexicana* groups.

There is evidence that cure is related to the type of cellular immune reaction provoked by the microorganism. Those with a Th1 reaction will do better than those with a Th2 reaction. Interferon production is also quite important because of its ability to induce parasite destruction by macrophages. Unfortunately, too much of an immune reaction can be hazardous to the patient, as is the case in mucocutaneous disease. In this condition, an excess of cytokines like interferon-γ and TNF-α overwhelms the production of interleukin (IL)-10. The result of this imbalance is an extremely destructive inflammatory reaction despite a small number of microorganisms present in tissue. The other pole (analogous to the bipolar spectrum of leprosy) is represented by cases of diffuse cutaneous leishmaniasis, where poor cellular responses results in abundant parasites.

Enteric Amebiasis

Entamoeba histolytica is best known as a cause of gastrointestinal disorders, mainly colitis and liver abscesses. However, the possibility of cutaneous disease does exist, either as the only manifestation (the so called primary cutaneous amebiasis) or associated with involvement of other organs, most frequently the large bowel and rectum. Cutaneous disease has been reported in different countries around the world, with an important number of cases seen in Mexico. Life cycle includes two states: cyst, which is the infective form, and trophozoites. The transmission pathway is through the orofecal route. Inoculation in humans occurs by ingestion of amoebic cyst, and their ability to infect the intestinal mucosa depends on the interaction of lectins on the surface of the ameba with mucin glycoprotein on the intestinal epithelium. Invasion of the mucosa is facilitated by the ability of the protozoa to destroy human defensive cells, such as neutrophiles, T lymphocytes, and macrophages. To do so, the ameba has a system that is analogous to the human complement pathway, including a pore formation protein (amebopore). The ameba itself counters with a mechanism that allows it to elude the host alternative complement system. After invading the colonic mucosa they may reach the blood stream and subsequently invade other organs, including the liver, lung, pleura, pericardium, and even the brain.

E. histolytica can cause significant cutaneous disease, either by continuity or by external inoculation with contaminated hands. Cutaneous amebiasis is most frequently seen in adults. Both sexes are equally affected. The incidence varies: in a series of 5,097 patients with invasive disease from South Africa, only

2 had cutaneous disease. Up until 1981, the Hospital General de Mexico reported a case of cutaneous amebiasis for every 3,000 dermatology patients.

The most common locations are those implicated in propagation by continuity, that is, the perianal regions, the perineum, the genitalia, and the groin. The penis can be inoculated during anal intercourse. Lesions by external inoculation can be located elsewhere, that is, the abdominal wall. The classical lesion consists of a very painful ulcer that enlarges rapidly, reaching a large diameter, with interposing normal areas. The ulcers become wider and deeper, with erythematous borders that then become violaceous and later necrotic. The shape is round or oval at the beginning and then becomes irregular. The base is covered by exudates including pus.

On histology, the characteristic finding is that of an ulcer, with a mixed infiltrate of lymphocytes, neutrophils, and eosinophils. Areas of necrosis, as well as extravasated erythrocytes, are commonly observed. Trophozoites are invariably present, measuring 20 to 50 μm, staining basophilic, with nuclei measuring 4 to 7 μm. Commonly they will show erythrophagocytosis. Granulomas are usually absent. The diagnosis is based on the finding of the microorganisms on biopsy. Touch preparations and wet drop preparations from the pus may also be used. Patients should be evaluated for other sites of involvement. Serology testing may be used for confirmation. Treatment is based on the use of oral or IV metronidazole, 250 to 750 mg every 12 to 8 hours for a 10-day period. Alternatives include the use of diloxanide, tinidazole, emetine hydrochloride, and pentamidine.

Free-Living Amebas

Free-living amebas, also known as amphizoic amebas, are an important cause of acute and subacute meningoencephalitis. Species capable of causing central nervous system (CNS) involvement include *Naegleria* spp., *Acanthamoeba* spp., *Balamuthia* mandrillaris and, most recently, *Sappinia diploidea*. Until 1990, *Acanthamoeba* was the only species known to cause skin disease along with CNS involvement, especially in immunosuppressed patients. However, since the initial report by Vivesvara in 1980, a new species was identified as an important cause of granulomatous meningoencephalitis. First classified under the *Leptomyxes* families, later it was renamed *B. mandrillaris*. What makes this microorganism so special to dermatology is the occurrence of a rather typical cutaneous lesion preceding the CNS involvement by months. This finding is very important, because it may allow an early diagnosis even before neurological involvement. The prompt diagnosis is essential for treatment of this otherwise invariably fatal disease.

Until 2003, nearly 100 cases of *B. mandrillaris* had been reported worldwide. Many come from the Americas and there are additional reports from Asia, Australia, and Europe. Cutaneous involvement is not always reported. The first description of the classical centrofacial lesion was done by Reed in Australia. The disease seems to be acquired from contact with contaminated water or soil. As in cases of *Naegleria* and *Acanthamoeba*, swimming in ponds and lakes seems to be a common history. Surprisingly, the first environmental isolation in relation to a clinical case was from soil coming from a flower pot in the home of the affected child.

Around half of the cases are seen in patients under the age of 15. The initial cases were reported in immunocompromised patients, including those with AIDS, but, recently, most of the cases from South America, Asia, and Australia occurred in immunocompetent patients. It is interesting to note that up to 44% of the US cases reported to the Center for Disease Control and Prevention for *Balamuthia* testing had Hispanic ethnicity. Up to 45 cases of free-living ameba infection have been identified at the Instituto de Medicina Tropical "Alexander von Humboldt," at Hospital Nacional Cayetano Heredia, in Lima, Peru. 20 cases have been confirmed, by immunofluorescense test, as being caused by *Balamuthia* by immunofluorescence test.

Acanthamoeba and *Balamuthia* are very similar in morphology. A distinction can be made on the basis of culture isolation, differences in the cell wall of the cystic state and lately, on the basis of PCR analysis of amebic mitochondrial RNA. They both enter the skin through microabrasions. From there, the infection may be either contained in the skin for a while, or rapidly disseminate to the CNS either by continuity (nasal skin involvement) or by hematogenous spread. The classical skin lesion in *Balamuthia* cases is an asymptomatic plaque, mostly located on the central face (Fig. 9.7). The lesion may enlarge, giving origin to smaller satellite lesions, or progressing into a more infiltrative involvement of the whole facial area. One single lesion is more common than several, and lesions only ulcerate at a very late state. When the lesion occurs on the extremities the findings may seem less characteristic, and with a wider differential diagnosis, the diagnosis is likely to be overlooked. Some patients may develop regional lymphadenopathy. The natural history will go toward the development of neurological disease. This progression may take from 30 days to 2 years; with an average of 5 to 8 months. Cutaneous involvement precedes the CNS involvement as a rule. The CNS involvement will manifest initially as fever, headache, and photophobia. Later, other signs of intracranial hypertension, such as seizures, lethargy, and focal signs of motor or sensorial deficit will appear. The patient will enter a comatose state and die. As opposed to *Balamuthia*, *Acanthamoeba* cases occur more commonly in immunosuppressed patients, many with AIDS. Lesions tend to be more ulcerated, and the progression toward CNS involvement may be faster.

The histology of the skin lesion in *Balamuthia* is very consistent. It is characterized by an ill-defined granulomatous infiltrate with many giant cells, lymphocytes, and plasma cells. Neutrophils and eosinophils are seen in only one-third of the cases. One should actively look for the ameba. Scarce trophozoites can be seen in three-fourths of the cases, but their morphology can be easily confused with macrophages. Only the presence of the amoebic nucleus and nucleolus may allow its differentiation from a human cell. As opposed to *E. histolytica*, they do not phagocytize red blood cells.

In *Acanthamoeba* cases the biopsy usually shows multiple trophozoites, many situated along vascular structures. The most specific identification is based on immunofluorescent staining of the microorganism in skin or brain tissue, as well as immunofluorescence testing of the patient's serum. Recently, PCR testing has become available for *B. mandrillaris*.

The disease will have a fatal outcome unless therapeutic intervention takes place. The aim is to make early diagnosis when the disease is only confined to the skin to avoid its spreading to the CNS. Unfortunately, there is no therapeutic regimen

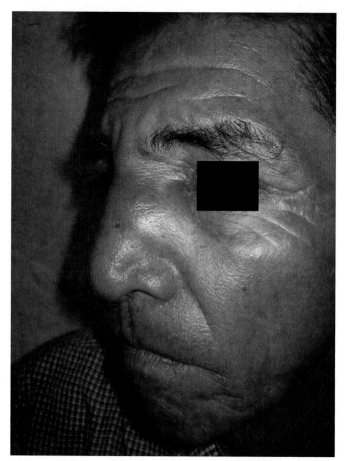

Figure 9.7. Balamuthiasis, plaque on the central face.

showing consistently good results. The cases reported in the literature as survivors have tried different modalities. Drugs used in *Balamuthia* include flucytosine, pentamidine, fluconazole, sulfadiazine, and a macrolide. Four additional unreported survivor cases from personal experience of one of the authors (F.B.P.) received amphotericin, albendazole, itraconazole, and fluconazole, with one of them also getting benefit from the surgical excision of the clinical lesion.

B. mandrillaris should be kept in mind when dealing with granulomatous lesions, with the morphology of a plaque occurring on the central face or elsewhere. If this infection is suspected, the pathologist should be alerted to look for the ameba or to use immunofluorescent testing (Laboratory of Parasitic Disease, Center for Disease Control and Prevention, Atlanta). Early intervention may give patients a hope for cure in an otherwise fatal disease. It is possible that at least some of the previous reported cases of midline lethal granulomas were nothing but free-living ameba cases where the causing agent was overlooked.

Trypanosomiasis

Only three members of this genus are capable of infecting humans: *Trypanosoma cruzi*, the cause of Chagas disease in the Americas; and *Trypanosoma brucei gambiense* and *Trypanosoma brucei rhodesiense*, the cause of human African trypanosomiasis.

Human African trypanosomiasis, or sleeping sickness, is transmitted to human hosts by bites of infected tse-tse flies, which are found only in Africa. The life cycle starts when the trypanosomes are ingested during a blood meal by the tse-tse fly from a human reservoir in the West African trypanosomiasis (*T. b. gambiense*) or an animal reservoir in the East African trypanosomiasis (*T. b. rhodesiense*). The trypanosome multiplies over a period of 2 to 3 weeks in the fly midgut; then, the parasite migrates to the salivary gland where they develop into epimastigotes. Humans are infected following a fly bite with inoculation of trypomastigotes.

A painful and indurated trypanosomal chancre appears in some patients 5 to 15 days after the inoculation of the parasite and resolves spontaneously over several weeks. Hematogenous and lymphatic dissemination is marked by the onset of malaise, headache, intermittent fever, rash, and weight loss. Lymphadenopathy is more common in West African trypanosomiasis with discrete, movable, rubbery, and nontender nodes. Cervical nodes are often visible, and enlargement of the nodes of the posterior cervical triangle (Winterbottom's sign) is a classic finding. Transient edema is common and can occur in the face, hands, feet, and other periarticular areas. Pruritus is frequent, and an irregular maculopapular rash is often present. This rash is located on the trunk, shoulders, buttocks, and thighs and consists of annular, blotchy erythematous areas with clear centers, called *trypanids*. Eventually, the parasitic invasion reaches the CNS, causing behavioral and neurological changes. A picture of progressive indifference and daytime somnolence develops (giving rise to the name sleeping sickness), sometimes alternating with restlessness and insomnia at night. The final phase includes stupor and coma, with high mortality. The most striking difference between the West African and East African trypanosomiasis is that the latter illness tends to follow a more acute course.

A definitive diagnosis requires detection of trypanosomes in blood, lymph nodes, CSF, skin chancre aspirates, or bone marrow. However, empiric treatment with subsequent symptomatic improvement is the usual confirmatory test in areas where diagnostic studies are not readily available. Treatment depends on type and stage of disease. Suramin, eflornithine, melarsoprol, and pentamidine are drugs that have proven efficacy.

American trypanosomiasis, or Chagas disease, is a zoonosis caused by the protozoan parasite *T. cruzi*. This parasite is found in the Americas from the southern United States to southern Argentina. Humans become involved in the cycle of transmission when infected vectors take up residence in the cracks and holes of the primitive wood, adobe, and stone houses common in Latin America. *T. cruzi* is transmitted among its mammalian hosts by bloodsucking triatomine insects, often called *reduviid bugs* (kissing bugs). The insects become infected by sucking blood from animals or humans who have circulating trypomastigotes. The ingested organisms multiply in the gut of the triatomines, and infective forms are discharged with the feces at the time of subsequent blood meals. Transmission to a second vertebrate host occurs when breaks in the skin, mucous membranes, or conjunctivae become contaminated with bug feces that contain infective parasites. *T. cruzi* can also be transmitted by transfusion organ transplantation and from mother to fetus during birth.

Acute Chagas disease occurs at least 1 week after invasion by the parasites. When the organisms enter through a break in the skin, an indurated area of erythema and swelling (chagoma), accompanied by local lymphadenopathy, may appear. The Romaña sign, which consists of unilateral painless edema of the palpebral and periocular tissues, occurs in cases of entry through the conjunctiva. These initial local signs may be followed by malaise, fever, anorexia, and edema of the face and lower extremities. Some patients may also develop a rash that clears in several days. Generalized lymphadenopathy and hepatosplenomegaly may develop. Severe myocarditis rarely develops. Neurological signs are not common, but meningoencephalitis occurs occasionally. Chronic Chagas disease becomes apparent years or even decades after the initial infection. Cardiac involvement is the most frequent and serious defined manifestation of chronic Chagas disease (approximately two thirds of cases) and typically leads to arrhythmias, cardiac failure, thromboembolic phenomena, and sudden death. The digestive forms of the disease lead to megaesophagus and/or megacolon in approximately one-third of chronic cases.

The diagnosis of acute Chagas disease requires the detection of parasites. Microscopic examination of fresh, anticoagulated blood or of the buffy coat is the simplest way to see the motile organisms. Chronic Chagas disease is usually diagnosed by the detection of IgG specific antibodies that bind to *T. cruzi* antigens. Treatment for Chagas disease is unsatisfactory, with only two drugs (nifurtimox and benznidazole) available for this purpose. Unfortunately, both drugs lack efficacy and often cause severe side effects.

HELMINTHS

Worm infections in humans and other animals are a significant contributor to the global burden of illness caused by infectious diseases in general. This group includes roundworms (nematodes), tapeworms (cestodes), and flukes (trematodes).

Nematodes

This phylum is the second largest phylum in the animal kingdom, with approximately 500,000 species. Members of this phylum are elongated with bilaterally symmetric bodies containing an intestinal tract and a large body cavity. Nematodes of medical importance may be broadly classified as either predominantly intestinal or tissue nematodes (some with lymphatic involvement). They are widely scattered around the world, especially in the tropics, and infect millions of people.

Filariasis

Filariasis are systemic infections due to different species of nematodes, all transmitted by mosquito bites, with hematogenous (rather than cutaneous, as in Onchocerciasis) spread of microfilariae. These parasites reside in lymphatic channels or lymph nodes, where they may remain viable for more than two decades. The symptoms are related to chronic inflammation of the lymphatic system. They commonly occur in tropical areas of the world. *Wuchereria bancrofti* and *Brugia malayi* are more common in Asia and tropical Africa. *Brugia timori* exists only on islands of the Indonesian archipelago. The symptoms are related to the stage of disease. During the hematogenous spread, microfilarias are abundant in blood, producing temporary migratory swelling on extremities that are self-limited and recurrent. Acute lymphangitis and lymphadenitis may affect the groin and axillae. Genital involvement includes acute orchitis, epididymitis, and funiculitis, which are very painful. They can also be recurrent, and evolve into fibrosis. Urticaria may be part of the clinical presentation. Late changes are due to obstruction of lymphatics, giving origin to different forms of elephantiasis, affecting the extremities and scrotum with massive edema. Diagnosis is made by the presence of microfilaria in blood smears, and serological testing. Treatment with diethylcarbamazine (DEC), 6 mg/kg daily for 12 days), remains the treatment of choice for the individual with active lymphatic filariasis, although albendazole (400 mg twice daily for 21 days) has also demonstrated macrofilaricidal efficacy. Ivermectin is also an option.

Loiasis

Caused by the filariae and microfilariae of *Loa loa*, loiasis is a disease of humans that results in skin and eye involvement. It is endemic in sub-Saharan Africa, from West to East equatorial countries. The vector is a deer and antelope fly (*Chrysops* spp.). Serving as intermediate host between human; it is in the fly that the microfilariae evolve into infective larvae and as such are then inoculated into the subcutaneous tissue of uninfected humans by another bite. Larvae mature into adult worms in the subcutaneous tissue, migrating to different parts of the body, where they will produce new microfilariae that eventually will be taken by another *Chrysops*, starting the cycle again. In a year's time, the proliferating mass of worms will reach a level capable of inducing symptoms.

The clinical manifestations are related to the migratory angioedema induced by moving worms. If the disease is present near joints, it will induce pain or itching. They are often located in the periorbital area. The lesions may last from days to weeks, giving the idea of a "fugitive swelling." At times, the microfilariae can be seen migrating under the skin or under the conjunctiva, causing severe conjunctivitis. Urticarial rashes may also develop. The allergic response induced by the worm may express as regional lymphedema, peripheral neuritis, or encephalitis, and eventually compromise the kidney, lungs, and heart.

A definitive diagnosis can be done by extraction of the worm from a subcutaneous nodule or from conjunctiva. Microfilariae can be detected in blood peripheral smears or from skin snips. A tentative diagnosis can be made on the basis of clinical findings with associated eosinophilia, leukocytosis, and increased levels of IgE. The Mazzotti test consists of the administration of a test dose of DEC, looking for the induction of intense itching, secondary to dying microfilariae. The treatment itself is based on the same drug, DEC, given on a 3-week oral course. One has to watch for severe meningoencephalitic reactions, which should be treated with steroids and antihistaminics. Ivermectin and albendazole are considered alternative therapies, although not exempt from the allergic reactions. Fatalities are more commonly associated to those allergic reactions due to high-dose therapy or worm rupture.

Onchocerciasis

Onchocerciasis is a chronic infestation of the skin with *Onchocerca volvulus*. This is a microfilarial nematode whose natural hosts are humans and the vectors are flies from the genus *Simulium*. The disease was first described in Africa and later in Central America.

Recently, some reports indicate the disease extends into the northern countries of South America. The transmission occurs when flies became infected by biting sick people. After a short period of maturation the microfilaria moves to the buccal apparatus of the insect and enters the skin of a noninfected human with the next blood meal. The infective forms become adults in 6 to 8 months, inside cutaneous nodules called *onchocercomas*, where they start to produce microfilarias. From then on, the infection propagates to all the tegumentary system. Worms move from one nodule to another to mate. Cutaneous involvement includes the characteristic onchocercomas. They tend to locate on the scalp in Central American patients and on extensor surfaces in the African patients. Many times the clinical picture is of itchy dermatosis. Other clinical presentations include acute and chronic papular forms, the lichenified unilateral form that Yemenites call sowda, facial erythema, facial lividoid discoloration, facial aging, and prurigo-like eruption on the buttocks and extremities. Later signs are extensive lichenification, dyschromia similar to vitiligo, elephantiasis of the extremities, and the scrotum, and the so called "hanging groin." Ocular involvement is related to the direct invasion of eye structures by the microfilaria, causing uveitis, conjunctivitis, keratitis, optical nerve atrophy, and glaucoma. All this may end up in complete and permanent loss of vision, hence the name "river blindness,"

Diagnosis is based on the clinical finding of onchocercomas and other characteristic skin changes. Scabies and papular urticaria induced by insect bites can be confused with the papular reactions seen in onchocerciasis. The skin snip is a useful confirmatory test, especially when taken from the iliac crest area. The amount of visualized microfilariae will give an idea of the parasitic load. A Mazzotti patch test with DEC will also serve as a diagnostic guide. ELISA and PCR testing are available, and a rapid format antibody card is being developed. Histological analysis of skin lesions will allow the identification of adult forms surrounded byfibrous or calcified tissue. Occasionally microfilaria may be identified in the surrounding tissue. Treatment for disease consists of the oral administration of ivermectin, which is extremely effective even as a single-dose therapy to kill the microfilariae; however, adult forms are resistant. Patient should receive repeated doses of ivermectin through the years to kill new microfilariae, thus keeping a low parasitic load. This scheme will prevent the development of blindness and improve skin symptoms. The role of symbiotic bacteria, *Wolbachia*, as a requirement for worm reproduction has given rise to the combined treatment of ivermectin and doxycycline, which seems very effective in decreasing the microfilariae mass more rapidly.

Dracunculiasis

Also known as Guinea worm, this parasitic infection is produced by *Dracunculus medinensis*, a nematode parasite of humans since early ages. The disease is prevalent in several countries of the sub-Saharan African continent. The population affected is among the most deprived in the world, and follows a dreadful cycle that repeats year after year during the harvest season affecting the adult labor force as well as children.

The life cycle starts with the elimination of eggs by a female worm extruding from an infected patient; each female may carry 3 million embryos. The larvae are then ingested by cyclopoid copepods, where they evolve into an infective organism. Humans are again exposed to the microorganism while drinking contaminated water containing *Cyclops*. When the crustaceans reach the stomach, the larvae are liberated. They then perforate the gastric mucosa, and after passing through the peritoneum, they finally locate in the subcutaneous tissues where a maturation process to male and female worms takes place. After a year, the female is fertilized and then migrates even more superficially until she can eliminate her eggs through the skin to reinitiate the cycle. The female can reach a length of 120 cm.

The disease will manifest itself only when the worms reach the maturation and fertilization period. The fertilized female will approach the skin surface while the patient is experimenting systemic symptoms such as nausea, vomiting, diarrhea, syncope, or dyspnea. The area of emersion will be preceded by pruritus and then a papule or a nodule will appear. If the area is located near a joint the process may become quite painful. They will evolve into a vesiculobullous lesion, associated with a strong burning sensation, and relieved by the immersion of the affected body area in water. The subsequent ulceration may become superinfected by pyogenic bacteria. If the worm ruptures inside the tissue it may cause a clinical picture of cellulites or eventually become calcified. Commonly affected areas will be the lower extremities, especially feet, although other areas can be affected as well. The average number of worms extruded at any given time is usually less than five, but as many as 20 at a time have been reported. The patient will become temporarily disabled, and obligated to stay in bed, which affects the economic situation of the household or causes failure to attend school in children or adolescents.

The presence of an extruding adult worm is obviously diagnostic. Also, a direct wet preparation from the lesion may reveal mobile larvae. Treatment consists of slowly extracting the worm by winding it around a stick, a process that may take several days. Oral treatments with mebendazole and metronidazole may facilitate the extraction of the worm.

Cutaneous larva migrans

Cutaneous larva migrans, also known as creeping eruption, is a disease produced by the third larval state of intestinal nematodes that parasitize dogs, cats, and other mammals. The disease has a wide distribution around the world and is commonly seen in the Southeastern United States, the Caribbean, Central and South America, Africa, India, and South East Asia. It is the most common parasitic disease of the tropics. Although frequently reported as a disease of the affluent tourist, it is highly prevalent in areas of poverty of the developing world. The most common species in the Americas is *Ancylostoma braziliensis* (hookworm of dogs and cats). *A. caninum* is found in Australia and *Uncinaria stenocephala* in Europe. Cattle hookworm such as *Butostotum phlebotomun* can also be a causative agent of cutaneous larva migrans. *Strongyloides stercoralis* produces a similar picture although the speed of migration is faster (thus the name larva currens) and commonly affects a different body area such as the buttocks. Even free-living soil nematodes such as *Pelodera strongyloides* can invade human skin, although with a more polymorphous clinical picture.

The infection is typically acquired while walking barefoot on sandy beaches frequented by stray dogs and becoming contaminated by their feces. Kids playing in sandboxes are also at risk. The larva feeds initially on soil bacteria, but as soon as it gets in contact with human skin, it will invade the stratum corneum with the aid of protease secretions, and will then begin its wandering cycle. Lacking the appropriate enzymatic armamentarium, it will not be able to go beyond the dermis as would have been the case in the definitive canine host.

The classical presentation will be a serpiginous lesion with an advancing edge, located most commonly on the feet, buttocks, hands, and knees. The trunk can also be involved if the patient was lying on the sand (Fig. 9.8). An itching, tingling, or burning sensation may be reported. The advancing border can extend several millimeters each day. Multiple pinpoint lesions can occur, especially in the gluteal areas. Secondary bacterial infections due to intense scratching are commonly seen in populations afflicted by poverty. The clinical course extends over weeks but rarely beyond 3 months. Spontaneous resolution usually takes place, but symptoms may force the patient to seek medical advice.

Peripheral eosinophilia can be seen. Although it is a clinical diagnosis, if a biopsy is taken one should look for the presence of a superficial and perivascular infiltrate of eosinophils. Rarely the larva will be seen on histological cuts, and most commonly at the stratum corneum level. The current therapies include topically applied thiabendazole, as well as the oral use of albendazole and ivermectin. In pregnant patients, cryotherapy may be another alternative. Differential diagnosis will include other parasites with migratory patterns, such as gnathostomiasis, loiasis, myasis, fascioliasis. Linear lesions from jellyfish attacks, blister

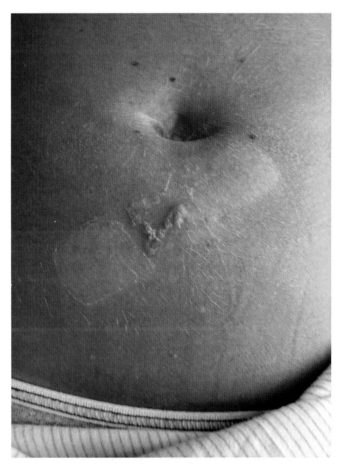

Figure 9.8. Cutaneous larva migrans.

beetle dermatitis, or phytophotodermatitis can also mimick these conditions.

The syndrome associated with *Strongyloides stercoralis* is known as larva currens. The migratory pattern is much faster than in regular larva migrans (up to 5 to 10 cm per hour). It is quite pruritic. Common locations include the buttocks, groin, and trunk. In the hyperinfection state, the lesions can adopt a more petechial to purpuric pattern. Thumbprint-shaped hemorrhages can be seen around the umbilicus. Strongyloidiasis may specifically affect those patients under immunosuppressive regimens, malnourished patients, or patients infected with HTLV-1.

Gnathostomiasis

Described by Owen in 1836, it is a parasitic infection produced by round worms of the *Gnathostoma* family. Different species have been described as causative agents, the most common being *G. spinigerum*. Other species include *G. turgidum, G. americanum, G. procyonis, G. miyasaki, G. binucleatum,* and lately *G. doloresi*. The highest incidence is reported in areas where eating raw fish is part of the local gastronomy, either as sashimi or ceviche. High prevalence areas in Asia include Thailand, Korea, Japan, and other countries in Southeast Asia. In the Americas, it has been reported in Mexico (Sinaloa and Acapulco), Ecuador (Guayaquil), and coastal areas of Peru. In fact, with more and more frequent intercontinental travel and tourism, gnathostomiasis is a disease that can now be seen throughout world. Series of cases have been reported in traveler clinics in the United States, United Kingdom, and France, and other case reports testify to worldwide distribution of the disease.

The infection is a zoonosis. The life cycle starts in the stomach of cats, where adult worms nest in the gastric mucosa. Other primary hosts include dogs, tigers, leopards, lions, minks, opossums, raccoons, and otters. Eventually, eggs reach the intestinal lumen and, carried in feces, they will reach the fresh water of a river. The egg will evolve into a first larval state and this in turn will infect the gastric mucosa of minute crustaceans (*Cyclops*). Inside this copepode, the larva will mature into a second and early third larval state. The copepode will then be ingested by a new temporary host, most commonly a fish. Other potential species harboring the infective larva may include frogs, snakes, chicken, or pigs. The worm will invade the gastric mucosa of the new host to later evolve into a late third larval state to finish as a cyst in the muscle tissue. This intermediate host will be at the same time ingested by the final host, the cat, as fishermen will throw away infected rotten fish in the beaches near a river. Once the contaminated flesh is ingested and digested, the larvae excyst into the stomach, penetrate the gastric wall, migrate through the liver, and travel to the connective tissue and muscles. After 4 weeks, they return to the gastric wall to form the tumor, where they mature into adults in 6 to 8 months. At 8 to 12 months after initial ingestion, the worms mate and eggs begin to pass into the feces of the host to begin a new cycle.

Humans get the infection by eating raw fish in several ways, classically in the form of sushi or sashimi in Asia, and ceviche (raw fish marinated in lime juice) in the Americas. Other potential sources of infection are shellfish (such as oysters) and undercooked meat from animals, such as pork and chicken, that are fed along with infected fish. Once the infected meat reaches the human stomach, the larva is liberated and rapidly perforates the gastric mucosa, 24 to 40 hours after initial ingestion. Some patients may then report epigastric discomfort. The parasite will reach the peritoneal space and either migrates through internal organs, such as the liver, or straight toward the subcutaneous fat. In the first case, the symptoms may simulate acute gallbladder disease, so the disease becomes relevant for surgeons in their differential diagnosis for a patient with acute right upper quadrant pain.

If the larva ends up in the subcutaneous fat, the classical presentation will be a migratory panniculitis. This event will take place about 4 weeks after the ingestion of the contaminated meat. It will consist of the appearance of a deeply seated, ill-defined nodule or plaque, located commonly in the abdominal wall, but potentially anywhere on the body. Sometimes, the area involved will have a "peau d'orange" appearance (Fig. 9.9).The lesion is easily confused initially with a deep bacterial abscess. It will be erroneously treated with antibiotics, and a temporary involution of the mass will occur. Then, a few days later, a similar lesion will recur a few centimeters beyond the original location (Fig. 9.10). These migratory episodes may continue for months or even years. A minority of cases may even have a more superficial, "larva migrans" type of presentation, either at the beginning of the process or at the end (Fig. 9.11). We have seen cases where the larva will move to a more superficial location near the epidermis after treatment with antiparasitic drugs. A more serious complication is pneumonia, which can result in a pleural or even pericardial effusion, due to its passing through the mediastinum. Also, there is always the possibility of migration of the parasite to the eye (which can cause uveitis, iritis, intraocular hemorrhage, increased intraocular pressure, or even retinal scarring and detachment). Migration to the CNS has also been reported. It can produce meningitis or meningoencephalitis. In Thailand, it is the most common parasitic infection of the CNS, where up to 6% of subarachnoid hemorrhages in adults and 18% of those in infants and children are due to gnathostomiasis.

The characteristic migratory pattern through the subcutaneous fat, so called "migratory panniculitis" should alert the physician about the possibility of gnathostomiasis. When associated with peripheral eosinophilia, as high as 50%, the suspicion

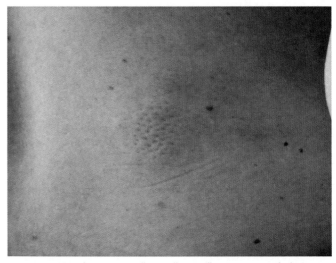

Figure 9.9. Gnathostomiasis "peau d'orange" appearance of a lesion at the time of first visit.

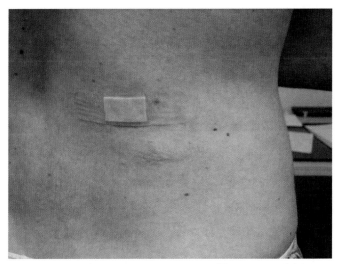

Figure 9.10. Gnathostomiasis: same patient of figure 9 a week later. Notice how the lesion has migrated from an area covered with a band-aid to a different site a few centimeters away.

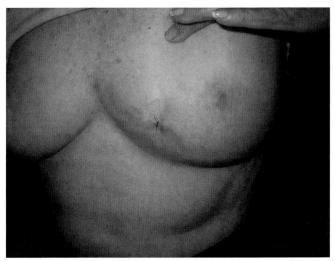

Figure 9.11. Gnathostomiasis with a superficial (cutaneous larva migrans pattern) and deep (panniculitis pattern) component.

should be high. Unfortunately, this finding in the peripheral blood is not always present. A skin biopsy is a very reliable method for confirming the diagnosis. Expected histological findings include a dense perivascular and interstitial eosinophilic infiltrate, mainly localized to the subcutaneous fat and dermis. Flame figures can be seen around collagen bundles in the dermis, similar to findings associated with eosinophilic cellulitis (Well's syndrome). This last entity, however, lacks the migratory course characteristic of gnathostomiasis. Of note, it is extremely difficult to see the worm on histology cuts, because the area of infiltration is large (up to several square cm in size) compared to the size of the larva, which is about 0.4 mm in diameter and 4mm in length. However, a curious observer may note that after medical therapy is given, the large areas may evolve into a small papule. If then the minute lesion is excised, the whole wandering larva may be seen on histologic cuts.

For diagnostic purposes, a history of eating raw fish, the clinical finding of a migratory panniculitis, and the presence of an eosinophilic panniculitis with associated dermatitis on biopsy should be enough criteria to make the diagnosis. A serological test has been developed in Thailand using immunoblotting of a 24 kDa protein extracted from *Gnatostoma* infective larva. This test will detect antibodies from any infection not older than 6 months. While diagnosing a recurrence, one should expect the migratory pattern to be present. In the differential diagnosis of migratory diseases one should include superficial and deep-seated parasites, such as *Ancylostoma* species (superficial larva migrans) and *Fasciola hepatica* (in cases of right upper quadrant location). Even though *Toxocara* presents most commonly as an acute pneumonia, it can also more rarely produce a migratory paniculitis. Myiasis can adopt a subcutaneous migratory pattern. A similar picture to gnathostomiasis can be seen in sparganosis. However, sparganosis most commonly will present as a fixed subcutaneous nodule, although a migratory pattern has also been reported.

Treatment is albendazole 400 mg to 800 mg for 14 to 21 days, or single doses of ivermectin 200 μg per kilogram repeated every two weeks until the clinical findings subside. Both treatments seem to be equally effective, but neither show 100% efficacy. Prevention is based on cooking or freezing of the potentially infected meat. Lemon juice, the classical ingredient in the preparation of ceviche, has no effect in eliminating the larva. Fish species responsible for the transmission of the disease varies from one area to the other, requiring a joint effort from physicians, biologists, and health officials to identify sources of infection for every region affected by the disease. People who like to prepare sushi at home are considered a high-risk group, as they lack the experience to select uninfected fish.

Trichinellosis

Seven species are recognized as causes of infection in humans (*Trichinella spiralis, Trichinella native, Trichinella nelsoni, Trichinella pseudospiralis, Trichinella britovi, Trichinella murrelli,* and *Trichinella papuae*). Most human infections are due to *T. spiralis,* which is found in carnivorous and omnivorous animals (pigs, rats, bears, foxes, dogs, cats, or horses) worldwide. Trichinellosis or Trichinosis develop after the ingestion of raw or undercooked meat (most commonly pork) contaminated with the infective larvae of *Trichinella* spp.

After the ingestion of infected meat by the host, encysted larvae are freed by acid-pepsin digestion in the stomach and then pass into the small intestine. Larvae invade the columnar epithelium at the bases of the villi and then develop into adult worms. After approximately 1 week, female worms release newborn larvae that migrate via the circulation to striated muscle. A cyst wall develops around the larvae and may eventually calcify. Larvae may remain viable in muscles for several years.

Clinical symptoms develop from the successive phases of parasite enteric invasion, larval migration, and muscle encystment. Small intestine invasion occasionally provokes diarrhea, abdominal pain, constipation, nausea, and vomiting. Symptoms due to larval migration and muscle invasion are much more common and usually begin to appear in the second or third week after infection. The migrating larvae produce a local and systemic hypersensitivity reaction, with fever and hypereosinophilia.

Symmetric periorbital and facial edema may be associated with hemorrhages in the subconjunctivae, retina, and nail beds (splinter hemorrhages). Some patients present with a rash that may be maculopapular or petechial. Headache, cough, dyspnea, hoarseness, or dysphagia sometimes also develops. Myositis with myalgias, muscle edema, and weakness are also common. The most frequently involved muscles include the extraocular muscles, the biceps, and the muscles of the jaw, neck, lower back, and diaphragm. Other symptoms may include myocarditis, pneumonitis, and encephalitis.

Trichinellosis should be suspected in a patient who develops periorbital edema, myositis, fever, and eosinophilia. Patients should be questioned thoroughly about recent consumption of poorly cooked meat, particularly pork or wild-animal meat, and about illness in other individuals who ate the same meat. Eosinophilia typically arises 10 days after infection, with total eosinophil counts of up to 40% to 80% of total white blood cells. Erythrocyte sedimentation rates are usually within the reference range. Creatine kinase, lactate dehydrogenase, and IgE levels are often elevated. A muscle biopsy requires at least 1 g of involved muscle. At the time of biopsy, initial preparation may be made by crushing a portion of muscle tissue between two slides and viewing it directly.

Serology results are not positive until 2 to 3 weeks after infection. They peak around the third month and may persist for years. Latex agglutination results are usually not positive for more than 1 year after infection. ELISA is 100% sensitive on day 50, with 88% of results remaining positive 2 years after infection.

Current antihelmintic drugs are ineffective against the larvae in muscle. Mebendazole (200–400 mg PO TID for 7 days) and albendazole (400 mg/day PO BID for 7–14 days), are active against enteric stages of the parasite. Jarisch-Herxheimer-like reactions have been described following the administration of antihelmintic medications. Fortunately, most lightly infected patients recover uneventfully with bed rest, antipyretics, and analgesics. Corticosteroid treatment can help reduce the immunologic response to the larvae and is beneficial for severe myositis and myocarditis. The most effective measure to eradicate Trichinella species is by adequate cooking to kill the parasite. Trichinella species can typically be killed by adequate cooking at 140°F (60°C) for 2 minutes. If no trace of pink in fluid or flesh is found, these temperatures have been reached.

Mansonelliasis

Three species routinely infect humans: *Mansonella streptocerca*, *Mansonella perstans*, and *Mansonella ozzardi*. Diagnosis of Mansonelliasis depends on demonstrating the microfilariae in thick or thin films of peripheral blood, skin snips, or biopsy specimens of skin.

Mansonella streptocerca is found mainly in the tropical forest of Africa and is transmitted by midges (*Culicoides*). Patients are usually asymptomatic but can develop pruritus, papular rashes, hypopigmented macules (that may be confused with leprosy), and inguinal adenopathy. DEC (2 mg/kg PO TID for 14–21 days) is effective in killing both microfilariae and adult worms. Ivermectin at a single dose of 150 µg/kg is also effective.

M. perstans is distributed across the center of Africa and in northeastern South America, and is transmitted by midges (*Culicoides*). Adult worms reside in serous cavities as well as in the mesentery and the perirenal and retroperitoneal tissues. Clinical manifestations may include fever, headache, arthralgias, fatigue, pruritus, and transient angioedema (similar to the Calabar swellings of loiasis). Mebendazole (100 mg PO bid for 30 days) and albendazole (400 mg PO bid for 10 days) have been reported to be effective. Ivermectin has no activity against this species. Allergic reactions have been reported from dying organisms.

M. ozzardi is restricted to Central and South America (Argentina, Bolivia, Brazil, Colombia, Ecuador, and Peru), and certain Caribbean islands. Vectors include midges (*Culicoides*) and blackflies (*Simulium*). Symptoms include fever, headache, arthralgias, hepatomegaly, adenopathy, papular rashes, and pruritus. DEC is ineffective with this species. Ivermectin at a single dose of 6 mg has been shown to be effective in treating this infection.

Enterobiasis (Pinworms)

This infection is more common in temperate countries than in the tropics, and humans are the only natural host for *Enterobius vermicularis*. In the United States, more than 40 million people are estimated to be infected with pinworms; schoolchildren account for a disproportionate number of cases.

The adult worms are approximately 1 cm long and dwell in the bowel lumen. The female worm migrates to the rectum after copulation and, if not expelled during defecation, migrates to the perineum, where on average of 10,000 eggs are released. The eggs become infective within hours and are transmitted through humans from hand to mouth passage. Self-infection results from perianal scratching and transport of infective eggs on the hands or under the nails to the mouth. Fecal–oral contamination via toys or clothes is a common method of infestation. Because of the ease of person-to-person spread, it is common among family members and institutionalized populations.

Perianal pruritus is the main symptom. The itching, which is often worse at night as a result of the nocturnal migration of the female worms, can lead to excoriation and bacterial superinfection. Heavy infections have been claimed to cause abdominal pain and weight loss. On rare occasions, pinworms invade the female genital tract, causing pruritus, vulvovaginitis and pelvic or peritoneal granulomas.

Diagnosis is made by examination of an adhesive cellophane tape pressed against the perianal region early in the morning. Serial examinations (3 or more) are advised. All affected individuals should be given a dose of mebendazole (100 mg once) or albendazole (400 mg once) with the same treatment repeated after 10 to 14 days. Because asymptomatic infestation of other members in a household is frequent, it may be reasonable to treat all household members simultaneously. Families should be informed that repeat infestations are common.

Cestodes

Members of this phylum are segmented worms. Cestodes, or tapeworms, can be divided into two major clinical groups. In the first, humans are the definitive hosts, with the adult tapeworms living in the gastrointestinal tract. In the second, humans are intermediate hosts, with larval stage parasites being present in tissues.

Cysticercosis

The pork tapeworm *Taenia solium* can cause two distinct forms of infection. The form that develops depends on whether humans are infected with adult tapeworms in the intestine or with larval cysts in tissues (cysticercosis). *T. solium* exists worldwide but is common in Latin America, sub-Saharan Africa, China, southern and Southeast Asia, and Eastern Europe.

Human cysticercosis develops after the ingestion of raw or undercooked pork meat contaminated with *T. solium* eggs. After ingestion of eggs by the intermediate host, the larvae are activated, escape the egg, penetrate the intestinal wall, and are carried to many tissues. The larvae have a predilection for striated muscle of the neck, tongue, and trunk. Within 60 to 90 days, the encysted larval stage develops. These cysts can survive for months to years. Autoinfection may occur if an individual with an egg-producing tapeworm ingests eggs derived from his or her own feces.

The clinical spectrum in cysticercosis is variable. Cysts can be found anywhere in the body but are most commonly detected in the brain, skeletal muscle, subcutaneous tissue, or eye. Symptoms depend on the number and location of cysts as well as on the extent of associated inflammatory responses and scarring. Neurological manifestations like seizures, hydrocephalus, and signs of increased intracranial pressure are common. When cysts develop at the base of the brain or in the subarachnoid space, they may cause chronic meningitis, communicating hydrocephalus, or strokes.

Diagnosis and treatment of cysticercosis depends on the site of involvement and the symptoms experienced. Cysts outside the CNS are usually not symptomatic. These eventually calcify, to be detected incidentally on plain radiographs of the limbs. For symptomatic cysts outside the CNS, the optimal approach is surgical resection. Medical therapy with praziquantel or albendazole may also be employed. Intestinal *T. solium* infection is treated with a single dose of praziquantel (10 mg/kg). However, praziquantel can evoke an inflammatory response in the CNS if concomitant cryptic cysticercosis is present.

Echinococcosis

Echinococcosis results when humans serve as intermediate hosts for cestodes of *Echinococcus* spp. This infection has two forms: hydatid or unilocular cyst disease, caused by *Echinococcus granulosus* or *Echinococcus vogeli*, and alveolar cyst disease, caused by *Echinococcus multilocularis*. *E. granulosus* is prevalent worldwide. *E. multilocularis* is found in Alpine, sub-Arctic, or Arctic regions, including Canada, the United States, central and northern Europe, and Asia. *E. vogeli* is found only in Central and South American highlands. Cysts develop in the intermediate hosts (sheep, cattle, humans, goats, camels, and horses for *E. granulosus*; and mice and other rodents for *E. multilocularis*) after the ingestion of eggs. When a dog ingests beef or lamb containing cysts, the life cycle is completed. Humans acquire echinococcosis by ingesting viable eggs with their food. Once in the intestinal tract, eggs hatch to form oncospheres that penetrate the mucosa and enter the circulation. Oncospheres then encyst in host viscera, developing over time to form mature larval cysts.

Symptoms are often absent and infection is detected incidentally by imaging studies. The liver (50%–70% of patients) and the lungs (20%–30% of patients) are the most common sites involved.

Some patients present with abdominal pain or a palpable mass in the right upper quadrant. Compression of a bile duct or leakage of cyst fluid into the biliary tree may mimic recurrent cholelithiasis, and biliary obstruction can result in jaundice. Rupture of a hydatid cyst may produce fever, pruritus, urticaria, eosinophilia, or anaphylactoid reactions. Pulmonary hydatid cysts may rupture into the bronchial tree or peritoneal cavity and produce cough, chest pain, or hemoptysis. A dangerous complication of cyst rupture is dissemination of protoscolices, which can form additional cysts. Rupture can occur spontaneously or at surgery. Other complications include involvement of bones, CNS, heart, and pelvis. Allergic reactions, including urticaria, asthma, and anaphylaxis are rare.

Diagnosis can be achieved by complementing imaging studies with specific ELISA and Western blot serology (available through the Centers for Disease Control and Prevention). Therapy is based on considerations of the size, location, and manifestations of cysts and the overall health of the patient. Optimal treatment of symptomatic cysts is obtained by surgical resection. An intermediate intervention for inoperable cysts is available, known as the *PAIR* (percutaneous aspiration, infusion of scolicidal agents, and reaspiration) procedure. For prophylaxis of secondary peritoneal echinococcosis due to inadvertent spillage of fluid during PAIR, the administration of albendazole (15 mg/kg daily in two divided doses) should be initiated at least 4 days before the procedure and continued for at least 4 weeks afterward.

Sparganosis

Sparganosis refers to the disease caused by the sparganum, second larval state of tapeworms of the genus *Spirometra* (mainly *Spirometra mansonoides*), a parasite of fish. The disease is prevalent in Asia, with some cases reported in North America plus sporadic cases seen in Australia, South America, and Europe. The definitive hosts are canids and felines, and the cycle includes larval states inside *Cyclops*, copepods, and amphibians. Humans get the infection by three routes: ingestion of contaminated amphibian meat, fish, or reptiles, drinking of water contaminated with infected *Cyclops*, and more rarely by the application of raw meat contaminated with plerocercoid over open wounds as folk remedies. The infection in humans will result in the development of a subcutaneous mass, where the plerocercoid will end up in a developmental form. Masses can be situated in deep structures or internal organs. The subcutaneous mass may have a migratory pattern, similar to what is seen in gnathostomiasis, a disease with a similar form of transmission. The diagnosis will be established by finding the worm in histological cuts of a subcutaneous mass, or even during surgery for acute abdominal pain. A more dramatic form with massive infiltration by multiple worms and high mortality rate has been associated with *Spirometra proliferum*.

Coenurosis

Coenurosis results when humans accidentally ingest coenurus (larval stage) of the dog tapeworm *Taenia multiceps, Taenia serialis,* or *Taenia crassiceps*, usually in contaminated fruits or vegetables. Larvae of these species may be inoculated directly into a child's conjunctiva and skin as the child plays on contaminated ground. This rare infection has been reported in Africa, and in North and South America. As in cysticercosis, involvement of the CNS, the eye, and subcutaneous tissue is most common. Surgical excision is the recommended therapy.

Trematodes

Members of this phylum share the classic, thick, oval leaf shape with variation in sizes. For clinical purposes this phylum could be divided according to the habitat in the infected host: blood flukes, hepatic flukes, intestinal flukes, and lung flukes. Human infection with trematodes occurs in many geographic areas and can cause considerable morbidity and mortality.

Schistosomiasis

Schistosomiasis or bilharziasis is the disease associated with infections by the flukes belonging to the genus *Schistosoma*. Humans get infected by coming into contact with water infested by the fluke. The disease is quite prevalent in the sub-Saharan African countries and Egypt. There are three species clearly associated with human beings: *Schistosoma hematobium*, *Schistosoma mansoni*, and *Schistosoma japonicum*. Whereas *S. hematobium* is associated with urogenital and late cutaneous schistosomiasis, *S. mansoni* and *S. japonicum* is associated with gastrointestinal disease. A very important group is the avian *Schistosoma* species associated with cercarial dermatitis. Human schistosomiasis is a disease of the fresh water cycle, whereas cercarial dermatitis of the avian type can occur either in fresh or salt water. The cycle requires that the eggs be eliminated in human urine or feces in order to reach the water and then infect an intermediate host, such as a snail. The cercariae, the infective larvae, will be produced inside the snail and then liberated into the water, where they can infect the human. The disease is acquired in the first and second decade of life, with a decline of the infection toward adulthood. The environmental impact of irrigation and hydroelectric projects will result in the development of new endemic areas.

The disease manifests itself by the immune response to invading and migrating larvae as well as to the presence of eggs in host tissue. Cercarial dermatitis refers to the clinical picture elucidated by the penetration of cercaria into the skin. In human schistosomiasis, it is most commonly seen in visitors to endemic areas rather than in permanent residents. That is not the case for avian cercarial dermatitis (swimmers itch), where anyone can be affected. This last form is self-limited, although symptoms will be similar for human and avian parasites. The clinical findings are those of an acute pruritic, papular rash at the site of the cercarial penetration, usually areas exposed to the water. The erythema and urticarial rash will be accompanied by a prickling sensation. The symptoms will peak at 2 to 3 days and resolve after 5 to 7 days, leaving post-inflammatory hyperpigmentation.

Acute schistosomiasis will appear 2 to 16 weeks after the cercarial phase. The symptoms will be similar to acute serum sickness, with fever, aches and pains, headache, fatigue, anorexia, diarrhea, and nausea (Katayama syndrome). Organomegaly can be seen. The disease usually lasts 2 to 3 weeks. It is caused by migration of the juvenile worm in the bloodstream. The worms will then reach their final destination, the venus plexus in the bladder, genital and groin areas in the case of *Schistosoma hematobium*, and mesenteric areas in cases of *S. mansoni*, and *S. japonicum*. The chronic visceral schistosomiasis will then manifest as symptoms related to the particular organ involved, that is, hematuria, obstructive uropathy, and hydronephrosis for *S. hematobium*. Diarrhea and bloody stools are more characteristic of *S. mansoni* and *S. japonicum* infection. Late cutaneous schistosomiasis will be produced as a reaction to chronic deposition of eggs in the dermis and subcutaneous tissue. It is commonly associated with *S. hematobium* infection. The clinical picture will be of clusters of pruritic papules, which then may coalesce into lichenified plaques. Classic locations include the anogenital areas, periumbilical areas, chest, and upper back. A zosteriform distribution may also be seen. Involvement of female genitalia is quite characteristic. Pruritus may lead to significant self-inflicted injury.

The diagnosis of cercarial dermatitis is based on the clinical history. It is based on the history of exposure to contaminated water of endemic areas associated with fever in the case of acute schistosomiasis, plus the presence of eggs in feces or urine and a positive serology. For chronic schistosomiasis, the diagnosis is based on the development of atypical pruritic lesions in patients residing in or traveling to endemic areas of *S. hematobium*. This last diagnosis can be corroborated by the presence of eggs in urine or in the biopsy of skin lesions accompanied by granulomatous reactions. Prevention of cercarial dermatitis is based on avoiding contact with contaminated water or the use of DEET as a repellent. Treatment of cercarial dermatitis and acute schistosomiasis should be directed toward treating the symptoms. Chronic schistosomiasis can be effectively treated with a single dose of praziquantel, or artemisine as an alternative treatment.

Fasciolasis

This infection occurs particularly in regions with intensive sheep or cattle production. Human cases have been reported in South America (high endemicity in Peru, Ecuador, and Bolivia), Europe, Africa, Australia, China, and Egypt. The predominant species is *Fasciola hepatica*, but in Asia and Africa an overlap with *Fasciola gigantica* has been reported.

Infection is acquired by ingestion of contaminated watercress, other aquatic plants, contaminated water, or food washed with such water. After ingestion, metacercariae excyst and penetrate the intestinal wall, peritoneal cavity, and Glisson capsule to reach the biliary system, where they mature into adult worms and deposit their eggs. These eggs are excreted in feces (about 4 months after infection) and then continue the cycle of infection in specific snails and encyst on aquatic plants.

The early phase of migration is characterized by fever, right upper quadrant pain, hepatomegaly, eosinophilia, and positive serologic findings. After migration to bile ducts, symptoms decline or disappear. Larvae sometimes also travel to ectopic body sites. Subcutaneous fascioliasis presents with painful or pruritic subcutaneous nodules, although this condition is rare.

Diagnosis of infection is based on a high degree of suspicion, geographic history, and finding of the characteristic ova in the feces. Eosinophilia occurs in 95% of acute stage infections, but may wax and wane during the chronic stage of infection. Magnetic resonance and computed tomography have been useful in detecting migratory tracts. New serologic tests may help in establishing the diagnosis. The drugs of choice are triclabendazole (10 mg/kg PO once) or praziquantel (25 mg/kg PO TID for 1 day).

Paragonomiasis

Paragonimus westermani is the most common lung fluke in humans. These species are endemic in Africa, Asia, and Central and South America. Humans acquire lung fluke infection when they ingest raw or pickled freshwater crabs or crayfish with encysted metacercariae. Once the organisms reach the small intestine, they excyst and penetrate the intestinal wall into the peritoneal cavity, traveling through the diaphragm to reach the pleural space and lungs. Mature flukes are found in the bronchioles, where they can live for 20 years or more. Eggs are expelled with sputum or swallowed and passed in human feces. The life cycle is completed in snails and freshwater crustacea.

Clinical manifestations include abdominal pain, diarrhea, and urticaria during the acute phase. These initial symptoms are followed by fever, dyspnea, chest pain, malaise, sweats, and dry cough followed by a productive cough with brownish sputum or hemoptysis. Chest examination may reveal signs of pleurisy. Extrapulmonary paragonomiasis can occur either from the migration of young or mature flukes to various organs or from eggs that enter the circulation and are carried to different sites. Subcutaneous paragonomiasis presents with migratory swelling or subcutaneous nodules in the lower abdominal and inguinal region containing immature flukes. Scrotal paragonomiasis may mimic epididymitis or an incarcerated hernia.

Paragonomiasis should be suspected in patients with eosinophilia and chest complaints. Diagnosis is confirmed by finding eggs in sputum, in feces, or pleural fluid. In extrapulmonary cases, serologic examination may be helpful. The drug of choice is praziquantel (25 mg/kg PO TID for 2 days).

PITFALLS AND MYTHS

One important myth in parasitology is to regard cutaneous larva migrans as a disease relevant only to tourist and leisure travelers. In fact, cutaneous larva migrans, along with tungiasis and papular urticaria, are extremely common in developing countries, and should be approached not only as mere medical curiosities but also as public health problems requiring the attention of local authorities and international health agencies.

A common misconception regarding American leishmaniasis is failure to recognize the important role that the immune system has in the pathogenesis of the disease. Most of the tissue destruction one can see in mucocutaneous leishmaniasis can be explained on the basis of marked cytokine imbalance seen in those patients, rather than a direct injury induced by the protozoa. Cure has been associated with a TH1 response, and increased production of IL-2 and gamma-interferon. Failure to cure, on the other hand, has been related to a TH2 response with excessive production of IL-4 and IL-10. Similarly, while TNF-α plays an important role in the destruction of the parasite, an excess of this cytokine is very much responsible for the associated tissue destruction that can be seen in mucocutaneous disease.

Another common pitfall in the care of leishmaniasis caused by *L. braziliensis* is failure to recognize the character of systemic disease and its potential for dissemination from just pure cutaneous disease. When dealing with cutaneous leishmaniasis of the New World, physicians are obligated to consider the possibility for mucocutaneous disease later. If any chance of *L. braziliensis* infection does exist, systemic treatment is obligatory. Although not 100% protective, systemic treatment will decrease the risk of developing mucocutaneous disease years later.

SUGGESTED READINGS

Textbooks

Canizares O, Harman R. *Clinical tropical dermatology*, 2nd edition. Boston, Blackwell Scientific, 1992.

Mandell GL, Bennett JE, Dolin R, eds. *Mandell, Douglas and Bennett's Principles and Practice of Infectious Diseases*, 5th edition. Churchill Livingstone, 2000.

Tyring S, Lupi O, Hengge U. *Tropical Dermatology*. Philadelphia: Elsevier, 2006.

Protozoa

Bravo F, Sanchez MR. New and re-emerging cutaneous infectious diseases in Latin America and other geographic areas. *Dermatol Clin* 2003;21(4):655.

Kichhoff LV. Agents of African Trypanosomiasis (Sleeping Sickness). In: Mandell GL, Bennett JE, Dolin R, eds. *Mandell, Douglas and Bennett's Principles and Practice of Infectious Diseases*, 5th edition. Churchill Livingstone, 2000, 2853–2858.

Kichhoff LV. Trypanosoma Species (American Trypanosomiasis, Chaga's Disease): Biology of Trypanosomes. In: Mandell GL, Bennett JE, Dolin R, editors. *Mandell, Douglas and Bennett's Principles and Practice of Infectious Diseases*, 5th Edition. Churchill Livingstone, 2000, 2845–51.

Maudlin I. African trypanosomiasis. *Ann Trop Med Parasitol* 2006;100(8):679–701.

Moncayo A, Ortiz Yanine MI. An update on Chaga's disease (human American trypanosomiasis). *Ann Trop Med Parasitol* 2006;100(8):663–677.

Singh S. New developments in diagnosis of leishmaniasis. *Indian J Med Res* 2006;123(3):311–330.

Helminths

Heukelbach J, Mencke N, Feldmeier H. Cutaneous larva migrans and tungiasis: the challenge to control zoonotic ectoparasitoses associated with poverty. *Trop Med Int Health* 2002;7(11):907–910.

Keiser J, Utzinger J. Emerging foodborne trematodiasis. *Emerg Infect Dis* 2005;11(10):1507–1514.

Pozio E, Gomez Morales MA, Dupouy-Camet J. Clinical aspects, diagnosis and treatment of trichinellosis. *Expert Rev Anti Infect Ther* 2003;1(3):471–482.

PART III: INFECTIONS IN SELECTED ECOSYSTEMS

10 | INFECTIONS IN THE DESERT

Joseph C. Pierson* and David J. DiCaudo*

Deserts make up over one-fifth of the earth's land surface. These areas have traditionally been defined as regions with low precipitation, <10 inches (<250 mm) annually. Potential evapotranspiration, in conjunction with precipitation levels, may more accurately delineate desert regions as it reflects the amount of water the atmosphere removes from the earth's surface. For example, the Tucson, Arizona area, which slightly exceeds 10 inches of rainfall annually, experiences evaporation that can be eight times higher than that amount. Nonpolar deserts are typically hot, have low humidity, and are characterized by extremes of their diurnal temperature range (high during the daylight, relatively low during the nighttime). The terrain of these dry regions is often dominated by sand and rocky surfaces with sparse vegetation.

There are two main infectious diseases of dermatologic significance that occur primarily in, or adjacent to the arid desert regions of the globe: Old World cutaneous leishmaniasis and coccidioidomycosis. The former is limited to the Eastern Hemisphere, while the latter is limited to the Western Hemisphere. There is a striking absence of either disease occurring naturally in the opposite hemisphere, and they are discussed separately here.

EASTERN HEMISPHERE: OLD WORLD CUTANEOUS LEISHMANIASIS

Leishmaniasis is a protozoal infection transmitted by the bite of a sandfly. The three main clinical syndromes are cutaneous, mucocutaneous, and visceral infections. The cutaneous leishmaniasis (CL) presentation is most common, with the World Health Organization estimating 1.5 million cases each year. CL is further classified by geography: Old World (eastern hemisphere) and New World (western hemisphere) subtypes, each transmitted by a different genus of the sandfly vector, which cause infection by different *Leishmania* protozoa species with variable behavior. New World (western hemisphere) leishmaniasis occurs in tropical and subtropical regions. The more common Old World CL is seen most frequently in desert regions throughout the Middle East, Central and Southwest Asia, and elsewhere in Asia, Africa, and the Mediterranean regions. It is transmitted by the *Phlebotomus* genera sandfly vector. The identified parasites harbored by the *Phlebotomus* sandfly in Old World CL are primarily *Leishmania major* and *Leishmania tropica,* and less

commonly *Leishmania aethiopica* and *Leishmania infantum* in Ethiopia and the Mediterranean, respectively.

Old World CL is the most important unique skin infection afflicting those who reside or travel in desert environments of the eastern hemisphere. Lesions present clinically following an incubation period of weeks to months. Although CL typically heals spontaneously, it can cause disfiguring active lesions or scarring. The diagnosis should be considered in any individual who presents with chronic persistent skin lesions and a history of being in an endemic region in the months before presentation. Although commonly referred to as the "Baghdad boil" over the last century, the city with the highest incidence now is actually Kabul, Afghanistan. Primary prevention of the disease-transmitting sandfly bite remains the most critical step in reducing the impact of CL worldwide. No standardized effective vaccine currently exists. Traditional methods of diagnosis and treatment have been well described in texts over the past several decades. However, there are major advances in both diagnostic techniques and therapeutic options that will be emphasized in this chapter.

History

Written descriptions typical of Old World CL appeared as early as the second or third millennium B.C. The *Leishmania* protozoa were discovered in 1885 by a British investigator, Major Cunningham from a "Delhi boil." Definitive proof that the protozoa caused the disease was established by other British physicians, Colonel Leishman and Colonel Donovan in 1903. Old World CL received significant global interest during World Wars I and II, when thousands of international soldiers were afflicted with the disease.

> In some cities infection is so common and so inevitable that normal children are expected to have the disease soon after they begin playing outdoors, and visitors seldom escape a sore as a souvenir. Since one attack gives immunity, Oriental sores appearing on an adult person in Baghdad brands him as a new arrival … *Introduction to Parasitology,* 1944

Numerous pseudonyms have been used to describe Old World CL by both laymen and clinicians alike (Fig. 10.1).

Epidemiology

Old World CL occurs predominantly in the eastern hemisphere in areas highlighted in the map in Figure 10.2. Inhabitants

---

* Eastern Hemisphere: Old World Cutaneous Leishmaniasis by Joseph C. Pierson
* Western Hemisphere: Coccidioidomycosis and the Skin by David J. DiCaudo

of both rural desert and urban areas are at risk. World Health Organization data show Kabul, Afghanistan, had 67,500 cases of the disease in 2003 – amounting to one-third of infected individuals in that country.

There is no racial predilection. Incidence may be higher in men from occupational exposures, and also perhaps because they have more uncovered skin than females in endemic regions, whose attire is often more concealing due to religious customs. The disease can afflict patients of any age, although those very young and very old may be more prone to complications of the disease due to reduced immunity.

Transmission: Sandfly Vector and *Leishmania* Lifecycle

The 2-mm long female *Phlebotomus* sandfly vector is a poor flyer, vulnerable to gusts of wind, and moves via a series of short hops (Fig. 10.3). Because of their small size, the sandflies are capable of passing through standard untreated mosquito netting. Ecosystems with feces, manure, rodent burrows, and leaf litter heighten sandfly breeding activity. It is typically most capable of transmitting leishmaniasis in the warmer nights during the spring through autumn months.

In Old World CL caused by *L. major*, transmission is zoonotic (typical of most *Leishmania* species) via the *Phlebotomus papatasi* sandfly. The reservoir hosts for the *Leishmania* parasite are mainly rodents and dogs, and also equines, opossum, sloth, and monkeys. Humans are actually incidental hosts. In *L. tropica*, transmission is anthroponotic via the *Phlebotomus sergenti* sandfly. Humans are the reservoir, and no known animal reservoir exists (Fig. 10.4).

When an infected sandfly bites a human, the leishmaniasis promastigotes are injected into the skin. Once phagocytized by mononuclear cells, they become amastigotes, where their

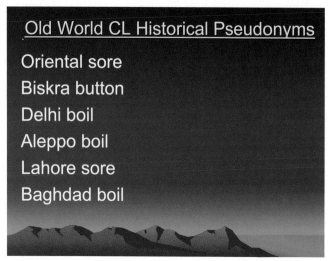

Figure. 10.1. Old World cutaneous leishmaniasis pseudonyms.

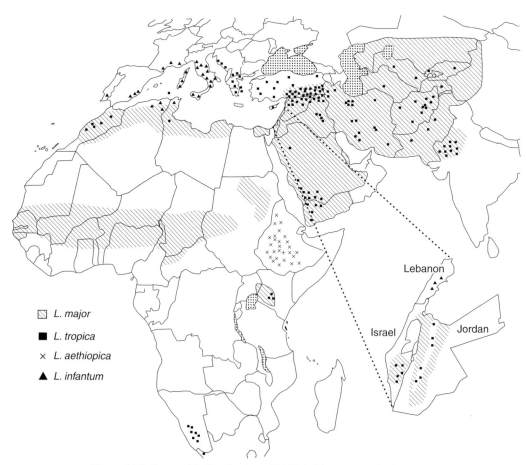

Figure. 10.2. Geographic distribution of Old World cutaneous leishmaniasis.

intracellular presence disrupts normal cellular immunity. It is during the amastigote phase that a subsequent sandfly may ingest the parasite, which develops into a promastigote form again within the insect vector. The pathogen can persist locally in its host following clinical cure, a reflection of the elusive durability of the parasite despite host immune mechanisms.

Prevention

Currently, the three components of prevention of leishmaniasis are (1) suppression of the host (usually rodent or dog)

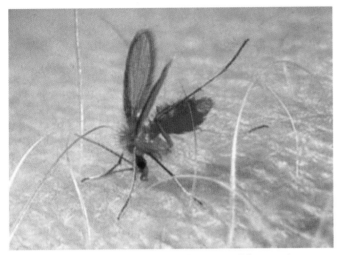

Figure. 10.3. *Phlebotomus sp.* sandfly, the vector of the parasite responsible for Old World cutaneous leishmaniasis.

reservoir, (2) suppression of the sandfly vector, and most importantly, (3) personal protective measures.

Host suppression can be done systematically where high rates of Old World CL due to the zoonotic transmission of *L. major* are seen. Bulldozing of rodent burrows and euthanizing of infected dogs can be helpful. Another approach is insecticide treatment of reservoir hosts, by pumping the agent into rodent burrows or by using delmethrin-treated dog collars.

The sandfly vector within living areas can be reduced by area environmental insecticide spraying. This may be beneficial in urban areas, though it is often impractical or ineffective in rural areas where dwellings are more dispersed.

The critical personal protective measures include limiting outdoor activity during nocturnal hours, permethrin-treated clothing with long-sleeved shirts tucked into trousers, which in turn, are tucked into socks or boots, the application of topical insecticides, permethrin-treated bed nets, and bedside fans. The permethrin-treated clothing will maintain efficacy through numerous washings. Exposed skin applications of diethyltoluamide (DEET) concentrations of 25% to 35% are recommended for those above 12 years. Sandfly bed nets are a finer mesh (smaller hole diameter: 18 holes/square in.) than standard mosquito bed nets, which may be warm for the sleeping occupant. Soaking the bed nets in permethrin should improve their effectiveness. In the absence of appropriate netting material, bedside fans may protect individuals by the limiting the approach of the relatively awkward flying vector.

There is no effective prophylactic medication, nor currently licensed effective vaccine. A killed *Leishmania* promastigote combined with BCG vaccine has been tested. It should be noted that individuals infected by one species of

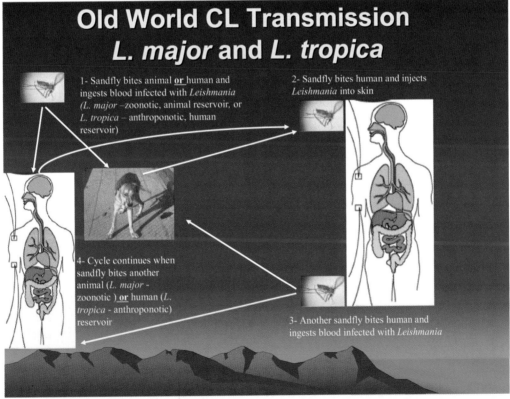

Figure. 10.4. Old World cutaneous leishmaniasis transmission cycle.

Leishmania are generally immune to reinfection from that specific species.

Clinical Presentation

The time range from the entry of the *Leishmania* amastigote within a human macrophage to the appearance of clinical lesions can vary from several days to years, but incubation is usually 2 to 12 weeks. Although the widely described lesion is a painless volcano-like ulceration with rolled borders, it can be a polymorphic "great imitator" disease and clinicians should keep the broad list of differential diagnoses in mind when evaluating suspected cases (Fig. 10.5).

The diversity in both incubation period and clinical appearance results from the variable interplay between the virulence of the infecting protozoa and the host immune response. Ultimately, uncomplicated cases in immunocompetent hosts tend to heal with variable degrees of scarring months to over a year later.

Classically, an individual with a history of endemic region exposure in the preceding 2 to 12 weeks initially presents with one or several inflammatory macules, papules, nodules, or plaques on exposed skin sites. They may recall transient papules typical of arthropod bite reactions weeks or months earlier. Individuals with significant outdoor nocturnal exposures in endemic regions may experience hundreds of such sandfly bite reactions. Ulceration, which may become "volcano-like" with rolled borders, can occur early or later in the progression of the disease process. Crusting, scaling, and concentric rings of desquamation may be seen. As a bacterial infection is often initially suspected, there may be a prior history of failure to respond to systemic antibiotic treatment, although this may clear any element of secondary bacterial infection. The lesions typically do not itch or hurt, although pain may occur if large, overlying joints are subjected to trauma or secondarily infected. Underlying neural involvement can rarely cause diminished sensation of lesional skin. Orientation along skin tension lines and lesion grouping are commonly seen. Satellitosis of smaller papules and nodules, proximal subcutaneous nodules in a lymphangitic sporotrichoid pattern, and regional adenopathy are seen in a significant minority of cases. These changes suggest cutaneous dissemination. In general, patients do not complain of systemic symptoms and are not febrile. A summary of the clinical findings that should raise the suspicion of a diagnosis of CL has been described by Kubba (Fig. 10.6). See Figures 10.7 to 10.11 for representative cases of CL.

Among the myriad atypical lesions that may be seen in localized cases of Old World CL are psoriasiform, verrucal, zosteriform, erysipeloid, and eczematous presentations. An olecranon bursitis underlying psoriasiform Old World CL has been seen in U.S. service members. *L. aethiopica* may rarely cause a diffuse Old World CL pattern in Africa in those who fail to mount an appropriate immune reaction.

Post-kala-azar dermal leishmaniasis is not a primary form of Old World CL, but rather a phenomenon seen in those recovering from visceral leishmaniasis in Africa and India. Symmetrical macules, papules, and nodules are seen on the face (which can cause a leonine facies), and less commonly on the trunk and extremities.

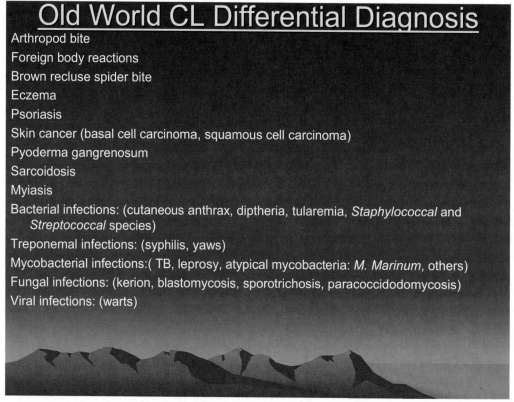

Old World CL Differential Diagnosis

Arthropod bite

Foreign body reactions

Brown recluse spider bite

Eczema

Psoriasis

Skin cancer (basal cell carcinoma, squamous cell carcinoma)

Pyoderma gangrenosum

Sarcoidosis

Myiasis

Bacterial infections: (cutaneous anthrax, diptheria, tularemia, *Staphylococcal* and *Streptococcal* species)

Treponemal infections: (syphilis, yaws)

Mycobacterial infections:(TB, leprosy, atypical mycobacteria: *M. Marinum*, others)

Fungal infections: (kerion, blastomycosis, sporotrichosis, paracoccidodomycosis)

Viral infections: (warts)

Figure. 10.5. A partial list of the differential diagnosis of Old World cutaneous leishmaniasis.

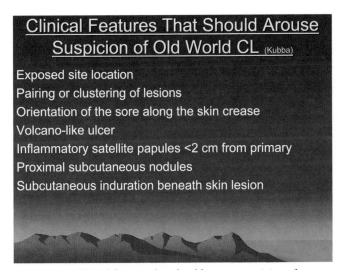

Figure. 10.6. Clinical features that should arouse suspicion of a diagnosis of Old World cutaneous leishmaniasis.

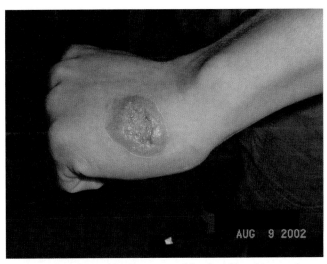

Figure. 10.7. Volcano-like ulceration of the dorsal hand in a patient with cutaneous leishmaniasis.

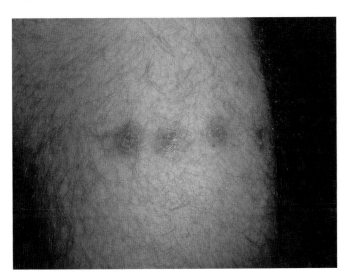

Figure. 10.8. Linear array of crusted papules corresponding to sites of earlier sandfly bites in a patient with cutaneous leishmaniasis. (Courtesy of Dr. Glenn Wortmann).

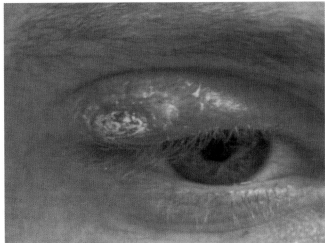

Figure. 10.9. Crusted ulceration of the upper eyelid in a patient with cutaneous leishmaniasis. (Courtesy of Dr. Peter Weina).

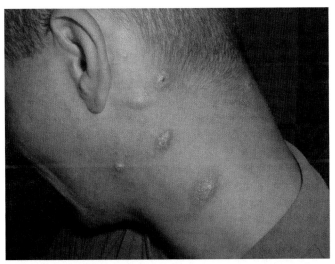

Figure. 10.10. Multiple crusted papules and plaques of the neck with accompanying visible regional adenopathy in a patient with cutaneous leishmaniasis. (Courtesy of Dr. Peter Weina).

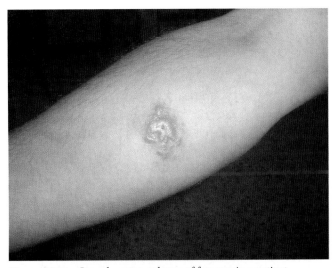

Figure. 10.11. Granulomatous plaque of forearm in a patient with cutaneous leishmaniasis. A punch biopsy with tissue impression "touch prep" smears would be the procedure of choice for the cytologic diagnosis of nonulcerative lesions.

Cases of mucocutaneous spread of Old World CL due to *L. major* and *L. aethiopica* are debatable as these could be instances of direct extension of skin lesions, rather than metastatic spread of the organism.

Scarring occurs in a centrifugal fashion within months of reaching maximum lesion size, but this may take nearly 2 years. The resulting scar is characteristically atrophic and depressed. However, dyspigmented, violaceous, and hypertrophic scarring can be seen. Permanent scarring that can be disfiguring in cosmetically significant areas can be psychologically devastating for patients, while scarring overlying critical joint areas can limit mobility.

Leishmaniasis recidivans is a late recurrence of the disease process at the site of a healed lesion, usually within 2 years, but sometimes more than a decade later. It is usually due to *L. tropica* in Old World CL, often appears as psoriasiform or lupus vulgaris-like "apple-jelly" papular or nodular lesions beginning at the periphery, and is notoriously treatment resistant.

Systemic spread of Old World CL is extremely rare, but was reported in several US troops following Operation Desert Storm in 1991 from *L. tropica* infection. Systemic spread, when it occurs, is more likely to occur in immunocompromised individuals, such as those infected by human immunodeficiency virus (HIV).

Diagnostic Procedures

When inflammatory lesions from a patient with exposure in endemic region promptly resolve with an empiric course of antibiotics, this generally excludes a diagnosis of Old World CL. For persistent lesions, laboratory testing of tissue specimens from suspected cases serves to confirm the diagnosis of CL and can exclude other disease processes. As early therapeutic interventions may reduce subsequent disfiguring or restrictive scarring, a simple diagnostic procedure with high sensitivity and specificity is ideal. Dermal scraping tissue smears and punch biopsy with tissue impression "touch prep" smears are widely employed. Both techniques yield specimens on glass slides. However, the quality of tissue samples submitted with either procedure can vary with the diligence and experience of the clinician, and even when optimal, the sensitivity for both techniques can be a modest 70% to 75%. In addition to sample quality variability, which is operator dependent, the diligence and experience of the microscopist can vary and further impact diagnostic yield.

Dermal scraping of suspected *Leishmania* lesions for tissue smears may be optimal when the lesion is ulcerative or the overlying crust is easily removed, yielding the underlying ulceration. Stepwise instructions and images of the procedure are shown in Figures 10.12 and 10.13. Dermal scraping tissue smears may have a better diagnostic yield than punch biopsy tissue specimens since the latter have a more dense tissue background.

Punch biopsies are recommended for nonulcerative lesions. In addition, the advantage of performing a punch biopsy in leishmaniasis diagnosis is that the specimen can simultaneously be examined for other diseases in the differential diagnosis. This is particularly important for atypical lesions, papules, nodules, and plaques. The punch should be obtained from an active bor-

Dermal Scraping Technique for *Leishmania* Tissue Smears

1. Anesthetize the area with a local agent such as lidocaine 1% with epinephrine 1:10^5 (unless the latter is contraindicated).
2. Obtain 2 to 4 tissue smears by horizontally scraping the base of the ulceration with a # 10 or #15 blade (this may require removal of the overlying crusted debris). The <u>dermal</u> tissue is then thinly applied in a circular fashion to a nickel-sized (approx. 2 cm) area in the center of the slide.
3. As the dermal tissue is required for pathologic visualization, minimize blood, keratin, pus, and crusted debris on slide.
4. Dermal tissue for ancillary PCR testing can be inserted into a small container of 70-100% ethanol. Overlying crusted debris may also be submitted for PCR analysis.

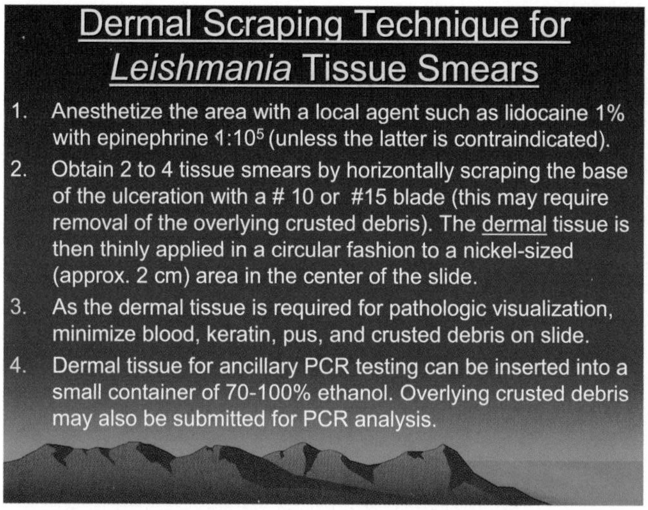

Figure. 10.12. Instructional steps for collection of dermal scrapings for *Leishmania* tissue smears.

Collection of Dermal Scrapings for Tissue Smears and PCR
Minimize blood, keratin, pus, and crusted debris on slides

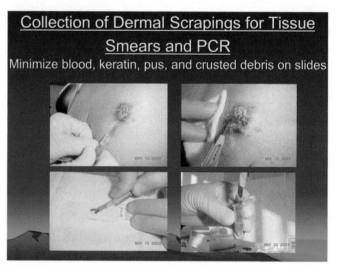

Figure. 10.13. Sequential photographs of the performance of dermal scraping collection for tissue smears and PCR. (Courtesy of Dr. Glenn Wortmann).

der, the excess blood is blotted, and then the cut edge rolled onto a glass slide creating the tissue impression smear.

Another option for obtaining specimens from papular or nodular lesions is through needle aspirates. A needle aspirate can be obtained by injecting preservative-free saline (0.1 mL) into a lesional border of intact skin, and then aspirating while moving the needle back and forth under the skin. A slit-skin smear technique for slide preparation is also used in some countries.

Slides obtained by any of the above techniques are stained with Giemsa and examined under oil immersion. The diagnostic feature is the finding of the nucleus and rod-shaped kinetoplast of the amastigote within the vacuoles of macrophages (Fig. 10.14). Amastigote kinetoplast visualization is critical in differentiation from *Histoplasma capsulatum*.

Formal histology of punch biopsy specimens submitted for H&E sections will reveal inflammation with lymphocytes, macrophages, and plasma cells in the dermis. Necrotizing granulomas may also be seen. Upper dermis macrophages may reveal the engulfed amastigotes, which usually stain well with H&E or Brown-Hopps modified tissue Gram's stain. The latter stain accentuates the kinetoplast and produces minimal background staining and maximum contrast. Oil immersion observation with a 100x objective is necessary, and multiple tissue sections may need to be reviewed before identification of the parasite (Fig. 10.15).

A portion of punch biopsy or needle aspirates can be sent for microbiologic culture identification. Specimens are inoculated for cultures on Novy-MacNeal-Nicolle biphasic or Schneider's insect media. Culture allows *Leishmania* speciation via subsequent isoenzyme electrophoresis. This requires specialized

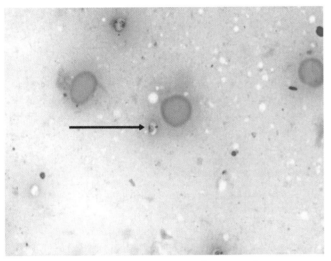

Figure. 10.14. A tissue impression smear illustrating the characteristics of an amastigote, with thin cell membrane, cytoplasm, nucleus, and kinetoplast *(arrow)* (Giemsa stain; original magnification, _1000). (Courtesy of Mr. Ron Neafie).

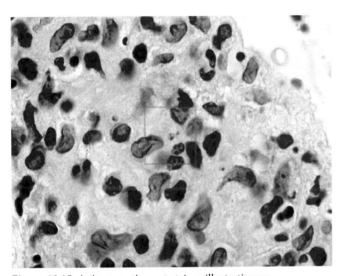

Figure. 10.15. A tissue section cut at 4μm illustrating an amastigote, with thin cell membrane, cytoplasm, nucleus, and kinetoplast *(arrow)* (hematoxylin and eosin stain; original magnification, _1000). (Courtesy of Mr. Ron Neafie).

laboratories and strong microbiologist skills. The main disadvantage is that results may take several weeks.

Delayed-type hypersensitivity (Montenegro) skin testing to *Leishmania* antigens is not available in the United States or Canada. This intradermal testing is performed as a diagnostic adjunct in many endemic countries, but is not standardized, and cannot distinguish between acute and remote infections.

The exciting key diagnostic advance in leishmaniasis is the use of polymerase chain reaction (PCR)–based amplification technology, which detects *Leishmania* nucleic acid sequences. Tissue collection for PCR testing is very simple, even for the novice, and more importantly, it has the highest sensitivity, and is highly specific. It will likely become the gold standard wherever available.

PCR testing is ideally performed from fresh tissue specimens (such as the tissue debris obtained from dermal scraping – see Fig. 10.13) merely inserted into 70% to 100% ethanol, but can also be done on paraffin-embedded tissue. In addition to the simplicity of specimen collection, results are available within hours, the sensitivity is >90%, and it is relatively inexpensive. Kinetoplast, telomere, nuclear DNA, and ribosomal RNA amplification targets have been used.

Delayed-type hypersensitivity (Montenegro) skin testing to *Leishmania* antigens is not available in the United States or Canada. This intradermal testing is performed as a diagnostic adjunct in many endemic countries, but is not standardized, and cannot distinguish between acute and remote infections.

Serologic immunodiagnosis is useful only for visceral leishmaniasis.

Free diagnostic assistance in the United States for civilian providers is available through the Centers for Disease Control and Prevention (CDC): phone 770–488–4475, online http://www.dpd.cdc.gov/dpdx/HTML/DiagnosticProcedures.htm

For U.S. military providers, diagnostic assistance is available through Walter Reed Army Institute of Research: phone 301–319–9956, online http://www.pdhealth.mil/leish.asp

Pathology assistance is available through the Armed Forces Institute of Pathology: online http://www.afip.org/

Treatment

The goal of any treatment options used in Old World CL is to reduce subsequent disfiguring or mobility-limiting scarring. As CL is a self-resolving process, no treatment is an option. This is particularly true for patients infected by *L. major*, whose lesions are small, few in number, and at concealed locations such as the trunk and proximal extremities, especially if they are in the resolution phase. There are several newer physical modalities and topical and oral therapeutic options that can be utilized in the majority of patients requiring treatment. In general, as opposed to New World CL, only a small minority of Old World CL patients eventually need aggressive systemic therapy. A suggested algorithm for the treatment of Old World CL is shown below (Fig. 10.16). Note the lower threshold for aggressive therapy of Old World CL due to the *L. tropica* parasite because of its tendency for therapeutic recalcitrance. Regardless of the *Leishmania* specific therapy employed, identification and treatment of secondary bacterial infection plays an important role.

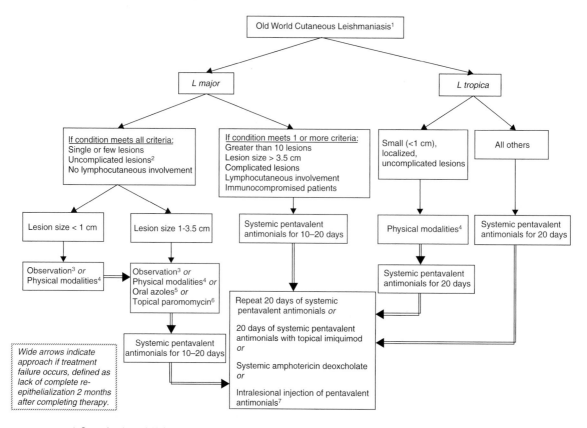

1. Secondary bacterial infections should be treated prior to using any physical methods, but this may be done concurrently with systemic treatments.
2. Lesions are considered "complicated" if they are located on the hands, feet, over joints, or in cosmetically important areas. Also consider if located above a bursa, sporotrichoid extension with subcutaneous nodules, multiple daughter modules, or regional adenopathy > 1 cm in size.
3. Depending on patient wishes. *L major* typically resolves within one year if left untreated.
4. Physical modalities include heat (ThermoMed™) or cryotherapy (liquid nitrogen) on aneshetized skin. Regimen used for cryotherapy is two 30-second freeze-thaw cycles. Can be used in pregnancy; use with care in darkly-skinned individuals (particularly cryotherapy) due to risk of permanent hypopigmentation. Avoid treatment directly over blood vessels and nerves, implanted metal, or in those with a pacemaker (specifically, ThermoMed™).
5. Ketoconazole, itraconazole, and fluconazole have all been used.
6. In the U.S., paromomycin capsules can be compounded into a topical formulation.
7. In some circumstances, pentavalent antimonials may be directly injected into skin lesions (although this is currently not indicated in the U.S. IND protocols).

Figure. 10.16. A treatment algorithm for the treatment of Old World cutaneous leishmaniasis caused by *L. major* and *L. tropica*. (Courtesy of Dr. Naomi Aronson).

The traditional physical modality treatment option of Old World CL, particularly for smaller lesions, is cryotherapy with liquid nitrogen. The recommended regimen is two 30-second freeze–thaw cycles, which can be repeated in 3 weeks. Liquid nitrogen treatment should be used with particular caution in dark-skinned patients because of the risk of permanent hypopigmentation.

A newer physical modality tool is the ThermoMed™ device (Fig. 10.17). It is a portable, battery-operated United States Food and Drug Administration (FDA)–approved device that delivers localized heat via radiofrequency (50°C × 30 seconds). Although simple to operate, it should only be used by individuals properly trained in its use. Local anesthetic is injected into the area before treatment. Treatment on the face, over large blood vessels or nerves, implanted metal, or in patients with pacemakers should be avoided. A prominent bullous response is often elicited in the ThermoMed™-treated area (Fig. 10.18). Topical application of gentamicin antibiotic ointment (an aminoglycoside that may also have some anti-*Leishmania* activity)

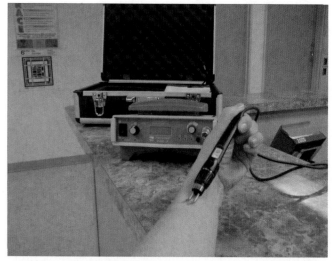

Figure. 10.17. ThermoMed™ device showing prongs of hand piece that are applied to the *Leishmania* lesions. (Courtesy of Dr. Naomi Aronson).

for several days following this localized heat therapy may reduce secondary infection risk.

The results of a controlled study in 2002 suggest that oral fluconazole 200 mg daily for 6 weeks speeds healing in Old World CL. Subsequent experience with this agent, and other azole antifungals, itraconazole, and ketoconazole, has yielded mixed results. Reports of success with systemic azole antifungal treatment of Old World CL have been primarily limited to the *L. major* species. Liver function screening and monitoring should be performed if these agents are utilized.

Topical paromomycin (aminosidine) formulations, an aminoglycoside antibiotic, hold great promise as an option for uncomplicated cases of Old World CL due to *L. major*. When the agent is mixed with methylbenzonium chloride, an efficacy of 74% was reported in the treatment of CL due to *L. major*; however, local discomfort can occur. In the United States, a paromomycin sulfate 15% with gentamicin sulfate 0.5% formulation (WR279396) has shown positive responses in healing times and subsequent scar cosmesis in phase II placebo-controlled studies. Owing to its simplicity for both the patient and the provider, coupled with the absence of blistering and dyspigmentation that may be seen with ThermoMed™ or cryotherapy treatments, if a paromomycin formulation of equal or better efficacy is eventually FDA approved, it would be an attractive alternative to the physical modalities described earlier. Currently in the United States, some pharmacies can compound paromomycin (15% paromomycin phosphate with 10% urea in white soft paraffin), which can be applied twice daily for 3 to 4 weeks. Compounding pharmacies in the United States can be located at http://iacprx.org/referral_service/index.html

Aggressive systemic treatment of Old World CL is reserved for specific scenarios as outlined in the algorithm. The standard for aggressive systemic treatment of Old World CL remains a parenteral pentavalent antimony (PVA) agent. Pentostam (sodium stibogluconate) is the agent used in the United States. In addition to relatively simple lesions that do not respond to earlier measures, larger Old World CL lesions (>3.5 cm diameter for *L. major*, >1cm for *L. tropica*), numerous lesions, lymphocutaneous manifestations, and the presence of disease in an immunocompromised patient all may merit parenteral PVA treatment. Also, patients with "complicated" lesions of the hands and feet, cosmetically conspicuous involvement of areas such as the face, involvement overlying joints or bursa, or the presence of multiple satellite "daughter" lesions are appropriate candidates for PVA treatment.

Pentostam (sodium stibogluconate) is only available in the United States via an approved investigational new drug (IND) protocol within the military (Walter Reed Army Medical Center in Washington D.C., phone 202–782–1663/8691 and Brooke Army Medical Center, San Antonio, TX, phone 210–916–5554) or the CDC Parasitic Drug Services section (phone 404–639–3670) free of cost to civilian physicians for parasitologically confirmed cases. The dosage regimen is 20 mg/kg/day for 10 to 20 days, with an overall efficacy ranging from 45% to 100%. It is recommended that the outpatient administration occur via a steel butterfly needle inserted into the antecubital vein each day to eliminate the risk of device-related infections. A timeline for the occurrence of side effects with this regimen is shown in Figure 10.19. Common side effects are reversible elevations of pancreatic and hepatic enzyme levels, arthralgias, and myalgias. The musculoskeletal side effects are the most common reason for early discontinuation of therapy. Although severe cardiac problems are rare, note that a >0.5-second prolongation of the QT interval is an indication to stop therapy temporarily.

Other PVA agents are used around the world, including Glucantime (meglumine antimoniate) in Europe. Although PVA in the form of Pentostam is only delivered intravenously in the United States, intramuscular and intralesional protocols are used in endemic areas. The intralesional route is advantageous because of reduced side effects and decreased cost, but can be painful.

Amphotericin B deoxycholate therapy, 0.5 to 1 mg/kg/day for 14 to 30 days to a cumulative dose of 1 to 2 gm, is reserved for Old World CL PVA treatment failures. It has a well-documented risk of nephrotoxicity and infusion-related allergic reactions.

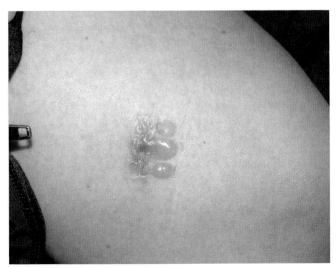

Figure. 10.18. ThermoMed™ -treated area yielding representative second-degree burn change.

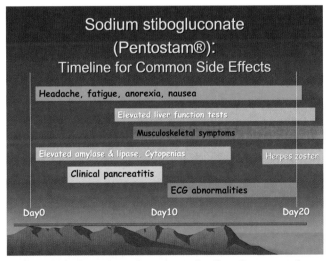

Figure. 10.19. Chronology of common side effects during a 20-day course of parenteral Pentostam

Miltefosine, an antineoplastic agent, has been used successfully to treat various forms of leishmaniasis in both hemispheres of the world. In a 2007 comparative study, oral miltefosine, 2.5 mg/kg/day for 28 days was as successful in treating Old World CL as a PVA agent and no patients showed serious side effects.

Published reports of successful treatment of Old World CL with photodynamic therapy have appeared in recent years. A 2006 series of five patients who underwent a regimen of δ-aminolevulinic acid in a water-in-oil emulsion applied to lesions, followed by irradiation once weekly for a month showed excellent results with no scarring (Ghaffarifar). Only mild local inflammatory reactions occurred at the treated areas.

Other oral agents, including allopurinol, dapsone, rifampicin, both oral and intralesionally injected zinc sulfate, and topical imiquimod have been used to treat Old World CL, either alone or in combination with a PVA, with variable results.

Regardless of therapeutic intervention (or nonintervention), complete healing and re-epithelialization of lesions with no recurrence 6 months later is considered a clinical cure of CL. In 2007, a systematic review of published randomized controlled trials of Old World CL concluded that studies thus far were highly variable in quality and methods, and provided weak evidence for the treatment of Old World CL. It is clear that well-designed, double-blinded, controlled studies are strongly needed.

Follow-up

Patients should be followed up for up to 6 to 12 months after apparent clinical healing. Relapse can occur and is most likely in the first few months after initial clearing. Patients should monitor healed sites for evidence of ulceration, scabbing, scaling, induration, new lesions, or increase in scar size. Reactivations often occur at sites of trauma of even minimal degree, the Koebner phenomenon (isomorphic response). Because of this, elective surgery and tattoo placements should be delayed for 12 months.

Reinfection from the same species causing Old World CL is unlikely for the remainder of the individual's lifetime, but occurs in a very small percentage of patients.

A diagnosis of any type of leishmaniasis precludes blood donation in the United States for the remainder of the patient's life as in the following document:

http://www.militaryblood.dod.mil/library/policies/downloads/03–08.pdf

WESTERN HEMISPHERE: COCCIDIOIDOMYCOSIS AND THE SKIN

Deserts of the New World are the habitat of *Coccidioides species*, the fungi that cause coccidioidomycosis. The organisms live in the soil and produce arthroconidia, which are dispersed by the wind. Suitable hosts, such humans, dogs, and horses, acquire pulmonary infection through the inhalation of the air-borne arthroconidia. The infection is virtually always acquired from an environmental source; person-to-person transmission does not occur.

Most cases of coccidioidomycosis are asymptomatic. A minority of patients develop a febrile, influenza-like respiratory illness. Extrapulmonary dissemination occurs in <1% percent of patients. Though only a relatively small percentage of patients experience severe symptoms, coccidioidomycosis is nevertheless a significant cause of morbidity, since the infection is so widely prevalent in endemic areas. Occasional deaths do occur, particularly in patients with risk factors.

History

Since the initial description of coccidioidomycosis in 1892, the skin has provided particularly important clues to the diagnosis. The first reported case was discovered as the result of striking cutaneous manifestations. The patient, an Argentine soldier, presented with cutaneous nodules that clinically resembled tumor-stage mycosis fungoides. Skin biopsy revealed distinctive organisms, which are now known to be the fungal spherules of *Coccidioides*. In the 1930s, the skin provided another clue to a milder expression of the disease. At that time in the San Joaquin Valley of California, erythema nodosum was considered an important sign of "Valley Fever," a self-limited respiratory illness caused by coccidioidomycosis. Over the past half-century, as the desert Southwest transformed into a popular destination for tourism and for migration, coccidioidomycosis became an increasingly important disease. In current times, cutaneous signs continue to be exceedingly useful clues to the diagnosis of coccidioidomycosis.

Epidemiology

Coccidioides species are found in arid regions of the New World from the western United States to Argentina. Areas with hot, dry summers, few winter freezes, low annual rainfall, and alkaline soil are particularly suitable for growth of the organism within the soil. Central and southern Arizona and the San Joaquin Valley of southern California have the highest incidence rates of coccidioidomycosis in the world. In California, the species *Coccidioides immitis* is identified as the causative organism. Outside California, the species *Coccidioides posadasii* (sometimes designated *C. immitis var. posadasii*) is responsible for nearly all infections. Both species produce clinically similar signs and symptoms.

In endemic areas, exposure to air-borne dust is a well-documented risk factor for infection. Clusters of cases have been associated with archeological excavations and with military exercises. Epidemics have occurred in association with dust storms, earthquakes, and droughts. Over the past decade, Arizona has been experiencing an epidemic attributed to a prolonged drought. From 1996 to 2006, the incidence in Arizona increased more than four-fold.

Both healthy and immunosuppressed patients are at risk for coccidioidomycosis. Occasionally, severe infections can develop even in healthy persons with no risk factors. Risk factors for severe disease and dissemination include genetic predisposition, immunosuppression, or pregnancy. Filipinos and African-Americans appear to be genetically predisposed to a markedly increased risk of severe coccidioidomycosis. Immunosuppressed patients, including acquired immunodeficiency syndrome (AIDS) patients and transplant recipients, have a particularly high risk of fulminant disease and dissemination.

Diagnosis

The lungs are the primary site of infection in nearly all cases. Chest radiographs commonly show pulmonary infiltrates,

Table 10.1: Cutaneous Manifestations of Coccidioidomycosis

Reactive skin lesions (without organisms)

Erythema nodosum

Acute exanthem

Erythema multiforme-like eruptions

Sweet's syndrome

Interstitial granulomatous dermatitis

Skin lesions with identifiable organisms

Disseminated cutaneous coccidioidomycosis

Primary cutaneous coccidioidomycosis

lung nodules, hilar lymphadenopathy, and/or pleural effusion. Excluding the respiratory system, the skin is the most common organ to demonstrate clues to the diagnosis of coccidioidomycosis. The organisms may be directly identifiable within the skin, or the skin may display important *reactive* signs of the pulmonary infection (Table 10.1).

Erythema Nodosum

Erythema nodosum is one of the most common and characteristic manifestations of coccidioidomycosis. Women are more likely than men to develop erythema nodosum in association with the infection. One to three weeks after the onset of the illness, patients present with tender red subcutaneous nodules, most often involving the legs (Fig. 10.20). Skin biopsies demonstrate a septal granulomatous panniculitis with no evidence of organisms. Erythema nodosum appears to reflect a strong cell-mediated response against the pulmonary infection and thus is believed to be associated with a generally good prognosis. The tender nodules resolve spontaneously as the pulmonary symptoms subside.

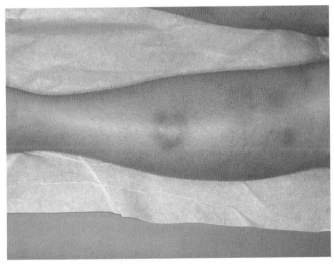

Figure 10.20. Erythema nodosum. Tender red subcutaneous nodules developed on the legs 1 week after the onset of pulmonary coccidioidomycosis.

Acute Exanthem

An acute exanthem commonly occurs very early in the course of the illness, often within the first 48 hours. In some cases, the onset even precedes the development of respiratory symptoms. The generalized eruption may be morbilliform, macular, papular, urticarial, or target-like (Fig. 10.21a & b). The acute exanthem closely resembles an allergic drug reaction, erythema multiforme, a viral exanthem, or generalized allergic contact dermatitis. Associated pruritus ranges from being minimal to severe. An enanthem sometimes accompanies the eruption. Skin biopsies demonstrate a nonspecific pattern of spongiotic dermatitis or mild interface dermatitis. The exanthem persists for days or weeks, and then subsides spontaneously. Desquamation of the palms ensues in some cases. Because the acute exanthem occurs so early in the course of the illness, the initial Coccidioides serologies may be falsely negative. Serologic testing may be repeated in 2 weeks, if necessary, to allow time for seroconversion.

Erythema Multiforme-like Eruptions

For many decades, erythema multiforme has been cited as a common reactive manifestation of coccidioidomycosis; however, review of the literature fails to reveal histopathologic

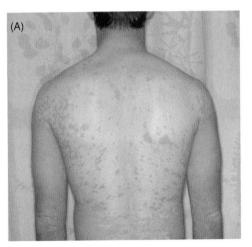

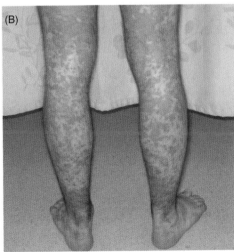

Figure 10.21. A & B. The acute exanthem of coccidioidomycosis. The eruption began within 48 hours of the first respiratory symptoms.

confirmation of the association. Both the acute exanthem and Sweet's syndrome may produce annular or target-like lesions, which clinically mimic erythema multiforme. Cases previously designated as erythema multiforme may actually have represented examples of these other two entities. Regardless of whether true erythema multiforme is associated, erythema multiforme-*like* eruptions (with annular or target-like features) remain an important clinical clue to the diagnosis of coccidioidomycosis.

Sweet's Syndrome

Sweet's syndrome (acute febrile neutrophilic dermatosis) is associated with a variety of underlying systemic disorders. Only recently has this eruption been recognized as a reactive manifestation of pulmonary coccidioidomycosis. Despite the paucity of reported cases, Sweet's syndrome is a common reactive manifestation of the infection in the experience of the author. Early in the course of the illness, patients present with painful edematous red papules and plaques, often with pustular features (Fig. 10.22). Annular and target-like lesions are sometimes evident. Fever and peripheral blood leukocytosis are frequently associated. Skin biopsies reveal marked subepidermal edema and dense neutrophilic dermal infiltrates with abundant leukocytoclastic debris. In skin biopsy specimens, no organisms are identifiable by microscopy or by culture. The cutaneous signs and symptoms resolve as the pulmonary symptoms improve. Recognition of underlying coccidioidomycosis is particularly important, so that patients do not receive inappropriate treatment with immunosuppressive therapies. Though idiopathic Sweet's syndrome is frequently treated with systemic corticosteroids, such immunosuppressive therapies are best avoided in patients with coccidioidomycosis.

Interstitial Granulomatous Dermatitis

An immunologically induced granulomatous dermatitis occurs in association with a variety of underlying systemic diseases, such as systemic vasculitides, connective tissue diseases, lymphoproliferative disorders, and infections. In such cases, the granulomatous inflammation appears to be a reactive phenomenon, occurring in the absence of detectable organisms. Histopathologically (and sometimes clinically) the eruptions resemble granuloma annulare or necrobiosis lipoidica. In a recent case series of five patients, interstitial granulomatous dermatitis was described as a reactive manifestation of pulmonary coccidioidomycosis. Despite the small number of reported cases, this eruption appears to be a relatively common manifestation of coccidioidomycosis in the experience of the author. Early in the course of the illness, patients develop scattered plaques and coalescing papules on the trunk and extremities (Fig. 10.23a & b). Skin biopsies reveal interstitial granulomatous dermal infiltrates,

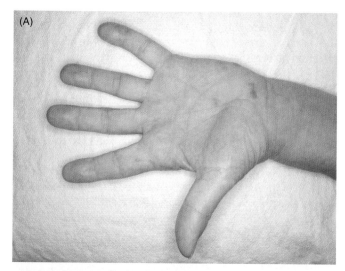

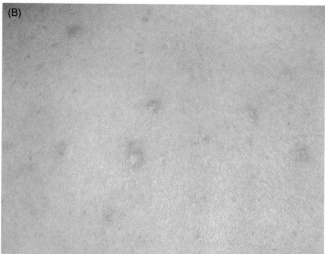

Figure 10.23. A & B. Interstitial granulomatous dermatitis associated with pulmonary coccidioidomycosis. **A.** Scattered smooth red papules developed on the extremities on the first day of fever in this elderly man. **B.** Edematous pink papules on the back. The patient's cutaneous eruption was the first sign of illness in this otherwise asymptomatic woman with coccidioidomycosis.

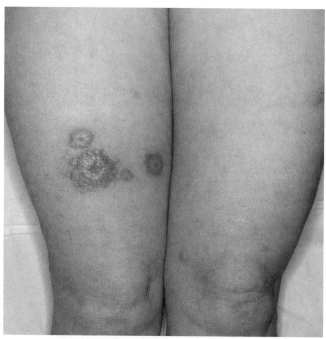

Figure 10.22. Sweet's syndrome associated with pulmonary coccidioidomycosis. Edematous plaques accompanied the patient's respiratory symptoms on the first day of illness.

which resemble granuloma annulare. In contrast to typical idiopathic granuloma annulare, neutrophils, karyorrhectic debris, and subepidermal edema may also sometimes be conspicuous. The eruption resolves as the pulmonary symptoms subside. Reactive granulomatous dermatitis must be distinguished from disseminated infection by microscopic examination and culture of skin biopsy specimens.

Disseminated Infection

In nearly all cases, the lungs are the primary site of infection in coccidioidomycosis. In less than 1% of cases, dissemination to other organs occurs. The skin is the most common site of dissemination. Other important sites of involvement include the meninges and bones. Disseminated skin lesions usually arise within the first few weeks or months of the illness. Most patients with disseminated infection have fever and appear acutely ill. Occasionally, however, patients may present with disseminated skin lesions after an apparently asymptomatic primary lung infection. In the skin, the clinical appearance of disseminated lesions is strikingly diverse. Solitary or multiple papules, nodules,

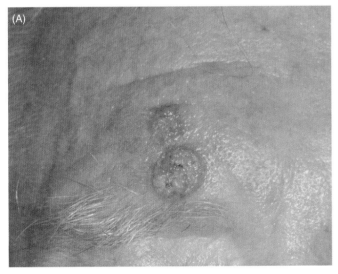

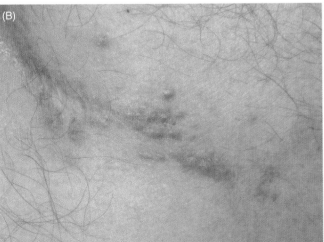

Figure 10.24. A & B. Disseminated coccidioidomycosis. **A.** Ulcerated plaques on the forehead in an otherwise healthy patient with no risk factors. **B.** Red-brown nodules and scar-like plaque involving the axilla in an immunosuppressed patient taking prednisone.

verrucous plaques, and abscesses may occur (Fig. 10.24a & b). In the skin, the organisms sometimes establish a chronic nidus of infection, which persists despite the apparent resolution of the pulmonary infection. Unusual cases of disseminated coccidioidomycosis may resemble tumor-stage mycosis fungoides, lepromatous leprosy, or lupus vulgaris.

Skin biopsy confirms the diagnosis. Histopathologic examination frequently reveals pseudoepitheliomatous hyperplasia and ulceration. A granulomatous and/or suppurative inflammatory infiltrate fills the dermis. Eosinophils are sometimes numerous. The organisms are usually evident in standard H&E-stained sections. Special fungal stains, such as methenamine silver stain or periodic acid-Schiff (PAS) stain, may also assist in revealing the organisms. In tissue sections, the spherules of *Coccidioides sp* are usually readily distinguished from other fungi because of their large size (10 to 80 microns). Mature spherules of *Coccidiodes sp* contain numerous distinctive endospores (Fig. 10.25). In some cases, immature *Coccidioides sp* spherules on the smaller end of the spectrum may be difficult to differentiate from *Blastomyces* or *Cryptococcus*. For such cases, in situ hybridization is available to differentiate these three different fungi. Culture is also a useful technique for confirmation of disseminated coccidioidomycosis. Cultured skin biopsy specimens commonly yield growth of *Coccidioides sp* in as early as 2 to 5 days.

Primary Cutaneous Coccidioidomycosis

Primary cutaneous coccidioidomycosis is much rarer than disseminated skin lesions. The literature contains only approximately 20 reported cases. Primary cutaneous infection may occur by direct inoculation into the skin through a splinter injury, laceration, or other trauma. Multiple cases have occurred among agricultural workers and laboratory technicians. The infection typically presents as an ulcer or nodule at the site of inoculation. In a pattern resembling sporotrichosis, secondary foci of infection sometimes arise along the distribution of lymphatics. Fever and regional lymphadenopathy may be associated. The microscopic appearance is identical to that of disseminated

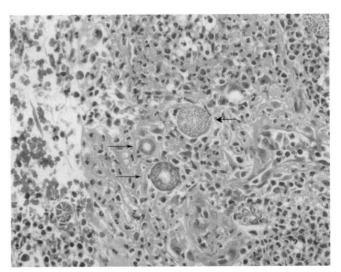

Figure 10.25. Skin biopsy specimen confirming disseminated coccidioidomycosis (hematoxylin-eosin, 400x). *Coccidiodes sp* spherules of varying sizes (small arrowheads). The largest spherule (large arrowhead) contains numerous endospores.

coccidioidomycosis. Clinical correlation is needed to distinguish a primary cutaneous infection from a disseminated infection.

Serologic testing

Serologic testing is an important tool in establishing the diagnosis of coccidioidomycosis. Both qualitative and quantitative serologic tests are commonly used. One of the most widely used qualitative tests, enzyme immunoassay, yields rapid results with high sensitivity. Because occasional false positives do occur, positive results are typically confirmed by a more highly specific quantitative technique, such as complement fixation or quantitative immunodiffusion. The antibody titer offers both diagnostic and prognostic information. High antibody titers (such as 1:16, 1:32, or greater) are often seen in severe infections, especially in cases of dissemination. The antibody titer is useful in assessing the course of the disease. Titers typically decrease and disappear within months or a couple years of an acute infection. Potential pitfalls in the interpretation of serologies are discussed subsequently.

Therapy

For patients with coccidioidomycosis, the dermatologist's primary role is to assist in the identification of diagnostic clues. Nevertheless, an awareness of current treatments is also relevant for the practicing dermatologist, especially in endemic areas. Decisions regarding treatment are based on the severity of the pulmonary infection, the presence of dissemination, and the existence of risk factors. In low-risk patients with mild self-limited respiratory symptoms, systemic antifungal therapy is frequently not necessary. Most patients improve spontaneously. Patients with severe respiratory illness and those with disseminated infection do routinely require antifungal therapy. Azoles and/or amphotericin B are the primary medications employed at this time. Current treatment recommendations are detailed in the article by Dr. Galgiani and collaborators, referenced here. An infectious disease specialist or primary care physician typically manages treatment. Serial antibody titers offer useful information regarding the patient's response to therapy. With successful treatment, antibody titers typically diminish and disappear over a period of months or several years. Efforts are currently underway to develop an effective vaccine.

Pitfalls and Myths

Serologic tests present a potential diagnostic pitfall. In contrast to serologic tests for many other infectious diseases, IgG antibodies for *Coccidioides sp* typically suggest an acute infection, rather than a remote past infection. In acute coccidioidomycosis, it is common for IgG antibodies to be present, regardless of whether IgM antibodies are detectable. The IgG antibody titer typically diminishes as the patient recovers from the infection. Thus, any titer, even a titer of 1:2, often signifies a true infection. Serologic testing also presents the potential pitfall of false-negative results early in the course of the illness. Dermatologists must recognize that several of the early reactive cutaneous manifestations of coccidioidomycosis may erupt before the development of detectable antibodies in the serum. If the initial serologies are negative, repeating the tests in 2 weeks may be helpful in documenting seroconversion.

Another important potential pitfall is the failure to consider coccidioidomycosis in *nonendemic* areas. Many persons from other regions of the country (and from throughout the world) may be exposed to the organism during a vacation in the Southwest. After an incubation period of 1 to 3 weeks, the infected patient may develop symptoms after he or she has returned home. If the local physician is unfamiliar with the signs of coccidioidomycosis, the diagnosis may be missed. Obtaining a travel history is obviously important to consider the possibility of coccidioidomycosis. Even in a nonendemic area, dermatologists can play a crucial role in the recognition of this fascinating infection.

SUGGESTED READINGS

Eastern Hemisphere: Old World Cutaneous Leishmaniasis

Al-Jawabreh A, Schoenian G, Hamarsheh O, et al. Clinical diagnosis of cutaneous leishmaniasis: a comparison study between standardized graded direct microscopy and ITS1-PCR of Giemsa-stained smears. *Acta Trop* 2006;99(1):55–61. Epub 2006 Aug 22.

Alrajhi AA, Ibrahim EA, De Vol EB, et al. Fluconazole for the treatment of cutaneous leishmaniasis caused by Leishmania major. *N Engl J Med* 2002;21;346(12):891–895.

Aronson NE. Leishmaniasis in American Soldiers: Parasites from the Front. In: Scheld M, Hooper D, Hughes J, eds. *Emerging Infections.* 7th edition. Washington DC: ASM, 2007.

El-On J, Livshin R, Even-Paz Z, et al. Topical treatment of cutaneous leishmaniasis. *J Invest Dermatol.* 1986;87(2):284–288.

Ghaffarifar F, Jorjani O, Mirshams M, et al. Photodynamic therapy as a new treatment of cutaneous leishmaniasis. *East Mediterr Health J* 2006;12(6):902–908.

Herwaldt BL. Leishmaniasis. *Lancet* 1999;354(9185):1191–1199.

Khatami A, Firooz A, Gorouhi F, et al. Treatment of acute Old World cutaneous leishmaniasis: A systematic review of the randomized controlled trials. *J Am Acad Dermatol* 2007 [Epub ahead of print].

Kubba R, Al-Gindan Y, el-Hassan AM, Omer AH. Clinical diagnosis of cutaneous leishmaniasis (oriental sore). *J Am Acad Dermatol* 1987;16(6):1183–1189.

Magill AJ. Epidemiology of the leishmaniases. *Dermatol Clin* 1995; 13(3):505–523.

Magill AJ. Cutaneous leishmaniasis in the returning traveler. *Infect Dis Clin North Am* 2005;19(1):241–266, x-xi.

Murray HW, Berman JD, Davies CR, et al. Advances in leishmaniasis. *Lancet* 2005;366(9496):1561–1577.

Panagiotopoulos A, Stavropoulos PG, Hasapi V, et al. Treatment of cutaneous leishmaniasis with cryosurgery. *Int J Dermatol* 2005;44(9):749–752.

Rahman SB, Bari AU, Mumtaz N. Miltefosine in cutaneous leishmaniasis. *J Coll Physicians Surg Pak* 2007;17(3):132–135.

Reithinger R, Coleman PG. Treating cutaneous leishmaniasis patients in Kabul, Afghanistan: cost-effectiveness of an operational program in a complex emergency setting. *BMC Infect Dis* 2007 30;7:3.

Safaei A, Motazedian MH, Vasei M. Polymerase chain reaction for diagnosis of cutaneous leishmaniasis in histologically positive, suspicious and negative skin biopsies. *Dermatology* 2002; 205(1):18–24.

Weina PJ, Neafie RC, Wortmann G, et al. Old world leishmaniasis: an emerging infection among deployed US military and civilian workers. *Clin Infect Dis* 2004;39(11):1674–1680. Epub 2004 Nov 9.

Willard RJ, Jeffcoat AM, Benson PM, et al. Cutaneous leishmaniasis in soldiers from Fort Campbell, Kentucky returning from Operation Iraqi Freedom highlights diagnostic and therapeutic options. *J Am Acad Dermatol* 2005; 52(6):977–987.

Wortmann G, Hochberg L, Houng HH, et al. Rapid identification of Leishmania complexes by a real-time PCR assay. *Am J Trop Med Hyg* 2005;73(6):999–1004.

Zimmo S. Desert dermatology. *Clin Dermatol* 1998;16(1):109–111.

Western Hemisphere: Coccidioidomycosis and the Skin

Chang A, Tung RC, McGillis TS, et al. Primary cutaneous coccidioidomycosis. *J Am Acad Dermatol* 2003;49(5):944–949.

DiCaudo DJ. Coccidioidomycosis: a review and update. *J Am Acad Dermatol* 2006;55(6):929–942.

DiCaudo DJ, Connolly SM. Interstitial granulomatous dermatitis associated with pulmonary coccidioidomycosis. *J Am Acad Dermatol* 2001;45(6):840–845.

DiCaudo DJ, Ortiz KJ, Mengden SJ, et al. Sweet syndrome (acute febrile neutrophilic dermatosis) associated with pulmonary coccidioidomycosis. *Arch Dermatol* 2005;141(7):881–884.

DiCaudo DJ, Yiannias JA, Laman SD, et al. The exanthem of acute pulmonary coccidioidomycosis: Clinical and histopathologic features of 3 cases and review of the literature. *Arch Dermatol* 2006;142(6):744–746.

Galgiani JN, Ampel NM, Blair JE, et al. Coccidioidomycosis. *Clin Infect Dis* 2005;41(9):1217–1223.

Harvey WC, Greendyke WH. Skin lesions in acute coccidioidomycosis. *Am Fam Physician/GP* 1970;2(3):81–5.

Quimby SR, Connolly SM, Winkelmann RK, et al. Clinicopathologic spectrum of specific cutaneous lesions of disseminated coccidioidomycosis. *J Am Acad Dermatol* 1992;26(1):79–85.

11 | INFECTION IN THE TROPICS

Marcia Ramos-e-Silva, Paula Pereira Araújo, and Sueli Coelho Carneiro

INTRODUCTION

Infectious diseases in the tropics, such as leishmaniasis, sleeping sickness (African trypanosomiasis), malaria, and Chagas' disease, which generate a devastating impact on humanity, are frequently referred to as neglected diseases, and affect mainly poor people.

According to the World Health Organization (WHO), there are around 530 million people – or almost one-tenth of the world population – suffering from some of these so-called neglected diseases. The number of people at risk for infection, however, is much greater. 40% of the world's population is at risk of acquiring malaria; 25% of the Latin American population is in danger of acquiring Chagas' disease; 55 million Africans are exposed to sleeping sickness, and leishmaniasis threatens another 350 million people around the world.

Affecting the skin, they are called dermatoses of the tropical and subtropical area, dermatoses of the poor (a term used by James Marshall), dermatoses of the developing and underdeveloped countries; and also dermatoses of malnutrition, illiteracy, sun radiation, humidity, and insect bites.

Tropical dermatosis is a difficult term to define, according to Canizares. Simmons stated that a tropical disease is one that "by virtue of its etiology, occurs, either exclusively or predominantly, in a tropical or subtropical region, where though not strictly endemic, it is either autochthonous or in residence, since it has been repulsed from other areas by hygienic measures."

The factors that most influence the development of tropical dermatoses are climatic, ecological, human, cultural, and socioeconomic factors.

Presently, tropical dermatoses occur mostly in the southern hemisphere, but are reappearing in the northern hemisphere; these recent changes in geography and epidemiology are caused by migration, opening of the international borders, transportation facilities, and also by acquired immunodeficiency syndrome (AIDS). By depleting the immune system, AIDS also increases the incidence of several infectious diseases. These changes are giving rise to a new specialty called *Migration Medicine.*

In Brazil and in many other countries, tourism has always been common and lately off-track tourism is increasing, with foreigners going to areas with very beautiful landscapes. These tourists can get bitten by different species of mosquitoes and flies, and also come into contact with contaminated water, soil, and animals.

The WHO listed, as its prime targets, six diseases that it considered major threats to the populations living in the tropics: filariasis, leishmaniasis, leprosy, malaria, schistosomiasis, and trypanosomiasis. Of these, only malaria does not produce cutaneous manifestations Therefore, dermatological knowledge is very important since early diagnosis and proper treatment can often be life saving.

The knowledge of these diseases is of utmost importance because the so-called tropical dermatoses are becoming more frequent worldwide because of tourism, migration, opening of international borders, and human immunodeficiency virus (HIV) infection. For this reason, they can be seen in any part of the globe and there has been a change in geography and epidemiology of tropical dermatoses. Thus, dermatologists of the entire world must be alert to and aware of the diseases foreign visitors can bring back to their countries.

A careful history can often locate the site of a possible infection and may suggest its nature. Viral infections occur in epidemics, more often in school-age children who had a recent contact with infected persons. Adults should be asked for the history of previous exposure to infections, occupation, social pursuits and hobbies, contact with animals, any kind of recent travel, insect bites, history of intravenous drug misuse, sexual activity, blood transfusion, and intake of herbal and "natural" medicines. Superficial mycoses (*tinea nigra* and *piedra*) typically occur more often in young adults in tropical climates. Subcutaneous mycoses (chromoblastomycosis, mycetoma, sporotrichosis, and lobomycosis) described in the tropical and subtropical regions of South America mainly affect young male and rural workers. Inoculation seems to occur by trauma. Paracoccidioidomycosis is endemic to Central and South America. Chagas' disease occurs in the rural areas of Latin America, being known as a "poverty disease." Leishmaniasis is a zoonosis associated primarily with forest occupations.

In this chapter, we will discuss some of the infections observed in the tropics, especially those seen in Brazil. There are infections, such as tuberculosis and leprosy, more frequently occuring in tropical areas that, because of their great importance, are discussed in separate chapters or together with other groups of diseases such as *tinea versicolor* and candidiasis.

HISTORY

The tropical infections seen in Brazil were enriched by the research of many Brazilian dermatologists. Several discoveries related to some of these diseases were made in Brazil and have been aiding the specialty in the world with several original reports, especially in this specific area of the infectious–contagious and tropical diseases. Alexandre Cerqueira, in 1891, described tinea nigra palmar; Gaspar Viana, in 1911, discovered *Leishmania brasiliensis* and was the first to use an effective medication, tartar emetic, for leishmaniasis. Together with Aragão, in 1912, he also discovered the etiologic agent of granuloma venereum, *Calymmatobacterium granulomatis*. Adolpho Lutz in 1908 described paracoccidioidomycosis and Floriano de Almeida in 1930 identified its etiologic agent as being the fungus *Paracoccidioides brasiliensis*. Parreiras Horta presented the original report on piedra nigra in 1911; and Olympio da Fonseca Filho and Arêa Leão, in 1928, identified the fungus *Piedraia hortai* as being its agent. In 1914 Max Rudolph, a German researcher living in Brazil, identified the brown to black color fungus of chromomycosis in the tissues and was also able to cultivate it in Sabouraud's agar. Jorge Lobo described the disease, lobomycosis, which takes his name in Recife in the Northeast of Brazil, although this disease is restricted to the North of Brazil. Montenegro's test, an intradermal test performed for the diagnosis of leishmaniasis, was idealized by João Montenegro in 1926, while the first mention of polarity of the several clinical forms of leprosy was made in 1938 by Francisco Rabello. In 1945, Flaviano Silva presented the first case of anergic leishmaniasis.

VIRUS

In tropical areas, viruses are frequent agents of exanthematic diseases, particularly in children. Most exanthemas are transient and harmless but some are potentially very dangerous. Viruses have an enormous capability of dissemination, because they present very frequent mutations and are capable of infecting men as well as animals. Changes to the tropical environment, such as deforestation and disorderly urbanization, rising population density, with poor health and living standards, result in direct exposure of humans to viral agents, thus increasing their frequency significantly.

In many cases, exanthema is the main marker of the disease, while in others it may appear merely as an incidental clinical manifestation. In exanthematous disorders the clinical manifestations are varied and depend on the infectious agent. When seeing a patient with exanthema, the examiner should check for general physical signs, such as dehydration, evidence of weight loss, anemia, jaundice, edema, oral temperature, enlargement of the liver or spleen, and alterations in lymph nodes. A thorough and careful examination of the skin should be carried out to detect any nodules, rashes, or insect bites. In addition, the oral mucosa and throat should be inspected for evidence of enanthema or ulceration, the conjunctiva for petechiae, and the nails for splinter hemorrhages.

Hemorrhagic Fevers

Hemorrhagic viruses are common in tropical regions of Old World countries. Tourism, migration, and contamination of animals can all act as reservoirs for the disease. There are also many important factors for dissemination of these agents to new areas and continents. The constant human incursions into areas where there is circulation of viruses and presence of vectors and animal reservoirs perpetuate the possibility of viral infection dissemination. Among the agents of the so-called hemorrhagic fevers, the producers of dengue, yellow fever, Lassa fever, South American hemorrhagic fevers, Ebola, West Nile, and Barmah Forest viruses are outlined.

Dengue Fever

Dengue is considered as the disease with greatest morbidity and mortality rate transmitted by arthropods. Epidemics have been reported in tropical and subtropical regions of Asia, Africa, and America. The first case of hemorrhagic dengue was described in Cuba in 1981 and 8 years later, a new case occurred in Venezuela. Several factors are responsible for the emergence and maintenance of the disease in those regions, mainly population growth and uncontrolled urbanization, with inadequate basic sanitation and care with water. Plane travel, migrations, and the deterioration of public health programs also contribute to the dissemination of dengue.

The dengue virus is an arbovirus (arthropod-borne viruses), of the family *Flaviviridae*, genus Flavivirus, like the yellow fever virus, with four distinct serotypes. Flavivirus are capable of replicating in different organisms, like man and mosquito, with an enormous capacity to adapt to the environment, allowing the preservation of these viruses in nature.

The main vector of the disease is the adult female of the *Aedes aegypti* mosquitoes, whose feeding habit is predominantly by day in the surroundings of homes and whose reproduction occurs in clean water. After biting individuals with viremia, the mosquito is infected and transmits, by a new bite, the virus to other susceptible individuals, thus establishing a transmission cycle. The environmental factors that favor this cycle include temperature (15°C–40°C) and moderate and high latitude and altitude. Conditions of the host such as immunological status, type of virus (mainly the serotype), vector, adult female density, feeding frequency, and others are also of fundamental importance in the transmission chain.

Crossover immunity between the different serotypes may last for a few weeks so that an individual may present with sequential infections. Re-infection by a different serotype can lead to dengue hemorrhagic fever.

Dengue has a short incubation period, between 5 and 8 days. After this period, it may present with sudden onset, fever, chills, frontal headache, retro-orbital pain, arthralgias, anorexia, nausea, and vomiting. The severe and often protracted aching arthralgia has given rise to the pseudonym of "break bone fever." Systemic complications include epistaxis, lymphadenopathy, and hepatomegaly.

The typical cutaneous feature is a transient mild flush-like macular rash over the nape of the neck and face that will last up to 5 days. Petechiae or purpura may also be seen. Difficult-to-control pruritus may be present. Fever appears usually in up to 6 days, beginning in the convalescent phase, and may last for weeks, with asthenia and depression.

The more severe hemorrhagic form of dengue occurs when an individual who has had a previous episode of dengue fever is re-infected by a second serotype. The clinical presentation is abrupt with fever, nausea, and vomiting. Petechiae and purpura appear on the second or third day. Hemoconcentration and thrombocytopenia can lead to digestive hemorrhages, metrorrhagias, gingival hemorrhage, and epistaxis. Hepatomegaly, hematemesis, and abdominal pain indicate a worse prognosis, with probable evolution to a shock syndrome. This syndrome appears between the third and seventh day of the disease with unrest and abdominal pain and evolves to lethargy and circulatory insufficiency, with hypotension, cyanosis, accelerated pulse, and cold sweats. Metabolic acidosis and disseminated intravascular coagulation occur and, in case of lack of therapeutic support, death can occur in 4 to 6 hours.

In some tropical countries, dengue is an endemic disease. In northern Brazil, 40% of patients presenting with fever and exanthema can be expected to have positive serology for acute dengue fever, with other viral exanthematic diseases (measles, rubella, parvovirus, oropouche, and mayaro) accounting for 26%. Dengue is rarely seen in urban settings where the mosquito vector is unable to thrive. However, between 2001 and 2002, an urban epidemic of dengue fever occurred in the city of Rio de Janeiro, and an outbreak of hemorrhagic dengue fever occurred 2 years later in Nicaragua, in which 26 cases of hemorrhagic dengue fever were recorded.

The treatment of dengue is nonspecific and essentially symptomatic. Depending on the severity of disease, volume expanders and oxygen therapy may be necessary. In severe cases of dengue, hemorrhagic fever mortality can reach 50%.

Person-to-person contamination does not occur. Therefore, vector control of mosquitoes is the most important prophylactic measure to control spreading of the disease. An efficient vaccination against dengue is difficult to achieve, since the four viral serotypes are present in most countries, and a future infection with another serotype can predispose to hemorrhagic dengue.

Yellow Fever

It is generally believed that the yellow fever virus was brought from Africa during the slave traffic, together with its vector. It is endemic in Equatorial, Central, and South America, and in Africa. In South America, infection is often related to deforestation and the subsequent encroachment of reclaimed land for agriculture. Yellow fever is not found in Asia. The disease continues to expand nowadays, including regions thought to be free of the disease, mainly in Africa. The virus is still present at low levels of infection in some tropical areas of Africa and America and may eventually give rise to an epidemic.

Yellow fever is caused by an arbovirus of the Flavivirus family (Flavus means yellow in Latin) and is maintained in a transmission cycle that involves monkeys and hematophagous mosquitoes. The mosquito vectors are species of *Aedes* and *Haemagogus* that can transmit the disease to humans.

Following inoculation by the hematophagous insect vector, the virus replicates itself in local lymph nodes with subsequent hematogenic dissemination and replication in tissues of the lymph, spleen, bone marrow, kidney, heart, and the gastrointestinal tract, mainly hepatocytes, leading to an intense jaundice. Severe yellow fever is further complicated by thrombocytopenia and clotting disorders. Renal involvement includes renal insufficiency, albuminuria and, in more severe cases, acute tubular necrosis. In the heart, myocarditis and alterations to the blood flow system can occur, leading to arrhythmia. For those patients who develop jaundice, the overall mortality rate is between 20% and 50%.

Yellow fever has a short incubation period between 3 and 6 days. The clinical spectrum of the disease varies greatly from a self-limiting, mild prodromal illness to fulminant liver necrosis and death. However, the classical clinical picture begins abruptly with fever, chills, intense cephalea, lumbar pain, myalgias, nausea, vomiting, and gingival hemorrhages or epistaxis of mild intensity. A classical finding is bradycardia despite high temperatures (Faget's sign). Approximately 3 days later, corresponding to the end of the virus circulation phase, remission of symptoms occurs. However, about 24 hours after the clinical improvement, in severe cases, the fever reappears as do the remaining symptoms of abdominal pain, intense prostration, and jaundice. Oliguria and albuminuria may also occur. This phase is due to the presence of circulating antibodies. The onset of liver failure, gastrointestinal bleeding, disseminated intravascular coagulation, and hepatic encephalopathy indicates a progressive worsening of the patient's prognosis. In laboratory analysis, there may be a rise of hepatic enzymes, leukopenia, thrombocytopenia, albuminuria, alterations of the coagulogram and electrocardiogram. In severe cases, the mortality can reach 40% and is usually due to hepatorenal failure. In the remaining cases, convalescence can last up to 2 weeks with intense asthenia.

For the diagnosis, the following should be considered: clinical findings, the epidemiologic history of recent travel, immunization, and professional activity exercised. The specific diagnosis depends on viral isolation in the blood, demonstration of serous viral antigens, or the detection of the RNA of the virus by PCR during the viremia phase. Serologically, the discovery of positive IgM in the blood collected after 7 to 10 days from beginning of the manifestations confers 95% sensitivity for the diagnosis.

There is no antiviral treatment for yellow fever. Case management is supportive. Therefore, prevention is the key to control, which is provided through yellow fever vaccinations. The yellow fever vaccine is highly efficacious and probably provides lifetime protection in most persons but should nevertheless be administered every 10 years.

West Nile Virus

West Nile virus (WNV), isolated for the first time in Uganda in 1937, is an RNA virus, of the *Flaviviridae* family, genus *flavivirus*, and is an important etiologic agent of meningoencephalitis. Two viral strains were identified. Strain I has a ubiquitous distribution (Africa, India, Europe, Asia, the Middle East, and North America) and was considered responsible for the more recent encephalitis epidemics. The strain II viruses were identified only in Sub-Saharan Africa. Birds are the natural reservoir. The infection is transmitted to humans by *Culex*, *Ochlerotatus*, and *Aedes* spp. mosquitoes and occurs during the period of active mosquito feeding.

In 2002, the spreading of WNV in the United States resulted in the largest arbovirus meningoencephalitis documented in the western hemisphere. Clinical manifestations include sudden onset of high fever, malaise, anorexia, photophobia, myalgia, lymphadenopathy, arthralgia, and neurological dysfunction producing an encephalitic manifestation, with multiple and generalized convulsions. The skin eruption is characterized by punctate, erythematous, maculopapular eruptions, most pronounced on the extremities.

The diagnosis of WNV infection is established by IgM-capture enzyme-linked immunosorbent assay (ELISA). Treatment is similar to that for a meningoencephalitis patient. There is no specific antiviral therapy.

Barmah Forest Virus

Barmah Forest virus (BFV) is an emerging mosquito-borne alphavirus. Many mosquito species can act as vectors for the disease, such as *Ochlerotatus vigilax*. BFV has only been described in Australia.

The infection is characterized by fever, arthralgias, myalgias, lethargy, anorexia, and rash. The rash is erythematous, maculo-papular, vesicular, or purpuric, involving trunk, limbs, and face. The diagnosis is made by detection of Barmah Forest–specific Ig-M by enzyme-linked immunosorbent assay (ELISA) method. Most cases can recover in weeks, but arthralgias, myalgias, and lethargy may continue for at least 6 months in about 10% of patients.

Marburg and Ebola

The Marburg and Ebola viruses contain RNA differing from their close relatives, *Rhabdoviridae* and *Paramyxoviridae*, and thus constitute a different family: *Filoviridae*. Both cause severe hemorrhagic fevers. The natural reservoirs for Marburg and Ebola viruses remain unknown.

Marburg virus was originally identified after a laboratory worker became infected following experiments using green monkeys (*Cercopithecus aethiops*). Since then, sporadic cases have been observed in Zimbabwe, South Africa, and Kenya.

The Ebola virus was responsible for two major epidemics, with an 88% mortality rate, in Zaire and Sudan in 1976. Since then, other epidemics have occurred in the Congo, Uganda, and other countries in Central Africa. It comprises four subtypes or genotypes: Zaire, Sudan, Reston, and Ivory Coast. The first two are responsible for several epidemics and serious cases of hemorrhagic fever. The third is only recognized in monkeys of the Philippines, while only a single case is known for the Ivory Coast type.

Humans are the only known source of infection. These diseases are easily transmitted by direct contact with body fluids or even clothes from the index case. Mortality is high.

Marburg and Ebola virus infections have a short incubation period of approximately 6 days, but can exceed 2 weeks. Clinically, there is acute onset of high fever, headache, generalized myalgia, prostration, odinophagia, abdominal pain, nausea, vomiting, and intense watery diarrhea. Development of a maculopapular rash, centripetal, without itch, with varied degrees of erythema, and with desquamation may occur on the fifth to seventh day of the disease. However, the characteristic clinical finding is hemorrhage, mainly gastrointestinal bleeding and mucocutaneous and pulmonary hemorrhages. Leukopenia, thrombocytopenia, proteinuria, and increased levels of hepatic enzymes and amylases are observed.

The serologic diagnosis includes finding of IgM and IgG, through ELISA and immunofluorescence, with the antibodies detectable after the first week of the disease. The virus can be isolated in guinea pigs after inoculation of blood from sick patients.

There is no specific treatment. Despite improvements in the management of circulatory collapse and disseminated intravascular coagulation the mortality figures remain high (50%–80%) even in treated cases. Strict isolation of cases and quarantine are essential to curtail any potential epidemic of these deadly diseases.

Lassa Fever

Lassa fever occurs in West Africa. It is caused by an arenavirus that is phylogenetically related to the viral agents of Argentinian and Bolivian hemorrhagic fevers and is transmitted to humans via the urine of the peridomicile rodent, *Mastomys natalensis*. The endemic regions are near forests with low population densities.

Lassa fever may clinically present 7 to 14 days after the infection. The onset may be insidious and the disease may even be subclinical. There is fever, chills, headache, sore throat, retro-orbital pain, myalgias, severe body pains, conjunctivitis, oral ulcers, and pharyngitis with tonsillar patches. A generalized petechial rash and facial edema may also occur. Shock occurs as a result of hemorrhage due to thrombocytopenia that contributes to a mortality rate of more than 20%. In pregnancy, the infection presents with greater severity, especially in the last trimester, when mortality is approximately 40%.

Lassa fever can be treated with ribavirin, which may be employed at any time of the disease and also as postexposure prophylaxis. Ribavirin is not indicated during pregnancy. Special care should be taken in the handling of the patients' blood and excreta. Prevention of Lassa fever relies on rodent control.

South American Hemorrhagic Fevers (Argentina, Bolivia, Venezuela, and Brazil):

The South American hemorrhagic fevers are similar in presentation to Lassa fever but present with more overt disease. They are caused by viruses of the *Arenaviridade* family. In Argentina, the virus involved is Junin, while in Bolivia it is Machupo, in Venezuela the Guanarito, and in Brazil the Sabia virus. The cycles of these viruses are relatively simple, being maintained through rodents, where they can be found in blood, urine and in the throat. There can be maternal–fetal transmission, perpetuating the virus through generations and generations of rodents. The true mechanism of human infection is not well established. Possibilities include the ingestion of food and inhalation of materials contaminated with excretes from infected animals and penetration through the skin or contact with blood from sick patients. The incubation period varies from 7 to 16 days. Clinically, it begins with fever and progressive indisposition, altered mental state, tremors, and central nervous system signs. There is marked thrombocytopenia leading to petechiae and widespread hemorrhage. Exanthema is less common. Etiologic diagnosis is made through viral isolation or serological findings.

Ribavirin is the treatment of choice. Hyperimmune globulin has also been used. Healthcare workers who have nursed the patient(s) should also be offered prophylactic ribavirin therapy. Once recovered from illness, patients should avoid intimate contact for at least a month because a persistent detectable viremia is present, and there is a risk of disease transmission during this period.

A live attenuated vaccine is available for the Argentinean hemorrhagic fever that provides some cross-protection against the Bolivian hemorrhagic fever virus.

SUPERFICIAL MYCOSES

White Piedra

Described the first time in 1865 by Beigel, white piedra is a rare infection of the hair cuticle, caused by the *Trichosporon beigelii* yeast. Its distribution is universal, but with clear preference for tropical and temperate climates, being common in South America. In Brazil, a high incidence in the North region is observed. There is no preference for sex or age-group. Poor hygiene commonly plays a role in the picture. The agent can be found in soil, air, water, vegetables, as well as on the surface of the body of animals such as monkeys and horses and as components of the normal human skin flora and oral mucosa, but the specific transmission media remains unknown.

Clinically, asymptomatic, easily detachable, softened nodules characterize it, with colorations varying from white to light brown. It is adherent to the hair shaft, and forms a refractive, irregular transparent sheath along the hair. Genitals, armpits, beards, and mustaches are the most involved sites. Infection of the scalp, eyebrows, and eyelashes is less frequent but can also occur. The underlying skin may show erythemato-desquamative lesions, with ill-defined borders, associated with humidity and pruritus. Wood's lamp does not reveal fluorescence.

Diagnostic differentiation should be carried out with black piedra, pediculosis, nodular axillary trichomycosis, and abnormalities of the hair shaft. In the genital area, involvement of the underlying skin may place dermatophytoses, candidiasis, and severe erythrasma in the differential diagnosis.

Diagnosis is made through microscopic examination of the hair, the finding of nodules made of mycelium elements and arthroconidea perpendicular to the hair surface. Culture of hair in Sabouraud's agar reveals growth of a white-yellowish colony, similar to wax, with a rough to cerebriform relief, comprising hyaline septated hypha, arthroconidia, and blastoconidia. Treatment of choice is cutting the hair, and in the case of recurrence, use of topical antifungal medication such as ketoconazole, ciclopirox olamine, and zinc pyrothione, among others.

Black Piedra

Black piedra is also an infection of the hair shaft, but the fungus *Piedraia hortae* causes it. Tropical areas have a higher incidence, mainly in Africa, Asia, and Central America, with soil being the most probable infection source. Humans, monkeys, and other primates can be affected, and women have a higher incidence of black piedra. During growth, the fungus tends to destroy the cuticle layer and penetrate deeply into the cortical hair region. Around the shaft, strongly adherent hardened nodules form, with sizes ranging from a few millimeters to 150 mm, but these are usually asymptomatic (Fig. 11.1). The scalp, contrary to white piedra, is the preferred site.

Clinical and direct mycological examination of the hair shaft with potassium hydroxide at 10% to 15% confirms the diagnosis. It reveals a mass of brown arthroconidia and ascie, which are structures of the sexual reproduction phase. Culture of nodules inoculated in Sabouraud glucose at 2% reveals slow growing, elevated black colonies that are very adherent to the medium, with a central groove and a flat periphery. The colony is formed by a net of brownish, branched, and septated hypha with clamidoconidia. Therapy is cutting the hair, along with the use of topical antifungals.

Tinea Nigra

Tinea nigra or superficial phaeohyphomycosis is a skin infection caused by the fungus *Hortaea werneckii* (formerly *Exophiala werneckii*), that dwells in soil and leaves. The microorganism remains confined to the horny layer and, normally does not stimulate an inflammatory response. It is endemic in tropical regions of the Caribbean, Asia, Africa, and South and Central America and begins with fungal inoculation after local trauma, mainly in women, before the second decade of life and in those with hyperhidrosis.

The clinical findings are characteristic, with the onset of a well-delineated, nondesquamate macular lesion. It is usually single, brownish, with larger intensity of the pigmentation in the periphery and is not usually accompanied by local symptoms (Fig. 11.2). Its most common location is the sole or palm, although sites such as the neck, thorax, and other areas of the body can also be affected.

The direct mycological examination reveals olive green or brownish irregular septated hypha and yeast elements. The culture shows slow growth, and is composed of yeasts that have an olive or black color and a shiny, mucus-like aspect. With maturation of the culture, a black or grayish aerial mycelium emerges. For identification of the agent, some biochemical tests may be necessary, such as assimilation of KNO_3 and thermal tolerance.

Among the differential diagnoses, the melanocytic lesions assume a prevailing role. Other pigmentation causes such as Addison's disease, syphilis, and postinflammatory hyperpigmentation should also be eliminated.

Spontaneous remission is rare, and for its treatment keratolytic substances, such as salicylic acid, and topical antifungal

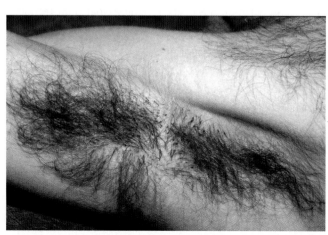

Figure 11.1. Black piedra.

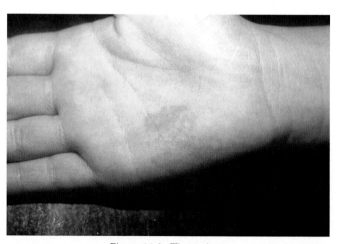

Figure 11.2. Tinea nigra.

agents, such as ketoconazole, miconazole, and itraconazole can be used.

SUBCUTANEOUS AND DEEP MYCOSES

Sporotrichosis

Sporotrichosis is the most common and less severe of the deep mycoses. It is caused by the dimorphic fungus *Sporothrix schenckii,* which lives in nature, usually associated with plants. Of universal occurrence, it is more common in tropical and subtropical regions and is considered endemic in South and Central America, as well as in Africa. It affects mainly healthy young patients, usually under 30 years of age. It appears after traumatic inoculation of the fungus in the skin or in the subcutaneous tissue and can, sometimes, occur by inhalation. Zoonotic transmission may occur through scratches from animals, like cats and rodents. In felines, the fungus can be demonstrated in cutaneous lesions and nasal or oral cavities, besides the possibility of disseminated infection. Factors such as alcoholism, diabetes mellitus, neoplasia, use of immunosuppressant agents, and HIV predispose to acquisition of the infection.

Several clinical forms (Figs. 11.3 and 11.4) have been suggested based on the virulence of the agent, size of the inoculum, depth of the inoculation, and host conditions. The lymphocutaneous form is the most common and is characterized by the appearance of hardened papules 2 to 4 cm in diameter, which appear 7 to 30 days after inoculation. These papules evolve into nodules with posterior ulceration, and new lesions appear along the lymphatic pathway. Light systemic symptomatology may occur, and regional lymphadenomegaly of the upper and

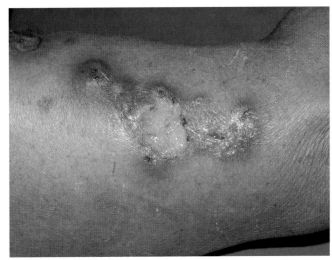

Figure 11.4. Sporotrichosis in a patient with multiple myeloma.

lower limbs is common. A second form described is the fixed cutaneous form because the lesions are restricted to the inoculation area and do not demonstrate lymphatic dissemination. The lesions may resemble a folliculitis or present as an acneiform, ulcerous, gummy, verrucous, or papillomatous aspect. It occurs mainly on the face, neck, trunk, and lower limbs. The disseminated form occurs by hematogenic dissemination. The fungus spreads from a cutaneous or pulmonary focus, and appears as lesions on the skin and in multiple organs. This picture is associated with states of immunodeficiency such as in infection by HIV, neoplasia, tuberculosis, organ transplants, and diabetes mellitus. Another form has no cutaneous lesions and occurs by inhalation or hematogenic dissemination of deep inoculums. Osteoarticular manifestations with monoarthritis or tenosynovitis, pulmonary involvement resembling tuberculosis, and ocular and even genital lesions can occur. Meningitis can arise, especially in HIV-positive patients.

Other infections such as leishmaniasis, tuberculosis, chromomycosis, and paracoccidioidomycosis should be excluded before making the final diagnosis. Supplementary examinations should be carried out. The elements of *S. schenckii,* in pus or tissues, are small in size and scarce, which makes observation through the microscope difficult. Histopathological examination reveals a granulomatous and not very specific formation with epithelial hyperplasia. Asteroid bodies can be seen and represent the fungal elements surrounded by eosinophilic radial protein material, but these are also nonspecific.

S. schenckii is a dimorphic fungus and its two phases, filamentous and yeast-like, are obtainable from culture, which is helpful in identification. The filamentous phase is obtained by cultivating the pus at 25°C and, after 3 to 5 days, white, star-shaped colonies grow, which turn a blackish color later on. The cultures show delicate septated and branched hypha, isolated or in groups with conidia displayed as flower petals. The yeast forms in cultures at 37°C, and shows white creamy colonies, comprising yeast elements in boat-shaped cigar or globular form.

Spontaneous resolution of sporotrichosis has been described. In spite of this, treatment is requested in most cases. The medication of choice is itraconazole, in dosages of 100 to 200 mg/day for 3 to 6 months, resulting in cure rates between 90% and 100%.

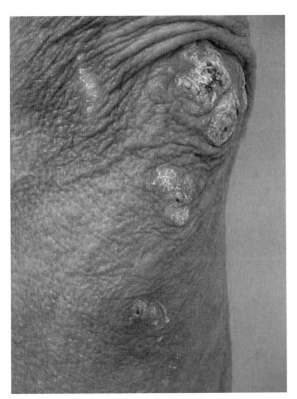

Figure 11.3. Sporotrichosis on the elbow.

For disseminated cases or in HIV-seropositive patients, the use of amphotericin B is preferred, changing to itraconazole later for maintenance. A saturated solution of potassium iodide remains a low-cost therapeutic option, but should be sustained for up to 4 weeks after clinical cure.

Chromoblastomycosis

This polymorphic mycosis involves the skin and subcutaneous tissues. It is a disease of urban distribution, with greater incidence in tropical and subtropical regions of hot and wet climates of Latin America, Africa, and Asia. It also mainly affects male farmers. There are five different agents; all are dematiaceous (meaning dark brown or black color) fungi: *Phialophora verrucosa, Fonsecaea pedrosoi, Fonsecaea compacta, Cladosporium carrionii,* and *Rhinocladiella aquaspersa.*

Fungal inoculation occurs by trauma, most frequently unilaterally and in the lower limbs. The initial lesion is a papule or nodule that ulcers and extends by contiguity, for months or years, assuming two clinical types: tumors or plaques (Figs. 11.5 and 11.6). The tumor form comprises hard dry nodules, on a smooth or verrucous surface, sometimes covering extensive areas. In such cases, microabscesses can be seen on the borders. The initial lesion can also extend itself, leaving a central cicatricial area, covered by smooth and shiny skin, with slightly squamous or finely verrucous, raised borders. Different types of lesions have been

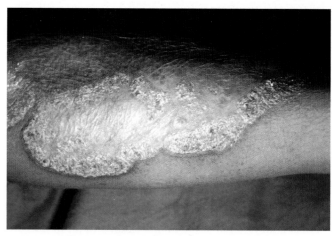
Figure 11.6. Chromoblastomycosis of the forearm.

described, resembling those of psoriasis, tuberculosis, syphilis, or mycetoma.

In pus or histological sections, any of the five agents present as a group of dematiaceous, globular structures with thick walls. Some elements may be septated in one or more planes. They are the typical moriform bodies, which are fumagoid or sclerotic, and characterize the mycosis. The colonies have a relatively slow growth and are velvety cotton-like with varied colors ranging from olive green to brown and black. Differentiation of the five species of agents of mycosis is made on the basis of the morphology of the fructification apparatus.

Chromoblastomycosis is considered a difficult to treat disease because of the varied response depending on the involved species. Options include surgery, itraconazole 100 to 200 mg/day for 12 to 24 months, 5-fluorocytosine, amphotericin B, and cryosurgery, among others.

Mycetoma

Mycetoma is the name given to a group of mycoses acquired through traumatic inoculation, whose etiologic agents are fungi (eumycetoma) or aerobic actinomycetes (actinomycetoma). They organize themselves in the tissues in an agglomerate of hypha or bacterial filaments called grains. The primary focus of infection is the subcutaneous tissue. The grains can present with varied texture, size, and coloration and such characteristics can aid in the causal agent's definition. *Actinomadura madurae*, for instance, is correlated to white-yellowish and soft grains, while *Nocardia brasiliensis* is correlated to white and soft grains of less than 1 mm. *Madurella mycetomatis*, however, generates black and firm grains.

Mycetoma agents are saprophytes in nature. Some species enjoy worldwide distribution, while others are more limited geographically. Infection is more common in tropical and subtropical regions with high rainfall affecting mainly the masculine sex. *Nocardia brasiliensis* mycetoma is the most common in the Americas. Eumycotic mycetoma has been reported with less frequency.

Clinically, mycetomas present as volume increases in certain areas, where abscesses fistulize, draininga purulent secretion with grains visible to the naked eye. They are usually located in the limbs and progresses by contiguity. The mycosis evolves with

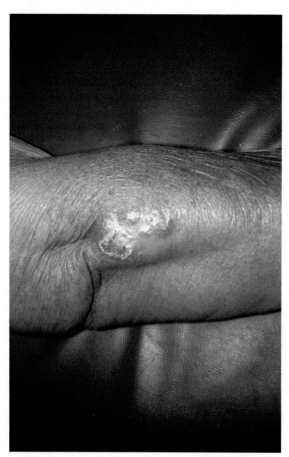
Figure 11.5. Chromoblastomycosis on the elbow.

periods of remission and recurrence, until becoming an enormous tumor that deforms the member. Nodules, fistulae, and scars can be seen in the skin that covers the tumor. The infection can extend to the muscles, fascia, bones, and tendons. The lower limbs are the main sites affected and asymmetry is the rule (Figs. 11.7 and 11.8).

The grain should be observed by the naked eye, under the microscope, and, if necessary, Gram-stained to allow better characterization, as well as in histological sections. Identification of fungi is based on the characteristics of the colonies and in the micromorphology they present in the cultures. In contrast, identification of the actinomycetes is made by the study of their morphology, of the chemical components of the cell wall, and by other physiologic evidences.

Mycetomas are chronic lesions that can evolve into incapacitation. Treatment should be based on identification of the etiologic agent. Therefore, for cases of bacterial nature, use of antibiotics such as sulphones and amikacin are indicated. In cases of fungal etiology, itraconazole and amphotericin B are the main medications of choice. Some cases are very resistant and difficult to treat, requiring amputation.

Lobomycosis

Lobo's mycosis or keloidal blastomycosis, also known as Jorge Lobo's disease, is a chronic, polymorphic, and localized deep mycosis, caused by a fungus, *Lacazia loboi*, whose habitat in nature is unknown. Jorge Lobo described it in the northeast of Brazil in a patient from the Amazon region. It has been described in the intertropical regions of South America, and in countries such as Brazil, Colombia, Suriname, Venezuela, Peru, French Guyana, Guyana, Ecuador, and Bolivia. In Central America, it has been observed in Costa Rica, Panama, and Mexico. Inoculation seems to be via trauma. Its incubation period is 1 to 2 years, and it affects mainly male rural workers in a proportion of ten men to every one woman.

The lesions are keloid-like and may also resemble vegetations, infiltrations, nodules and, sometimes, ulcers or gummae (Figs. 11.9 and 11.10). Preferred locations are ears and lower and upper limbs. Lesions have pinkish or brownish color, are smooth or with small scales or crusts, and slow growing. They are also usually asymmetrical and confined to a single region or are confluent, sometimes covering large areas. More seldom, lesions are macular or gumma-like. Pruritus may occur, but there is no systemic symptomatology. When lymph nodes are involved, they are hard and there is no flotation. The patient maintains good general health.

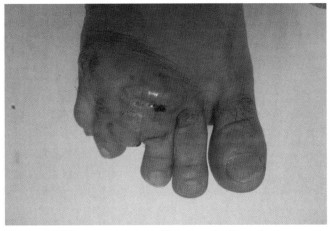

Figure 11.7. Mycetoma (courtesy Thais Dresch, Rio de Janeiro, Brazil).

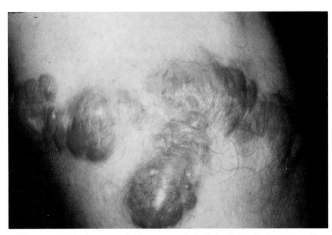

Figure 11.9. Lobomycosis (courtesy Arival de Brito, Belem, Brazil).

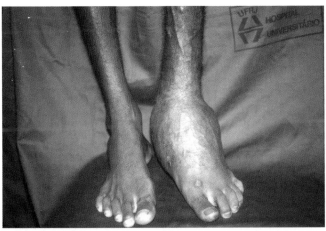

Figure 11.8. Mycetoma (Courtesy of Nurimar Fernandes, Rio de Janeiro, Brazil).

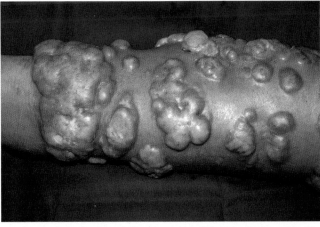

Figure 11.10. Lobomycosis (courtesy Arival de Brito, Belem, Brazil).

Differential diagnosis includes leprosy and leishmaniasis, as well as keloids.

In tissue sections and especially in exudate, *Lacazia loboi* is seen as spherical elements or in lemon form with thick walls and more or less uniform size. In exudate or in histological sections with Grocott's stain, it is possible to observe the characteristic form of the fungus: cells presenting a protuberance and, at the opposite pole, a small cicatricial depression. These cells present gemmulation in the lateral chain. The richness of parasite forms in the dermis is remarkable, being separated from the epidermis by a Grenz zone. Culture of *Lacazia loboi* has not yet been achieved.

There is no consensus on treatment, but some options may be prescribed such as clofazimine, either isolated or in conjunction with itraconazole. Keloid lesions do not respond well to drug therapy and, therefore, one should consider the possibility of their surgical removal.

Paracoccidioidomycosis

Paracoccidioidomycosis is a systemic mycosis of great interest for Latin American countries (from Mexico to Argentina), where it is endemic. It is caused by inhalation of the dimorphic fungus *Paracoccidioides brasiliensis*, and presents in a heterogeneous distribution, with areas of low and high endemic density. The main factor for infection risk is working with soil contaminated by the fungus, such as agriculture, earth moving, soil preparation, and gardening, among others. Tabagism and alcohol addiction are additional factors. Contrary to other systemic mycoses, paracoccidioidomycosis is not usually related to immunodepression, but there are cases associated with HIV infection, neoplasia and, more rarely, organ transplantion. An association with tuberculosis is reported in up to 12% of the cases.

The infection is acquired mainly in the first two decades of life, with a peak incidence between 10 and 20 years. Presentation of clinical manifestations or evolution of the disease is uncommon in this group, occurring with greater frequency among adults between 30 and 50 years as reactivation of a latent endogenous focus. The rate of onset in adults varies, with a ratio of 10 to 15 men for each woman. During childhood, however, the distribution is equal between sexes.

The clinical picture is variable, the disease therefore being classified in different clinical forms. After inhalation of the fungus, there may be development of pulmonary forms that may or may not regress or that spread by hematologic dissemination. The acute/subacute juvenile form prevails in children and adolescents, but can eventually affect individuals up to 35 years. It is characterized by a faster evolution, with the patients seeking medical care in 4 to 12 weeks after onset of the disease. The main manifestations of the disease are fever, digestive manifestations, lymphadenomegaly, osteoarticular involvement, hepatosplenomegaly, and cutaneous lesions (ulcerated lesions, with verruciform or papulonodular aspect). Possible complications are obstructive jaundice, intestinal subocclusion or occlusion, vena cava compression syndrome, diarrhea with malabsorption syndrome, ascites, adrenal involvement (asthenia, weight loss, arterial hypotension, skin hyperpigmentation, abdominal pains), and central nervous system involvement (headache, motor deficiency, convulsions, alterations of behavior and/or level of consciousness).

The chronic or adult form is responsible for more than 90% of the cases and occurs, most commonly, between 30 and 60 years, with a greater prevalence in males. The disease progresses slowly and silently, and can take years until diagnosed. Pulmonary manifestations are present in 90% of the patients. It is called unifocal presentation when it is restricted to a single organ, with the lungs being the only affected site in up to 25% of the cases. There may be coughing, dyspnea, and mucopurulent expectoration with chest X-ray showing bilateral infiltration, predominantly of the lower third. Usually, however, the disease is multifocal, affecting lungs, mucosa and skin. The so-called moriform stomatitis of Aguiar-Pupo is considered characteristic. These are lesions of the mouth and/or oropharynx with sialorrhea, odinophagia, hoarseness, and evidence of fine granulation with hemorrhagic dots on the surface. Cutaneous lesions are papular, ulcer-crusted, or vegetating and may also present with hemorrhagic dots on their surface (Figs. 11.11–11.13).

The golden standard for the diagnosis is the finding of fungal elements suggestive of *P. brasiliensis* in the examination of fresh saliva or other clinical specimens (lesion smear; lymph node aspirate) and/or fragments of biopsy of organs supposedly involved (Fig. 11.14). The cells are spherical, with refringent

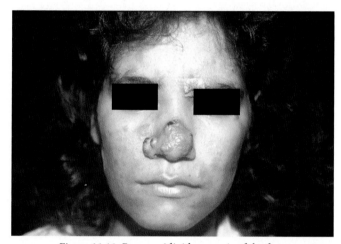

Figure 11.11. Paracoccidioidomycosis of the face.

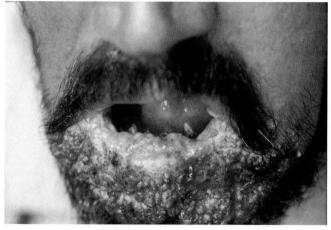

Figure 11.12. Paracoccidioidomycosis – vegetating lesion on the lower lip.

100%. Specific anti-*P. brasiliensis* antibody titer is related to the severity of the clinical forms being higher in the acute–and subacute forms of the disease.

P. brasiliensis is sensitive to most antifungal drugs. For mild to moderate cases, the best choice is itraconazole, at doses of 200 mg/day for up to 24 months. The drugs to be used in severe cases are intravenous amphotericin B or trimethoprin-sulfamethoxazole. The cure criteria in PCM are clinical (disappearance of symptoms of the disease), radiological (stabilization of the image pattern of pulmonary cicatricial images), and immunological (with negative titers in double immunodiffusion).

PROTOZOA

Chagas' disease

Described in 1909, by Carlos Chagas, Chagas' disease or trypanosomiasis americana, is caused by *Trypanosoma cruzi*, a human parasite that also affects domestic and wild animals. Transmission occurs through bites of a vector animal, the triatominae, "barbeiro" or reduviid bug (Fig. 11.15). Chagas' disease occurs in rural areas of the tropical Americas, being the main cause of cardiac problems in some countries. In Latin America it is considered a disease of the poor population, living in adobe homes, which is a favorable environment for the vector. Age, sex, and race do not influence disease incidence, despite the acute phase being more common in children. Dermatologists must be attentive for early signs of the disease, occurring at inoculation sites, so that treatment can be started immediately and to avoid future complications.

Two transmission cycles are known for this parasite in nature: forest and domestic. The first occurs among wild animals and the triatominae. Marsupials, rodents, monkeys, rats, and rabbits are the main reservoirs. The domestic cycle results from invasion of uninhabited areas by man. Transmission occurs when the infected vector bites animals living in the periphery of the houses. The trypomastigote form that circulated in the peripheral blood of vertebrates undergoes a transformation in the vector's organism, changing to the epimastigote form and multiplies itself, passing later to metacyclic trypomastigotes in the digestive

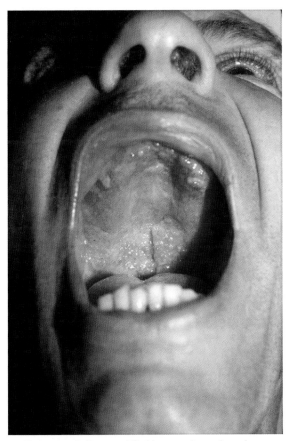

Figure 11.13. Paracoccidioidomycosis on the palate.

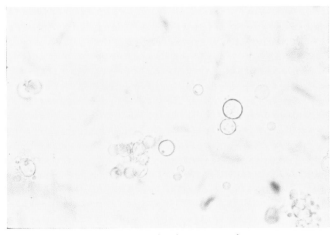

Figure 11.14. Paracoccidioidomycosis – direct exam.

walls with single or multiple budding. Presence of a ship's steering wheel aspect due to the multiple budding is typical. The culture presents slow growth, resulting either in the filamentous or yeast form of the fungus. Specific serologic tests are important not only as help to the diagnosis, but also for allowing an assessment of the host's response to the specific treatment. Presently, several methods are available, as double immunodiffusion (ID), counter immunoelectrophoresis (CIE), indirect immunofluorescence (IFI), immunoenzymatic test (ELISA), and immunoblot (IB), which reach a sensitivity and specificity between 85% and

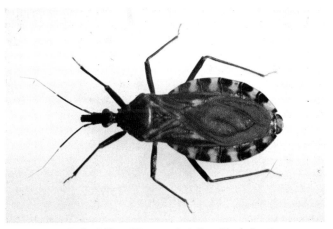

Figure 11.15. Reduviid bug (Courtesy Luís Rey, Rio de Janeiro, Brazil – with permission of Springer-Verlag).

system of the triatominae. The latter then invades the domiciles seeking sources for its sole food, which is the blood. The main species of this arthropod are *Triamota infestans* (Argentina, Bolivia, Brazil, Chile, Paraguay, Peru and Uruguay), *Rhodnius prolixus* (Colombia, Guyanas, Surinam, Venezuela, and Central America), and *Panstrongylus megistus* (Brazil). Transmission occurs through stools of the triatominae, which usually defecates while feeding. Other forms of transmission are reported such as vertical transmission, transfusion, congenital, accidental andoral.

Most of the infected individuals remain asymptomatic. When symptoms appear, there is an incubation period of approximately one week. The acute Chagas' disease is more frequently seen in children and begins with inflammatory lesions at the site of the inoculation. This can be in the skin or in the conjunctiva. When penetration occurs through the ocular mucous membrane, there is a periorbital edema, known as *Romaña's sign* (Fig. 11.16). This picture, also known as primary ophthalmo–lymph node complex, will manifest after 5 to 10 days of the agent's penetration and is unilateral, accompanied by conjunctivitis, dacrioadenitis, and satellite adenitis.

The inoculation chagoma denotes that the entry site was the skin and it is a macular or papulonodular erythematous violet, hard and painless lesion that may ulcerate. This initial lesion tends to regress in 3 weeks. Satellite lymphadenitis is also usually present. Other signs of acute disease are fever, indisposition, migraine, myalgia, hepatosplenomegaly, and maculopapular, morbiliform, or urticariform cutaneous rashes (schizotrypanids).

The phases that follow can produce megaesophagus, megacolon, and heart involvement. The latter, at its turn, can manifest as myocarditis, arrhythmias, and complete heart blockade, typically the right and left anterior bundle branches being affected more frequently.

The methods, which may assist in the diagnosis, will depend on the phase of the disease. In the acute phase, direct search of the protozoon (Fig. 11.17) and search for anti-*T. cruzi* IgM antibodies by indirect immunofluorescence and PCR are used. In the chronic phase, serological tests of indirect hemoagglutina-

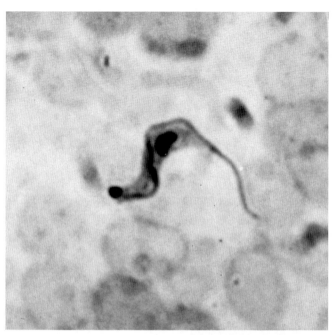

Figure 11.17. *Trypanosoma cruzi* in blood (Courtesy Luís Rey, Rio de Janeiro, Brazil – with permission of Springer-Verlag).

tion, indirect immunofluorescence, and ELISA are the methods with better results.

Therapeutics are unsatisfactory. Even when correct, the treatment does not alter the serological reactions or the heart function in the chronic phases, in spite of usually curing the patient in the acute phase. The two main drugs are benzonidazole and nifurtimox. Both are active against the circulating and tissue forms and should be administered between 30 and 90 days. For patients with stable chronic disease, the treatment should include antiarrhythmics and control of the affected systems, with diets, laxatives, and surgical procedures. The prevention of the disease involves sanitary education of the population and the use of insecticides. Vaccines are being studied but are not yet available.

Mucocutaneous or Tegmental Leishmaniasis

Leishmaniases are anthropozoonoses including a set of diseases with an important clinical spectrum and epidemiologic diversity. The World Health Organization (WHO) estimates that about 350 million people are exposed to the risk with approximately two million new cases per year. It has a worldwide distribution, being considered a public health problem in 88 countries, distributed in four continents (America, Europe, Africa and Asia). In the American Continent there are records of cases from the extreme south of the United States to the north of Argentina, except for Chile and Uruguay. It is considered by the WHO as one of the six most important infectious diseases, for its high rate of detection and capacity of producing deformities.

In Brazil, in 1895, Moreira identified for the first time the existence of the endemic boil of the tropical countries, the so-called endemic "Bahia boil" or "Biskra boil." In 1909, Lindenberg found leishmania forms in cutaneous and nasopharyngeal ulcers in workers of deforestation areas in the interior of the state of São Paulo. Splendore, in 1911, diagnosed the mucosal form of the disease and Gaspar Vianna named the parasite *Leishmania*

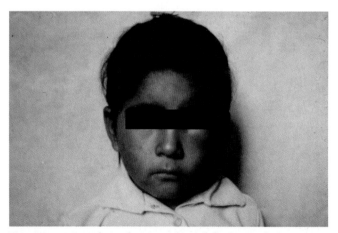

Figure 11.16. Inoculation lesion on the eyelid – Romaña's sign (Courtesy João Dias & Luís Rey, Rio de Janeiro, Brazil – with permission of Springer-Verlag).

brazilienses, and was the first to use an effective drug, emetic tartar, for its treatment. In 1922, Aragão demonstrated the role of the Phlebotomus in the transmission of the disease and Forattini, in 1958, found parasitized wild rodents.

Leishmania belongs to the *Trypanosomatidae* family of protozoa. It is an obligatory intracellular parasite of the mononuclear phagocytic system, with two main forms: flagellated, leptomonas or promastigote, observed in the digestive tube of the vector insect, and aflagellated leishmania or amastigote, found in the tissues of the vertebrate hosts. In the Americas 11 dermotropic species of Leishmania are recognized and eight species described only in animals, all belonging to the subgenus Viannia and Leishmania. The three principal species are *L. (V.) braziliensis, L. (V.) guyanensis* and *L. (L.) amazonensis*.

The vectors are insects called *phlebotominae*, belonging to the Dyptera order, family *Psychodidae*, subfamily *Phlebotominae*, genus *Lutzomyia*, known popularly, depending on the geographical location, as straw mosquito, tatuquira, and birigui, among others. The reservoirs can be wild animals (as rodents and marsupials), synanthropic (species that, undesirably, cohabit with humans, such as rats, cockroaches, flies, mosquitoes, fleas, hematophagous bats, pigeons, and others) and domestic (canines, felines, and equines, considered accidental hosts of the disease).

Transmission occurs through the bite of infected transmitter insects. There is no person-to-person transmission. There is no preference for sex, race, or age. However, most of the cases occur in men with ages between 20 and 40 years. In the countries of the Old World, the cutaneous form of leishmaniasis, the Orient boil, is more frequently observed in children. The incubation period of the disease in humans lasts on average, 2 to 3 months, but can vary from 2 weeks to 2 years.

Epidemiological analyses suggest that in the last decades there were changes in the transmission pattern of the disease. It was initially considered a wild animal zoonosis that, occasionally, affected people in forests. Later, the disease started to appear in rural zones, already practically deforested, and in periurban areas. The existence of three epidemic profiles is noted. The first is forest, where transmission occurs in the areas of primary vegetation (zoonosis of wild animals). The second is occupational, associated with the disordered exploration of the forest and deforestation (anthropozoonosis) and the third is rural or periurban. In periurban areas or "colonization areas" the vector has adapted to the peridomicile area (zoonosis of residual forests and/or anthropozoonosis).

Transmission cycles vary according to the geographical area, involving a diversity of parasite species, vectors, reservoirs, and hosts. *Leishmania (Leishmania) amazonensis* is present in areas of primary and secondary forests of the Legal Amazon (Amazonas, Pará, Rondônia, Tocantins, and Maranhão) and also in the states of the following regions of Brazil: Northeast (Bahia), Southeast (Minas Gerais and São Paulo), Midwest (Goiás) and South (Paraná). It causes localized cutaneous ulcers and, occasionally, some individuals can develop a classic picture of diffuse cutaneous leishmaniasis. *Leishmania (Viannia) guyanensis*, in Brazil, is apparently limited to the north region (Acre, Amapá, Roraima, Amazonas and Pará), extending into the Guyanas. It is found mainly in dry land forests (areas that are not flooded in the rainy period) and causes predominantly single or multiple ulcerated cutaneous lesions, with the multiple lesions being consequences of simultaneous bites of several infected mosquitoes or secondary

lymphatic metastases. Mucosal involvement is very rare for this species. The disease affects mainly young and adult males in their productive phase. Individuals infected commonly work in the so-called work fronts, which are areas associated with deforestation, virgin forests, and military exercises. In endemic areas children with the disease may be seen. *L. (Viannia) braziliensis* is the most important species, not only in Brazil, but also in all Latin America, with a wide distribution from Central America to the north of Argentina and throughout Brazil. The lesions can occur in eyelids or in areas usually covered by clothes, suggesting that the transmission often occurs inside the houses. The disease in humans is characterized by a cutaneous ulcer, single or multiple, whose main complication is the metastasis by hematogenic spread to the mucous membranes of the nasopharynx, with corresponding destruction of those tissues. Likewise, the remaining species have their own characteristics regarding transmission cycles.

As they are introduced into the skin, the promastigotes encounter the cells of the immune system, as T and B lymphocytes, macrophages, Langerhans cells, and mastocytes. Through a mechanism not yet totally clarified, the parasite adheres to the surface of the macrophages and Langerhans cells passing into the intracellular media, and changes into the amastigote form, characteristic of parasitism in mammals. The leishmanias develop defense mechanisms capable of subverting the microbicide capacity of the macrophages, enabling them to survive and to multiply until the rupture of the cell, when they are released to infect other macrophages, thereby spreading the infection. Then there is release of antigenic particles that will be presented to the immune system. The location of amastigotes inside macrophages makes the control of the infection dependent on the cell-mediated immune response.

Even with the diversity of Leishmania species, the spectrum of clinical manifestations of the disease depends not only on the species involved, but also on the infected individual's immunologic condition. The cutaneous leishmaniasis (CL) represents the most frequent clinical manifestation. In CL, the lesions are exclusively cutaneous. These lesions are prone to healing and present more frequently as single lesions, or in small numbers. In more rare cases, the lesions can be multiple, characterizing the form called disseminated cutaneous leishmaniasis. In CL, the cellular immunity is preserved, thus enabling verification by the positivity for the cutaneous test with leishmanin, intradermal reaction of Montenegro (IDRM), and other in vitro tests. CL can be caused by all the dermotropic species of *Leishmania*, but some particular characteristics have been attributed to the different species. Thus, the lesions caused by L. (L.) amazonensis have more infiltrated borders, containing abundant parasites. In the lesions caused by species of the subgenus Viannia, there is a reduced number of macrophages and parasites.

Some authors suggest a clinical classification based on criteria such as physiopathogeny of the site of the vector bite, aspect, and location of the lesions (including nonapparent infections), and lymph node leishmaniasis. The nonapparent infection, without clinical manifestation, is characterized by positive results in serological tests and intradermal reaction of Montenegro in seemingly healthy individuals, inhabitants of areas of transmission of leishmaniasis, with negative previous history and absence of suggestive cutaneous scars of mucocutaneous or cutaneous leishmaniasis. Lymph node leishmaniasis involves the discovery of located lymphadenopathy in the absence of tegmental lesion.

It can precede the tegumentary lesion and should be differentiated from the lymphangitis or satellite lymphadenomegaly.

CL develops with a typical painless ulcer and is frequently located on exposed areas of the skin, that are round or oval, measuring from several millimeters to a few centimeters. It also has an erythematous base, which is infiltrated and of firm consistency, with well-delineated, elevated borders, and a red bottom with rough granulations. The associated bacterial infection can cause local pain and produce a seropurulent exudate. Other types of lesions are vegetating, papillomatous, and humid (of soft consistency). Or, the lesions can be verrucous with a dry rough surface that can include small crusts and desquamation. These two can be primary or develop initially as ulcers. In nontreated cases, the lesions tend to spontaneously resolve over a period of months to a few years, but can also remain active for several years and coexist with mucous lesions. When the lesions heal, they leave atrophic depressed scars, with hypo- or hyperpigmentation and fibrous areas. CL presents with varying clinical forms. The cutaneous form primarily affects the skin with an ulcer type lesion. These lesions can be single or multiple (up to 20 lesions). They have a tendency to spontaneously remit and respond well to treatment. In the North of Brazil, the multiple lesions are frequently caused by *L. (V.) guyanensis*. The disseminated form of leishmaniasis is relatively rare, being observed in approximately only 2% of the cases. The two species recognized as agents of this syndrome are *Leishmania (V.) braziliensis and Leishmania (L.) amazonensis*. The disease is characterized by the emergence of multiple papular lesions of acneiform aspect, affecting several body segments, and frequently involving the face and trunk. The number of lesions may reach hundreds. The natural history of the disease in these patients begins with one or several localized lesions with the classic characteristics of ulcers of a granular base and elevated borders. The satellite adenomegaly observed in more than half of these cases in the localized form is rarely detected in patients with the disseminated form and, if present, it is discrete. Later, after the development of the primary lesions, a phenomenon of dissemination of the parasite through the blood or lymph systems occurs. This happens within only a few days, sometimes even in 24 hours, causing lesions distant from the original place of the bite.

Concurrent mucosal onset has been observed in up to 30% of the patients and systemic manifestations, such as fever, general indisposition, muscular pains, weight loss, and anorexia, among others, can also appear. The finding of the parasite in the disseminated form is low, when compared with the diffuse form. The titers of serum anti-*Leishmania* antibodies are high and the response in IDRM is variable. Most of the patients require one or more additional rounds of treatment. Regarding the response to specific treatments, it can be stated that it presents satisfactory results, although rounds of treatment. In HIV-positive individuals, ulcerated lesions affecting several corporal segments prevail. This rare form of presentation is a sign of possible of co-infection with HIV and that should alert the physician to investigate for infection of this virus.

The diffuse cutaneous form, in Brazil, is caused by *L. (L.) amazonensis*. It is rare, severe, and occurs in patients with anergy and specific deficiency to antigens of *Leishmania* in the cellular immune response. Insidiously, a single lesion, appears, which develops slowly into plates and multiple nonulcerated nodulations in vast areas of the skin. The response to therapy is poor or absent and IDRM is usually negative. The cutaneous forms should be differentiated from other diseases such as syphilis,

leprosy, tuberculosis, atypical mycobacterioses, paracoccidioidomycosis, histoplasmosis, lobomycosis, sporotrichosis, and chromoblastomycosis, among others.

It is considered that 3% to 5% of the cases of CL develop mucosal lesions. Clinically, mucocutaneous leishmaniasis is expressed by locally destructive lesions in the mucous membranes of the upper airways. The classic form is secondary to the cutaneous lesion and it is believed that the metastatic mucosal lesion occurs by hematogenous spread or lymphatic dissemination. Patients with multiple cutaneous lesions and extensive lesions of more than 1 year duration, located above the waist, are the group with greater risk of developing metastases to the mucosa. The lesion is usually painless and begins in the cartilaginous anterior nasal septum, near the nasal entrance. This allows for easy visualization of the lesion. The etiologic causative agent of mucocutaneous leishmaniasis in Brazil is *L. (V.) braziliensis;* however, cases attributed to *L. (L) amazonensis and L (V.) guyanensis* have also been mentioned. This form of the disease is strongly positive for IDRM. However, due to the scarcity of parasites, it is difficult to confirm their presence They have a difficult therapeutic response, which demands greater doses of drugs, and results in a more frequent recurrence (7.5%) than in the cutaneous form (4.3%). It is also more susceptible to the infectious complications and can result in death in 1% of cases.

The mucocutaneous form (Figs. 11.18–11.26) has nasal obstruction, the elimination of crusts, epistaxis, dysphagia, odynophagia, hoarseness, dyspnea, and coughs as the main physical symptoms. There are rarely complaints of nasal itching and pain. In the mucous membranes of the nose, perforation or

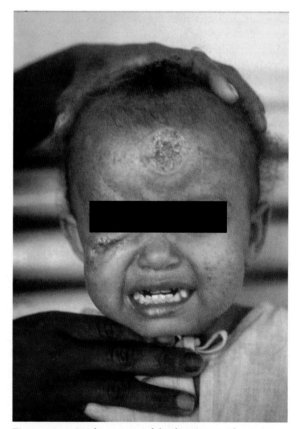

Figure 11.18. Leishmaniasis of the face (sister of patient in Fig. 11.18).

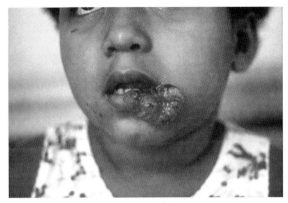

Figure 11.19. Leishmaniasis – vegetating lesion on the lower lip (sister of patient in Fig. 11.17).

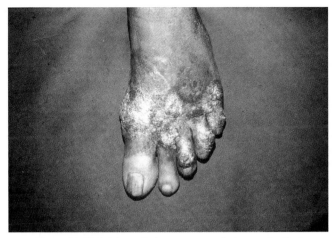

Figure 11.22. Leishmaniasis – verrucous lesion on the foot.

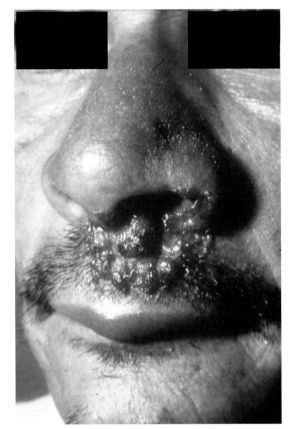

Figure 11.20. Leishmaniasis on the nose and upperlip.

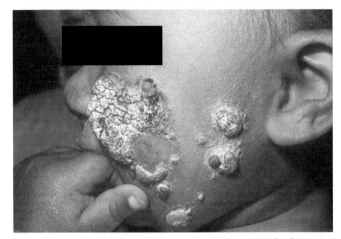

Figure 11.23. Leishmaniasis – verrucous lesion on the face.

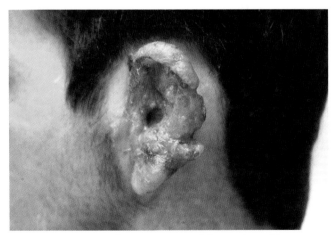

Figure 11.24. Leishmaniasis – partial destruction of the ear.

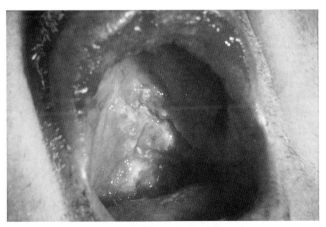

Figure 11.21. Leishmaniasis of the palate.

even destruction of the cartilaginous septa may occur and in the mouth, perforation of the soft palate can occur. In chronic and advanced lesions, mutilations with partial or total loss of the nose, lips, and eyelids may occur, causing deformities and consequent social stigma. The differential diagnosis includes paracoccidioidomycosis, squamous cell carcinoma, basal cell carcinoma, lymphoma, rhinophyma, lepromatous leprosy, tertiary syphilis, rhinosporidiosis, entomophthoromycosis, traumatic perforation

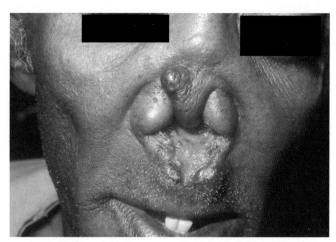

Figure 11.25. Leishmaniasis – total destruction of the nose.

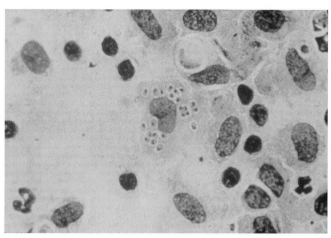

Figure 11.27. Leishmaniasis – leishmania inside a macrophage.

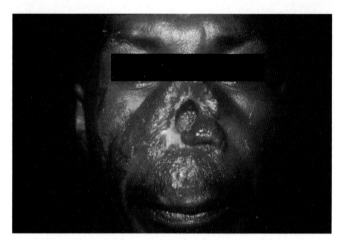

Figure 11.26. Leishmaniasis – also destruction of the nose.

or use of drugs, allergic rhinitis, sinusitis, sarcoidosis, Wegener's granulomatosis, and other rarer diseases.

In the occurrence of typical lesions of leishmaniasis, the clinical and epidemiological diagnosis can be accomplished, especially if the patient originates from endemic areas or was present in places with cases of leishmaniasis. The clinical–epidemiological diagnosis can be complemented by positive IDRM and eventually by therapeutic response. Direct demonstration of the parasite is the procedure of first choice because it is faster, of lower cost, and can be easily executed (Fig. 11.27). Finding the parasite is inversely proportional to the length of time the cutaneous lesion has been there. For example finding the parasite after having the lesion for a year is rare. The isolation by cultivation in vitro is a method that allows the subsequent identification of the species of involved leishmania. The intradermal tests (IDRM or leishmanin test) are based on the visualization of the response of late cellular hypersensitivity. Intradermal reaction usually remains positive after treatment or healing of the treated cutaneous or spontaneously cured lesion. It can be negative in weak-reacting individuals and in those treated previously. It can also be negative in the first 4 to 6 weeks after the appearance of the cutaneous lesion. Patients with mucosal disease present with exacerbated IDRM, with several centimeters of induration and with vesiculation in the

center of the reaction. There is also the possibility of ulceration and local necrosis. In the diffuse cutaneous form IDRM is usually negative. Other methods like the detection of circulating antibodies or PCR can also be used.

The drugs of first choice in the treatment of the leishmaniases are the pentavalent antimonials. There are two types of pentavalent antimonials that can be used, the antimoniate of N-methylglucamine and sodium stibogluconate. The latter is not marketed in Brazil. The pentavalent antimonials are drugs considered as leishmanicides, because they interfere in the bioenergetics of the amastigote forms of leishmania. It should not be administered in pregnant women and there are restrictions to the use of antimonials in patients over 50 years and in patients with cardiopathies, nephropathies, hepatopathies, and Chagas' disease. In the case of unsatisfactory response with pentavalent antimonials, the drugs of second choice are amphotericin B and pentamidines.

The criterion for cure is clinical, with a regular follow-up for 12 months being indicated. Cure is defined by the epitheliazation of the ulcerated lesions and total regression of the infiltration and erythema. Recurrence is defined as reappearance of the lesion in any part of the body 1 year after clinical cure. Measures to prevent leishmania infection include use of repellents when exposed to environments where the vectors can usually be found, avoidance of areas of exposure in vector activity periods (sunset and night) and in areas of occurrence of *L. umbratilis,* avoidance of exposure during the day and the night, use of mosquito nets of fine mesh, screening of doors and windows, environmental handling through cleaning of back yards and land, and finally altering the environmental conditions that help the survival of the vector's immature forms.

PITFALLS AND MYTHS

There are still many habits and superstitions in Brazil that can influence control of these diseases and the fear that they instill.

The use of toothpicks made of vegetable fragments for cleaning of teeth, the habit of chewing vegetable leaves to pass time, and the use of plant leaves for anal hygiene are hypotheses for contamination with P. *brasiliensis*, which is the agent for South American blastomycosis.

There are certain tribes of Indians in the Amazon that consider piedra as an indispensable decoration for the hair. Tinea corporis is still treated with pen ink in certain places in the interior of Brazil. There is also a belief that if herpes zoster reaches both sides of the body and crosses the median line or closes a circle around the body, that the patient will soon die. This belief causes unnecessary fear.

The construction of houses in deforested areas, still close to the forest, where the children play with reservoir animals, domestic or wild, and are continuously exposed to the vectors, can lead to diseases like leishmaniasis, yellow fever, and malaria. The bad habit of leaving old tires in back yards for children to play with allows rain water or other sources to fill them, making them nurseries for Aedes, which is a vector of dengue and yellow fever.

The wattle and daub houses, where reduviid bugs hide in crevices, facilitate infection with Chagas' disease.

Besides superstitions and habits, there are also many regionalisms regarding those diseases that should always be taken into consideration when examining patients from those areas.

SUGGESTED READINGS

Amato VS, Tuon FF, Siqueira AM, et al. Treatment of mucosal leishmaniasis in Latin America: systematic review. *Am J Trop Med Hyg* 2007;77(2):266–274.

Anderson RC, Horn KB, Hoang MP, et al. Punctate exanthema of West Nile Virus infection: report of 3 cases. *J Am Acad Dermatol* 2004;51:820–823.

Bailey MS, Lockwood DN. Cutaneous leishmaniasis. *Clin Dermatol* 2007;25(2):203–211.

Barros MB, Schubach Ade O, do Valle AC, et al. Sporotrichosis with widespread cutaneous lesions: report of 24 cases related to transmission by domestic cats in Rio de Janeiro, Brazil. *Int J Dermatol* 2003;42:677–681.

Borges-Pereira J, de Castro JA, da Silva AG, et al. Seroprevalence of Chagas disease infection in the State of Piaui, 2002. *Rev Soc Bras Med Trop* 2006;39(6):530–539.

Brasil. Ministério da Saúde. Secretaria de Vigilância em Saúde. Departamento de Vigilância Epidemiológica. Manual de Vigilância da Leishmaniose Tegumentar Americana/Ministério da Saúde, Secretaria de Vigilância em Saúde, Departamento de Vigilância Epidemiológica. 2 ed. Brasília: Editora do Ministério da Saúde, 2007. Available at: http://bvsms.saude.gov.br/bvs/publicacoes/07_0454_M.pdf Last accessed Sep 22, 2008.

Brito AC, Quaresma JAS. Lacaziose (doença de Jorge Lobo): revisão e atualização. *An Bras Dermatol* 2007;82(5):475–476.

Carneiro SC, Cestari T, Allen SH, et al. Viral exanthems in the tropics. *Clin Dermatol* 2007;25(2):212–220.

CDC. Imported dengue – United States, 1997 and 1998. *MMWR* 2000; 49:248–253.

Cofré G J. Avances en exantemas virales. *Rev Chil Dermatol* 1998;14:5–10.

Costa RO. Micoses subcutâneas e sistêmicas. In: Ramos-e-Silva M, Castro MCR. eds. *Fundamentos de Dermatologia*. Rio de Janeiro: Atheneu, 2009: 861–873.

De Lima Barros MB, de Oliveira Schubach A, Galhardo MC, et al. Cat-transmitted sporotrichosis epidemic in Rio de Janeiro, Brazil: description of a series of cases. *Clin Infect Dis* 2004;38:529–535.

Depoortere E, Kavle J, Keus K, et al. Outbreak of West Nile virus causing severe neurological involvement in children, Nuba Mountains, Sudan, 2002 *Trop Med Int Health* 2002; 9(6):730–736.

Dias JC, Prata A, Schofield CJ. Chagas' disease in the Amazon: an overview of the current situation and perspectives for prevention. *Rev Soc Bras Med Trop* 2002;35(6):669–678.

Dore A, Auld J. Barmah Forest viral exanthems. *Australas J Dermatol* 2004;45:125–129.

Elsayed S, Kuhn SM, Barber D, et al. Human case of lobomycosis. *Emerg Infect Dis* 2004;10(4):715–718.

Fahal AH. Ycetoma: a thorn in the flesh. *Trans R Soc Trop Med Hyg* 2004;98:3–11.

Figueiredo LTM. Viral hemorrhagic fevers in Brazil. *Rev Soc Bras Med Trop* 2006;39(2):203–210.

Figueiredo RMP, Thatcher BD, Lima ML, et al. Doenças exantemáticas e primeira epidemia de dengue ocorrida em Manaus. *Rev Soc Bras Med Trop* 2004;37:476–479.

Flexman J, Smith D, Mackenzie J, et al. A comparison of the diseases caused by Ross River virus and Barmah Forest virus. *Med J Aust* 1998;169:159–163.

Fonseca BAL, Figueiredo Ltm. Dengue. In: Focaccia R. ed. Veronesi. *Tratado de Infectologia*. Atheneu SP, Brasil 2004. 343–356.

García de Marcos JA, Dean Ferrer A, Alamillos Granados F, et al. Localized Leishmaniasis of the oral mucosa. A report of three cases. *Med Oral Patol Oral Cir Bucal* 2007;12(4):E281–E286.

Goddard LB, Roth AE, Reisen WK, et al. Vector competence of California mosquitoes for West Nile virus. *Emerg Infect Dis* 2002;8:1385–1391.

Granato CFH. Febres Hemorrágicas de etiologia viral. In: Schechter M, Marangoni DV. eds. *Doenças infecciosas: conduta diagnóstica e terapêutica*. Rio de Janeiro: Guanabara Koogan. 1998:154–157.

Guedes ACM, Santos SNMB. Dermatoviroses. In: Ramos-e-Silva M, Castro MCR. eds. *Fundamentos de Dermatologia*. Rio de Janeiro: Atheneu. 2009: 973–1001.

Hay R. Fungal infections. *Clin Dermatol* 2006;24(3):201–212.

Johnson KM. Marburg and Ebola viruses In: Mandel GL. Douglas Jr. RG, Benett JE. eds. *Principles and Practice of Infectious Diseases*. New York, Churchill Livingstone. 1990:1303–1306.

Kauffman CA, Hajjeh R, Chapman SW. Practice guidelines for the management of patients with sporotrichosis. For the Mycoses Study Group. *Infectious Diseases Society of America. Clin Infect Dis* 2000;30:684–687.

Koga T, Matsuda T, Matsumoto T, et al. Therapeutic approaches to subcutaneous mycosis. *Am J Clin Dermatol* 2003;4:537–543.

Lacaz CS, Porto E, Martins JEC, et al. Esporotricose e outras micoses gomosas. In: Lacaz CS, Porto E, Martins JEC, Heins-Vaccari EM, Melo NT, eds. *Tratado de micologia médica*. 9th ed. São Paulo: Sarvier; 2002:233–247.

Machado ES, Braga Mda P, Da Cruz AM, et al. Disseminated American muco-cutaneous leishmaniasis caused by Leishmania braziliensis braziliensis in a patient with AIDS: a case report. *Mem Inst Oswaldo Cruz* 1992;87(4):487–492.

Machado-Pinto J, Pimenta-Gonçalves MP. Dermatoses por protozoários. In: Ramos-e-Silva M, Castro MCR. eds. *Fundamentos de Dermatologia*. Rio de Janeiro: Atheneu, 2009: 1039–1041.

Marques SA, Cortez DB, Lastória JC, et al. Paracoccidioidomicose: freqüência, morfologia e patogênese de lesões tegumentares. *An Bras Dermatol* 2007;82(5):411–417.

Martins FSV, Setúbal S, Castineiras Tmpp. Dengue. In: Schechter M, Marangoni DV. *Doenças infecciosas: conduta diagnóstica e terapêutica*. Rio de Janeiro Guanabara Koogan. 1998:157–164.

Matte SMW, Lopes JO, Melo IS, et al. Cromoblastomicose no Rio Grande do Sul: relato de 12 casos. *Rev Soc Bras Med Trop* 1997;30:309–311.

Menezes VM, Soares BG, Fontes CJ. Drugs for treating paracoccidioidomycosis. *Cochrane Database Syst Rev* 2006(2):CD004967.

Ministerio de Salud. Direción de Vigilancia Epidemiologica. Situacion epidemiológica del dengue en Nicarágua. Manágua. MINSA 2005; Boletim Epidemiológico no 5:12.

Monath TP. Flavivirus yellow fever, dengue and St. Louis encephalitis. In: Mandel GL,Douglas Jr. RG, Benett JE. eds. *Principles and Practice of Infectious Diseases*. New York Churchill Livingstone. 1990:1248–1251.

Monath TP. Yellow fever: an update. *Lancet Infect Dis* 2001;1(1) 11–20.

Moncayo A, Ortiz Yanine MI. An update on Chagas disease (human American trypanosomiasis). *Ann Trop Med Parasitol* 2006;100(8):663–677.

Morris-Jones R. Sporotrichosis. *Clin Exp Dermatol* 2002;27:427–31.

Nelson JSB, Stone MS. Update on selected viral exanthems. *Curr Opin Pediatr* 2000;12:359–364.

Paniago AM, Aguiar JI, Aguiar ES, et al. Paracoccidioidomycosis: a clinical and epidemiological study of 422 cases observed in Mato Grosso do Sul. *Rev Soc Bras Med Trop* 2003;36(4):455–459.

Paniz-Mondolfi AE, Reyes Jaimes O, Davila Jones L. Lobomycosis in Venezuela. *Int J Dermatol* 2007;46(2):180–185.

Peters CJ. Doenças Infecciosas – Infecções causadas por virus transmitidos por artrópodes e roedores. In: Kasper FL, Fauci AS, Longo DL, Braunwald E, Hauser SL, Jameson JL. eds. *Harrison Medicina Interna*. Rio de Janeiro McGraw-Hill Interamericana do Brasil. 2006:1218–1232.

Peters CJ. Doenças Infecciosas – Vírus Marburg e Ebola. In: Kasper FL, Fauci AS, Longo DL, Braunwald E, Hauser SL, Jameson JL. eds. *Harrison Medicina Interna*. Rio de Janeiro McGraw-Hill Interamericana do Brasil. 2006:1232–1234.

Peterson LR, Marfin AA. West Nile Virus: A primer for the clinician. *Ann Intern Med* 2002;137:173–179.

Pinto Dias JC. The treatment of Chagas disease (South American trypanosomiasis). *Ann Intern Med* 2006;144(10):772–774.

Puig L, Pradinaud R. Leishmania and HIV co-infection: dermatological manifestations. *Ann Trop Med Parasitol* 2003;97(Suppl 1): 107–114.

Ramos-e-Silva M, Fernandes NC. Parasitic diseases including tropical. In: Parish LC, Brenner S, Ramos-e-Silva M. eds. *Women's Dermatology: from infancy to maturity*. Lancaster: Parthenon, 2001: 291–302.

Ramos-e-Silva M, Vasconcelos C, Carneiro S, Cestari T. Sporotrichosis. *Clin Dermatol* 2007;25(2):181–187.

Ramos-e-Silva M. Diseases of the oral cavity caused by protozoa. In: Lotti, TM, Parish LC & Rogers III RS. eds. *Oral Diseases. Textbook and Atlas*. Berlin: Springer-Verlag; 1999:122–125.

Ramos-e-Silva M. Facial and oral aspects of some venereal and tropical diseases. *Acta Croatica Dermato Venereologica*: 2004;12(3):173–180.

Ramos-e-Silva M, Saraiva LES. Paracoccidioidomycosis. *Dermatol Clin* 2008;26:257–269.

Restrepo A. Treatment of tropical mycoses. *J Am Acad Dermatol* 1994;31:S91–S94.

Sayal SK, Prasad GK, Jawed KZ, et al. Chromoblastomycosis. *Indian J Dermatol Venereol Leprol* 2002;68(4):233–234.

Schwartz RA. Superficial fungal infections. *Lancet* 2004;364(9440): 1173–1182.

Scott LA, Stone MS. Viral exanthems. *Dermatol Online J* 2003;9:4.

Setúbal S. Febre amarela In: Schechter M, Marangoni DV. eds. *Doenças infecciosas: conduta diagnóstica e terapêutica*. Rio de Janeiro Guanabara Koogan. 1998:152–154.

Shikanai-Yasuda MA, Telles Filho Fde Q, Mendes RP, et al. Guidelines in paracoccidioidomycosis. *Rev Soc Bras Med Trop* 2006;39(3):297–310.

Silva JP, de Souza W, Rozental S. Chromoblastomycosis: a retrospective review of 325 cases in the Amazonic Region (Brazil). Mycopathologica 1990;143:171–175.

Silveira FT, Lainson R, Corbett CE. Clinical and immunopathological spectrum of American cutaneous leishmaniasis with special reference to the disease in Amazonian Brazil: a review. *Mem Inst Oswaldo Cruz* 2004;99(3):239–251.

Singh S, Sivakumar R. Recent advances in the diagnosis of leishmaniasis. *J Postgrad Med* 2003;49(1):55–60.

Taborda VBA, Taborda PRO, McGinnis MR. Constitutive melanin in the cell wall of the etiologic agent of Lobo's disease. *Rev Inst Med trop S Paulo*, 1999;41(1):9–12.

Teixeira AR, Nascimento RJ, Sturm NR. Evolution and pathology in Chagas disease – a review. *Mem Inst Oswaldo Cruz*. 2006; 101(5):463–491.

The Centers for Disease Control and Prevention. Available at: http://www.cdc.gov/ncidod/dvbid/westnile/birdspecies.htm Last accessed Sep 22, 2008.

The IX International Meeting on Paracoccidioidomycosis, Aguas de Lindoia, SP, Brazil, October 2–5, 2005. Abstracts. *Rev Inst Med Trop Sao Paulo*. 2005;47 Suppl 14:2–64.

Tong S. Spatiotemporal variation of notified Barmah Forest virus infections in Queensland, Australia, 1993–2001. *Int J Environm Health Res* 2005; 15(2):89–98.

Welsh O, Vera-Cabrera L, Salinas-Carmona MC. Mycetoma. *Clin Dermatol* 2007;25(2):195–202.

Zaitz, C, Ramos-e-Silva M. Tropical pathology of the oral mucosa. In: Lotti, TM, Parish LC & Rogers III RS. eds. *Oral Diseases. Textbook and Atlas*. Berlin: Springer-Verlag; 1999:129–147.

12 | AQUATIC DERMATOLOGY

Domenico Bonamonte and Gianni Angelini

HISTORY

The field of aquatic dermatology owes its development both to modern man's extreme mobility around the globe and to a growing attention to skin diseases provoked by the aquatic environment. Aquatic dermatoses are frequently observed in fishermen, scuba divers, sailors, boatmen, bay watchers, swimming pool attendants, swimming instructors, and workers at aquariums, saunas, and Turkish baths, apart from bathers. The different forms of dermatoses can be caused by either biotic or nonbiotic (physical and chemical) agents.

The seas, rivers, lakes, ponds, swimming pools, and aquariums are populated by a myriad of animal and vegetable organisms. During the course of evolution, multitudes of aquatic species have developed both defensive and offensive mechanisms against their predators, in the form of stings and bites that often include a venomous apparatus. These self-protective mechanisms are also used against humans. Many species of marine vertebrates and invertebrates produce biotoxins, most of which serve to capture prey for food (e.g. the toxins produced by Coelenterates). These toxins can also have a simple defense function, like those present on the dorsal spines of the scorpionfish or the spine under the stingray's tail. From a chemical standpoint, the biotoxins identified up to now are amino and phenol derivatives with a low molecular weight, choline esters, or other more complex peptides or proteins. The dermatological manifestations induced by marine organisms can be associated with systemic reactions. These are sometimes of a severe nature leading to shock, and even death. In this context, it should be borne in mind that about 5% of fatal accidents occurring during underwater activities are due to accidental contact with aquatic organisms that do not attack man. This fact is even more significant when one considers that the mean total number of deaths worldwide caused by shark attacks is 6 per year. Diseases caused by aquatic biotic organisms can arise due to three different pathogenic events: toxic-immune, toxic-traumatic, and traumatic. Traumatic lesions (e.g. an encounter with an electric fish or shark) are not of dermatological concern and so will not be dealt with in this chapter.

DERMATITIS FROM COELENTERATES

Coelenterates or Cnidari (from the Greek *knidi* = nettle) are animals with a simple symmetrical radial structure. Because of the symptoms they cause they are also known as "sea-nettles."

The Coelenterates *phylum* is abundantly present in tropical and subtropical seas. Of the 9000 identified species, about 100 are known to be harmful to humans.

These belong to the Scyphozoa, Anthozoa, and Hydrozoa classes (Table 12.1). These species share the same type of offensive organule, production of biotoxins, and inoculation mechanism used to capture their prey.

On the surface of the body and tentacles, Coelenterates have a myriad of microscopic organules, variously known as cnidoblasts, cnidocytes, "urticant cells" or "sting capsules." Cnidocytes

Table 12.1: The Phylum of Toxic Coelenterates

1. Scyphozoa (jellyfish)	
Species:	*Pelagia noctiluca*
	Rhizostoma pulmo
	Cyanea capillata
	Chrysaora quinquecirrha
	Chironex fleckeri
	Aurelia aurita
2. Anthozoa	
Order:	Actinidae (sea anemones)
Species:	*Anemonia sulcata*
	Actinia equina
	Adamsia palliata
	Calliactis parasitica
	Condylactis aurantiaca
Order:	Scleractinia (corals)
Order:	Sagartidae
Species:	*Sagartia elegans*
3. Hydrozoa	
Order:	Siphonophora
Species:	*Physalia physalis*
	Physalia utriculus
	Velella velella
Order:	Leptomeduse (hydroids)
Order:	Milleporina
Species:	*Millepora alcicornis* (stinging corals: not true coral)

contain special globe-shaped bodies in the cytoplasm called *nematocysts* that contain a very long, thin, spiral-shaped filament. On contact with a foreign body, due to stimulation of their external receptors (cnidocilia), the cnidocytes eject their nematocysts. When these penetrate the body of the prey, the filament is extruded and toxin is injected. Apart from physical contact with the prey, a specific chemical stimulus produced by the prey is needed to cause expulsion of the nematocysts. The whole expulsion process lasts less than 3 milliseconds.

The nematocysts vary in corpuscle shape and size, filament length, and morphology according to species. They also contain various biologically active toxic substances. The chemical structure of these is not known for all species. It was in 1902, in the course of studying the toxins of the sea anemone, that Richet, the French physiologist, discovered the phenomenon of anaphylaxis which later won him the Nobel Prize in 1913.

From the tentacles of the actinia *Anemonia sulcata,* Richet isolated three different components: hypnotoxin (that induces somnolence and respiratory paralysis), thalaxin (that has an urticant action and causes cardiac arrest), and congestin (that causes anaphylaxis). As well as these, various other substances have been isolated in Coelenterates (including tetramine, histamine and 5-hydroxytryptamine), which cause these animals to be classified as venomous or actively toxic. Apart from some rare exceptions (the Palythoa genus of the Zoantharia family), these same organisms are not poisonous if ingested, because the protein toxins are inactivated by heat and then innocuously digested by the proteolytic bowel enzymes. The skin effects (burning, erythema and edema) are caused by tetramine, histamine, and 5-hydroxytryptamine. Some of the cytotoxic effects are attributable to damage to the cell membrane due to the toxic actions on the mitochondria. Some species of anemones produce protease inhibitors that can act against trypsin and chemotrypsin. In other cases, commonly in the Caribbean anemones, effects of the toxins are brought about by blockage of the potassium channels or glutamate receptor antagonism.

Reactions to jellyfish

Jellyfish are the most frequent cause of adverse reactions to marine animals. There are about 150 million cases of jellyfish stings reported each year. The pathogenic mechanism of such reactions can be toxic or allergic. In the latter case they may be either humoral or cell-mediated. Jellyfish venoms are difficult to work with and are sensitive to pH, temperature, and chemical changes. The toxins produced by the nematocysts include substances with an enzymatic action, compounds of quaternary ammonium, catecholamines, histamine, and its release substances; serotonin and quinine-like substances.

In the Mediterranean, there are 11 species of jellyfish, six of which are harmful to humans. Among the six, the most common and toxic is *Pelagia noctiluca,* a small jellyfish whose entire body and tentacles are covered with cnidocytes.

Reactions to jellyfish can present with different clinical–morphological pictures and pathogenic mechanisms (Table 12.2). The most common forms are localized toxic urticarial reactions. Instant pain is followed by an immediate skin eruption, which is characterized by figured urticarial lesions lasting from a few minutes to several hours depending on the severity of the damage. Blistering, hemorrhagic, or necrotizing manifestations can

Table 12.2: Skin and Systemic Reactions to Jelly Fish

1. Local reactions: toxic reactions, angioedema, recurrent reactions, persistent delayed reactions, reactions at a distance

2. Local sequelae: cheloids, dyschromia, atrophy, scarring, gangrene

3. Systemic reactions: asthenia, ataxia, muscle cramps, paraesthesia, vertigo, fever, vomiting

4. Fatal reactions: toxic reactions (immediate cardiac and respiratory arrest, delayed renal failure), anaphylaxis

5. Reactions after ingestion: pain and abdominal cramps, urticaria

6. "Indirect" dermatitis from Coelenterates: "dermatitis from nudibranchs,"* dermatitis from antigenic substances in the water**

* Nudibranchs (Mollusks) feed on the tentacles and nematocysts of Physalia. These nematocysts are not digested but migrate and are stored in the dorsal papillae. Swimmers coming in contact with these "armed" Nudibranchs can be stung by the nematocysts.
** when strong storms are blowing nematocysts can detache from the tentacles of jellyfish and cause a dermatitis ("dermatitis caused by nematocysts" without any contact with the coelenterate).

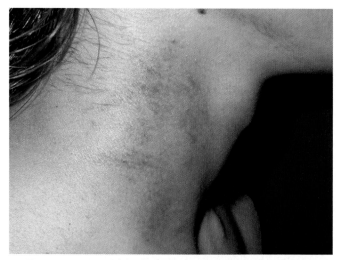

Figure 12.1. Figured erythematovesicular reaction to jellyfish.

also be observed (Figs. 12.1–12.3). Even diffuse urticarial reactions together with anaphylaxis (laryngeal edema, collapse) can be frequent.

There have been cases of recurrent linear skin eruptions that resulted from a single isolated sting and onset did not occur until after a variable time interval (up to many months in some cases). These delayed reactions appear 4 to 7 days after contact, are of granulomatous type, and can persist for months. Histopathological examination shows a dense dermal cell infiltrate, similar to that seen in delayed hypersensitivity reactions. Apart from toxic reactions, there can also be allergic type reactions mediated by specific IgG or IgE antibodies. These antibodies persist for several years and can cross-react. Jellyfish-induced dermatitis can leave scarring outcomes in the form of keloids, dyschromia, scar tissue, subcutaneous atrophy, and gangrene (Fig. 12.4).

In cases where the eyes come into contact with the animal, photophobia, pain, and burning may develop. Chemosis, corneal ulceration and palpebral edema, iritis, increased intraocular

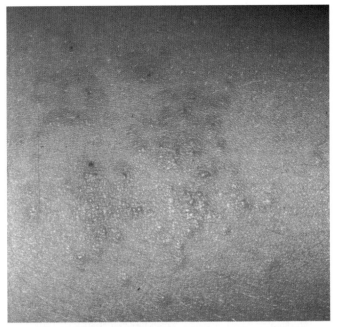

Figure 12.2. Figured erythematovesicular reaction to jellyfish.

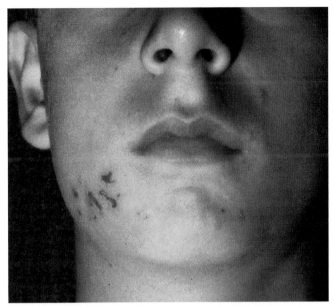

Figure 12.4. Figured scabs due to a reaction to jellyfish.

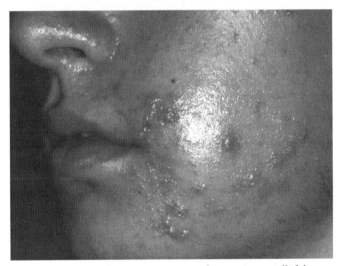

Figure 12.3. Erythemato-vesico-pustular reaction to jellyfish.

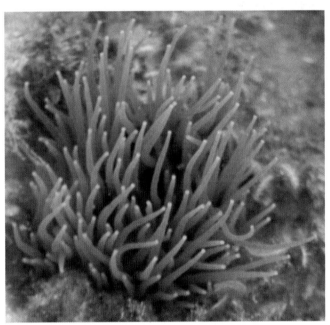

Figure 12.5. *Anemonia sulcata*.

pressure, mydriasis, and reduced accommodation can also occur. These ocular lesions can be followed by anterior synechiae and unilateral glaucoma in some cases.

Some jellyfish widely present in Southeast Asia and Australia (i.e. *Chironex fleckeri* and *Chiropsalmus quadrigatus*) can provoke extremely severe systemic reactions that can even be fatal. Among the causes triggering these reactions, a cardiotoxin, which acts on the calcium channels, has been identified. A hemolytic toxin has also been described. *Chironex fleckeri* venom is able to produce a transient hypertensive response followed by cardiovascular collapse in anesthetized rats; boiling of the venom abolished therefore this cardiovascular activity.

Reactions to actinias

Actinias, belonging to the Anthozoa class and also known as "sea anemones" because they resemble the flower, cover seabeds with their tentacles. They are iridescent and may be a reddish, orange, or purple color. They are extremely variable in shape. They generally live attached to the seabed like carnivorous flowers on a thick stem, while the long, slender tentacles emerging from the apex oscillate gently in the water, creating elegant figures. The actinia most commonly found in the Mediterranean is *Anemonia sulcata* (Fig. 12.5). This sea anemone is diffusely present in shallow waters and up to depths of 10 meters.

Particular attention has been paid by researchers to the toxins produced by sea anemones because they have a greater stability than those produced by other Coelenterates. There are more than 800 species of sea anemones. 40 of these 800 have been studied from a toxicological standpoint. They produce large quantities of three different classes of toxins: (1) toxins of 20 kDA with a cytolytic action (known as actinoporins); (2) neurotoxins of 3 to 5 kDA that can inactivate the sodium channels; (3) neurotoxins of 3.5 to 6.5 kDA whose action is exerted on the potassium channels. Apart from the well-known toxins (hypnotoxin, thalaxin, congestin, equinatoxin) isolated from various species of actinias, some peptides from *Anemonia sulcata* and *Condylactis aurantiaca* have been individuated and characterized. These peptides induce paralysis in crustaceans, fish, and mammals. Newer peptide toxins, produced by the anemone *Stichodactyla gigantea*, have recently been discovered. A few of these new toxins show amino acid sequences that are homologous to the epidermal growth factor (EGF) of mammals. Apart from their structural homology, these toxins also seem to have functions comparable to EGF. This discovery suggests that the phylogenetic origin of EGF could have been as a toxin and that this toxic function could have been lost during the course of evolution.

Sea anemones can induce the same skin picture that is seen in jellyfish stings. In our experience, these reactions present with much more severe symptoms than those provoked by jellyfish. This is likely due to patients coming into closer contact with sea anemones when patients are sitting or lying on the rocks where the anemones are attached (Figs. 12.6 and 12.7). These lesions are generally much more extensive and have many more bizarre pathognomonic figures. From a morphological standpoint along with being erythematoedematous, the lesions are often vesicular or blistering (Fig. 12.8) and sometimes even necrotizing. Edema is often severe and can feature an angioedematous picture. Some isolated cases of allergic IgE-mediated reactions to certain species of anemones have caused anaphylactic shock, and acute renal failure.

This disorder lasts from 15 to 20 to 30 days and can be associated with extreme subjective (intolerable pain and burning) and systemic symptoms (malaise, asthenia, and muscle cramps) (Table 12.3). Dyschromic or scarring sequelae (Fig. 12.9) are also much more frequent after contact with sea anemones than with jellyfish.

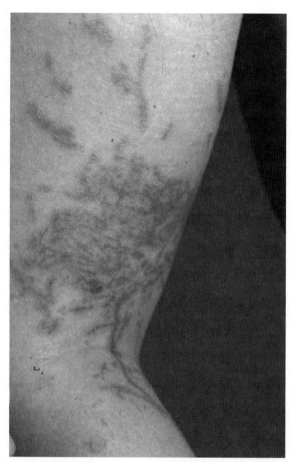

Figure 12.7. Figured erythematovesicular dermatitis from *Anemonia sulcata*.

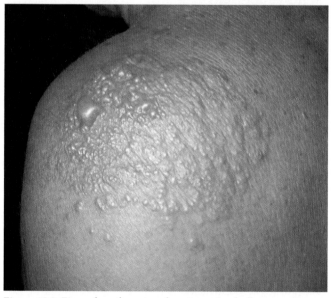

Figure 12.8. Figured erythemato-edemato-vesico-bullous reaction from *Anemonia sulcata*.

Table 12.4 shows some principles of treatment regarding reactions to Coelenterates. In nations with a high incidence of reactions to Coelenterates, protective measures are often adopted for preventative purposes. However, none of these measures have been shown to be efficacious. A wetsuit leaves some skin areas

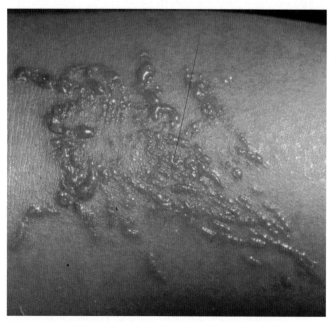

Figure 12.6. Figured erythemato-edemato-vesico-bullous reaction due to *Anemonia sulcata*.

Table 12.3: Differential Characteristics between Reactions to Jellyfish and Sea Anemones

	Reactions to Jellyfish	Reactions to Sea anemones
Incidence	Frequent	Less frequent
Type of contact	Generally superficial	Generally very close
Method of contact	Brushing while swimming	Sitting or lying on the rocks
Sites	All sites	Especially posterior face of the thighs, back, and volar surface of the wrists
Extension of dermatitis	Slight	Extensive
Morphology of the lesions	Figured, mainly linear figures	More bizarre and arabesque-like
Clinical lesions	Erythema, edema, rarely blisters and necrosis	Erythema, severe edema, frequent blisters and necrosis
Local symptoms	Pain, burning	Intolerable pain and burning sensations
Systemic symptoms	Possible	Virtually constant
Clinical course	Few days	15–30 days
Sequelae	Infrequent	Frequent

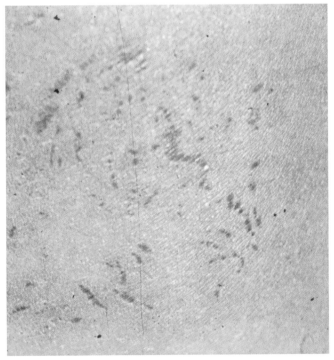

Figure 12.9. Figured atrophic and dyschromic reaction to a sea anemone sting.

Table 12.4: Principles of Treatment of Reactions to Coelenterates

Local Treatment

Vinegar, alcohol, ammonia, urine, and salt water as hot as can be tolerated.

Avoid the use of fresh water because it activates the nematocysts. Avoid showers until the nematocysts toxins have been neutralized.

Wear gloves to remove tentacles. For this purpose a paste made of salt water and bicarbonate or flour or talcum powder can be used. The tentacles can be removed with a knife or sharp tool. If none of the above powders are available dry sand can be used. Wash the affected part with sea water.

In severe cases apply a hemostatic band above the dermatitis when a limb is affected.

Administer local anesthetics and corticosteroids.

Systemic Treatment

Corticosteroids, antihistamines, epinephrine, cardiotonic drugs, calcium gluconate, analgesics (aspirin, fenacetin, codeine).

exposed, while a mesh of protective nets is too wide to prevent the passage of smaller Coelenterates. Recently, by exploiting the ability of the clownfish (genus: *Amphiprion*) to live unharmed within the tentacles of sea anemones, a lotion has been formulated using the mucous that coats the clownfish. This topical medication seems to be able to prevent most contact reactions to jellyfish.

Sagartia, a sea anemone that lives symbiotically at the base of sponges, causes severe skin and systemic reactions among fishermen who collect sponges with their bare hands ("sponge fisherman's disease" or "maladie des pécheurs d'éponges nus"). The onset of symptoms occurs a few minutes after contact with the sea anemone and includes burning and itching, followed by erythematovesicular manifestations that are initially erythematous and then turn purple. This picture can also be associated with systemic symptoms (headache, vomiting, fever, and muscle spasms).

Sea bathers' eruption

This affliction is observed in Florida, Mexico, and the Caribbean. It is linked to several Coelenterates, including the larvae of the jellyfish *Linuche unguiculata* and the sea anemone *Edwardsiella lineata.* This dermatitis develops as a result of bathing in sea water, scuba diving, or windsurfing. It can present during or after bathing, with papules (Figs. 12.10 and 12.11) that evolve into pustules, blisters, and wheals. The patient will also report malaise, fever, nausea, headache, abdominal pain, and diarrhea. It generally affects covered areas. Removal of bathing attire and showering immediately after bathing limits the extent of the dermatitis, which evolves spontaneously over the course of two weeks. From a pathogenic standpoint, sea bathers' eruption can be of either a toxic or allergic nature, as demonstrated by the findings of specific IgG in some subjects. This disorder must be differentiated from dermatoses induced by algae (observed in Hawaii, in both fresh and salt water) and cercariae (in fresh water, manifesting on uncovered skin areas).

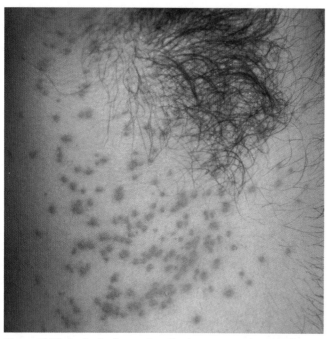

Figure 12.10. Sea bather's eruption: Erythemato-papulo-vesicular dermatitis.

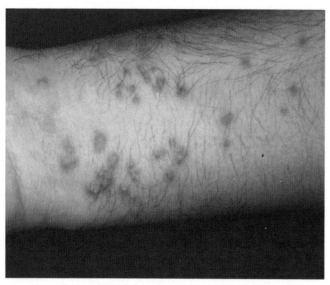

Figure 12.11. The same case as in Fig. 12.10.

Reactions to physaliae, corals, and hydroids

The Physalia genus includes two species: *Physalia physalis* ("sea caravel" or "Portuguese man-of-war"), the most common species, which is present in the tropical Atlantic and the Mediterranean, and *Physalia utriculus*, which is in the Indo-Pacific and south of Japan. The tentacles of a Portuguese man-of-war can be as long as 10 meters. Stings from these species cause extremely intense, unbearable pain that radiates from the affected area and is accompanied by intense burning. The clinical picture features linear erythematous-edematous and vesiculobullous lesions. A few minutes after contact, there is onset of the so-called "physalia syndrome" consisting of systemic symptoms, including anguish, lipothymia, myalgias, dyspnea, vomiting, bradycardia, and hypothermia. The affliction may resolve benignly in a few days or may lead to coma, particularly in tropical areas.

Skin lesions caused by corals can be of various types. Toxic reactions due to contact with the nematocysts are relatively rare and generally mild, whereas wounds caused by their sharp cutting points are quite frequent. These wounds rapidly evolve into painful ulcerations or cellulitis and heal very slowly.

Hydroids, belonging to the Hydrozoa class, are small polyps that form colonies 5 cm high. They are Coelenterates and are prevalent in tropical and subtropical waters. They can provoke immediate (contact urticaria) or delayed (papulous eruptions with a hemorrhagic or zosteriforme evolution developing 4 to 12 hours after contact) reactions.

DERMATOSES DUE TO ECHINODERMS

Echinoderms are animals with symmetrical pentameric rays. Of the 6000 known species, 80 are poisonous or venomous. They are subdivided into five classes according to their shape: Echinoids (sea urchins), Asteroids (starfish), Ophiuroidea (sea serpents), Holothuroidea (sea cucumbers) and Crinoidea (sea lilies). Except for the Holothuroidea, all the other Echinoderms have a rigid endoskeleton made of calcareous stone.

Reactions to sea urchins

Sea urchins are widespread in the Mediterranean (one of the most common is *Paracentrotus lividus*) and frequently induce reactions of both immediate and delayed type after contact with their spines. These spines are sharp and very fragile. At the moment of contact they penetrate the skin and break off. The fragments are then left inside the wound and are difficult to extract.

Immediate reactions. Skin penetration by sea urchin spines causes an immediate fiery burning pain that can persist for some hours, followed by reddening, excoriation, and edema of the body part affected (Fig. 12.12). In some cases the lesions will bleed abundantly. The patient may develop torpor and muscle pain. Secondary infections are quite common, and usually lead to rejection of the spines. The dermatitis generally resolves in 1 to 2 weeks unless the spines remain inside the skin. For this reason it is essential to remove all the fragments of the spines completely. Treatment also consists of applying water as hot as can be tolerated on the edematous, painful lesions.

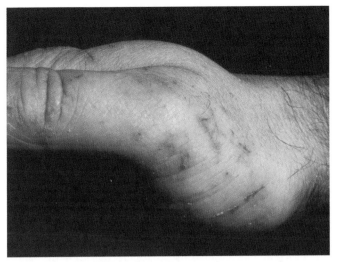

Figure 12.12. Abrasions from sea urchin spine pricks.

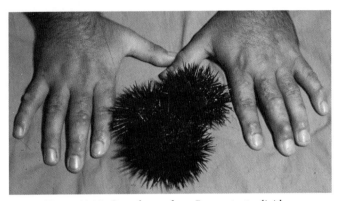

Figure 12.13. Granulomas from Paracentrotus lividus.

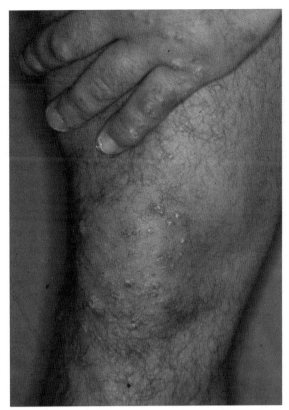

Figure 12.14. Granulomas from Paracentrotus lividus.

Granulomas from sea urchins. This well-known delayed type reaction develops 2 to 3 months after the original contact and can persist for very long periods, although spontaneous healing is also possible. The resulting nodular lesions have a hard, parenchymatous consistency and range from 4 to 5 mm to 1 to 2 cm in diameter. They may be bright or dark red (Figs 12.13 and 12.14). It is possible to elicit a delayed allergic reaction by injecting an extract of the spines in a water–alcohol solution intradermally.

There may be various histopathologic granulomatous findings in the nodular lesions. These types of granulomas may be foreign body, sarcoidal, tuberculoid, or necrobiotic. Albeit rarely *Mycobacterium marinum* has been identified in some granulomas caused by sea urchins, suggesting a possible causal role of this germ in determining the infiltrate. In about 30% of cases, the infiltrate is not of a granulomatous type but is instead characterized by a nonspecific chronic inflammation or suppurating type dermatitis. The nodular lesions are treated with intralesional injections of corticosteroids or liquid nitrogen.

Chronic traumatic lymphedema of the hands. This is another type of diffuse delayed reaction on the back of the hands that consists of a peculiar chronic scleredema. This form of trauma is found in fishermen. It is caused by repeated penetration of the sea urchin spines, constriction of the wrists by the wetsuit, and the low water temperature. It manifests in the form of a

hard edema of the back of the hands and sometimes, also the forearms. Initially the edema is recurrent, but over the years it becomes persistent, very hard, and clearly delineated. It will persist for many years even after retirement from the working activity (Fig. 12.15). The scleredema can be associated with sea urchin granulomas, functional limitations of movement of the wrists and fingers, dystrophic alterations of the nails. And sometimes scleredema can also be associated with acrocyanosis, cigarette paper atrophy of the damaged skin, joint dysmorphisms, and lymphographic alterations of the affected limb. This chronic professional scleredema must be differentiated from deliberate, self-provoked lesions created with various repeated mechanical stimuli (hemostatic bands, occlusive bandaging, traumas) for economic gain (generally pertaining to a retirement fund) or due to psychiatric problems. It must also be differentiated from acute or chronic lymphedema of other natures (lymphatic aplasia, recurrent erysipelas, deep thrombophlebitis, angioedema, cold urticaria, filariasis, venous obstruction, complications of surgical procedures, or radiotherapy for breast cancer or other tumors).

Reactions to starfish

Starfish (about 2000 species) have spines that can secrete toxins that spread throughout the water. These are saponins with a hemolytic, antibiotic action that can irreversibly block neuromuscular transmission. In the presence of many such animals, contact with the surrounding water can therefore induce a papulo-urticarial reaction.

Some starfish, like *Acanthaster planci* (or "crown of thorns"), can inflict a painful sting that may cause granulomatous lesions.

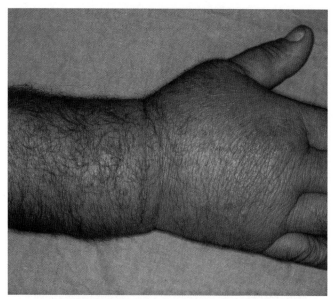

Figure 12.15. Intense chronic traumatic scleredema of the hands and forearms in a fisherman.

The spines of *A. planci* can easily penetrate through gloves and thin-soled shoes.

DERMATOSES FROM MOLLUSKS

The Mollusks *phylum* includes about 45,000 species that are present all over the world. Some of their biotoxins are urticant while others are much more toxic. There are three main classes: Lamellibranchs (bivalves), Gasteropods (conidae), and Cephalopods (octopus, squid, sepia).

Cephalopods *(Octopus vulgaris)* can inflict small bites with their sharp bony beaks, and cause a lacerated star-shaped wound with edematous margins. The wound causes a burning pain that can spread to the whole limb and bleeds abundantly. Above all, during the summer, the Australian coasts are populated by a small octopus *(Hapalochlaena maculosa,* also known as the "blue-ringed octopus" because it has two blue rings on the yellowish-brown background of the body), whose bite may be fatal because of muscle and respiratory paralysis. A bite from the more toxic tropical and subtropical Conidae (shells: *Conus aulicus, C. geographus, C. gloria maris)* can induce intense burning and pain, ischemia and cyanosis, and even death after coma and cardiac arrest. For preventive purposes, gloves must be worn and the shells should be picked up only by their wide, posterior extremity and dropped immediately if the animal extends its rod-like shaft.

LESIONS FROM ARTHROPODS

Unlike poisonous land arthropods, marine arthropods do not contain toxins. The harmful effects of crustaceans (crabs, prawns, lobster, limpets) are thus purely mechanical (lacerated wounds), and caused by the action of the claws of these large animals. Dermatitis of the hands has been reported in lobster fishermen.

This is a pruriginous eruption complicated by hyperkeratosis and ragade-like fissures. The pathogenic mechanism may occur at various stages including: trauma during manoeuvres while cleaning the lobster, contact with seawater, and the sensitizing action of some seasonal algae.

DERMATITIS FROM SPONGES

Sponges (Poriphera), stationary animals attached to the seabed or riverbed, have always been known not to be completely innocuous. In fact, various toxins have been isolated. Sponge fishing is carried out in the Mediterranean, Florida, Cuba, and the Bahamas and hence are the areas where dermatoses from sponges can be observed. When the sponge is detached or its branches are broken off, the fisherman feels a burning, pricking sensation. In a few hours, pain, edema, rigidity of the hands, erythema, and blisters develop. The dermatitis resolves within about 2 days. Sometimes, a multiforme erythematous eruption may also appear. Some of the sponges colonizing the Red Sea *(Latruncula magnifica* or "red sponge"), the coasts of Florida *(Tedania ignis* or "fire sponge," *Fibula nolitangere* or "touch me-not-sponge," *Microciona prolifera),* and Australia *(Tedania anhelans)* are particularly toxic.

Other sponges can induce traumatic dermatitis because of contact with the skeletal spikes made of silicone dioxide or calcium carbonate. Gloves must be worn when handling live sponges.

DERMATITIS FROM ALGAE AND BRYOZOANS

Dermatitis from algae

About 30,000 species of algae have been identified in salt and fresh waters. Those producing biotoxins belong to the classes: Cyanophyceae (among the Prokaryotes) and Dinophyceae (among the Eukaryotes).

Lyngbya majuscola, a cyanophycea seaweed, causes dermatitis epidemics ("bather's itch") among Hawaiians on the Island of Oahu and in Australia in the northern area of Moreton Bay (Queensland). In this last locality it seems that no less than 34% of the inhabitants have reported symptoms that could be correlated with exposure to the alga. The toxins mainly incriminated are lyngbyatoxin A and debromoaplisiatoxin. A few minutes after swimming, intense itching and burning develop, followed by bullous lesions that leave painful erosions, especially at the level of the genitals and the anal and perianal regions. The eruption involves all zones covered by the swimming costume, and must be differentiated from "bather's eruption." Contact allergy to *Sargassum muticum,* a brown alga in European seas that proliferates massively from March to October, has been reported.

Prothothecosis

Skin prototothecosis is an exceptional opportunistic infection by *Prototheca,* an achlorotic mutant of the green seaweed *Chlorella.* The affliction is mainly linked to the species *P. wickerhamii.* More than 80 cases of prototothecosis have been reported worldwide, but the infection is particularly common in tropical areas and the southeastern United States.

The natural habitat of *Prototheca* is the mucilage of trees and waste waters but it can also be found in cats, dogs, seawater, lakes, and ponds. Protothecosis affects the cutaneous and subcutaneous layers. The incubation time is unknown, but is probably some weeks or months. Clinically, protothecosis may manifest in three forms: (1) cutaneous lesions; (2) olecranon bursitis, which occurs in 25% of cases; and (3) systemic protothecosis. A local or systemic immunosuppressive factor is found in half of the cases. A few cases of peritonitis due to *P. wickerhamii* in peritoneal dialysis have been reported.

There is no specific skin picture. Most cases manifest with papulous or eczematous lesions at the entry site, which is generally the face or limbs. The lesions have a slow evolution, with a centrifugal extension. Other possible lesions are blisters, cellulitis, verrucous nodules, pustules, plaques, and ulceration.

Diagnosis is not easy, and is based on the search for the microorganism in the tissues, confirmed in culture (Sabouraud dextrose agar). Histological examination shows numerous organisms among the collagen fibers, adnexa, and epidermis; in sections stained with hematoxylin-eosin (H&E) they appear intensely basophilic with a clear halo.

Treatment is also quite difficult, especially in immunocompromised patients, who are more susceptible. Rarely, the infection can resolve spontaneously. Localized lesions should be surgically excised. In some cases oral ketoconazole, itraconazole, intravenous amphotericin B, or a combination of amikacin and tetracycline have given good results.

Dermatitis from Bryozoans

Bryozoans ("sea moss") are invertebrate animals that for a long time were mistakenly identified as algae and corals because their colonies, attached to the seabed, assemble to form either coral-like masses encrusting various substrates or free masses appearing as fine threads forming a branching shape resembling algae. Those responsible for contact dermatitis are mainly *Alcyonidium gelatinosum, Alcyonidium hirsutum, Alcyonidium topsenti,* and *Electra pilosa*. *A. gelatinosum* is widespread in the northern hemisphere and, in particular, in the Atlantic Ocean, Baltic Sea, North Sea, Arctic Ocean, and the English Channel. Dermatitis due to Bryozoans is quite disabling in fishermen. It was first reported in the North Sea (named "Dogger Bank itch" after the Dogger Bank in the North Sea). It starts with an allergic mechanism and recurs each summer. The distribution of the eczema might well be due to an additional photoallergic reaction. Fishermen come in contact with "sea moss" when they pull the nets on board, filled not only with fish but also other marine organisms. The dermatitis presents with dry lesions or acute exudative manifestations. The hands and forearms are first affected by direct contact, and then the face and neck by airborne contact through drops of water containing the allergenic matter. The dermatitis can also become generalized. In the case of *A. gelatinosum* the allergen is 2-hydroxy-ethyldimethylsulfoxone. Prick tests are made with fragments of freshly collected live Bryozoans, sea water containing the allergen, and aqueous and acetone extracts of "sea moss."

DERMATOSES FROM AQUATIC WORMS

These organisms are classified in the *phyla* of the Platyhelminths, Nemertines, Nematodes, and Anellids. Some salt and fresh water species contain biotoxins.

Dermatitis from cercariae

Dermatitis from cercariae ("swimmer's itch" or schistosomial dermatitis) is due to skin penetration by cercariae of the Schistosomatidae family (Platyhelminths). The skin picture of dermatitis caused by nonhuman schistosomes is different from that of visceral and skin schistosomiasis, or bilharziosis, caused by human schistosomia.

It is most often caused by *Trichobilharzia ocellata, Trichobilharzia stagnicolae, Gigantobilharzia huronensis,* and *Schistosomatium douthitti*. The intermediate hosts, that is, mollusks, belong to the species Lymnaea, Physa, Planorbis, and Stagnicola. Dermatitis from cercariae is common everywhere, and apart from swimmers, it can affect subjects working with fresh irrigation waters, farmhands, and rice pickers. The probability of developing swimmer's itch increases with the days of water use and at locations with onshore winds. Similarly, the severity of episodes increases with the time spent in the water and at the same locations. Three different pictures have been identified, according to the definitive host involved. Dermatitis from fresh water cercariae, for which the definitive host is a bird, has also been reported in swimmers in rapids and, in Italy, in female rice pickers in the Padania Plain. Nowadays, technological changes in rice growing have made this form an exceptional observation.

Dermatitis from sea water cercariae has a sea bird as the definitive host, and has been reported in the United States, Australia, and Hawaii. In workers in oriental rice fields (India, Malaysia, China) and in East Africa, dermatitis from fresh water cercariae has been observed. The definitive hosts for these cercarial are buffalos, sheep, and goats. The clinical manifestations develop because of a hypersensitivity phenomenon in allergic subjects and involve the epidermis because cercariae seem to be unable to cross the papillary dermis. Initial itching is followed by an urticarial eruption that resolves in about half an hour, leaving maculae; after several hours these transform into very pruriginous papules. The dermatitis resolves in 1 to 2 weeks but may be complicated by abrasions due to scratching and secondary infection featuring the formation of pustules.

Individual protection is essential as a preventive measure (wearing protective clothing and washing carefully), as well as environmental clean-up (molluscicides). Dermatitis from cercariae must be differentiated from "bather's itch" and dermatitis from algae (Table 12.5).

Onchocercosis

Onchocercosis, or onchocerciasis, is an infection by *Onchocerca volvulus,* a thread-like nematode that parasitizes only humans and the gorilla. The adult worms live in the dermis and subcutaneous tissues. Some are free while others gather in masses surrounded by a fibrous capsule (onchocercomas). The disease is transmitted by the females of the diptera of the *Simulium* genus (black fly) that deposit eggs on plants and rocks washed by rapid

Table 12.5: Differential Diagnosis among Dermatitis from Cercariae (DC), Bather's Eruption (BE), and Dermatitis from Algae (DA)

	DC	BE	DA
Localization	Ubiquitous	Atlantic Coast	Hawaii
Etiology	Cercariae	Larvae of cnidari	Algae
Type of water	Especially fresh	Salt	Fresh and salt
Skin sites	Exposed	Covered-exposed	Covered

running waters (torrents, rivers, waterfalls). Mobile larvae hatch from the eggs and live in running waters, growing into adult insects. Simulids become infected by stinging a parasitized individual, and then transmit the larvae to another host, again by stinging.

Onchocercosis is present in Sub-Saharan Africa (Senegal, Congo), Saudi Arabia, Yemen, and Central and South America (Mexico, Guatemala, Venezuela, Colombia, and Brazil).

The organs affected are the skin, lymphatic apparatus, and the eyes. The skin manifestations start with intense, diffuse itching that can persist for a long time, caused by migration of the microfilaria and lysis of adult worms. Males and juvenile worms migrate through the host tissue, thanks to the production of matrix-degrading metallo- and serine proteinases in excretory-secretory worm products; the enzymes may be essential for migration of the mobile stages. After incubation for 3 to 36 months, an acute, pruriginous erythemato-papulous exanthema appears (with elements measuring 1–3 mm in diameter) in various sites: the trunk and lower limbs in the African form, lower limbs in the Saudi Arabia and Yemen forms, and the head and chest in the American form. This is followed by a chronic phase of diffuse lichenification, with a possible hypertrophic and verrucous appearance. In a later phase, onchodermatitis presents with hypotrophy or atrophy and hypoachromic lesions, leading to the typical "leopard-skin" picture. The late onset skin form manifests with onchocercomas, nodular single or multiple lesions generally measuring 2 to 5 cm, mobile against the underlying planes, but no evolution to ulceration and suppuration. Involvement of the eye (conjunctivitis, irreversible keratitis, uveitis, iridocyclitis, chorioretinitis, blindness) is observed in cases where the head is affected or in long-standing infections (10–15 years).

Widespread lymphadenopathy is possible. Laboratory tests show eosinophilia, increased total IgE and ESR. Histopathology reveals microfilaria extended or twisted inside the papillary and superficial dermis among the collagen fibers. Microfilaria can also be found in the epidermis and above all in onchocercomas, where adult worms are also visible. Among the immunological tests, it is important to search for direct antibodies against the specific antigen OV-16; these antibodies are present in the circulation even before there is any evidence of microfilaria in the dermis.

The etiological treatment of choice is based on a combination of ivermectin and albendazole. Onchocercomas can be surgically removed.

Reactions to leeches

Leeches are segmented fresh water worms of the Hirudinea class and Anellida *phylum*. These slender invertebrates, 5 to 7 cm long, attach themselves to the skin and suck blood until they are engorged, doubling their volume and then fall off. Their saliva has local anticoagulant and fibrinolytic and anesthetic properties so the victim bleeds abundantly but feels no pain. They live in ponds and rivers and feed off the blood of vertebrates, especially mammals. Leeches can also live in the sea and earth (in the tropical rainforests). Man can be attacked in summer months when entering infested waters.

With its bite the leech injects an anticoagulant, hirudin, as well as other unknown antigenic substances. In nonsensitized subjects the wound bleeds and heals slowly. In allergic subjects urticarious, bullous, and necrotic reactions, and sometimes even anaphylaxis can develop.

Dermatitis from Polychaetes

The Polychaetes class of the Anellida *phylum* includes some species that are widespread in the seas, such as *Hermodice caruncu-lata* (the "dogworm" of dark, rocky depths), which is ubiquitous in the Mediterranean, and *Aphrodite aculeata* (the "sea mouse" of sandy and muddy sea bottoms). These worms have bristles on their surface, which provoke an intensely itchy, painful erythemato-edematous reaction if they penetrate the skin. If a joint is affected, there may be painful swelling and functional limitation. Unless they are removed (with a sticking plaster) the spines can give rise to a purulent, granulomatous swelling. The mechanical effect of the bristles ("bristle worm dermatitis") can be associated with a toxic reaction to an as yet unidentified biotoxin with cardiorespiratory effects.

Dermatitis from contact with bait

Fishermen using rods can develop a peculiar contact dermatitis, albeit rarely. This affects the finger pads, perionychium, and nails of the left hand and manifests with desquamation, ragades, and onycholysis (Fig. 12.16). This painful dermatitis is provoked by a sea worm used as bait. It develops 10 to 24 hours after contact, and resolves with suspension of the use of the bait.

This dermatitis, also known as "escavenite," has been described in Italy, France, and Spain and has been attributed to some anellida, namely, *Nereis diversicolor* (Fig. 12.17) and *Lumbrinereis impatients*. When the bait is fixed on the hook, the coelomic fluid of the anellid impregnates the fisherman's fingers causing the clinical picture, which can be defined as a protein contact dermatitis.

Dermatitis from Nematodes

Larva migrans cutanea

This dermatosis, also known as "creeping eruption," is caused by Nematode larvae, including the species *Ancylostoma brasiliense*, *Ancylostoma caninum* and *Uncinaria stenocephala*, the natural parasites of dogs and cats. The affliction is frequently observed in tropical and subtropical areas. In Europe and in temperate zones cases due to local contact are less frequently observed. Man is an occasional host in the parasite's life cycle. The larva

with topical thiabendazole suspension at 10% in eucerine or 2% in dimethyl sulfoxide (DMSO). In extensive forms the same drug can be administered orally at doses of 20 to 50 mg/kg/day for 7 to 10 days. Some valid alternatives are albendazole (400 mg/day for 3 to 7 days) and ivermectin (0.2 mg/kg in a single oral administration).

DERMATITIS FROM FISH

There are 250 species of venomous fish, equipped with glandular structures or apparatus that can secrete toxic substances. These serve to paralyze prey and can be inoculated by biting or stinging. Humans can be accidental victims of these animals both in the water, generally due to a defensive reaction by the animal, and outside the water, due to clumsy handling.

Venomous fish belong to two classes, the Chondrichthyes (fish with a cartilaginous skeleton) and Osteichthyes (fish with a bony skeleton) (Table 12.6).

The Chondrichthyes are known as rays. They have a flat rhomboid or trigonal shape and a long tail with one or more spines on the dorsal surface. They vary from a few centimeters to several meters in length. Rays generally live in sandy or muddy waters, half-hidden under a thin layer of sand. The venomous apparatus is in the caudal spine, a caduceus formation situated in the proximal part of the tail. Glandular and ductal structures are present inside the spine, which can secrete and inoculate toxic substances.

Accidents normally occur when the subject inadvertently steps on the body of the ray or falls in the water onto the animal. Pressure induces it to arch its tail and violently project the spine

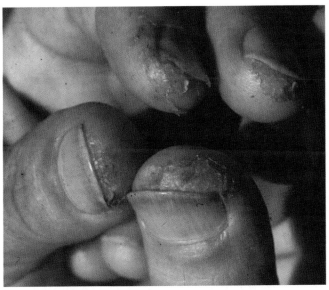

Figure 12.16. Protein contact dermatitis to bait.

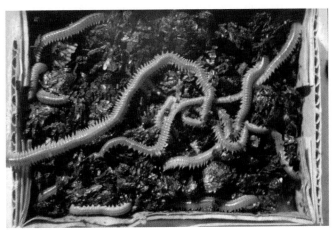

Figure 12.17. *Nereis diversicolor*.

is unable to pass through the dermis, probably lacking the necessary enzymes, and migrates within the epidermis or between the epidermis and the dermis. This migration lasts a limited time and the larva generally dies within one month. Its progress varies from a few millimeters to a few centimeters per day, except for "*larva currens*" (*Strongyloides stercoralis*) that moves 10 cm a day. The sites most often affected are the feet, hands, and buttocks, which are the body parts most likely to come into contact with earth contaminated by dog and cat feces. The incubation time varies and can even be a few months. In general, 24 to 48 hours after the time of larval penetration, an erythematous-papulous lesion forms at the site of entry, and one or more snaky tunneling formations extend out of it. The linear lesion is about 2 to 4 mm wide, bright red, and slightly raised above the skin plane. The affliction resolves spontaneously. Atypical clinical presentations, with vesiculo-bullous or frankly bullous lesions, are possible as well. Histologic isolation of the larva is very difficult because the larva generally lies beyond the visible lesion. Cryotherapy with liquid nitrogen or carbon snow, applied beyond the margins of the visible migration line, is generally efficacious in moderately severe disease. Good results are obtained

Table 12.6: Fish that Induce Toxic Reactions

1. Class:		Chondrichthyes
Order:		Rays (stingrays or trigoni)
Family:		Dasyatidae
Species:		*Dasyatis pastinaca*
		Dasyatis violacea
		Dasyatis centroura
2. Class:		Osteichthyes
A. Family:		Trachinidae (weeverfish)
Species:		*Trachinus araneus*
		Trachinus draco
		Trachinus vipera
		Trachinus radiatus
B. Family:		Scorpaenidae (scorpionfish)
Species:		*Scorpaena porcus*
		Scorpaena scrofa
		Scorpaena ustulata
		Scorpaena dactyloptera
C. Family:		Muraenidae (moray eels)
Species:		*Muraena helena*

against the victim, most often at the level of the foot or leg. The poison, consisting of substances with a protein structure (serotonin, 5-nucleotidase, phosphodiesterase), acts on the cardiovascular, respiratory, and neurological systems. The wound caused by the spine of a stingray is wide and lacerated.

Venomous Osteichthyes belong to the Trachinidae family (weeverfish) and Scorpoenidae family (scorpionfish). The toxicity of Muraedinae (moray eels) is still under debate.

Weeverfish are relatively small fish measuring 10 to 50 cm present along the coasts of the Mediterranean and the Northeast Atlantic (European coasts). All species have spines connected to cells that secrete toxic substances. Weeverfish live in shallow waters half-hidden under the sand. Accidents are due to treading on the animal or careless handling.

Scorpionfish are the most actively toxic fish. These brightly colored fish live near the bottom of the sea (they prefer a rocky seabed) and have a plump body, large fins, and venomous spines. Contact with these fish generally occurs during deep-sea fishing and scuba diving.

The clinical symptoms of stings from a venomous fish are typical (Fig. 12.18). There is constant, immediate, and extremely violent pain. This is even worse in the case of a sting from a weeverfish. The pain radiates all along the limb within 30 minutes and persists for 12 to 48 hours. In all cases it is so severe that the victim suffers malaise, functional impotence of the limb, and lipothymia. The appearance of the wound is falsely reassuring. Stings from a stingray have lacerated edges whereas those from a weeverfish are pointed. The sting is followed by a violent inflammatory reaction with ischemic necrosis, pallor, cyanosis, and blood-serum bullous lesions. Then there is onset of a hard, painful edema with lymphangitis and satellite lymphadenitis. The tearing pain can bring on anguish, tachycardia, dyspnea, and hypotension, and even syncope and death. Neurological signs include vertigo, contracture and muscle spasms, convulsions, and delirium. In the Mediterranean the outcome is invariably good. Immediate treatment must be administered at the site of the event (Table 12.7).

Contact with moray eels generally occurs when capturing the animal and pulling it on board. There is strong, burning local pain after a bite from a moray eel, which may be accompanied by dyspnea and shock.

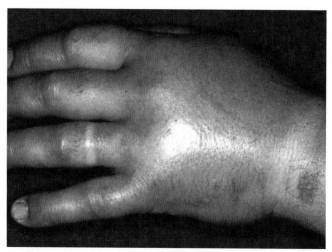

Figure 12.18. Weeverfish lesion with intense edema of the arm.

Table 12.7: Principles of Treatment for Reactions to Fish

Wash the area with sea water.

Open the wound and remove fish spine residues.

Use a hemostatic band if a limb is affected.

Immerse the limb in water as hot (45°C) as can be tolerated for 30–90 minutes.

If the face or trunk is involved, apply warm compresses or rinse the wound with hot water. Heat inactivates the heat-sensitive component of the toxins.

Systemic treatment in an intensive care unit.

Fish with an electrical defense mechanism

The Torpenidae family includes fish with kidney-shaped electrical organs arranged on each side of the back. These organs can produce electric shocks up to 200 volts. In an emergency, the torpedo ray uses higher voltage and amperage. Repeated shocks gradually lose their power. Contact is again during capture or handling the animal, and may be direct or mediated by the metal harpoon. In general, the shock induces only a slight stupor.

DERMATOSIS DUE TO AQUATIC BACTERIA

Infection by *Mycobacterium marinum*

Mycobacterium marinum is a slow-growing (10–28 days) photochromogenic bacterium belonging to group I of Runyon's classification. It grows best at a temperature of 25°C to 32°C. *M. marinum* is present in temperate salt and fresh water, and causes disease in fish and humans. In the latter case the infection usually manifests as "swimming pool granuloma" and "aquarium granuloma."

In swimming pools, the bacillus is most likely to be found at the water entry tubes and on the walls. It can be destroyed by high concentrations of chlorine (10 mg/L). The form of granuloma incurred is generally localized to the elbows and knees.

Aquarium granulomas can be occupational (aquarium sales staff or workers) or nonoccupational (when cleaning an aquarium in the home). The sites affected are the hands and forearms. There is usually only one lesion initially. It presents as a reddish or reddish-blue nodule with a soft consistency and a diameter of up to 5 to 6 cm (Fig. 12.19). This initial lesion may undergo ulceration or colliquation, and turn into an open wound. It can also present a verrucous surface. There are rarely disseminated lesions except in immunosuppressed subjects. Sporotrichoid forms are common, featuring various nodules along lymphatic drainage lines (Fig. 12.20). There may be mild involvement of the regional lymph nodes. The infection may resolve spontaneously after a few months but can persist for many years.

The incubation time is 2 to 3 weeks. *M. marinum*, antigenically correlates with *M. tuberculosis* and does not confer immunity, so re-infection is possible. A firm diagnosis is based on culture of the mycobacterium from biopsy or aspirate samples in Löwenstein–Jensen culture medium. The culture is positive in

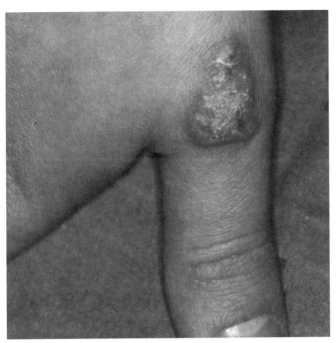

Figure 12.19. Fish tank granuloma.

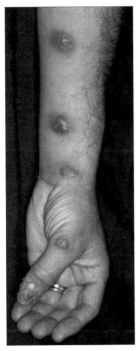

Figure 12.20. Sporotrichoid
fish tank granuloma.

70% to 80% of cases. Intradermal tests with PPD of *M. marinum* yield positive results.

Searches for the bacillus in samples taken from the lesions or biopsy samples stained with the Ziehl–Neelsen method are nearly always negative. The bacillus can sometimes be isolated in dead fish in the aquarium, or in the filter. Histopathological analyses show an aspecific inflammatory infiltrate in the first months, while older lesions are usually characterized by a granulomatous structure.

A strong clinical suggestion of *M. marinum* infection warrants initial empirical treatment to prevent progression to a deep-seated infection. The treatment should preferably be preceded by an antibiogram. The most efficacious drugs are minocycline, tetracycline, rifampicin, isoniazid, sulfamethoxazole, and clarithromycin. Polytherapy is sometimes necessary.

In recent years, we have observed 11 cases of granulomas from aquariums, all of a professional nature. 6 patients presented with a single lesion and 5 nodular lesions with a sporotrichoid arrangement. 3 of these had an ulcerative evolution. All the cases were caused by trauma of the hands during maintenance of an aquarium. In all cases, specific PPD was positive, while culture gave positive results in only nine cases. Apart from one case that was successfully treated with rifampicin and isoniazid and another with clarithromycin, all other cases resolved with minocycline therapy.

Erysipeloid

Also known as Baker-Rosenbach's erysipeloid, this is an acute infection that rarely becomes chronic. It is induced by *Erysipelothrix rhusiopathiae*, a gram-positive nonsporogenous, nonmobile bacterium that usually has elongated filaments. Infection is frequent in pigs, horses, sheep, turkeys, and other animals as well as in freshwater and seawater fish. For this reason, it is most frequently observed in fishermen and butchers. The complaint has also been reported in housewives who suffered a puncture wound from fish gills or chicken bones.

The onset of erysipeloid is generally observed in the later summer months, when infection of animals is most common. After about 3 days from contagion, a dark erythematous skin patch develops at the site of the inoculation, with an irregular centrifugal extension and distinct, raised polycyclic margins. The sites most often involved are the hands and forearms. In 10% of cases, fever develops. Pain and itching may also be present. The skin patch reaches a maximum diameter of 10 cm and spontaneously resolves within 2 to 3 weeks. Rarely, generalized skin pictures have been described, as well as systemic forms with endocarditis. The disease leaves no immunity, so re-infection is possible. The bacterium responsible can be cultured after biopsy in the margin of the skin lesion, or in the blood in systemic forms. One week's treatment with penicillin and tetracycline should cure the disease.

PITFALLS AND MYTHS

Various skin eruptions caused by marine biotic agents can develop, each with a specific clinical–morphological picture. Such pictures may also mimic other forms of dermatosis. Generally, from the clinical–differential diagnosis standpoint, the most important element is the clinical history. In fact, in the great majority of cases the history will reveal a close contact with biotic agents while bathing in a sea, river, or lake. Another important point is the time of onset of the complaint, especially if it is during or immediately after a visit to an exotic area. Again, with regards to clinical history, any manipulation of a fish tank is an important point. Details on working activities are also useful, especially involving cases of sailors, fishermen, scuba divers, or patients pursuing amateur aquatic activities and hobbies, such as fishing.

Aquagenic complaints caused by biotic agents have a polymorphic morphology. Lesions can be strictly localized or widespread all over the skin. In most cases, there are subjective symptoms, like itching, burning pain, and sometimes systemic signs with involvement of internal organs. In fact, the toxins of aquatic agents can wreak havoc on several organ systems simultaneously. A list of the most common skin complaints from which a differential diagnosis from aquagenic dermatitis caused by biotic agents can be made is shown in Table 12.8.

Forms of urticarial contact dermatitis are most often induced by Coelenterates. In localized forms, which are often linked to contact with jellyfish, differential diagnoses with urticaria is relatively easy. However, it is much more difficult in diffuse forms, which are more frequently induced by sea anemones. In the latter case, urticaria from various causes and cold urticaria (that could be secondary to swimming in cold waters) both need to be excluded. However, it must be borne in mind that in common urticaria the wheals last for a few hours ("short-lived" lesions) whereas dermatitis manifestations caused by Coelenterates are not only extremely figured but also last for several hours or even days.

In cases involving the face (lips and eyelids) and hands, Coelenterates can induce pictures that mimic angioedema. Apart from the clinical history, evidence that the dermatitis is due to Coelenterates includes a bright red erythema, the simultaneous presence of blistering-bullous lesions, and the longer persistence of the symptoms. Finally, unlike urticaria or angioedema, dermatitis caused by Coelenterates can leave the skin atrophic or scarred.

Erysipeloid, a relatively rare disease, and occupational chronic traumatic scleredema must be differentiated from other acute or chronic forms of lymphedema, such as recurrent erysipelas, angioedema, deep thrombophlebitis, and chilblains. All these afflictions are accompanied by a specific set of subjective and objective symptoms and signs. In particular, erysipelas is accompanied by septic fever with an acute onset, intense pain, and satellite adenopathy. Fishermens' scleredema, on the other hand, features a very slow evolution over time and is irreversible.

The erythematous-edematous-vesicular or erythematous-pustular pictures provoked by contact with Coelenterates sometimes pose problems of differential diagnosis with contact dermatitis and contagious impetigo, respectively. Contact dermatitis is linked to chemical causes that are present in the living or working environment. It is strictly related to contact of the skin area involved with the harmful substance, and has a chronic, recurrent course. Impetigo shows pustulous or more often bullous lesions and is generally observed in the pediatric age group and affects particular sites (i.e. the periorifices and hands). It may be accompanied by satellite adenopathy and fever. In doubtful cases, microbiological examination of the pus will confirm or exclude the presence of cocci.

Dermatitis caused by contact with Coelenterates can sometimes present with erythemato-bullous lesions. Clearly, in these cases a differential diagnosis is with physical (burns) or chemical (topical drugs, photosensitizing plants) causes. The more figured nature of the clinical manifestation will make the diagnosis of dermatitis induced by Coelenterates more likely.

Isolated granuloma from *M. marinum* clinically mimics the papulo-verrucous lesions induced by *M. tuberculosis* or *M. bovis* (verrucous tuberculosis). Amateur or professional manipulation of fish tanks will favor a diagnosis of *M. marinum* whereas granuloma due to *M. bovis* is observed in workers on farms, in those milking cows, and in veterinary surgeons. An intradermal test with mycobacteria may be positive in both diseases. Culture of tissue biopsies or aspirate from the lesions will dispel any doubt. In fact, *M. marinum* is photochromogenic, and grows in 3 to 4 weeks in Löwenstein–Jensen medium. Moreover, it develops at a temperature of 31°C to 32°C rather than at 37°C. Histopathologic examination is also diagnostic. Unlike the constant, classic tubercular picture of verrucous tuberculosis, in cases of fish tank granuloma, there is no evidence of caseous necrosis, giant cells are rarely present, and the infiltrate is often aspecific.

In the more common sporotrichoid variant, fish tank granuloma must be differentiated from sporotrichosis. Both complaints are characterized by nodulous-granulomatous lesions with a possible ulcerative evolution, arranged as "a rosary" along a lymph tract. Culture reveals *Sporothrix schenckii* in the case of sporotrichosis, in which the intradermal reaction to the mycobacterium will be negative. The site for fish tank granuloma is the upper limbs whereas sporotrichosis is more commonly localized on the lower limbs. "*Ex adiuvantibus*" therapeutic criterion is also very useful.

Granulomas caused by sea urchins need to be differentiated from granulomas caused by other foreign bodies. The clinical history reveals occupational or amateur fishing for sea urchins. Sea urchin granulomas are almost always localized on the hands, and sometimes the knees or elbows.

There are two important points to be remembered. Firstly, although many aquagenic complaints can resolve spontaneously, it is essential not to underestimate them. Even if they are of an apparently modest entity, they can be accompanied by serious systemic symptoms, including anaphylactic and life-threatening reactions. In all cases immediate intervention with appropriate treatment is necessary, especially bearing in mind that most such "accidents" with aquatic agents happen far away from the nearest hospital facility. First aid locally followed by admission to a hospital as soon as possible is vital in many cases.

From the medical standpoint, the complex problems arising due to marine organism toxins have yet to be entirely elucidated. Even the clinical manifestations are often unknown to the public and sometimes even the clinician, especially in "imported" forms.

Table 12.8: Skin Diseases That Mimic Aquagenic Dermatitis Induced by Biotic Agents

Urticaria

Angioedema

Erysipelas

Contact dermatitis

Contagious impetigo

Localized bullous dermatitis

Verrucous tuberculosis

Granulomas caused by foreign bodies

Sporotrichosis

In conclusion, in the presence of strange, uncommon, and unfamiliar clinical pictures with skin eruptions, the possibility of an etiology involving contact with marine biotic agents should always be entertained.

SUGGESTED READINGS

Anderluh G, Macek P. *Cytolytic peptide and protein toxins from sea anemones* (Anthozoa: Actiniaria). *Toxicon* 2002;40:111–124.

Angelini G, Bonamonte D. *Aquatic dermatology*. Berlin: Springer-Verlag, 2002.

Angelini G, Bonamonte D. Dermatoses acquatiques Méditerranéennes. *Nouv Dermatol* 1997;16:280–286.

Angelini G, Meneghini CL, Vena GA. Secrétan's syndrome: an artefact edema of the hand. *Contact Dermatitis* 1982;8:345–346.

Angelini G, Vena GA, Meneghini CL. Occupational traumatic lymphedema of the hands. *Dermatol Clinics* 1990;8:205–208.

Angelini G, Vena GA. *Dermatologia acquatica*. Milano: Lepetit, 1991.

Angelini G, Vena GA. *Dermatologia professionale e ambientale*. Vol. 1. ISED, Brescia, 202–246, 1997.

Angelini G. Occupational aquatic dermatology. In: Kanerva L, Elaner P, Wahlberg JE et al. ed. *Handbook of Occupational Dermatology*. Berlin: Springer, 234–247, 2000.

Antensteiner G. Dangerous marine animals. *Wien Med Wochenschr* 1999;151:104–110.

Barnett JH, Estes SA, Wirman JA et al. Erysipeloid. *J Am Acad Dermatol* 1983;9:116–123.

Boulware DR. A randomized, controlled field trial for the prevention of jellyfish stings with a topical sting inhibitor. *J Travel Med* 2006;13:166–171.

Brown TP. Diagnosis and management of injuries from dangerous marine life. *Med Gen Med* 2005;28:5.

Burnett JW, Calton GJ, Burnett HW. Jellyfish envenomation syndromes. *J Am Acad Dermatol* 1986;14:100–106.

Burnett JW, Calton GJ, Morgan RJ. Venomous Coelenterates. *Cutis* 1987;39:191–192.

Carme B. Filariasis. *Rev Prat* 2007;57:157–165.

Chao SC, Hsu MM, Lee JY. Cutaneous protothecosis: report of five cases. *Br J Dermatol* 2002;146:688–693.

De La Torre C, Toribio J. Sea-urchin granuloma: histologic profile. A pathologic study of 50 biopsies. *J Cutan Pathos* 2001;28:223–228.

De La Torre C, Vega A, Carracedo A et al. Identification of *Mycobacterium marinum* in sea-urchin granulomas. *Br J Dermatol* 2001; 145.114–116.

Fisher AA. *Atlas of Aquatic Dermatology*. Grune and Stratton, New York, 1978.

Fisher AA. Toxic and allergic cutaneous reactions to jellyfish with special reference to delayed reactions. *Cutis* 1987;40:303–305.

Giretti F, Cariello L (eds). *Gli animali marini velenosi e le loro tossine*. Padova: Piccin, 1984, 165.

Isbister GK, Hooper JN. Clinical effects of stings by sponges of the genus tedania and review of sponge stings worldwide. *Toxicon* 2005;46:782–785.

Jeanmougin M, Janier M, Prigent F. Eczéma de contact avec photosensibilité à *Alcyonidium gelatinosum*. *Ann Dermatol Venereol* 1983;110:725–726.

Jeanmougin M, Lemarchand-Vénencie, Hoang XD. Eczema professionnel avec photosensibilité par contact de Bryozoaires. *Ann Dermatol Venereol* 1987;114:353–357.

Johnson RP, Xia Y, Cho S et al. *Mycobacterium marinum* infection: a case report and review of the literature. *Cutis* 2007;79:33–36.

Kokelj F. Patologia da meduse. In: Veraldi S. Caputo R eds. *Dermatologia di importazione*. Milano: Poletto Ed., 286–296, 2000.

Leimann BC, Monteiro PC, Lazera M et al. Protothecosis. *Med Mycol* 2004;42:95–106.

Lim YL, Kumarasinghe SPW. Cutaneous injuries from marine animals. *Singapore Med J* 2007;48:e25–e28.

Mansson T, Randle HW, Maudojana RM et al. Recurrent cutaneous jellyfish eruptions without envenomation. *Acta Dermatovener* 1985;65:72–5.

Nagata K, Hide M, Tanaka T et al. Anaphylactic shock caused by exposure to sea anemones. *Allergol Int* 2006;55:181–184.

Osborne NJ, Shaw GR, Webb PM. Health effects of recreational exposure to Moreton Bay, Australia waters during a *Lyngbya majuscola* bloom. *Environ Int* 2007;33:309–314.

Osborne NJ, Webb PM, Shaw GR. The toxins of *Lyngbya majuscola* and their human and ecological health effects. *Environ Int* 2001;27:381–392.

Perez Melon C, Camba M, Tinajas A et al. *Prototheca wickerhamii* peritonitis in patients on peritoneal dialysis. *Nefrologia* 2007;27:81–82.

Portier P, Richet C. Sur les effects physiologiques du poison des filaments pécheurs et des tentacules des Coelentérés (hypnotoxine). *CR Acad Sci* (Paris) 1902;134:247.

Reed KM, Bronstein BR, Baden HP. Delayed and persistent cutaneous reactionsto Coelenterates. *J Am Acad Dermatol* 1984;10:462–466.

Romagnera C, Grimalt F, Vilaplana J, et al. Protein contact dermatitis. *Contact Dermatitis* 1986;14:184–5.

Veraldi S, Arancio L. Giant bullous cutaneous larva migrans. *Clin Exp Dermatol* 2006;31:613–614.

Verbrugge LM, Rainey JJ, Reimink RL et al. Prospective study of swimmer's itch incidence and severity. *J Parasitol* 2004;90:697–704.

Wong DE, Meinking TL, Rosen LB, et al. Seabather's eruption. Clinical, histologic and immunologic features. *J Am Acad Dermatol* 1994; 30:399–406.

PART IV: INFECTIONS IN SELECTED PATIENT POPULATIONS

13 | SKIN INFECTIONS IN HIV PATIENTS

Joseph S. Susa and Clay J. Cockerell

Treating cutaneous infections requires that the provider be aware of the spectrum of challenges that may be faced in an immunosuppressed patient. An unusual infection or even a common infection that is recalcitrant to treatment may be a clue that can suggest a diagnosis of immunosuppression or HIV infection. In a patient who has already been diagnosed, it becomes important to realize that immunosuppression can modify the course of common diseases. Unusual presentations, resistance to traditional treatments, increased risks of a more aggressive course, disease progression, and complications are all common challenges in this population subset. Although the epidemiologic incidence of opportunistic infections has decreased with the onset of highly active antiretroviral therapy (HAART), the clinician still must be familiar with the presentation of infections that occur more frequently in immunosuppressed patients as well as the possibility of other unusual infections that need to be considered in the differential diagnosis of a cutaneous infection for HIV positive patients. Certain dormant infections, such as mycobacterial disease or varicella zoster, may flare up following the initiation of HAART in what is known as the immune reconstitution inflammatory syndrome (IRIS). The detection of opportunistic infections also provides a clue to the degree of immunosuppression since certain infections are associated with decreased CD4 levels. Several cutaneous infections can also be AIDS defining. Worldwide, and in the individual patient with advanced immunosuppression, these infections can result in significant morbidity and even death. It is the purpose of this chapter to survey the more common cutaneous infections seen in patients with HIV infection.

HISTORY

Before AIDS was formally described, a trend of increasingly unusual infections began being reported on the continent of Africa, and in 1981 in the United States, case reports involving cohorts of gay men who were developing Kaposi's sarcoma (KS) and *Pneumocystis carinii* pneumonia began coming to the attention of the medical personnel due to a disease that would eventually become known as acquired immune deficiency syndrome (AIDS). AIDS then clinically became defined by a cellular immunodeficiency and by the numerous opportunistic infections that started becoming its inevitable consequence. In 1983, the etiologic virus, later termed the human immunodeficiency virus (HIV), was isolated. During the initial years of the epidemic, the natural course of the disease included a morbidity and mortality of stunningly high rates. By 1984, there had been 7699 AIDS cases and 3665 AIDS deaths in the United States alone. KS and

other cutaneous manifestations such as bacillary angiomatosis and disseminated fungal infections were the predominant visible markers of HIV infection during this time period.

Initial treatments were only limited to the management of infections or other complications secondary to the disease. In 1987, azidothymidine (AZT) became the first approved antiretroviral drug to treat HIV by the U.S. Food and Drug Administration (FDA). Later, additional reverse transcriptase inhibitors were approved and by the mid-1990s, multidrug combination therapy had demonstrated an ability to delay disease progression and prolong life in HIV positive patients. Pharmacologic advances have continued to improve, and new classes of drugs like protease inhibitors and fusion inhibitors have also now been introduced. Several novel therapeutic approaches also continue to be tested. The combination of multiple drugs and of different classes of antiviral drugs is known as highly active antiretroviral therapy or HAART. Introduction of HAART has markedly decreased the incidence of opportunistic infections in these patients. While certain cutaneous manifestations of HIV such as bacillary angiomatosis have decreased, others, including zoster, dermatophyte infections, and recalcitrant folliculitis have actually become more frequent. With slowed disease progression and prolonged survival, recognizing the cutaneous manifestation of HIV will take on additional importance with regard to quality of life concerns and as a marker of disease progression and immunosuppression.

ACUTE EXANTHEM OF HIV INFECTION

Within days of acquiring the HIV infection and before complete seroconversion (which can up take 6 weeks), 25% to 80% of patients will have prodromal symptoms known as *acute retroviral syndrome* or *seroconversion illness*. Systemic symptoms can include lympadenopathy, fatigue, fever, headache, nausea, diarrhea, and night sweats. Cutaneous findings include a viral exanthem that is characterized by a morbilliform eruption with pink oval to round macules and papules affecting the trunk, chest, back, and extremities. Approximately 25% will also have mucosal ulcerations. The usual clinical course is resolution within 4 to 5 days without sequelae. Rarely, a more severe form of acute HIV infection characterized by pneumonitis, esophagitis, meningitis, abdominal pain, and melena can develop. These patients may demonstrate more severe cutaneous manifestations such as oral ulceration, urticaria, alopecia, desquamation of palms and soles, and even Stevens–Johnson syndrome. These patients are also more prone to secondary co-infections with candida spp. and herpes viruses. The prognosis in these patients is poorer than for those without symptoms or those having only mild symptoms. Early institution of antiretroviral therapy helps rapidly resolve symptoms of acute retroviral syndrome and preserve CD4 counts.

Herpes simplex virus

Infections with HSV types 1 and 2 can result in recurrent, painful grouped vesicles with an erythematous base localized mainly on the lips genital and perianal areas. HSV-1 is most commonly associated with oral lesions, whereas HSV-2 is most commonly associated with genital lesions. However, there is considerable overlap between the two viruses. Sometimes, ulceration takes place without well-defined vesicles ever being noted clinically. It is possible to establish the specific diagnosis by means of polymerase chain reaction (PCR), biopsies, and/or viral cultures. Culture from tissue can be positive even if a swab and Tzank preparation is negative. PCR, however, has a two- to four-fold higher sensitivity in diagnosing genital ulcer disease when compared to viral cultures. Distinction between HSV-1 and -2 can be achieved with culture and PCR techniques.

While the immune system is intact, the course of disease is similar to that found in noninfected individuals. If left untreated, these lesions may enlarge and become persistent, confluent ulcerations that show slow healing and often become secondarily infected with bacteria. In immunosuppressed patients, the lesions more commonly become persistent. With deterioration of immune status due to onset or advanced stages of AIDS, lesions of herpes simplex become clinically atypical. These atypical features can be roughly divided into three forms: chronic ulcerative herpes simplex, generalized acute mucocutaneous herpes simplex, and systemic herpes simplex. Chronic ulcerative herpes simplex exhibits recalcitrant, painful ulcerations occurring at the usual sites (perioral and perigenital regions) that enlarge, deepen, and become confluent (Fig. 13.1). Nonhealing ulcers that persist for greater than 1 month, with or without therapy are recognized as AIDS-defining lesions.

An aggressive therapeutic approach should be used with these patients, as they may be poorly responsive to the standard treatment and HSV infection increases the probability of HIV transmission and shedding. Oral acyclovir in doses of up to

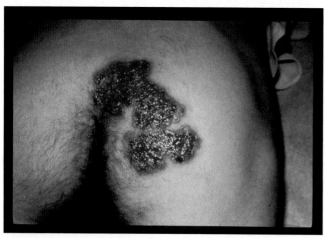

Figure 13.1. Large and confluent Herpes virus infection in an HIV-positive male.

400 mg five times a day for 10 days should be used for primary infections. Alternatively, valcyclovir given in doses of 1g twice daily may be preferential to acyclovir given its lower dosing requirements. For suppressive therapy, 800 mg of acyclovir can be given 2 to 3 times daily to prevent HSV reactivation. In severe cases, hospitalization for administration of high-dose intravenous acyclovir may be required. Foscarnet is recommended in patients in whom acyclovir resistance is suspected.

Generalized acute mucocutaneous lesions of herpes simplex can occur following a localized skin lesion. The disseminated, vesicular lesions clinically resemble those of varicella or small pox. Patients exhibit high fever and other systemic symptoms. Death can occur without obvious visceral involvement. Systemic infection of herpes simplex is an exceedingly rare sequela even in AIDS patients. It usually follows outbreaks of oral or genital herpes. The most frequently involved internal organs are lungs, liver, adrenal glands, pericardium, and brain.

Herpetic whitlow manifests as a deep-seated, painful ulcer involving the volar aspect of distal phalanges. This form of herpetic infection most frequently occurs in young children who suck their fingers and in healthcare workers who perform oral examinations or procedures on a daily basis. Periungual infection may also occur. Herpetic folliculitis is a herpes simplex–inflicted inflammation of hair follicles that most commonly occurs on the face.

Varicella-zoster virus

The incidence of herpes zoster is higher in AIDS patients than in general population. The development of recrudescent varicella-zoster virus (VZV) infection in a patient at risk for HIV infection may be a sign of the presence of HIV and should alert the clinician to screen the patient for the disease. Primary infection, known as varicella or colloquially as chickenpox, produces crops of vesicles on an erythematous base, beginning on the head and spreading cetrifugally. In children or previously unexposed adults, primary infections can be more severe, causing extracutaneous diseases such as pneumonitis, pancreatitis, and encephalitis. It may even be fatal in some cases. The CDC recommends live, attenuated VZV vaccination for HIV-infected children and in adults with early stage HIV infection. If a known exposure occurs in a VZV-naive, immunocompromised patient, immunoglobulin should be administered as a prophylactic measure within 96 hours.

After primary infection, VZV exists in a dormant state in the neural dorsal root ganglia. With reactivation, the virus progresses downward through the nerve tracts of a solitary dermatome, leading to the characteristic zosteriform distribution of painful tense vesicles in the skin. In individuals who have HIV infection, the infection may be recurrent and severe, with more than one dermatome involved, and it may run a protracted course associated with residual postherpetic neuralgia and scarring. Disseminated herpes zoster is not as common but may be more common in HIV-infected individuals. Atypical presentations of VZV include verrucous zoster, follicular zoster, and ecthymatous or crusted zoster. Chronic lesions, also known as verrucous or ecthymatous zoster, can often be a presenting sign of HIV disease.

Occurrences of VZV are common after initiation of HAART as part of the IRIS. The diagnosis of VZV is largely based on its classical clinical presentation. Swabing for direct immunofluorescence is a rapid and effective way to diagnose atypical presentations. High doses of acyclovir (up to 800 mg five times daily for 7 days) are used to treat these patients. Systemic administration may be necessary. Famciclovir given in doses of 250 mg three times daily may improve patient compliance and decrease adverse side effects, while still providing the same efficacy supplied by acyclovir.

Cytomegalovirus

Cytomegalovirus (CMV) is the most common cause of serious opportunistic viral infection in patients who have AIDS, but cutaneous involvement is rare. In the skin, CMV can have diverse manifestations including ulcerations, keratotic verrucous lesions, hyperpigmented plaques, morbilliform eruptions, and palpable purpuric papules. The perianal region, perineum, and genitalia are frequent sites of involvement (Fig. 13.2). Because the mucocutaneous lesions caused by CMV do not have specific features, tissue biopsy or immunoglobulin titers (IgG and IgM) and viral cultures, are required for definitive diagnosis. The treatment of choice for CMV infection is intravenous ganciclovir 5 mg/kg every 12 hours. Foscarnet should be used if ganciclovir resistance is suspected. In those with CD4 counts <100 mm^3, valganciclovir prophylaxis can be given in doses of 900 mg by mouth every 24 hours.

Epstein–Barr virus

The primary infection of Epstein–Barr virus (EBV) is infectious mononucleosis. After primary infection, the majority of adults harbor latent EBV within B lymphocytes. With advanced immunodeficiency, EBV reactivation occurs, leading to oral hairy leukoplakia (OHL), Burkitt's lymphoma, or EBV-associated large cell lymphoma. OHL manifests as single or multiple white plaques on the lateral margins of the tongue with a verrucous surface. These plaques are often asymptomatic (Fig. 13.3). The presence of oral leukoplakia correlates with moderate to advanced immunodeficiency and has also been correlated with progression from HIV infection to AIDS. OHL will respond to systemically administered acyclovir and valcyclovir, or topical podophyllin. However, many clinicians elect not to treat patients because the lesions are asymptomatic and because recurrence

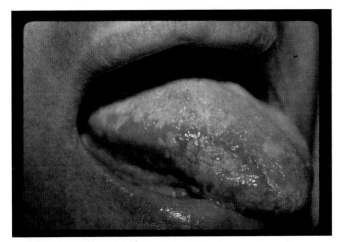

Figure 13.3. White verrucous plaques on the lateral aspect of the tongue typify oral hairy leukoplakia.

is common following discontinuation of treatment. OHL may regress with highly active antiviral therapy alone.

Poxvirus

Molluscum contagiosum (MC) is a common disease, present in 10% to 20% of AIDS patients. It is caused by *Molluscipoxvirus*, which is a member of the Poxvirus family. MC is transmitted by direct skin-to-skin contact and produces cutaneous lesions, and also more rarely mucosal lesions. In adults, it is most commonly transmitted by sexual contact. Molluscum contagiosum is characterized by dome-shaped, umbilicated, translucent, 2 to 4 mm papules that develop on any part of the body but especially on the face and genital areas. In AIDS patients, these lesions are widespread, may be larger than 1 cm, and can become confluent and disfiguring (Fig. 13.4). Most patients who have extensive molluscum contagiosum associated with HIV infection have CD4+ counts well below 250 cells/mL. The diagnosis should be confirmed by histologic examination in any case that is questionable because it may resemble more serious infections such as cutaneous pneumocystosis, histoplasmosis, *Penicillium marneffei* infection, or cryptococcosis. Treatment options include cryotherapy, electrodessication, curettage, topical application of podophyllin, tretinoin, or imiquimod cream.

Human papillomavirus

The human papillomaviruses comprise over 120 genotypes. They cause a variety of warty lesions in the skin and mucous membranes including common verrucae, epidermodysplasia verruciformis (EDV), and condyloma accuminata. This family of viruses is the cause of cervical and anal intraepithelial dysplasias, bowenoid papulosis, cervical cancer, and anogenital squamous cell carcinoma.

Common types of warts that can be observed include filiform, flat, and plantar types. In patients with HIV, warts can be widespread and can develop in unusual locations, such as on the lips, tongue, and oral mucosa. EDV consists of a widespread papular eruption of pink-red, flat, wart-like lesions distributed mostly on sun-exposed areas of the skin. These can be related to an autosomal recessive impairment of cell-mediated immunity

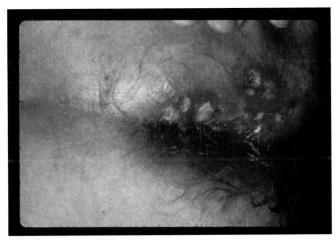

Figure 13.2. Erosions and ulcerations due to cutaneous CMV infection.

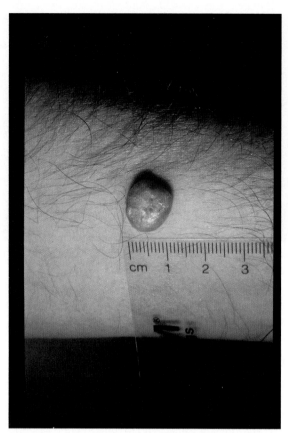

Figure 13.4. In immunosuppressed patients, lesions of molluscum contagiosum can be much larger than the typical 2 to 4 mm umbilicated papules usually seen.

to certain EDV associated HPV subtypes. EDV and common warts are often treated with cryotherapy, electrocauterization, or topically with caustic agents such as podophyllin, imiquimod, trichloroacetic acid, and 5-fluorouracil. Howevermost of these lesions are resistant to these modalities and require repeated treatments.

Condyloma accuminata are soft sessile lesions with finger-like projections. Imiquimod, podophyllotoxin solution or resin, 80% trichloroacetic acid, 5-fluorouracil injectable gel, interferon alpha, cidofovir, cryotherapy, electrocautery, thermocoagulation, laser, and excision are all treatment options.

Certain subtypes of HPV are considered to be high risk (16, 18, 31, 33, 35, 39, 45, 51 and others) and others to be low risk (6, 11, 12, 43, 44, 54, 61, 70, 72, and 81) for development of anogenital intraepithelial neoplasia and associated squamous cell carcinoma. Cervical, vulvar, and anal intraepithelial dyplasia may manifest as a flat condyloma with viral cytopathic effect but without raised warty lesions. A solution of 2% to 5% acetic acid is helpful in delineating HPV lesions (acetowhitening). Colposcopy or anoscopy may also reveal atypical vascular patterns in areas of intraepithelial dysplasia. HIV is associated with an increased incidence of high-grade dysplasia, and increases the risk of progression to invasive squamous cell carcinoma. HPV has been detected in more than 95% of cervical cancers and in more than 50% of anal cancers. Given the increased risk of HPV infection, cytologic screening for dysplasia via cervical and anal Papaniculou smears should be obtained regularly in HIV patients.

Human Herpes Virus 8

Human herpes virus 8 (HHV-8) was originally known as Kaposi's sarcoma (KS)–associated herpes virus, owing to its original discovery in KS in AIDS patients. Its discovery changed the thinking that KS was a low-grade sarcoma and introduced the concept that KS is actually a diffuse vascular hyperplasia in response to a viral infection. Early lesions appear as violaceous or sometimes even yellowish-green ecchymotic macules. In time, these can enlarge and become confluent, forming papules, plaques, nodules, and tumors. These lesions are violaceous, red, pink, tan, and eventually become brown-purple (Fig. 13.5). The morphology of these lesions defines three clinical stages as patch, plaque, or tumor. Lesions are usually unilateral at the onset of disease and progress to become bilateral over time. Oral mucosal involvement presents as violaceous plaques (Fig. 13.6). Lymphedema of the involved areas may be present and is secondary to confluent lesions involving the lymphatics vessels and lymph nodes. Extracutaneous KS is also frequently encountered in the lymph nodes, gastrointestinal tract, and lungs. Diagnosis is generally based on the finding of violaceous skin lesions in the appropriate clinical setting in conjunction with concordant histological findings. HHV-8 is also associated with other malignancies including primary

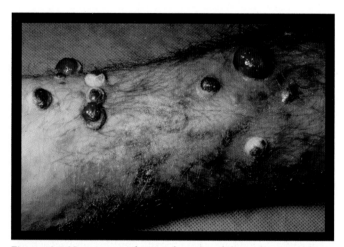

Figure 13.5. Numerous violaceous-brown nodules and tumors of Kaposi's sarcoma.

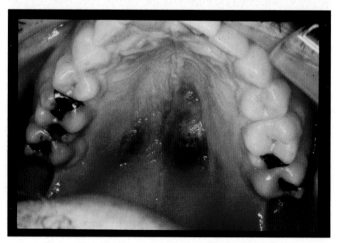

Figure 13.6. Oral mucosal plaque of Kaposi's sarcoma.

effusion lymphoma and the plasma cell variant of Castleman's disease. Angiolymphoid hyperplasia with eosinophilia is also HHV-8 associated.

BACTERIAL INFECTIONS

Folliculitis

Bacterial folliculitis is common in HIV-infected patients, and appears as a widely distributed acneiform rash with papules and pustules. Recurrent bacterial folliculitis may serve as a clue for underlying HIV infection. It is important to screen these patients for possible HIV infection. Folliculitis may be more severe than typical cases and present as a plaque-like folliculitis in HIV patients. Most cases of folliculitis are caused by *Staphylococcus aureus*. However, other organisms such as *Staphylococcus epidermidis* and *Pseudomonas aeruginosa. Micrococcus spp.*, gram-negative bacteria such as *Acinetobacter baumanni*, dermatophytes, pityrosporum yeast, or demodex mites can also be etiologic. Patients with HIV often have risk factors for contracting methicillin-resistant *Staphylococcus aureus* (MRSA). Such risk factors include intravenous drug use, hospitalization, men who have sex with men, frequent use of antibiotics, or incarceration. Hospitalized patients are at an increased risk of contracting nosocomial infections. Bacterial folliculitis in HIV-infected patients is often resistant to standard treatment, and prolonged use of systemic antibiotics may be required. Risk factors for drug-resistant or unusual organisms should also be considered when deciding on a treatment plan. Patients with HIV may also get eosinophilic pustular folliculitis, or Ofuji's disease, which is an acneiform eruption of uncertain etiology characterized by folliculitis with numerous eosinophils on biopsy and intractable itching. Treatment with HAART, as well as with corticosteroids and antihistamines, may reduce lesions. Empiric treatment with antimicrobial, antifungal, or antimite therapy has also been shown to alleviate symptoms.

Impetigo, abscesses, cellulitis, and necrotizing fasciitis

Impetigo, a superficial intraepidermal bacterial infection, is usually caused by group A β-hemolytic *Streptococci* or *S. aureus*. It is seen most commonly on the face, shoulders, and axillary or inguinal areas. The infection begins with painful red macules. These macules later become vesicles and pustules that contain purulent fluid. These soon rupture and give rise to the characteristic honey-colored crust. When impetigo produces painful plugged folliculitis, it is known as *impetigo of Bockhart*. Patients with HIV are at an increased risk of soft tissue and deep-seated bacterial infections such as cellulitis and abscesses due to MRSA. By direct extension, these can lead to pyomyositis or necrotizing fasciitis, which would manifest as diffuse, red, warm, tender areas in the skin, and can be associated with severe toxemia. Frequently these abscesses are polymicrobial. Excision and drainage of pyogenic abscesses has been reported as an effective treatment modality in community-acquired MRSA cases containing abscesses, even in the absence of antibiotic treatment.

Mycobacterial infections

HIV-infected individuals are susceptible to a number of mycobacterial infections that can produce a wide variety of cutaneous infections. Since the presenting lesions of cutaneous infections have nonspecific morphology, tissue biopsy and culture are requisite for diagnosis. Clinical suspicion is important since mycobacterial cultures can take up to 6 weeks to perform. PCR for Mycobacterium tuberculosis or atypical mycobacterial infections may accelerate the diagnosis.

Infections with *M. tuberculosis* may be the result of a primary infection at the site of broken skin that results in a local verrucous lesion. However, it can also be the result of a systemic disseminated infection. Many manifestations of cutaneous tuberculosis such as scrofuloderma, lupus vulgaris, and orofacial tuberculosis represent host reactions to tuberculosis infection. These manifestations require intact cellular immunity and do not occur at significantly increased rates in the setting of HIV.

Cutaneous miliary tuberculosis, however, occurs in the setting of advanced immunosuppression when active tuberculosis spreads secondarily to the skin. This presentation occurs most frequently when the CD4 count is less than 200 cells/mL. Lesions of miliary tuberculosis may occur as macules, papules or nodules with small vesicles. Cutaneous tuberculosis is treated with the same regimens as pulmonary or extrapulmonary disease.

Cutaneous infection by *Mycobaterium avium-intracellulare* occurs in the setting of profound immunosuppression and may present as a variety of skin lesions including erythematous papules, pustules, nodules, ulcers, abscesses, folliculitis, panniculitis, plaques, verrucous lesions, or draining sinuses.

The patient with HIV may be susceptible to a variety of other less common mycobacterial infections as well. Case reports have documented infection by *Mycobaterium kansaii, Mycobaterium genavense, Mycobaterium marinarum,* and *Mycobaterium leprae*. The incidence of infection by *Mycobaterium leprae*, the organism responsible for the various manifestations of leprosy, does not seem to be increased in the setting of HIV.

Bacillary angiomatosis

Bacillary angiomatosis (BA) is an infection which may appear at first impression to be a vascular neoplasm. The disease is caused by infection by *Bartonella henselae* or *Bartonella quintana* and presents in advanced stages of HIV when the CD4 count is less than 200 cells/mL. While once considered a hallmark of HIV, this disease has now become uncommon. Perhaps this is related to the effects of HAART or as a result of antibiotic prophylaxis with trimethoprim–sulfamethoxazole against *Pneumocystis*. The earliest and most common lesions appear as discrete pinpoint red-purple papules that resemble pyogenic granulomata (Fig. 13.7). These lesions may ulcerate and become crusted. Another variant consists of subcutaneous nodules that may extend into the underlying skeletal muscle and bone. Patients who have BA may have systemic signs and symptoms, including fever, chills, night sweats, and weight loss. In advanced cases, the liver and spleen may also be involved. Because the clinical presentation of this infection can easily be confused with pyogenic granuloma, biopsy should be performed if the diagnosis is suspected. Bacillary angiomatosis responds to treatment with macrolide antibiotics such as erythromycin, clarithromycin, and azithromycin or

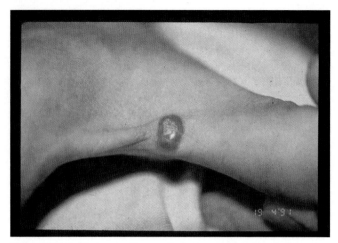

Figure 13.7. Solitary vascular papule that resembles a pyogenic granuloma. Biopsy proved that this lesion was actually bacillary angiomatosis.

doxycycline. A 2- to 3-month course of erythromycin (500 mg/ QID) or doxycycline (100 mg BID) is effective against BA. Recurrence is common.

SEXUALLY TRANSMITTED DISEASE

The accurate diagnosis of sexually transmitted diseases (STDs) is of exceptional importance in individuals at high risk for HIV infection because their presence increases the risk of transmitting and acquiring HIV infection. Studies have demonstrated that, in some populations, the pattern of HIV acquisition parallels that of STDs.

Syphilis

A high prevalence of syphilis, active as well as latent, has been found among AIDS patients in the United States. In HIV-infected patients, the infection begins as it does for immune competent hosts. There is a single chancre that occurs at the site of inoculation, although recent studies have reported multiple chancres that can be aggressive and slower to heal. Chancres are described as 1- to 2-cm, painless, nonpurulent, round to oval ulcers with raised, indurated borders. Secondary syphilis may occur in a number of forms in patients who have HIV infection. It can range from the classic papulosquamous form with involvement of palms, soles, and mucous membranes to unusual forms such as verrucous plaques, extensive oral ulcerations, alopecia, keratoderma, deep cutaneous nodules, or widespread gummata (Fig. 13.8).

Malignant syphilis, or lues maligna, is a rare, ulcerating, widespread form of secondary syphilis. Papulopustular lesions enlarge into sharply bordered ulcers that can be associated with fever, malaise, and ocular disease. Cases of malignant syphilis have been rising and mostly affect those with the lowest CD4 counts.

Syphilis may progress faster from secondary to tertiary disease in HIV-seropositive patients than in noninfected individuals. Those with CD4 counts below 350 mm are at a 4-fold higher risk for neurosyphilis. Early central nervous system (CNS)

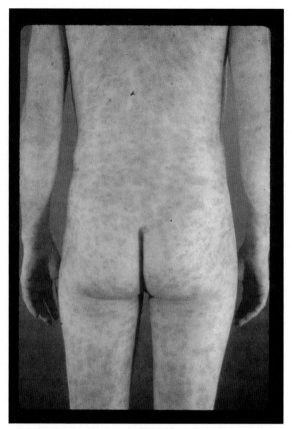

Figure 13.8. Extensive macular and subtle popular eruption of secondary syphilis. Polymorphous presentations have earned syphilis the title of "The great masquerader."

relapse and unresponsiveness to treatment can also be more common in HIV-infected individuals.

Co-infection with syphilis and HIV is somewhat common, and shares risk factors for transmission. Therefore it is recommended that all patients with syphilis should undergo screening for HIV. Serologic negativity may not rule out secondary syphilis in HIV-infected individuals as false-negative serologic studies can be seen with both the FTA-ABS and VDRL tests. This is due to the because of loss of antibody production in advanced HIV. If there is a discrepancy between clinical suspicion and serologic tests, skin biopsy for demonstration of spirochetes by special stains may be necessary to establish the diagnosis. Dark field microscopy will also directly visualize the organisms. Current treatment involves a single dose of long-acting benzathine penicillin (2.4 million units IM) or ceftriaxone (1g daily for 8–10 days).

Other Sexually Transmitted Diseases

Although granuloma inguinale, alternately called *donovanosis*, is a relatively uncommon STD in the United States and other developed countries, this condition is quite common in certain hotspots such as South Africa, Papua New Guinea, Brazil, India, and among aborriginal Australians. It is caused by the gram-negative rod *Calymmatobacterium granulomatis* and manifests clinically as vegetating lesions on the penis associated with pseudobuboes in the inguinal crease. HIV-positive patients may present with ulcers that are slow to respond to treatment and cause extensive local tissue destruction. Culture and skin biopsy for identification of the safety pin-shaped organisms (Donovan bodies) is required to establish the diagnosis. Current first-line CDC-recommended treatments are either doxycycline 100 mg orally twice a day or trimethoprim–sulfamethoxazole (800 mg/160 mg) orally twice a day for 3 weeks.

Lymphogranuloma venereum (LGV) is a disease caused by *Chlamydia trachomatis* that is uncommon in HIV-infected patients in the United States, but is endemic in some developing nations. It presents as a generalized lymphadenopathy with vulvar or penile edema with recurrent ulcerations and erosions. Inguinal lymph nodes may be fluctuant or may form draining sinuses. Diagnosis for LGV is presumptive based on clinical findings, and can be confirmed by serologic testing or PCR confirmation. Those thought to be infected with LGV should be started on a course of 100 mg of doxycycline twice daily for 21 days.

FUNGAL INFECTIONS

Candidiasis

Recurrent or persistent oral candidiasis may be the initial sign of HIV infection in many individuals and has been shown to be a predictor of progression from HIV infection to AIDS. Most commonly, infections are caused by *Candida albicans*, but infections with nonalbicans species including *Candida glabrata, Candida tropicalis, Candida parapsilosis, Candida krusei,* and *Candida dubliniensis* are becoming more frequent. The most common clinical presentation is that of thrush. Thrush is a painful, whitish exudate present on the tongue or buccal mucosa that can easily be scraped away. Candida is also implicated in causing angular cheilitis, chronic paronychia, onychodystrophy, distal urethritis, and persistent intertriginous infections. Esophageal candidiasis is an AIDS-defining condition. Disseminated cutaneous lesions present as clusters of asymptomatic pustules on an erythematous base or as nodules with central necrosis. Systemic dissemination can produce candidal septicemia, brain abscesses, and meningitis. Invasive, chronic, or recurrent disease should be treated with oral fluconazole (100 mg/d) after a single loading dose of 200 mg, or itraconazole (100 mg two times per day). Fluconazole resistance has recently emerged, probably as a result of prolonged azole prophylaxis. If disseminated disease or resistance occurs, amphotericin B can be used.

Dermatophytosis

Cutaneous dermatophytosis is more common in patients with HIV than in the general population and can be extensive and severe. In any individual with extensive T*inea corporis* or *Trichopyton rubrum*, the possibility of underlying HIV infection should be considered. Tinea coporis, often caused by *Trichophyton rubrum,* can present as a widespread dermal infection with multiple fluctuant erythematous ulcerative nodules seen mostly on the extremities (Fig. 13.9). Infection of the hair follicle with secondary rupture is known as Majocchi's granuloma and will present as firm violaceous folliculocentric nodules. Subungual proximal superficial onychomycosis, which is rarely seen in the HIV negative population, appears as white plaques under the proximal nail. Diagnosis can be established by skin scraping and direct visualization with

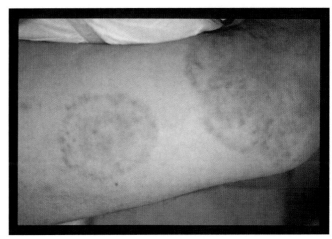

Figure 13.9. Sharply demarcated patch and annular plaque of tinea corporis, likely caused by *Trichophyton rubrum.*

potassium hydroxide preparation, or by skin biopsy with special stains or culture. If topical treatment is not successful, systemic therapy, such as terbinafine for onychomycosis, may be needed. Deep dermal infections may require systemic treatment with oral fluconazole or itraconazole.

Pneumocystosis

Pneumocystis jiroveci, previously known as *Pneumocystic carinii,* is most often associated with pneumonia that occurs when the CD4 count is significantly depressed. It is an AIDS-defining illness, and it may rarely involve the skin in patients who use aerosolized pentamidine for prophylaxis of *P. jiroveci* pneumonia. The lesions are friable reddish papules or nodules, most often in the ear canal or nares. Small translucent molluscum contagiosum–like papules, bluish cellulitic plaques, and deeply seated abscesses have also been observed. Extrapulmonary disease is treated with the same regimens as for Pneumocystis pneumonia.

Cryptococcus

The most common opportunistic fungal infection to affect the skin in HIV-seropositive patients is cryptococcosis. However, with the increased use of HAART the incidence has decreased considerably. Cutaneous involvement may be seen with disseminated disease and is an AIDS-defining and life-threatening condition. Cryptococcus usually occurs when the CD4 count is less than 100 cells/μL. Umbilicated papules similar to molluscum contagiosum, nodules, pustules, ulcers, and erythematous papules are all common manifestations (Fig. 13.10). If cutaneous cryptococcus is diagnosed, a thorough investigation for extracutaneous disease should be undertaken to initiate early life-saving treatment. Cutaneous cryptococcus can be treated with fluconazole (200–400 mg/d) or itraconazole (400 mg/d). Disseminated disease is treated with amphotericin B plus flucytosine.

Histoplasmosis

Histoplasmosis is a frequent opportunistic infection in patients with HIV/AIDS. The infection begins with a flu-like illness, and cutaneous lesions represent hematogenous dissemination that

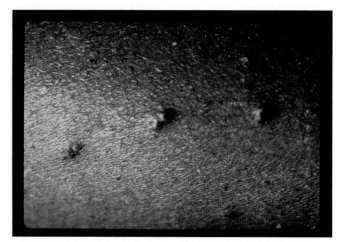

Figure 13.10. Crusted umbilicated papules in a cutaneous Cryptococcus infection.

usually manifests after the CD4 cell count falls below 150 cells/mL. A variety of lesions are seen including nodules, vesicles, erythematous scaly plaques, necrotizing lesions mimicking pyoderma gangrenosum, purpura, petechiae, and pustules with or without ulceration (Fig. 13.11). Biopsy with histologic confirmation is an important method of diagnosis because histoplasmosis can be difficult to culture and serologic tests for histoplasmosis may be falsely negative in HIV-infected patients. Treatment consists of 2 weeks of amphotericin B followed by itraconazole. Primary prophylaxis with itraconazole 200 mg/day is given to HIV-infected individuals with CD4 counts less than 150 cells/μL.

Coccidiomycosis

Coccidiomycosis is an infection endemic to the southwestern United States and arises from inhalation of arthroconidia. Initial symptoms are nonspecific and include fever, malaise and a flu-like illness that begins 1 to 3 weeks after infection. Up to 50% of patients will have an associated inflammatory skin manifestations such as erythema nodosum, erythema multiforme-like reaction, or toxic erythema. In a small percent of individuals, the infection will progress beyond pulmonary disease. The majority of HIV patients have CD4 counts below 250 cells/μL at the time progressive disease occurs. Skin is the most common site for disseminated disease to present. Common cutaneous lesions include morbilliform eruptions, violaceous or ulcerating plaques, papules, and pustules. If a patient has cutaneous disease, a search for other systemic manifestations should be initiated. Diagnosis can be established by culture, serology, or histology. HIV patients with nonmeningeal, pulmonary, and disseminated disease should be treated initially with amphotericin B (0.6 – 1.0 mg/kg/day). AIDS patients and any patient with disseminated disease should be placed on lifelong azole therapy. Secondary prophylaxis with either fluconazole 400 mg/day (first line) or itraconazole 200 mg twice daily is recommended as standard of care when patients respond to initial treatment.

Aspergillosis

Invasive aspergillosis is rare in AIDS, but when present, has a very poor prognosis. It occurs predominantly in patients with advanced HIV with leukopenia and neutropenia. CD4

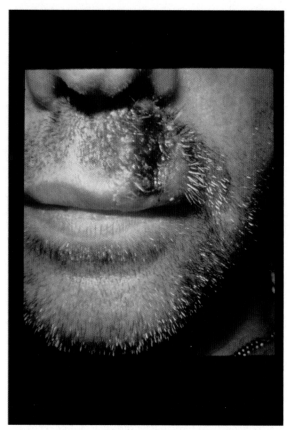

Figure 13.11. An ulcerated erythematous plaque is one of many possible presentations of cutaneous histoplasmosis.

lymphopenia has been identified as an important risk factor for HIV-1–associated aspergillosis, and CD4 cell counts less than 50 cells/μL have been reported in the majority of cases. Other factors that may predispose patients to infection include extended use of high-dose corticosteroids, exposure to broad-spectrum antibacterial therapy, or previous underlying lung disease.

Paracoccidiomycosis

Paracoccidioides brasiliensis is an important chronic, progressive, systemic deep mycosis that is endemic in South America. The usual course involves predominantly the pulmonary system with lymphadenitis, although mucocutaneous sites can become secondarily involved. The disease is most commonly acquired by inhalation of airborne conidia produced in the mycelial phase of this dimorphic fungus. Direct inoculation of either skin or oral mucous membranes is a less common route of infection that accounts for uncommon cases of cutaneous lesions without pulmonary involvement.

Penicilliosis

Penicilliosis is due to the dimorphic fungus *Penicillium marneffei*, and is the third most common opportunistic infection in HIV-infected patients of countries of southeast Asia and southern parts of China. The majority of cases of penicilliosis are seen in patients with CD4 counts <50 cells/μL. The most common clinical presentation is fever, cough, weight loss, anemia, and disseminated papular skin lesions (Fig. 13.12). Umbilicated papules present over the

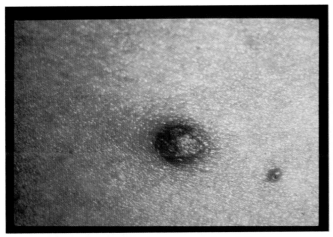

Figure 13.12. Papular eruption of penicillosis.

face, pinnae, extremities, and occasionally the genitalia. Diagnosis can be established by fungal isolation from blood culture or other specimens, or by histopathologic demonstration of organisms on biopsy or by Wright-stained scrapings. Treatment is with amphotericin B 0.6 mg/kg/day IV for 2 weeks, followed by oral itraconazole solution in a dose of 400 mg daily for a subsequent duration of 10 weeks. Simultaneous administration of treatment for penicilliosis and initiation of HAART may improve outcome. On completion of initial therapy, secondary prophylaxis with oral itraconazole 200 mg daily should be given for life.

Other Fungal Infections

Blastomycosis and sporotrichosis have also been observed in HIV-seropositive patients albeit rarely. Mucocutaneous lesions associated with systemic fungal infections consist of pustules, ulcers, papules, and nodules and less often as patches or plaques. Since mucocutaneous fungal infections assume a number of morphologies that may mimic other disorders including HSV infection, cellulitis, or molluscum contagiosum, a tissue biopsy of the lesion should be performed for histologic evaluation and confirmatory microbiologic cultures. The HIV-associated disseminated form of sporotrichosis can also involve the eyes, joints, lungs, liver, spleen, intestines, and meninges. Definitive diagnosis at any site requires culture isolation of *Sporothrix schenckii* from a normally sterile body site.

PARASITIC AND ECTOPARASITIC INFECTIONS

HIV-seropositive individuals may present with a wide variety of parasitic and ectoparasitic infections, including scabies, demodicidosis, acanthamebiasis, and leishmaniasis. These infections can manifest either as localized conditions or as disseminated disease. The clinical presentation may be unusual and the use of cultures and skin biopsies is essential to render an accurate diagnosis.

Scabies

The causative agent of scabies is the mite *Sarcoptes scabei*. Scabies is the most common ectoparasitic infection seen in the setting of

HIV. The clinical presentation can vary from discrete scattered pruritic papules and slight scale to a widespread papulosquamous eruption that resembles atopic dermatitis. A common clinical presentation is that of hyperkeratotic plaques present on the palms, soles, trunk, and extremities in addition to intense pruritus that is worse at night. Contacts are almost always infected. In HIV-infected patients who have CD4 cell counts less than 150 cells/mL, or in patients who have advanced peripheral neuropathy and diminished sensation, scabies infection may be severe and have a much greater number of mites than normal. This presents as crusted or "Norwegian" scabies. In rare cases, complications from a scabetic infection could include secondary bacteremia and sepsis. The diagnosis can be confirmed by microscopic examination of scrapings for mites or ova. Topical treatments include permethrin and benzyl benzoate. Ivermectin can be given orally.

Demodicidosis

The causative agent of demodicidosis is the mite *Demodex*. It presents as a persistent pruritic follicular eruption of the face, trunk, and extremities. Demodicidosis has also been associated with the pathogenesis of rosacea-like dermatoses, perioral dermatoses, and blepharitis. Diagnosis is by clinical and pathologic correlation, since Demodex are normal skin fauna.

Acanthamebiasis

Acanthamebiasis caused by several species of the free-living amoebae Acanthamoeba sp. can have an aggressive course in the setting of immunosuppression. The cutaneous presentation is that of painful red to violet nodules that ulcerate and arefrequently located on the trunk and extremities (Fig. 13.13). HIV-positive patients are at risk for granulomatous amoebic encephalitis or disseminated amoebic disease, which are both of which life threatening conditions. Cutaneous lesions may serve as a source for these more serious infections. Acanthameobic keratits is not increased in HIV. The organism is identified histologically. Treatment is not standardized but a case that involved only the skin was treated successfully with intravenous pentamidine,

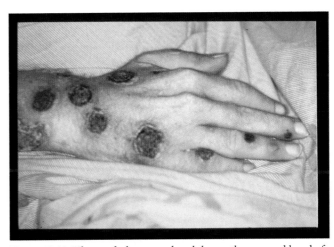

Figure 13.13. Ulcerated plaques and nodules on the arm and hand of an HIV-positive patient. These lesions would have started as deep red to violet nodules or pustules.

topical chlorhexidine gluconate, and 2% ketoconazole cream, followed by oral itraconazole.

Leishmaniasis

Leishmaniasis is more difficult to treat when associated with HIV infection. Amastigotes persist for years in macrophages and actually accelerate compromised immunity in hosts by increasing viral HIV replication. Leishmaniasis has three classifications: cutaneous, mucocutaneous, and visceral (also known as *kala-azar*). Cutaneous leishmaniasis lesions in immunosuppressed patients mirror those seen in immunocompetent. The skin lesions present as scaly lichenified depigmented plaques. Nonulcerated nodules on the extensor surfaces of the limbs overlying the joints have also been described. Mucocutaneous disease begins with single or multiple lesions that eventually heal. These lesions can be painful and disfiguring. Given the prevalence of HIV infection in the Americas, the incidence of leishmaniasis in these patients is surprisingly low.

PITFALLS AND MYTHS

There are many cutaneous manifestations of HIV/AIDS that are not infectious. HIV is associated with an increase in certain malignancies such as leukemias and lymphomas that may present as ulcerated nodules that mimic infections. Patients with HIV may be taking multiple medications and are at an increased risk for drug reactions. Drug reactions can have varied morphologies but may resemble a viral exanthem.

Since immune suppression commonly alters the course of a disease and the body's host response, treatment regimens should be modified to each patient according to published guidelines. In general, HIV-positive patients may require prolonged treatments and sometimes, increased dosages of medications.

SUGGESTED READINGS

Adal KA, Cockerell CJ, Petri WA. Cat scratch disease, bacillary angiomatosis, and other infections due to Rochalimaea. *N Engl J Med* 1994 May 26;330(21):1509–1515.

Alessi E, Cusini M. The exanthem of HIV-1 seroconversion syndrome. *Int J Dermatol.* 1995;34(4):238–239.

Alvar J, Canavate C, Gutierrez-Solar B, et al. Leishmania and human immunodeficiency virus coinfection: the first 10 years. *Clin Microbiol Rev* 1997;10(2):298–319.

Aly R, Berger T. Common superficial fungal infections in patients with AIDS. *Clin Infect Dis* 1996; 22:S128–S132.

Barbagallo J, Tager P, Ingleton R, et al. Cutaneous tuberculosis: diagnosis and treatment. *Am J Clin Dermatol* 2002;3(5):319–328.

Celum C, Levine R, Weaver M, et al. Genital herpes and human immunodeficiency virus: double trouble. *Bull World Health Organ* 2004;82(6):447–453.

Chin-Hong PV, Palefsky JM. Human papillomavirus anogenital disease in HIV-infected individuals. *Dermatol Ther* 2005;18:67–76.

Conant MA. Immunomodulatory therapy in the management of viral infections in patients with HIV infection. *J Am Acad Dermatol* 2000; 43(1 Pt 2):S27–30.

Elston DM. Community-acquired methicillin resistant *Staphylococcus aureus*. *J Am Acad Derm* 2007;56:1–16.

Huselbosch HJ, Claessen FA, van Ginkel CJ, et al. Human immunodeficiency virus exanthem. *J Am Acad Dermatol* 1990;23:483–486.

Marrazzo J. Syphilis and other sexually transmitted diseases in HIV infection. *Top HIV Med* 2007;15:11–16.

Millikan LE. Role of oral antifungal agents for the treatment of superficial fungal infections in immunocompromised patients. *Cutis* 2001;68(1 Suppl):6–14.

Osborne GEN, Taylor C, Fuller LC. The management of HIV-related skin disease. Part I: infections. *Int J STD AIDS* 2003;14:78–88.

Pappas PG, Rex JH, Sobel JD, et al. IDSA guidelines for treatment of candidiasis. *Clin Infect Dis* 2004;38:161–189.

Paredes R, Laguna F, Clotet B. Leishmaniasis in HIV-infected persons: a review. *J Int Assoc Physicians AIDS Care* 1997;3(6):22–39.

Partridge JM, Koutsky LA. Genital human papillomavirus infection in men. *Lancet Infect Dis* 2006;6:21–31.

Piketty C, Kazatchkine MD. Human papillomavirus-related cervical and anal disease in HIV-infected individuals in the era of highly active antiretroviral therapy. *Curr HIV/AIDS Rep* 2005; 2(3):140–145.

Ramdial P, Mosam A, Dlova NC, et al. Disseminated cutaneous histoplasmosis in patients infected with human immunodeficiency virus. *J Cutan Pathol* 2002;29(4):215–25.

Ruhnke M. Mucosal and systemic fungal infection in patients with AIDS. *Prophylaxis and treatment*. Drugs 2004;64(11):1163–1180.

Sandler B, Potter TS, Hashimoto K. Cutaneous *Pneumocystis carinii* and *Cryptococcus neoformans* in AIDS. *Br J Dermatol* 1996;134(1):159–163.

Smith KJ, Skelton H. Molluscum contagiosum: recent advances in pathogenic mechanisms, and new therapies. *Am J Clin Dermatol* 2002;3(8):535–545.

Strick LB, Wald A. Diagnostics for herpes simplex virus: is PCR the new gold standard? *Mol Diagn Ther* 2006;10:17–28.

Tariq A, Ross JDC. Viral sexually transmitted infections: current management strategies. *J Clin Pharm Ther* 1999;24:409–14.

Venkatesan P, Perfect JR, Myers SA. Evaluation and management of fungal infections in immunocompromised patients. *Dermatol Ther* 2005;18(1):44–57.

Wheat J, Sarosi G, McKinsey D, et al. IDSA practice guidelines for the management of patients with histoplasmosis. *Clin Infect Dis* 2000;30:688.

14 | INFECTIONS IN ORGAN TRANSPLANT PATIENTS

Daniela Kroshinsky, Jennifer Y. Lin, and Richard Allen Johnson

Bacterial infections represent the major cause of morbidity in patients undergoing solid organ transplantation (SOT). Soft tissue infections from bacteria generally occur in the first month after transplantation when the skin is disrupted by the surgery itself or by indwelling catheters and lines. Incidence of wound infections in solid organ transplant patients ranges from 2% to 56%, depending on surgical technique, host characteristics, and antibiotic prophylaxis.

The skin flora is also the culprit when introduced to less tolerant tissue such as the transplanted organ itself. This can lead to pyelonephritis and cystitis in renal transplant recipients, cholangitis, and intra-abdominal abscesses in liver transplants, and bronchitis and pneumonia in the lung transplant recipient. Frequently, bacteremia ensues and may again come to the attention of a dermatologist as a subcutaneous abscess from hematogenous spread.

In the setting of immunosuppression, it is helpful to characterize pathogens by their pathophysiology:

(1) True pathogens – infection originating in skin and being typical of that which occurs in immunocompetent persons, albeit with the potential for more serious illness
(2) Sometime pathogens – extensive cutaneous involvement with pathogens that normally produce trivial or well-localized disease in immunocompetent patients
(3) Opportunistic pathogens – infection originating from a cutaneous source and caused by opportunistic pathogens that rarely cause disease in immunocompetent patients but that may cause either localized or widespread disease in compromised persons
(4) Indicators of visceral pathogens – cutaneous or subcutaneous infection that represents metastatic spread from a non-cutaneous site

With this framework, we will explore the common cutaneous bacterial pathogens.

HISTORY

The immunosuppressive regimens required to maintain organ viability in transplant patients puts these individuals at risk for infection. The skin is an organ that is easily infected, but can also be a window to internal infections. Early recognition and treatment of these infections can minimize long-term morbidity and mortality in this vulnerable population.

BACTERIAL DISEASE IN TRANSPLANTATION

Staphylococcus aureus

Staphylococcus aureus causes the majority of all pyodermas and soft tissue infections seen in solid organ transplant (SOT) patients. Although not one of the cutaneous resident flora, it colonizes the anterior nares in up to 30% of healthy individuals at any given time, and more than 50% of chronically ill individuals. The incidence of *S. aureus* nasal carriage is higher in SOT patients, as it is in other immmunologically compromised individuals, such as those with HIV disease, diabetes mellitus, or neutropenia.

Ensconced in the nares, *S. aureus* is able to colonize and infect superficial skin breaks such as around hair follicles, skin disruptions from secondary dermatologic disorders (i.e., eczematous dermatitis, herpetic ulcer, molluscum contagiosum), or via vascular access line and drainage tubes. The spectrum of pyodermas includes folliculitis, furuncles, carbuncles, abscess, impetigo, bullous impetigo, and ecthyma (Fig. 14b.1).

Once established in the skin, *S. aureus* is able to invade more deeply into the soft tissue with resultant infections such as cellulitis and necrotizing cellulitis (Fig. 14b.2). *S. aureus* can also reach the skin via dissemination from another source of infection. In this form of hematogenous seeding, the lesions can appear nonspecific as petechiae, hemorrhages, subcutaneous nodules, soft tissue infections, and pyomyositis. Systemic symptoms that would normally herald the onset of an infection, such as fever, may be masked if the patient is on steroids for immunosuppression.

S. aureus colonization has been associated with increased risk of soft tissue infection, especially in the first 2 months after transplantation. This has been well characterized in the liver transplant patients where pretransplant colonization with methicillin resistant *S. aureus* (MRSA) and methicillin-susceptible *S aureus* (MSSA) were independent variables for increased *S. aureus* infections (bacteremia, pneumonia, abscess, wound infection, sinusitis). MRSA has emerged as the leading cause of postoperative resistant infections in liver transplant patients in some hospitals. In some cases, colonization can be tied to use of urinary catheters, postoperative bleeding at the surgical site, and fluoroquinolone use in the months preceding transplantation. MRSA colonization has not been definitively tied to increased long-term morbidity or mortality. MRSA infection in liver transplant patients, however, has been associated with a higher rate of posttransplant complications and longer stays in the intensive care unit.

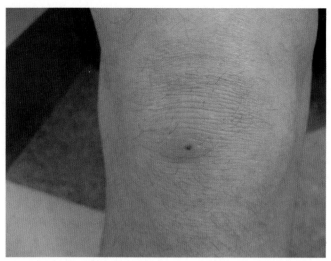

Figure 14b.1. Erythematous edematous warm fluctuant plaque with central erosion, consistent with an abscess; cultures grew MRSA.

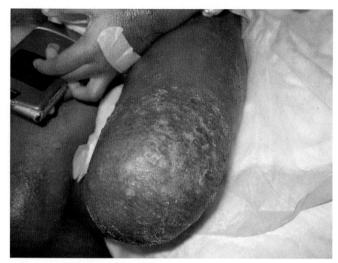

Figure 14b.3. Yellow crusted erosions in a child with a history of eczema, consistent with impetigo.

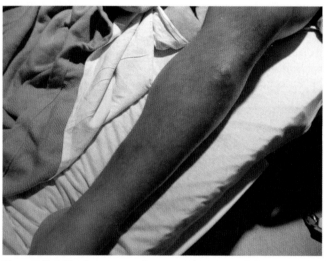

Figure 14b.2. Erythematous, edematous plaques consistent with cellulitis.

Treatment of *S. aureus* carriage with topical mupirocin has been successful in decreasing the rate of infections post cardiothoracic surgery. It is still unclear whether the same effect will be achieved for SOT patients for several reasons: (1) patients may be colonized in areas on the skin other than nares, (2) there is an increased rate of mupirocin-resistant *S. aureus*, and (3) many patients subsequently become recolonized. Decolonization of liver transplant patients has been reported with intranasal mupirocin three times daily with daily chlorhexidine baths.

Various strains of *S. aureus* are capable of producing a variety of toxins, which cause the clinical syndromes of staphylococcal scalded skin syndrome (SSSS), staphylococcal scarlet fever, and toxic shock syndrome (TSS). TSS is a febrile, multiorgan disease caused by the elaboration of staphylococcal toxins, characterized by a generalized scarlatiniform eruption, hypotension, functional abnormalities of three or more organ systems, and desquamation in the evolution of the exanthem. Cellulitis caused by strains of *S. aureus* that produce TSS toxins can be accompanied by the cutaneous and systemic findings of staphylococcal

scarlet fever or TSS. SSSS is characterized by fever, skin pain, and an erythematous or scarlatiniform rash with subsequent blister formation and superficial desquamation. It results from the elaboration of epidermolytic toxins from *S. aureus* and has been reported in SOT patients.

Standard perioperative antibiotics are administered to eradicate potentially active infections and cover skin flora. A first-generation cephalosporin is most commonly used. Cultures must always be taken, however, in STIs because of increased prevalence of MRSA and the potential for atypical organisms such as fungal and mycobacterium. Vancomycin or linezolid is employed where MRSA is of significant concern.

B-hemolytic streptococcus

Group A β-hemolytic streptococci (*Streptococcus pyogenes*) (GAS) commonly colonizes the upper respiratory tract, and secondarily infects (impetiginizes) minor skin lesions from which invasive infection can arise. Impetigo often appears as golden crusts with small vesicles and pustules (Fig. 14b.3). Certain strains of group A streptococci have a higher affinity for the skin than the respiratory tract and can colonize the skin, subsequently causing superficial pyodermas or soft tissue infections.

Other streptococci, such as Group B streptococci, commonly colonize the perineum and may cause soft tissue infections at this site. Morbidity and mortality are relatively high for group B streptococcus infections, with a high incidence of bacteremia.

S. pneumoniae can cause a range of infections including otitis media, sinusitis, and more rarely, cellulitis. Clinically, affected skin is characterized by bullae, brawny erythema, and a violaceous hue. Approximately 50% of cases are the result of pneumococcal bacteremia, often from a pulmonary source with an associated high morbidity. Transplant patients, especially pediatric patients who have the highest exposure risk, are also more likely to have recurrent disease, with a mean time of 5.4 months between the first and second infections.

Studies have demonstrated decreased pneumococcal antibody titers 3 months after transplantation secondary to the suppression of cell-mediated immunity. In the past, prophylaxis has been

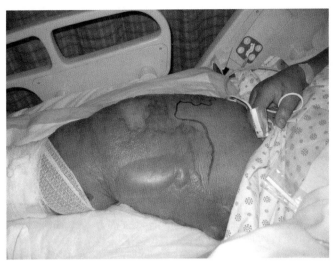

Figure 14b.4 Erthythematous, edematous, tender plaque consistent with bullous cellulitis.

controversial but recent studies suggest that the polyvalent poly-saccharide pneumococcal vaccine is safe and effective for patients with well-functioning allografts, and the conjugate vaccine is similarly efficacious in generating a functional antibody response.

Necrotizing fasciitis

Necrotizing fasciitis is a severe form of soft tissue infection extending into the subcutaneous fat and deep fascia. Immunosuppressed patients are particularly prone to this type of infection. Causes can be monomicrobial (i.e., Group A β-hemolytic *streptococcus)*, or polymicrobial (nongroup A *streptococcus* plus anaerobes). Transplant patients are also prone to infections caused by Pseudomonas, Klebsiella, and Serratia. Pain out of proportion to physical findings in a patient with evidence of a systemically toxic condition should raise the clinical suspicion of necrotizing fasciitis. Very rapidly, the clinical picture can change, with skin becoming erythematous to dusky and edematous, and with pain transforming into anesthesia. Cases in transplant patients often have subcutaneous emphysema, and finding gas on imaging can be helpful in making the diagnosis.

Necrotizing fasciitis arising in the setting of transplantation is classified as early (within ten days of transplantation) or late (greater than one year after transplantation). While the majority of cases are late, these infections tend to be less aggressive.

Treatment for necrotizing fasciitis includes early surgical debridement, antibiotics, and intensive care monitoring. Some success has been noted with intravenous γ-globulin use as well. The mechanism is thought to involve antibody-mediated neutralization of contributing superantigens and a reduction in circulating inflammatory cytokines. In the setting of a life-threatening infection, diminishing or temporarily halting immunosuppressive therapies can be considered.

Gram-negative bacilli

E. coli and other gram-negative bacilli (GNB) such as *Klebsiella pneumonia, Escherichia coli, Pseudomonas aeruginosa, Proteus mirabilis,* and *enterobacter* can rarely cause soft tissue infections, most notably occurring in patients with hepatic cirrhosis, nephritic syndrome, and immunosuppression. Spontaneous cellulitis secondary to gram-negative bacilli has been reported post transplantation, particularly in the setting of edema with no clear portal of entry. More than 80% have associated secondary bacteremia from sources such as pneumonia (48.9%) and central line infections (22.2%) and as such, blood cultures should be obtained when cellulitis arises in an SOT patient. Presentation can be characterized by cellulitis, bullous lesions, ulcers, abscesses, or extensive cutaneous necrosis with prominent vascular involvement on pathology (Fig. 14b.4).

Initial empiric coverage with gentamicin is helpful until cultures from the blood and skin biopsy return. The rate of mortality and graft loss is increased in patients with GNB infections, and can be as high as 60% in the presence of bacteremia.

Pseudomonas aeruginosa causes the necrotizing soft tissue infection ecthyma gangrenosum (EG), which occurs as a primary skin infection or as a complication of pseudomonal bacteremia. EG occurs commonly as a nosocomial infection, especially in immunocompromised patients. *P. aeruginosa* gains entry into the dermis and subcutaneous tissues via adnexal structures or in areas where epidermal integrity has been breached (pressure ulcers, thermal burns, and trauma). EG occurs most frequently in the axillae or anogenital regions but can arise at any cutaneous site. Clinically, EG first presents as an erythematous, painful plaque that then quickly undergoes necrosis. Established lesions show bulla formation, hemorrhage, necrosis, and surrounding erythema. If effective antibiotic therapy is not initiated promptly, the necrosis may often extend rapidly. Bacteremia occurs soon after the onset of EG, and may result in metastatic spread of *P. aerations* with subcutaneous nodules and abscesses. Intravenous antibiotic treatment is typically required. Of note, in one study of resistant *P. aerations*, ciprofloxacin susceptibility was inferior to that with imipenem, gentamicin, and tobramycin, emphasizing the need to obtain cultures for sensitivities and to offer initial double coverage in this susceptible population.

Vibrio vulnificus

Vibrio vulnificus is a naturally occurring marine, gram-negative rod, occasionally contaminating oysters and other shellfish. Either ingestion of raw seafood or exposure of open wounds to seawater can result in *Vibrio* bacteremia and soft tissue infections. The cutaneous lesions begin as erythematous plaques, rapidly evolving into hemorrhagic bullae and then into necrotic ulcers. Infection by the *Vibrio* species can lead to necrotizing fasciitis or fulminant sepsis in compromised hosts, and patients should be warned about eating uncooked seafood. Doxycycline 100 mg PO BID is the preferred treatment.

Bacillary Angiomatosis

Bacillary angiomatosis (BA) is characterized by angioproliferative lesions resembling pyogenic granulomas or Kaposi's sarcoma. It has been reported in cardiac, renal, and liver transplant patients with significant immunosuppression. BA is caused by infection with fastidious gram-negative bacilli of the genus *Bartonella*, namely, *Bartonella henselae* and *Bartonella quintana*.

Clinically, the cutaneous lesions of BA are red-to-violaceous, dome-shaped papules, nodules, ranging in size from a few mm up to 2 to 3 cm in diameter. While cutaneous involvement is the most common manifestation of Bartonella infection, the organism can also cause bacteremia, meningitis, neuroretinitis, endocarditis, necrotizing lymphadenitis, pneumonia, and peliosis hepatitis. The diagnosis should be suspected in patients with skin lesions, signs of systemic infection, and a history of cat exposure. The antibiotics of choice are erythromycin, doxycycline, or azithromycin continued for several weeks to months. Relapses are frequent if the duration of treatment is shortened.

Nocardiosis

Nocardia is an aerobic, ubiquitous environmental actinomycete that can cause a localized or disseminated, life-threatening infection called *nocardiosis* in the compromised host. While more than 50 species exist, the most common causative organism is *Nocardia asteroides*. Nocardia can cause a variety of clinical scenarios, most often as an opportunistic infection in persons with decreased immunity.

These gram-positive, weakly acid-fast bacteria can be directly introduced into the skin of immunocompromised patients or, more often, represent metastatic spread from a primary pulmonary infection. Primary cutaneous infection uncommonly occurs and can present nonspecifically as cellulitis, papules, nodules, pustules, abscesses, ulcers, granulomas, soft tissue infection, mycetoma, and sporotrichoid infection. It is most likely to be seen following trauma to the extremities or face, after exposure to soil or sand, or via inoculation during medical procedures.

Secondary cutaneous infection from a pulmonary focus is the most common type of cutaneous nocardiosis in the immunocompromised patient and can present as pustules, abscesses, or nodules. At least one-third of cases of pulmonary nocardiosis result in dissemination to other organs, with skin involvement being observed in 10% of the cases In the majority of transplant patients, cutaneous nocardiosis results in disseminated disease with involvement of other organs.

Isolation of *Nocardia* by culture is preferable but may take several days to grow. Trimethoprim–sulfamethoxazole (TMP-SMX) is the treatment of choice but SOT patients on prophylactic therapy for *P. carinii* have still been shown to acquire the disease. Minocycline, aminoglycosides, ceftriaxone, fluoroquinolones, imipenem, and linezolid have been reported as effective second-line therapeutics. Long-term therapy is important to prevent reactivation of quiescent disease.

Given the myriad of cutaneous findings associated with nocardiosis, a high level of suspicion must be maintained in the SOT patient, especially in the first year after transplantation when the risk of nocardia infection is highest.

SUGGESTED READINGS

Audard V, Pardon A, Claude O, et al. Necrotizing fasciitis during de novo minimal change nephrotic syndrome in a kidney transplant recipient. *Transpl Infect Dis* 2005;7(2):89–92.

Bert F, Bellier C, Lassel L, et al. Risk factors for Staphylococcus aureus infection in liver transplant recipients. *Liver Transpl* 2005;11(9):1093–1099.

Bonatti H, Mendez J, Guerrero I, et al. Disseminated bartonella infection following liver transplantation. *Transpl Int* 2006;19(8):683–687.

Chao CS, Tung DY, Wei J, et al. Necrotizing soft tissue infection in heart transplantation recipients: two case reports. *Transplant Proc* 1998;30(7):3347–3349.

Chapman SW, Wilson JP. Nocardiosis in transplant recipients. *Semin Respir Infect* 1990;5(1):74–79.

Cline MS, Cummings OW, Goldman M, et al. Bacillary angiomatosis in a renal transplant recipient. *Transplantation* 1999;67(2):296–8.

Cohen E, Korzets A, Tsalihin Y, et al. Streptococcal toxic shock syndrome complicating necrotizing fasciitis in a renal transplant patient. *Nephrol Dial Transplant* 1994;9(10):1498–1499.

Dardenne S, Coche E, Weynand B, et al. High suspicion of bacillary angiomatosis in a kidney transplant recipient: a difficult way to diagnose- case report. *Transplant Proc* 2007;39(1):311–313.

Garcia-Benitez V, Garcia-Hidalgo L, Archer-Dubon C, et al. Acute primary superficial cutaneous nocardiosis due to *Nocardia brasiliensis*: a case report in an immunocompromised patient. *Int J Dermatol* 2002;41(10):713–714.

George SJ, Rivera AM, Hsu S. Disseminated cutaneous nocardiosis mimicking cellulitis and erythema nodosum. *Dermatol Online J* 2006;12(7):13.

Hibberd PL, Rubin RH. Renal transplantation and related infections. *Semin Respir Infect* 1993;8(3):216–224.

Imhof A, Maggiorini M, Zbinden R, et al. Fatal necrotizing fasciitis due to *Streptococcus pneumoniae* after renal transplantation. *Nephrol Dial Transplant* 2003;18(1):195–197.

Kazancioglu R, Sever MS, Yüksel-Onel D, et al. Immunization of renal transplant recipients with pneumococcal polysaccharide vaccine. *Clin Transplant* 2000;14(1):61–65.

Kobayashi S, Kato T, Nishida S, et al. Necrotizing fasciitis following liver and small intestine transplantation. *Pediatr Transplant* 2002;6(4):344–347.

Koehler JE, Duncan LM. Case records of the Massachusetts General Hospital. Case 30–2005. A 56-year-old man with fever and axillary lymphadenopathy. *N Engl J Med*, 2005. 353(13): p. 1387–94.

Korzets A, Ori Y, Zevin D, et al. Group A Streptococcal bacteremia and necrotizing fasciitis in a renal transplant patient: a case for intravenous immunoglobulin therapy. *Nephrol Dial Transplant* 2002;17(1):150–152.

Kumar D, Rotstein C, Miyata G, et al. Randomized, double-blind, controlled trial of pneumococcal vaccination in renal transplant recipients. *J Infect Dis* 2003;187(10):1639–1645.

Linares L, Cervera C, Cofán F, et al. Epidemiology and outcomes of multiple antibiotic-resistant bacterial infection in renal transplantation. *Transplant Proc* 2007;39(7):2222–2224.

Merigou D, Beylot-Barry M, Ly S, et al. Primary cutaneous Nocardia asteroides infection after heart transplantation. *Dermatology* 1998;196(2):246–247.

Paterson DL, Gruttadauria S, Lauro A, et al. Spontaneous gram-negative cellulitis in a liver transplant recipient. *Infection* 2001;29(6):345–347.

Paterson DL, Rihs JD, Squier C, et al. Lack of efficacy of mupirocin in the prevention of infections with Staphylococcus aureus in liver transplant recipients and candidates. *Transplantation* 2003;75(2):194–198.

Peleg AY, Husain S, Qureshi ZA, et al. Risk factors, clinical characteristics, and outcome of Nocardia infection in organ transplant recipients: a matched case-control study. *Clin Infect Dis* 2007;44(10):1307–1314. Epub 2007 Apr 3.

Santoro-Lopes G, de Gouvêa EF, Monteiro RC, et al. Colonization with methicillin-resistant *Staphylococcus aureus* after liver transplantation. *Liver Transpl* 2005;11(2):203–209.

Schneider CR, Buell JF, Gearhart M, et al. Methicillin-resistant *Staphylococcus aureus* infection in live transplantation: a matched controlled study. *Transplant Proc* 2005;37(2):1243–1244.

Schutze GE, Mason EO Jr., Wald ER, et al. Pneumococcal infections in children after transplantation. *Clin Infect Dis* 2001;33(1):16–21.

Sligl W, Taylor G, Brindley PG. Five years of nosocomial Gram-negative bacteremia in a general intensive care unit: epidemiology, antimicrobial susceptibility patterns, and outcomes. *Int J Infect Dis* 2006. Jul;10(4):320–325.

Strauss G, Mogensen AM, Rasmussen A, et al. Staphylococcal scalded skin syndrome in a liver transplant patient. *Liver Transpl Surg* 1997;3(4):435–436.

Wiesmayr S, Stelzmueller I, Tabarelli W, et al. Nocardiosis following solid organ transplantation: a single-centre experience. *Transpl Int* 2005;18(9):1048–1053.

Woeste G, Zapletal C, Wullstein C, et al. Influence of methicillin-resistant *Staphylococcus aureus* carrier status in liver transplant recipients. *Transplant Proc* 2005;7(4):1710–1712.

Yoon TY, Jung SK, Chang SH. Cellulitis due to *Escherichia coli* in three immunocompromised subjects. *Br J Dermatol* 1998;139(5):885–888.

VIRAL DISEASE IN TRANSPLANTATION

Viral pathogens have emerged as the most significant microbial agents infecting solid organ transplant (SOT) recipients. Cytomegalovirus (CMV) is the most common opportunistic organism encountered during the 1- to 6-month posttransplantation period of maximal immunosuppression. Prophylactic regimens have been carefully developed to counter its virulence. Several other viruses manifest at mucocutaneous sites during this period, ranging from cosmetically disfiguring facial molluscum contagiosum virus (MCV) lesions to extensive common or genital warts due to human papillomavirus (HPV) to life-threatening or invasive HPV-induced squamous cell carcinoma. In the great majority of cases, viral opportunistic infection (OI) represents reactivation of latent viral infection, that is, herpes family of viruses or of subclinical infection with HPV or MCV.

Herpetoviridae (human herpesviruses)

The human herpesviruses (HHV) – herpes simplex virus (HSV) types 1 and 2, cytomegalovirus (CMV), varicella-zoster virus (VZV), Epstein-Barr virus (EBV), and human herpesvirus 6, 7, 8 (HHV-6, HHV-7, HHV-8) – share three characteristics that make them particularly effective pathogens in the compromised host: latency, cell association, and oncogenicity. *Latency* refers to the fact that once infected with the virus, the individual remains infected for life, with immunosuppression being the major factor responsible for reactivation of the virus from a latent state. These viruses are highly *cell associated*, rendering humoral immunity inefficient as a host defense and cell-mediated immunity paramount in the control of these infections. All herpes group viruses should be regarded as potentially oncogenic, with the clearest demonstration of this being EBV-related lymphoproliferative disease. Of the herpes group viruses, those with the greatest impact on the mucocutaneous tissues of the compromised host are HSV, VZV, CMV, HHV-8, and, to a lesser extent, EBV.

Herpes simplex virus (HSV) -1 and -2

The greater majority of HSV-1 and HSV-2 infections occurring in the compromised host are reactivations of latent infections of the oropharynx or genitalia. They typically occur within the first 3 months following transplantation, with up to 50% in the first 3 weeks. Pretransplant HSV seropositivity in SOT recipients is said to mirror that of the general population, with higher percentages seen in liver and kidney transplantees as compared to cardiac transplantees, given the lower mean age at transplantation in cardiac patients. In latency, viral genetic material persists in host tissues without the formation of virus particles or clinical infection. Reactivation results in disease manifestation or silent viral shedding. Risk factors for HSV reactivation include physical trauma, immunosuppression, severe illness with intubation, and surgical manipulation of the trigeminal root ganglion. The degree of reactivation is common, with 40% to 50% noted in some studies. In some instances, oral reactivation can be detected by polymerase chain reaction (PCR) with only 1 out of 12 patients demonstrating clinical disease.

Recurrent HSV is characterized by an itching or tingling sensation at the site, often before any visible alteration. Ulcerated, crusted lesions in perioral, anogenital, or digital locations are usually HSV in etiology, in spite of occasional atypical clinical appearances in SOT patients. With increasing immunosuppression, recurrent HSV infection may become persistent and progressive, forming large, deep ulcers. Large atrophic scars remain even after these lesions heal. Herpetic infection of one or more fingers can form large, painful whitlows. HSV can then be inoculated into nearly any site including the ears and toes. Local spread can occur from the oropharynx onto esophageal mucosa or lower respiratory tract and from the anogenital area to rectal tissue.

Primary HSV infection after organ transplantation is less common, but in the background of immunosuppression, it can have a more fulminant presentation such as acute liver failure in the liver transplant recipient. Both primary and reactivated HSV can result in dissemination to visceral organs. Disseminated HSV can involve the skin, or, of more concern, the viscera – particularly the lungs, liver, and brain. This is associated with significant morbidity and mortality. Reactivation is not associated with patient or allograft mortality except in the setting of CMV co-infection, which results in reduced patient and allograft survival. Rarely, HSV-negative recipients of an HSV-positive graft can develop fulminant HSV infections presenting as febrile illness in the absence of cutaneous lesions. As such, HSV should be included in the differential diagnosis of isolated febrile illnesses in the setting of HSV-negative SOT recipients. In addition, HSV hepatitis can present indirectly as disseminated intravascular coagulation with fever, abdominal pain, and elevated transaminases. Clearly, a high level of suspicion is warranted.

HSV can be diagnosed by isolation of the virus or identification of HSV antigen on lesional smears or biopsy specimens. If indicated, the isolate can be tested for sensitivity to various antiviral agents. Multinucleated giant epidermal cells on histopathology are indicative of HSV or VZV infection. A Tzanck smear looks for giant epithelial or adnexal cells, preferably multinucleated, after scraping the base of the lesions. This test is useful but is not always positive even in frank herpetic lesions; its reliability is completely dependent on the skill of the practitioner and microscopist. Lesional biopsy is helpful when it demonstrates giant epidermal cells, but cannot distinguish HSV from VZV infection. Viral culture of a lesion has a high yield in making the diagnosis. The PCR can detect VZV and HSV DNA sequences from a variety of sources including formalin-fixed tissue specimens.

Currently, three drugs are available for oral therapy of HSV infections: famciclovir, valaciclovir, and acyclovir. These agents can be given to treat primary or reactivated infection or prophylactically to suppress reactivation. Intravenous acyclovir (5 mg/kg every 8 hours) may be given for severe infections. Improved bioavailability of famciclovir and valaciclovir makes oral therapy with these agents preferable to oral acyclovir. Foscarnet, cidofovir, and trifluridine are administered intravenously for infections caused by acyclovir-resistant HSV. Cidofovir is a broad-spectrum antiviral medication with efficacy against HSV, human papilloma virus (HPV), VZV, EBV, HHV-6, -7, and –8, and pox-, polyoma-, and adenoviruses. Cidofovir gel has been effective as a topical therapy for acyclovir-resistant HSV infections. The use of chronic HSV suppression is controversial. In the management of chronic herpetic ulcers, immunosuppressive therapy should be reduced when possible. Fortunately, acyclovir resistance has not been as commonly seen in the transplant population as in the HIV population. In a study of acyclovir susceptibilities in 18 SOT patients after viral prophylaxis with either acyclovir or ganciclovir, all isolates were susceptible. Prophylaxis can be achieved with acyclovir, valacyclovir, or famciclovir.

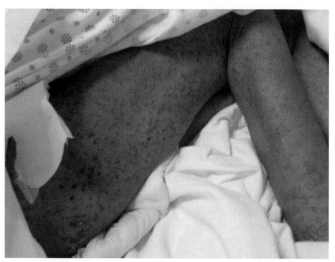

Figure 14v.1 Multiple vesicles and punched-out erosions in a patient with AIDS, concentrated over dermatome but extending over the entire body – consistent with disseminated zoster.

Varicella-zoster virus (VZV)

Varicella is the most contagious of the human herpes viruses. Two percent to 5% of adult SOT recipients are VZV seronegative, with a greater number of seronegative children. Primary VZV infection manifests as varicella (chickenpox) while reactivation of VZV in seropositive patients occurs from a dorsal root ganglion or cranial nerve ganglion and manifests as herpes zoster (HZ). In the compromised adult host, VZV disease is almost always due to reactivation. In these individuals, VZV can present as severe varicella, dermatomal HZ, disseminated HZ (sometimes without dermatomal HZ), and chronic or recurrent HZ (Figs. 14v.1 and 14v.2). The first manifestation of zoster is often pain and paresthesias in the dermatome that subsequently manifests as the classical grouped vesicles on an erythematous base. Disseminated HZ is defined as more than 20 lesions outside of two contiguous dermatomes, or systemic infection (hepatitis, pneumonitis, encephalitis, pancreatitis, and disseminated intravascular coagulation). Occasionally, in SOT patients, the dermatomal eruption may be bullous, hemorrhagic, necrotic, and can be accompanied by severe pain.

Rarely, reactivation of VZV can produce pain without any cutaneous lesions (zoster sine Herpe). The compromised host previously infected with VZV is still subject to exogenous reinfection with VZV. Overall, zoster occurs in 5% to 15% of SOT patients, usually within the first year post transplantation but later than HSV or CMV (median onset of 9 –14 months).

In this chronically immunosuppressed group, risk of dissemination is as high as 40%. Despite antiviral therapy, mortality rates range from 4% to 34%. The most common complications are cutaneous scarring (18.7%) and postherpetic neuralgia (PHN) (42.7%), defined as pain persisting for more than 6 weeks after the development of cutaneous lesions. In SOT patients, complications from reactivated VZV tend to be more severe, including progressive small-vessel encephalitis or central nervous system myelitis. Ophthalmic zoster has the highest incidence of serious complications, which include corneal ulceration, variable decrease of visual acuity, and retinal necrosis.

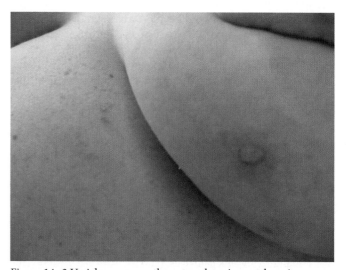

Figure 14v.2 Vesicles on an erythematous base in an otherwise healthy woman, consistent with primary varicella.

Viscerally disseminated HZ in a compromised host can be life threatening, involving the lung and liver. It manifests as fever, abdominal pain, disseminated intravascular coagulation, and hepatitis, with or without concomitant pancreatitis or pneumonitis, and is considered an emergency. The development of cutaneous lesions is often delayed, and PCR can be helpful in confirming the diagnosis in the absence of visible lesions.

In the immunocompromised patient, reactivated cutaneous VZV lesions can persist for months, in either the localized or the disseminated form, as chronic verrucous or ecthymatous VZV infection. The lesions consist of hyperpigmented and/or hyperkeratotic painful nodules often with central crusting, ulceration and/or bordering vesicles. Verrucous/ecthymatous VZV was first described in HIV patients, typically those with low CD4 counts (<100/mm^3). There are now reports in the literature of verrucous VZV following kidney transplantation on tacrolimus and prednisolone.

Primary VZV after SOT is rare and tends to present later, usually, within 3 years, depending on exposure. It is more commonly seen in the pediatric transplant population. Primary varicella in immunosuppressed children and adults can be severe, prolonged, and complicated by internal dissemination (pneumonia, hepatitis, encephalitis, and pancreatitis), disseminated intravascular coagulation, bacterial superinfection, and death.

The diagnosis of varicella and HZ can be made clinically, but as with HSV, the diagnosis can be confirmed by detection of viral antigen on a smear of the base of a lesion or in a biopsy. A positive Tzanck test confirms the diagnosis of either VZV or HSV. Isolation of VZV by culture is more difficult than isolation of HSV. Lesional biopsy is also helpful in establishing a diagnosis, especially in unusual manifestations of VZV infection such as ecthymatous or chronic verrucous lesions. The diagnosis can be confirmed by detection of VZV antigen on direct immunofluorescence testing. Immunoglobulin serologies are now routinely screened before transplantation and there are reported rates of 1.6% VZV serology-negative patients. It is important to note that a negative VZV serology does not necessarily preclude prior infection, and that these patients can still manifest herpes zoster.

The drugs approved for treatment of HSV are also effective for treatment of VZV infection: famciclovir, valaciclovir, and acyclovir. Intravenous acyclovir (10 mg/kg every 8 hours) is given for severe zoster or primary varicella. As with HSV infections, acyclovir-resistant strains can emerge following prolonged acyclovir treatment; most of these resistant strains respond to foscarnet, cidofovir, or trifluridine therapy.

The routine antiviral prophylaxis used for preventing CMV disease appears to reduce CMV-induced mortality but does not affect the incidence of zoster. Prophylactic regimens for zoster are not practical because of late onset of disease and low proportion of affected individuals.

Varicella vaccination in the SOT population has slowly been emerging as more evidence indicates its safety. Seropositive-bone marrow transplant (BMT) patients immunized with the vaccine had greater protection from varicella. Vaccination is currently recommended before transplantation in children and adolescents. Pretransplantation vaccination has been successful in inducing seroconversion, though transplantation must then be postponed for 3 months to avoid iatrogenic immunosuppression following vaccination. While live attenuated Oka strain vaccination is not FDA-approved for use in immunocompromised individuals because of the risk of potential disseminated varicella and isolated reports of acute graft rejection, the vaccine has been safely used post transplantation in adults and children. One study evaluating use post renal transplantation demonstrated no adverse effects and a 66% rate of seroconversion. Vaccination post transplantation can induce suboptimal immunogenicity, with protection waning each year after vaccination in some individuals. In these individuals, any subsequent disease is usually mild; alternatively, a second "booster" vaccine dose can be administered. Some series report maximal protection at 1 year post vaccination. In addition, postponing pediatric SOT live vaccinations until at least 1 year of age improves seroconversion and diminishes vaccine side effects, though some recommend starting the vaccination process at an earlier age and at a faster rate. Zostavax, the vaccine approved for zoster prophylaxis in immunocompetent adults aged 60 or older contains a significantly higher dose of live virus than the vaccine for varicella and has not been described or recommended for transplant patients. Unvaccinated, seronegative individuals should avoid exposure to individuals with varicella or zoster. Should contact occur, varicella-zoster immune globulin (VariZIG) should be administered within 96 hours of exposure, but may not have efficacy once clinical disease develops.

Ideally, a pretransplant program should assess individual immunity and vaccinate any susceptible individuals. In addition, immunization of household contacts and healthcare workers should take place.

Epstein-Barr virus (EBV)

EBV selectively infects cells of the B-lymphocyte lineage and certain types of squamous epithelium. The majority of adults have been infected with EBV and harbor the latent virus. Primary cutaneous EBV-associated posttransplant lymphoproliferative disorder (PTLD) is the most common severe manifestation of EBV in SOT patients. PTLD can present in several ways including isolated or multiple lymphoid tumors, an infectious mononucleosis-like pattern, generalized lymphadenopathy, and rapidly progressive and widespread disease. PTLD can be seen in any organ site and the incidence ranges depending on organ type from 1% of renal transplant patients to 5% of heart–lung transplant recipients. Disease localized to the skin is even rarer and the appearance is polymorphic: single or multiple erythematous nodules, ulcers, or morbiliform eruptions. At the onset, PTLD is polyclonal and often responds to a reduction of immunosuppression. The disease can become a rapidly progressive and ultimately fatal monoclonal disease. Predisposition to developing PTLD is intimately related to CMV infection and CMV D$^{+/}$ R$^-$ SOT patients are most susceptible.

Posttransplant cutaneous B-cell lymphoma, associated with EBV infection, is an uncommon complication of SOT. Findings are usually confined to the limited regions of the skin; systemic involvement is not common. Treatment is usually directed at the lesions, with surgery or radiotherapy.

Cytomegalovirus

Cytomegalovirus (CMV) is the major microbial pathogen in SOT patients. Pathogenicity is by (1) causing infectious disease syndromes, (2) augmenting iatrogenic immunosuppression via cytokine and chemokine production, and (3) contributing to graft failure. CMV infection occurs in 20% to 60% of all transplant recipients, the rate of infection being related to the serologic status of both the donor and recipient and the degree of immunosuppression. The CMV-seronegative recipients of organs from seropositive donors (CMV D$^{+/}$ R$^-$ patients) develop primary disease and represent the highest risk group. The highest incidence of immunosuppression and CMV disease is seen in heart–lung transplant recipients, followed by pancreas and kidney–pancreas, and finally kidney, heart, or liver transplants alone.

Seroprevalence studies of CMV infection indicate that 50% of the general population is infected by age 50 years. Primary infection is usually asymptomatic, but can produce symptoms of fever, pneumonitis, esophagitis, colitis, myalgias, leukopenia, thrombocytopenia, and transaminitis. Following primary infection, CMV enters a latent phase of infection, during which asymptomatic viral shedding in saliva, semen, and/or urine is extremely common. In the compromised host, CMV disease occurs via (1) primary CMV infection, (2) reactivation of latent CMV infection, or (3) re-infection with a new CMV subtype. As with the other members of the herpesvirus family, CMV disease usually represents reactivation of latent virus. This typically occurs in the first 3 months post transplantation when immunosuppression is most intense.

Reactivated CMV can cause hepatitis, pneumonitis, chorioretinitis, encephalitis, and colitis/esophagitis in transplant recipients. Cutaneous CMV infections are rare, presenting as nodules, ulcers, plaques, vesicles, petechiae/purpura, bullous lesions, or nonspecific maculopapular exanthems. Cutaneous ulcers and morbilliform eruptions are the most common presentation of cutaneous CMV involvement. Cutaneous manifestations may be seen in 10% to 20% of systemic CMV infections and are associated with a poor prognosis. This association has been postulated to be a marker of severe immune compromise as CMV generally does not replicate well in the dermis.

Chronic CMV infection predisposes the SOT patient to acute and chronic graft failure, as well as secondary immune deficiency and further risk of opportunistic infections.

Infection can be detected by a greater than four-fold increase in CMV IgG or on culture from urine, skin, respiratory secretions, or blood. Skin and other organ biopsy will demonstrate characteristic "owl-eye" inclusion bodies, or CMV can be demonstrated by immunoperoxidase staining of tissue. PCR is considered to be the "gold standard" of diagnostic methods, with a sensitivity of 95% to 100% but low specificity.

Treatment of choice for CMV is intravenous valganciclovir for 2 to 3 weeks. Prophylactic regimens can be used and the standard is ganciclovir (15 mg/kg TID × 14–90 days). Oral prophylaxis with both ganciclovir and valganciclovir is effective at decreasing the incidence of infection in the CMV $D^{+/}$ R^- SOT group. As a side benefit, the prophylactic regimen helps control other herpes virus family members such as HSV, VZV, and even EBV. More recently, late onset CMV infections occurring a year after transplantation suggest the need to alter the length of prophylaxis regimen to extend for a longer period. Doing so, however, has been shown to delay disease onset and elicit atypical presentations of disease. In addition, this practice may increase rates of viral resistance, and ganciclovir-resistant strains cause severe disease with increased graft loss and mortality. The reported incidence of ganciclovir-resistant infections in SOT patients on prophylactic regimens ranges from is up to 13%. Use of hyperimmune CMV globulin (CMVIG) alone does not provide sufficient prophylaxis in SOT patients, but can diminish the severity of disease in this patient population. It has demonstrated efficacy when used in combination with ganciclovir. For resistant virus strains, foscarnet 40 mg/kg IV every 8 hours is employed. Its use is limited by nephrotoxicity.

Human herpesvirus-8

Kaposi's sarcoma (KS) is a proliferation of endothelium-derived cells, first reported by Moritz Kaposi in 1872 as "idiopathic pigmented sarcoma of the skin." Classical KS occurs in men of Mediterranean or Eastern European origin. African KS was described in young patients from equatorial Africa. In the 1960s, a third variant of iatrogenic KS was described in patients on long-term immunosuppressive therapy but became most strongly associated with the HIV/AIDS epidemic as a marker of end-stage AIDS. The prevalence of KS in SOT is anywhere from 0.1% to 5%, depending on the type of immunosuppression, HHV-8 status of donor and recipient, and country of origin.

HHV-8 is a lymphotropic, oncogenic herpesvirus that was first detected in KS in 1994. HHV-8 has also been detected in other neoplasms such as body cavity–based lymphoma and Castleman's tumor. Reported cases of HHV-8 transfer from donor to recipient in heart and lung transplantations with resulting KS also strongly implicate this member of the herpesvirus family as the cause of SOT-associated KS.

The clinical course of SOT-associated KS may be quite variable with frequent occurrence of widespread cutaneous and visceral lesions. Early lesions of KS present as slight discolorations of the skin, usually barely palpable papules, and, if very early, macules. Over a period of weeks-to-months-to-years, these early lesions enlarge into nodules or frank tumors, and the color darkens to a violaceous, Concord grape color, often with a yellow-green halo. As lesions enlarge, epidermal changes may occur, showing a shiny, atrophic appearance if stretched, or, at times, hyperkeratosis with scale formation. In late lesions, tumor necrosis may occur with erosion or ulceration of the surface. Oral lesions are common, and may be the first site of involvement, occurring typically on the hard palate as a violaceous stain of the mucosa.

The course of KS depends upon restitution of immune function. Few patients die from complications directly related to KS. An occasional patient will develop KS lesions involving internal organs in the absence of any visible mucocutaneous involvement. Although the diagnosis of KS can usually be suspected clinically, in most instances histological diagnosis on a lesional punch biopsy specimen can be done.

In the management of KS, the initial therapeutic focus is reduction in immune compromise by changing immunosuppressive drug therapies. In particular, the addition of rapamycin as an immunosuppressant in place of other drugs such as cyclosporine has been associated with regression of KS. Localized cutaneous disease can be approached with application of an intralesional injection of vinblastine, cryotherapy, surgical excision, or radiation. Indolent, disseminated cutaneous KS is best treated with systemic immunotherapy or chemotherapy.

Molluscum contagiosum virus

MCV commonly infects keratinized skin subclinically, and can cause lesions at sites of minor trauma and in the infundibular portion of the hair follicle. Transmission is usually via skin-to-skin contact, occurring commonly in children and sexual partners. MCV infection is common in SOT patients with a reported 6.9% incidence in pediatric transplant patients.

Clinically, MCV infection presents as skin-colored papules or nodules, often with a characteristic central umbilicated keratotic plug. Lesions larger than one centimeter in diameter (giant molluscum), can be seen in the immunosuppressed population. In males, lesions are often confined to the beard area, the skin having been inoculated during the process of shaving.

Therapeutically, the most efficacious approach toward MCV infection is correction of the underlying immunodeficiency. Otherwise, treatment is directed at controlling the numbers and bulk of cosmetically disturbing lesions. Liquid nitrogen cryospray is the most convenient therapy, and usually must be repeated every 2 to 4 weeks. Imiquimod 5% cream has also demonstrated success in healthy and immunocompromised patients. The molecule binds Toll-like receptor 7, activating dendritic cells, macrophages, and monocytes, leading to Th1 cytokine production and local stimulation of both cell-mediated and innate immune responses. Side effects include an expected, mild erythema at the site of application, and while systemic immune stimulation has been reported, it has not been substantiated.

Human papillomavirus infections

Subclinical infection with human papillomavirus (HPV) is nearly universal in humans. With immunocompromise, cutaneous and/or mucosal HPV infection reemerges from latency, presenting clinically as verruca, condyloma acuminatum, squamous cell carcinoma in situ (SCCIS), or invasive squamous cell carcinoma (SCC). HPV colonizes keratinized skin producing common warts (verruca vulgaris, verruca plantaris) in many healthy individuals. The greater majority of sexually active individuals are subclinically infected with one or multiple HPV types. HPV-6 and -11 infect mucosal sites (genitalia, anus, perineum, oropharynx) and cause genital warts (condyloma acuminatum); HPV-16 and -18 have greater malignant potential and can cause precancerous lesions, squamous intraepithelial lesion (SIL), SCCIS, and invasive SCC. A significant number of SOT candidates are HPV-positive before transplantation. Chronic immunosuppression can increase the likelihood of progression to and persistence of clinical lesions. In addition, the incidence of these lesions increases as the duration and degree of suppression increases.

In SOT recipients and other compromised hosts, the initial morphology, number, or response to treatment of verrucae are not atypical. They are, however more often distributed over sun-exposed sites in adults. With time, verrucae can enlarge, become confluent, and become unresponsive to therapy. The incidence and severity of warts are related to the degree of immunosuppression, with previously acquired latent virus being reactivated with institution of immunosuppressive therapy. Warts are the most common skin finding in pediatric SOT population, affecting 53.8%. The prevalence in renal transplant patients increases with length of immunosuppression, from 11% in first year post transplantation, to as high as 92% in >5 years of immunosuppression. Verruca vulgaris and verruca plantaris appear as well-demarcated keratotic papules or nodules, usually with multiple tiny red-brown dots representing thrombosed capillaries; palmar and plantar warts characteristically interrupt the normal dermatoglyphics. The warts may be numerous and confluent, giving the appearance of a mosaic. Verruca plana, or flat warts, appear as well-demarcated, flat-topped papules, which lack the dots seen in other types of verrucae. When occurring in the beard area, hundreds of flat warts may be present. All types of verrucae may have a linear arrangement because of koebnerization or autoinoculation.

Condylomata acuminata or genital warts are usually asymptomatic, although voluminous lesions may be painful and may bleed. Lesions may be numerous and become confluent. Oropharyngeal HPV-induced lesions resemble anogenital condyloma, pink or white in color. Extensive intraoral condyloma acuminatum (oral florid papillomatosis) presents as multiple large plaques, analogous to anogenital giant condylomata acuminata of Buschke–Löwenstein, and can also transform to verrucous carcinoma.

In compromised patients, HPV-induced lesions have the potential for malignant transformation, particularly in sun-exposed areas of the body. Squamous cell carcinoma (SCC) arising in sites of chronic sun exposure occurs 36 times more frequently in renal transplant recipients than in the general population, some clearly arising within warts. HPV DNA is demonstrable within the tumors and is detected more frequently in SCC arising in transplant recipients than in immunocompetent individuals. Ultraviolet radiation in combination with immunosuppression can activate HPV. Rapidly enlarging hyperkeratotic verrucae should also be investigated for transformation to rule out squamous cell carcinoma.

As many as 23% of newly transplanted patients are anal HPV positive, with this number more than doubling in established SOT patients. HPV-induced anogenital in-situ and invasive squamous cell carcinoma (SCC) is also ten times more common in transplant recipients and HIV-infected individuals; these persons should be screened for in situ and invasive SCC with Pap test of the anus and cervix and lesional biopsy when indicated. The appearance of white micropapules or macules after the application of 5% acetic acid (white vinegar) to the anogenital epithelium or "acetowhitening," can be helpful in defining the extent of HPV infection.

Efficacy of treatment of verrucae vulgaris and condyloma acuminatum in SOT patients varies with the degree of immunocompromise, and can be very recalcitrant. In patients with early disease, these lesions should be managed as in the normal host. Cryotherapy remains a common choice but for extensive lesions, management includes bleomycin injections, topical salicylic acid, topical retinoids, laser ablation, curettage and dessication, cimetidine, podophyllotoxin, intralesional interferon, or a combination of the above. More recently, imiquimod has been introduced for condyloma, and studies suggest safe usage in SOT population. Topical and intralesional cidofovir has also demonstrated efficacy in SOT patients with HPV-associated skin lesions. The role of chemoprevention with systemic retinoids still awaits final determination. Management of patients with extensive warts should include avoidance of sun exposure, use of strong sunscreens, reduction in immunosuppressive therapy when possible, and careful observation for the development of malignant lesions. Prophylactic vaccination in transplant candidates may be of value to prevent primary HPV infection. In some cases, modification of the immunosuppressive regimen can help modify the size and number of warts in SOT patients. Ultimately, immunosuppressed patients may never completely clear their HPV, and lesions often recur.

PITFALLS AND MYTHS

The opportunity to identify an infection in the immunosuppressed population is often hindered by the subtlety of the skin findings and the absence of common signs of infection. Classically, skin infections are characterized by rubor, calor, tenderness, and/or edema of the affected areas. These signs and the clinical features of a rash can be reduced or absent in individuals who are unable to mount a full immune response to infection.

As such, it is important to vigilantly monitor the skin for any changes and to evaluate all new or changing lesions with skin culture, biopsy, and tissue stains as appropriate. Concern for a deep tissue infection warrants obtaining a sterile skin biopsy for tissue culture.

Obtaining a prompt diagnosis and rapid intervention may be hindered if biopsy is delayed because of concerns of breach in skin integrity or possible iatrogenic infection. The actual risk of this is very low when the skin is prepared appropriately with alcohol, iodine, chlorhexidine, or other skin cleansing agents and when the biopsy is performed properly with sterile equipment. When possible, obtaining tissue for biopsy or culture should take place from the most cephalad location possible to facilitate wound healing. Postprocedural wound care with newer topical antibiotic agents such as mupirocin or retapamulin will also minimize risk of subsequent infection in this patient population.

SUGGESTED READINGS

Alper S, Kilinc I, Duman S, et al. Skin diseases in Turkish renal transplant patients. *Int J Dermatol* 2005;44(11):939–941.

Ballout A, Goffin E, Yombi JC, et al. Vaccinations for adult solid organ transplant recipient: current recommendations. *Transplant Proc* 2005;37(6):2826–2827.

Barba A, Tessari G, Boschiero L, et al. Renal transplantation and skin diseases: review of the literature and results of a 5-year follow-up of 285 patients. *Nephron* 1996;73(2): 131–136.

Benson E. Imiquimod: potential risk of an immunostimulant. *Australas J Dermatol* 2004;45(2):123–124.

Boivin G, Erice A, Crane DD, et al. Acyclovir susceptibilities of herpes simplex virus strains isolated from solid organ transplant recipients after acyclovir or ganciclovir prophylaxis. *Antimicrob Agents Chemother* 1993;37(2):357–359.

Bonati H, Aigner F, De Clercq E, et al. Local administration of cidofovir for human papilloma virus associated skin lesions in transplant recipients. *Transpl Int* 2007;20(3):238–246.

Brown CL, Atkins CL, Ghali L, et al. Safety and efficacy of 5% Imiquimod cream for the treatment of skin dysplasia in high-risk renal transplant recipients: randomized, double-blind, placebo-controlled trial. *Arch Dermatol* 2005;141(8):985–993.

Capaldi L, Robinson-Bostom L, Kerr P, et al. Localized cutaneous posttransplant Epstein-Barr virus-associated lymphoproliferative disorder. *J Am Acad Dermatol* 2004;51(5): 778–780.

Chaves S, Lopes MH, de Souza VA, et al. Seroprevalence of antibodies against varicella-zoster virus and response to the varicella vaccine in pediatric renal transplant patients. *Pediatr Transplant* 2005;9(2):192–196.

Collart F, Kerbaul F, Damaj G, et al. Visceral Kaposi's sarcoma associated with human herpesvirus 8 seroconversion in a heart transplant recipient. *Transplant Proc* 2004;36(10): 3173–3174.

Cunha BA, Eisenstein LE, Dillard T, et al. Herpes simplex virus pneumonia in a heart transplant: diagnosis and therapy. *Heart Lung* 2007;36(1):72–78.

Dharancy S, Catteau B, Mortier L, et al. Conversion to sirolimus: a useful strategy for recalcitrant cutaneous viral warts in liver transplant recipient. *Liver Transpl* 2006;12(12):1883–1887.

Dunn DL, Matas AJ, Fryd DS, et al. Association of concurrent herpes simplex virus and cytomegalovirus with detrimental effects after renal transplantation. *Arch Surg* 1984;119(7): 812–817.

Eid AJ, Brown RA, Razonable RR. Toll-like receptor-2 Arg753Gln polymorphism and herpes virus infections in transplantation. *Transplantation*. 2006;82(10):1383–1385.

Euvard S, Kanitakis J, Cochat P, et al. Skin diseases in children with organ transplants. *J Am Acad Dermatol*. 2001;44(6): 932–939.

Euvrard S, Kanitakis J, Cochat P, et al. Skin diseases in children with organ transplants. *J Am Acad Dermatol* 2001;44(6):932–939.

Fehr T, Bossart W, Wahl C, et al. Disseminated varicella infection in adult renal allograft recipients: four cases and a review of the literature. *Transplantation* 2002;73(4):608–611.

Gardner LS, Ormond PJ. Treatment of multiple giant molluscum contagiosum in a renal transplant patient with imiquimod 5% cream. *Clin Exp Dermatol* 2006;31(3):452–453.

Geel AL, Landman TS, Kal JA, et al. Varicella zoster virus serostatus before and after kidney transplantation, and vaccination of adult kidney transplant candidates. *Transplant Proc* 2006;38(10):3418–3419.

Geel AL, Zuidema W, van Gelder T, et al. Successful vaccination against varicella zoster virus prior to kidney transplantation. *Transplant Proc* 2005;37(2):952–953.

Gilden DH, Kleinschmidt-DeMasters BK, LaGuardia JJ, et al. Neurologic complications of the reactivation of varicella-zoster virus. *N Engl J Med* 2000;342(9):635–645.

Gilson IH, Barnett JH, Conant MA, et al. Disseminated ecthymatous herpes varicella-zoster virus infection in patients with acquired immunodeficiency syndrome. *J Am Acad Dermatol* 1989;20(4): 637–642.

Gourishankar S, McDermid JC, Jhangri GS, et al. Herpes zoster infection following solid organ transplantation: incidence, risk factors and outcomes in the current immunosuppressive era. *Am J Transplant* 2004; 4(1):108–115.

Griffiths WJ, Wreghitt TG, Alexander GJ. Reactivation of herpes simplex virus after liver transplantation. *Transplantation* 2005;80(9):1353–1354.

Harwood CA, Perrett CM, Brown VL, et al. Imiquimod cream 5% for recalcitrant cutaneous warts in immunosuppressed individuals. *Br J Dermatol* 2005;152(1):122–129.

Hogewoning AA, Goettsch W, van Loveren H, et al. www.ncbi.nlm.nih.gov/sites/entrez?Db=pubmed &Cmd=ShowDetailView&TermToSearch=11168313& ordinalpos=5&itool=EntrezSystem2.PEntrez. Pubmed. Pubmed_ResultsPanel.Pubmed_RVDocSum Skin infections in renal transplant recipients. *Clin Transplant* 2001;15(1):32–38.

Hoppenjans WB, Bibler MR, Orme RL, et al. Prolonged cutaneous herpes zoster in acquired immunodeficiency syndrome. *Arch Dermatol* 1990;126(8):1048–1050.

Jeyaratnam D, Robson AM, Hextall JM, et al. Concurrent verrucous and varicelliform rashes following renal transplantation. *Am J Transplant* 2005; 5(7):1777–1780.

Johnson R, Stockfleth E. Imiquimod 5% cream for the treatment of cutaneous lesions in immunocompromised patients. *Acta Derm Venereol Suppl (Stockh)* 2003;(214):23–27.

Khan S, Erlichman J, Rand EB. Live virus immunization after orthotopic liver transplantation. *Pediatr Transplant* 2006;10(1):78–82.

Kovach BT, Stasko T. Use of topical immunomodulators in organ transplant recipients. *Dermatol Ther* 2005;18(1):19–27.

Lalezari J, Schacker T, Feinberg J, et al. A randomized, double-blind, placebo-controlled trial of cidofovir gel for the treatment of acyclovir-unresponsive mucocutaneous herpes simplex virus infection in patients with AIDS. *J Infect Dis* 1997;176(4): 892–898.

Luthy KE, Tiedeman ME, Beckstrand RL, et al. Safety of live-virus vaccines for children with immune deficiency. *J Am Acad Nurse Pract* 2006;18(10):494–503.

McGregor JM, Yu CC, Lu QL, et al. Posttransplant cutaneous lymphoma. *J Am Acad Dermatol* 1993;29(4):549–554.

Miller GG, Dummer JS. Herpes simplex and varicella zoster viruses: forgotten but not gone. *Am J Transplant* 2007;7(4):741–747.

Nalesnik MA, Makowka L, Starzl TE. The diagnosis and treatment of posttransplant lymphoproliferative disorders. *Curr Probl Surg* 1988;25(6):367–472.

Nebbia G, Mattes FM, Ramaswamy M, et al. Primary herpes simplex virus type-2 infection as a cause of liver failure after liver transplantation. *Transpl Infect Dis* 2006;8(4):229–232.

Neu AM. Indications for varicella vaccination post-transplant. *Pediatr Transplant* 2005;9(2):141–144.

Pandya A, Wasfy S, Hébert D, et al. Varicella-zoster infection in pediatric solid-organ transplant recipients: a hospital-based study in the prevaricella vaccine era. *Pediatr Transplant* 2001; 5(3):153–159.

Pariser RJ. Histologically specific skin lesions in disseminated cytomegalovirus infection. *J Am Acad Dermatol* 1983;9(6): 937–946.

Patel HS, Silver AR, Northover JM. Anal cancer in renal transplant patients. *Int J Colorectal Dis* 2007;22(1):1–5.

Razonable RR. Epidemiology of cytomegalovirus disease in solid organ and hematopoietic stem cell transplant recipients. *Am J Health Syst Pharm* 2005;62(8 Suppl 1):S7–13.

Razonable RR, Brown RA, Humar A, et al. Herpesvirus infections in solid organ transplant patients at high risk of primary cytomegalovirus disease. *J Infect Dis* 2005;192(8):1331–1339.

Robertson S, Newbigging K, Carman W, et al. Fulminating varicella despite prophylactic immune globulin and intravenous acyclovir in a renal transplant recipient: should renal patients be vaccinated against VZV before transplantation? *Clin Transplant* 2006;20(1):136–138.

Rodriguez-Moreno A, Sanchez-Fructuoso AI, Calvo N, et al. Varicella infection in adult renal allograft recipients: experience at one center. *Transplant Proc* 2006;38(8):2416–2418.

Roka S, Rasoul-Rockenschaub S, Roka J, et al. Prevalence of anal HPV infection in solid-organ transplant patients prior to immunosuppression. *Transpl Int* 2004;17(7): 366–369.

Rowshani AT, Bemelman FJ, van Leeuwen EMM, et al. Clinical and immunologic aspects of cytomegalovirus infection in solid organ transplant recipients. *Transplantation* 2005;79(4):381–386.

Safrin S, Berger TG, Gilson I, et al. Foscarnet therapy in five patients with AIDS and acyclovir-resistant varicella-zoster virus infection. *Ann Intern Med* 1991;115(1):19–21.

Schmook T, Nindl I, Ulrich C, et al. Viral warts in organ transplant recipients: new aspects in therapy. *Br J Dermatol* 2003;149 Suppl 66:20–24.

Slifkin M, Doron S, Snydman DR. Viral prophylaxis in organ transplant patients. *Drugs* 2004;64(24):2763–2792.

Stallone G, Infante B, Grandaliano G, et al. Sirolimus for Kaposi's sarcoma in renal-transplant recipients. *N Engl J Med* 2005;352(13):1317–1323.

Stockfleth E, Nindl I, Sterry W, et al. Human papillomaviruses in transplant-associated skin cancers. *Dermatol Surg* 2004;30(4 Pt 2): 604–609.

Stockfleth E, Nindl I, Sterry W, et al. Human papillomaviruses in transplant-associated skin cancers. *Dermatol Surg* 2004;30(4 Pt 2): 604–609.

Tan HH, Goh CL. Viral infections affecting the skin in organ transplant recipients: epidemiology and current management strategies. *Am J Clin Dermatol* 2006;7(1):13–29.

Verma A, Wade JJ. Immunization issues before and after solid organ transplantation in children. *Pediatr Transplant* 2006;10(5):536–548.

Waite E, Laraque D. Pediatric organ transplant patients and long-term care: a review. *Mt Sinai J Med* 2006;73(8):1148–1155.

Walker RC, Paya CV, Marshall WF, et al. Pretransplantation seronegative Epstein-Barr virus status is the primary risk factor for posttransplantation lymphoproliferative disorder in adult heart, lung, and other solid organ transplantations. *J Heart Lung Transplant* 1995; 14(2):214–221.

Weinberg A, Horslen SP, Kaufman SS, et al. Safety and immunogenicity of varicella-zoster virus vaccine in pediatric liver and intestine transplant recipients. *Am J Transplant* 2006;6(3):565–568.

15 | CANCER PATIENTS AND SKIN INFECTIONS

John C. Hall

The two basic components of cancer therapy have long been chemotherapy and radiation therapy. Both these modalities, especially chemotherapy, were based on the cytotoxic effect they exerted on cancer cells. Their cytotoxicity, of course, carried over to both rapidly dividing normal cells and nonmalignant host cells. The most commonly affected cells were those of the lymphatic and hematopoietic systems. Destruction of these cells, most notably the neutrophil, could leave the patient with less cancer, but it would also leave the patient with less immunity, and therefore, more susceptibility to infection. Death in these patients was frequently due to infection rather than malignancy.

Oncology has now progressed to the point that survival for extended periods of time can take place with control as opposed to eradication of the cancer. Although a patient is less immunocompromised with receptor blockers, monoclonal antibodies, tyrosine kinase inhibitors, antiangiogenic therapy, and therapies yet to be discovered, there is still immune suppression and a larger window of time for infections to develop. There is also a much larger number of patients for whom infection, not cancer, becomes the life-threatening event.

The seminal laboratory finding that is most often associated with these infections is decreased numbers of neutrophils. Also, most of these infections will occur when the neutrophil count is at its lowest. Improvement conversely occurs when the neutrophil count begins to return to normal. Prophylactic antibiotics are often used when the neutrophil count is drastically reduced.

Leukemia and lymphoma are more capable of interfering with neutrophil function and numbers. As a result, both of them are more likely to present with skin infections at the onset. Solid tumors, unless they have extensively invaded the bone marrow, however, are more likely to present with skin infections after chemotherapy has begun and the neutrophil count has been suppressed.

HISTORY

It has longed been recognized that a major cause of morbidity and mortality in cancer patients whether they are on or off therapy is infection. The skin is often the organ where these infections are first apparent.

An excellent example is with leukemia, bacteria, and *Staphylococcus aureus*, which are the commonest malignancy, the most common offending organism, and the most common offending bacteria respectively. In 1980, Sotman et al. examined 370 leukemia cases, 95% of which were granulocytopenic (WBC counts less than 1,000 μL), and found 9% with *Staphylococcus aureus* bacterial infection. The commonest sites for primary infection were the skin and lower respiratory tract.

EPIDEMIOLOGY

Since cancer patients cannot put up a sustained immune response, they tend to acquire whichever organism is present in their environment. An example of this is aspergillosis, which can be stirred up at hospital work sites by construction work. The change of organisms in the community greatly affects the infections these patients acquire just like in the general population. A recent example is cases of infection caused by coagulase-positive *Staphylococcus aureus* that have now been replaced by methicillin-resistant *Staphylococcus aureus* with a new genotype. This has not only changed the antibiotics used to treat cutaneous staphylococcus infections, but has also changed the nature of the infection itself with early abscess formation and the requirement for early surgical incision and drainage to treat cutaneous staphylococcus infections.

DIAGNOSIS

The clinical appearance of these infections may be altered from what is usually seen since a lack of immunity leads to florid growth of the infecting organism. This feature is useful when there is suspicion of an underlying cancer in a previously undiagnosed patient. Any infection that is poorly responsive to therapy (Fig. 15.1), unusually fulminant (Fig. 15.2), or present at a location or in a population that is highly unusual (Fig. 15.3) should be suspect (see Table 15.1). Chronic lymphocytic leukemia is the classic systemic malignancy associated with cutaneous infections. This probably occurs because of the relative frequency of this cancer, its occurrence in the elderly population, the prolonged course before treatment is necessary, and the prolonged course often seen after treatment is begun.

For patients in whom malignancy is already known, the index of suspicion of cutaneous infection rises since chemotherapy decreases the neutrophils in the peripheral blood. The most important principle to remember in these patients is that all tissue biopsy specimens should be sent for culture of acid-fast bacilli, fungi, bacteria in sterile saline as well as viral transport media for herpes simplex and herpes zoster. This should be done even if inflammatory conditions or solid tumors are suspected since the normal clinical signs that are usually thought of in these cases may be absent (Fig. 15.4).

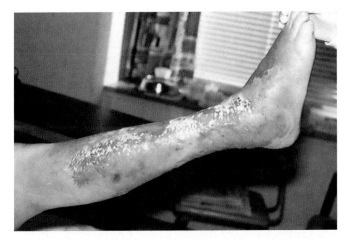

Figure 15.1. Severe cellulitis of the lower extremity poorly responsive to normal dosages of antibiotics that would be expected to be effective. The patient had widespread non–Hodgkin's lymphoma.

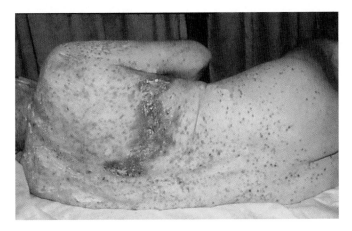

Figure 15.2. Severe herpes zoster infection with dissemination of the virus to involve all the skin in a patient with chronic lymphocytic leukemia.

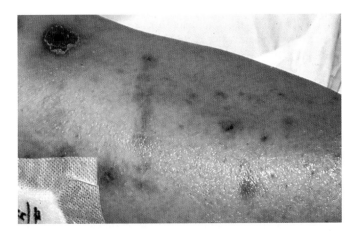

Figure 15.3. Aspergillosis in the skin or the pretibial in a patient with acute myelogenous leukemia. Pulmonary aspergillosis was also diagnosed. Rare cutaneous infection would cause concern for underlying malignant disease.

Table 15.1: Cutaneous Infections That May Be Indicative of an Underlying Cancer

Bacterial Infections

Streptococcus of Streptococcal (group A beta hemolytic) cellulitis: Consider if severe and recurrent and no other explanation is present such as poor circulation.

Viral Infections

Herpes Simplex: Consider if very severe, has run a prolonged course, or is disseminated over wide areas of the skin or internal organs.

Herpes Zoster: If it occurs more than once, is severe, and/or disseminates beyond a dermatomal distribution to become a generalized varicella.

Warts: If they disseminate over large areas of the body or if they appear destructive such as under the nail or over the genitalia. In these two locations, warts may actually become squamous cell cancer. Size over 1 cm is worrisome.

Fungal Infections

Aspergillosis: If the site is cutaneous and occupational exposure is not an issue.

Other organisms that do not usually cause skin infections: Most commonly Rhizopus and Mucor spp. A very long list of saprophytes is also included in this category.

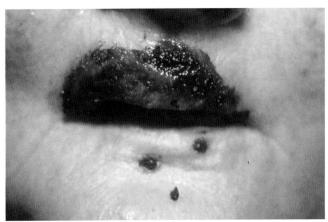

Figure 15.4. Severe necrotic lip lesion caused by herpes simplex in a patient with chronic lymphocytic leukemia. The severity of the infection has caused loss of the normally expected clinical setting of grouped vesicles on a red base.

THERAPY

The therapy for cutaneous infections in cancer patients is similar to the therapy for noncancer patients and the various chapters in this book can be consulted for more specific recommendations. However, some general guidelines can be used (See Table 15.2).

PITFALLS AND MYTHS

Although skin disease morphology may mimic an infection, at times it can actually be a malignancy. As may be expected, the

Table 15.2: Principles of Therapy in Cancer Patients with Cutaneous Infections

1. Therapeutic intervention usually must be continued until the neutrophil count is at least partially restored.

2. Medication dosage often needs to be higher and of a longer duration than in noncancer patients.

3. Local care such as surgical debridement can prevent dissemination and be lifesaving.

4. Therapeutic maneuvers are greatly altered when a noncutaneous nidus of infection is discovered. Therefore, these sites of infection should be searched for vigorously by the clinician.

5. Culture and sensitivity studies of fluids and tissue should help serve as a guide for therapy whenever possible. Specimens for these studies must be collected appropriately, and grown at an appropriate temperature on an appropriate culture media.

6. Staining methods should be used on tissue specimens whenever applicable to help identify potential pathogens. Sometimes polymerase chain reactions and antibody tests are indicated.

7. Prophylactic antibiotics are often given to cancer patients when the neutrophil count drops to a critical level.

Table 15.3: Skin Disease That Appears Infectious but Is Malignant

1. Lymphoma

2. Leukemia

3. Inflammatory breast cancer

4. Stewart–Treves syndrome

5. Angiosarcoma

6. Verrucous carcinoma

7. Lethal midline granuloma (nasal NK/T-cell lymphoma)

8. Squamous cell carcinoma

9. Keratoacanthoma

10. Cancer that is metastatic to the skin

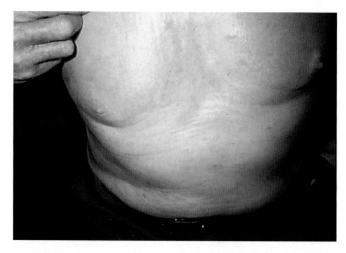

Figure 15.5. Cutaneous T-cell lymphoma (mycosis fungoides) mimicking a cellulitis on the right breast.

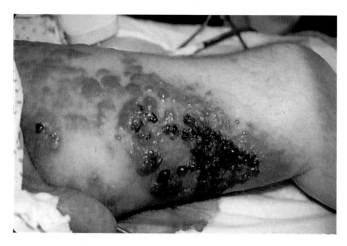

Figure 15.6. Metastatic B-cell lymphoma on the inner thigh. The tumors appear vesicular, seem in a dermatomal distribution, and arose rapidly to mimic a herpes zoster infection.

more vascular cancers look the most like infections due to their increased rubor, swelling, and sometimes increased warmth. Usually, the two most important clinical features are a lack of pain or tenderness and the chronicity of the malignancy. Both infection and cancer can be invasive and destructive. They can also be seen in toxic, febrile patients. Examples of skin malignancies that can mimic infection are given in Table 15.3.

Lymphoma of the skin can either be a metastatic process or a primary lymphoma of the skin, which is usually cutaneous T-cell lymphoma (CTCL). Lymphomas in the skin may have a surrounding acute inflammatory reaction of nonmalignant cells. This causes both clinical confusion with infection (Fig. 15.5) and histologic confusion with infection or other inflammatory processes. Therefore, a superficial biopsy will miss the primary pathology and make the diagnosis of infection seem more likely. Ways to avoid this pitfall include deep punch or ellipse biopsies as well as multiple biopsy attempts if the index for cancer is high. Skin biopsies can easily be repeated since these procedures have little or no morbidity or mortality associated. Special histologic stains may also be helpful in the diagnosis, especially T- and B-cell markers, where monoclonality is often associated with malignancy. Gene rearrangement studies can also be helpful when genetic defects are seen in the cancer. This can only be meaningfully achieved if a large enough number of cells are available for evaluation on the skin biopsy. Lymphoma in the skin can also mimic a vesicular eruption due to the fact that lymphedematous blebs or tumors on the skin mimic blisters (Fig. 15.6). Chronic draining ulcerative, fungating tumors can sometimes mimic a more chronic granulomatous infection (Fig. 15.7) such as deep fungal infections, maduromycosis, lupus vulgaris, or leishmaniasis. Sometimes, an elevated border can even cause confusion with a dermatophyte infection (Fig. 15.8).

Benign inflammation such as from another infection can mimic leukemia cutis because the cells are atypical and share some of the morphologic characteristics of leukemia. This is a very important differentiation. Leukemia when seen in the skin is a very poor prognostic sign. Breast cancer tends to mimic

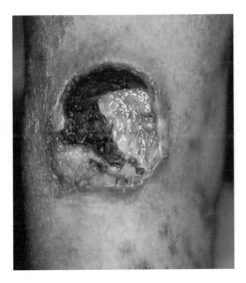

Figure 15.7. Cutaneous T-cell lymphoma on the anterior arm just proximal to the elbow with a chronic fungating, destructive ulcer mimicking a chronic granulomatous skin infection.

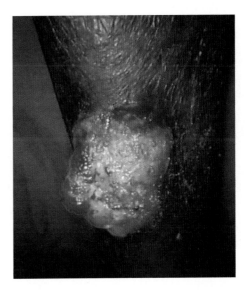

Figure 15.9. Verrucous tumor on the lower leg mimicking a wart but with a size much greater than 1 cm.

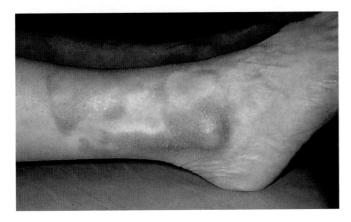

Figure 15.8. Cutaneous T-cell lymphoma on the medial malleolus with an elevated border and central clearing, suggestive of corporis.

infection both as primary inflammatory breast cancer and recurrent metastatic breast cancer. Primary disease is suspicious for infection when axillary lymphadenopathy due to local cancer spread clinically mimics an enlarged lymph node due to cellulitis. Both of these conditions show wide areas of bright red chest wall induration that can be tender and warm. Biopsy is required to make a correct diagnosis.

Stewart–Treves syndrome, which is an angiosarcoma that arises at sites of chronic lymphedema, occurs most notably at sites of mastectomies for breast cancer and axillary lymph node resections. This angiosarcoma is filled with blood vessels that give it a reddish-purple discoloration and also may have associated warmth and pain.

Angiosarcoma usually arises as a primary malignancy without lymphedema on the scalp and head of elderly men. Again, it can mimic an infection due to its great vascularity and redness.

Verrucous carcinoma can occur in three locations. On the bottom of the foot, it is referred to as *epithelioma cuniculatum*. On the genital area, it is referred to as *giant condyloma acuminatum*

of Lowenstein and Buschke. In the oral cavity, it is referred to as *florid oral papillomatosis*. Rarely, it has been reported in the larynx, nasal fossa, back, hands, and lower legs (Fig. 15.9). These tumors are locally aggressive and rarely metastasize. If metastasis does occur, it usually goes to local lymph nodes. It mimics a wart clinically and is most likely viral in origin. Clinically, it eventually becomes more destructive than a wart. Another clue that there is a malignancy is when the size of the lesion is greater than 1 cm. Subungual squamous cell carcinoma may also mimic a wart or arise in a wart especially in the location under the thumbnail. Occupational radiation exposure in physicians holding X-ray plates was once a common etiologic factor.

Lethal midline granulomas were originally thought to be a form of granulomatous vasculitis. They are very destructive midline facial lymphomas. The infection these lesions mimic is a chronic granulomatous infection such a tuberculous lupus vulgaris, deep fungi, or a zygomycosis. Since these lymphomas are chronic and slow growing, they are even more likely to be considered a chronic granulomatous infection. This cancer is often fatal and has been associated with Epstein-Barr virus.

Some malignancies such as squamous cell cancer also mimic slow-growing, chronic granulomatous infections. These infections can be very destructive locally just like malignancies. Location on chronically sun-exposed areas such as the face, ears, dorsal hands, balding scalp in men, and extensor forearms is most common. However, non–sun-exposed skin can also be involved. Long-standing granulomatous infections can develop over time into squamous cell cancer. A histologic pitfall is that epitheliomatous hyperplasia can mimic the overproduction of keratin and squamous cells in malignancies such assquamous cell cancer. Dyskeratotic cells, which are a characteristic sign of squamous cell cancer, can also be seen.

Keratoacanthoma was at one time thought to be a skin infection since there were anecdotal reports of spontaneous resolution. It is now believed, however, that it is a locally aggressive squamous cell cancer without evidence of metastasis caused by chronic sun exposure and occurring on sites of chronic sun

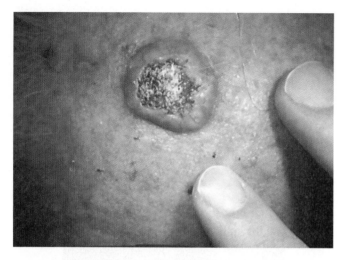

Figure 15.10. Keratoacanthoma of the forehead that grew to this size in a matter of weeks.

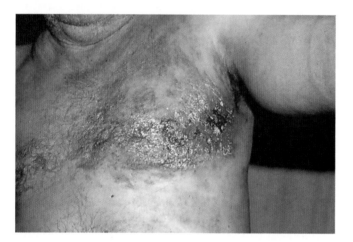

Figure 15.11. Metastatic lung cancer to the skin mimicking herpes zoster or bacterial cellulitis.

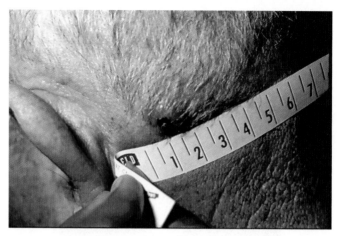

Figure 15.12. Lung cancer metastatic to the skin behind the ear. The central erosion has the clinical appearance of a bacterial furuncle.

Solid tumors metastatic to the skin usually do not have an infectious appearance or growth pattern. However, occasionally a solid tumor metastasis will grow quickly and have an erythematous appearance, therefore mimicking an infection (Fig 15.11). A malignancy can mimic a furuncle in clinical appearance when it erodes into the surface and is covered with a serous or hemorrhagic crust (Fig. 15.12).

There are two important points to remember. First, perform culture and sensitivities on all inflammatory and tumor-like skin lesions in cancer patients so that an infection will not be missed. Second, it is very important to make sure that biopsies are of appropriate depth so that a malignancy is not missed. It is not uncommon for a malignancy in the skin to have surrounding superficial tissue that is inflammatory and benign. In addition, if the suspicion for cancer is high, repeat biopsies should be done.

SUGGESTED READING

Sotman SB, Schimpff SC, Young VM: *Staphylococcus aureus* bacteremia in patients with acute leukemia. *AM J Med* 1980;69(6):814–818.

exposure such as the face (Fig. 15.10), extensor forearms, and hands. Its main confusion with infection relates to the fact that it grows very rapidly unlike squamous cell cancer, which it mimics histologically. It also has a verrucous or warty appearance, which can make differentiation from a viral wart very difficult.

Michelle R. Wanna and Jonathan A. Dyer

INTRODUCTION

The topic of infectious diseases of the skin in children is quite broad, and an exhaustive review in a single chapter is not possible. Those infections with particular importance to pediatric patients will be emphasized.

HISTORY

Cutaneous infections are a major cause of morbidity in the pediatric population. It is estimated that one in five children presenting to their primary care provider have at least one skin complaint, and cutaneous infections represent the largest portion of these complaints. Certain cutaneous infections are unique to or more common in the pediatric population. Most recently, the rise of community-acquired methicillin-resistant staphylococcus aureus (CA-MRSA) and its spread in the pediatric population has highlighted the ever-changing nature of the battle against infectious disease. This chapter will review such conditions.

GRAM-POSITIVE BACTERIA

Impetigo

Impetigo is the most common bacterial skin infection in children, and has two different clinical presentations: nonbullous and bullous. Since the 1980s, nonbullous impetigo, which accounts for at least 70% of the cases, has been caused primarily by *Staphylococcus aureus*. Those infections caused by group A β-hemolytic streptococci (GABHS) cannot be distinguished clinically, but most frequently occur in preschool age children. *Staphylococcus aureus* is the cause of bullous impetigo, and it is most commonly caused by phage group 2, type 71.

Nonbullous impetigo presents as a small vesicle or pustule on sites of prior trauma. This vesicle or pustule then ruptures and results in honey-colored papules and plaques predominantly on the face, neck, and extremities (Fig. 16.1). Children also often have regional lymphadenopathy. Untreated skin lesions may progress slowly, but typically resolve within a 2-week period.

Lesions of bullous impetigo usually occur on nontraumatized skin of the face, trunk, extremities, buttocks, and perineum. They begin as transparent, flaccid bullae that easily rupture, leaving a rim of scale surrounding shallow erosions (Fig. 16.2). Pathophysiologically, these are localized lesions of staphylococcal scalded skin syndrome (SSSS), induced by exfoliative toxin A.

Complications of nonbullous and bullous impetigo include cellulitis, sepsis, septic arthritis, osteomyelitis, and pneumonia.

Cases related to GABHS can result in lymphadenitis, lymphangitis, scarlet fever, guttate psoriasis, and acute poststreptococcal glomerulonephritis. A 2003 Cochrane review analyzed the treatment options for impetigo. Some patients were simply followed and not treated. In patients with limited skin involvement, topical treatments with mupirocin or fusidic acid were at least as effective as, and sometimes more effective than, oral antibiotic therapy. For those with more extensive disease, it was unclear whether oral or topical therapy was more effective, and in cases where oral treatment is warranted, local antibiotic-resistance patterns should be considered when choosing a macrolide, β-lactamase-resistant antibiotic, or cephalosporin. Treatment has no impact on the risk for poststreptococcal glomerulonephritis.

Ecthyma

Ecthyma is caused by GABHS and occurs commonly on the buttocks and lower extremities of children. The lesions begin in a manner similar to that of nonbullous impetigo. A small vesicle or pustule in a previously traumatized area becomes a shallow ulcer. An adherent crust then develops over several days, and healing occurs slowly over weeks, with scar formation. Antibiotics with gram-positive coverage and local wound care are adequate treatments.

Erysipelas

This condition is discussed in Chapter 1.

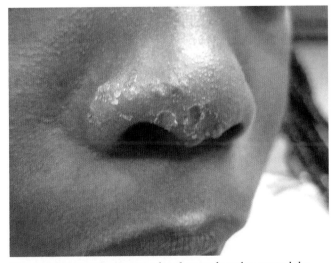

Figure 16.1. Impetigo. Honey-colored crusted patches around the nares.

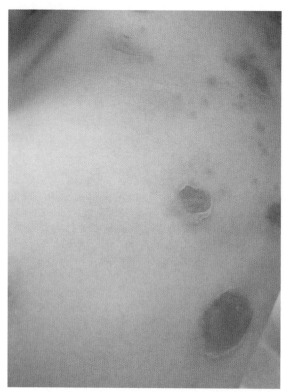

Figure 16.2. Bullous impetigo. Spreading circular superficial erosions, some with honey-colored crusts, others with remaining flaccid bullae roofs at the perimeter. Culture was positive for methicillin-sensitive *staphylococcus aureus*.

Perianal Streptococcal Dermatitis

Perianal streptococcal dermatitis occurs in children aged 6 months to 14 years, with a slight male predominance. The majority of cases are caused by group A β-hemolytic streptococci, although there are reports of streptococci and *S. aureus* as etiologic agents. The dermatitis manifests as a well-demarcated erythema, tenderness, and edema of the perianal area. Painful defecation, incontinence, constipation, anal fissures, blood-streaked stools, pruritus, and drainage may also be present. Vulvovaginitis and balanitis can be associated as well.

Some seasonality of disease with spring and winter predominance is noted, and pharyngeal streptococcal infections have been seen concurrently in more than 90% of cases. This suggests that the disease may be related to oral–perineal autoinoculation or gastrointestinal passage of organisms from the pharynx. Complications include disseminated infection, abscess, proctitis, myositis, and post-streptococcal glomerulonephritis. Infections may trigger guttate psoriasis, and poststreptococcal digital desquamation can also occur.

Swab cultures of the perianal area should be obtained, and some advocate obtaining cultures of family members and close contacts as familial transmission and day care outbreaks have been reported. Urinalysis should also be obtained in suspected cases to rule out glomerulonephritis with repeat testing following the course of treatment. Local resistance patterns should be considered when selecting antibiotic therapy, but a 2- to 3-week course of penicillin V, a macrolide, amoxicillin, amoxicillin/clavulanic acid, or clindamycin is appropriate. Topical antibiotics and antiseptics can also be useful in speeding resolution. Eradication should be ensured with posttreatment swab culture.

Blistering Dactylitis

Blistering distal dactylitis is characterized by 10- to 30-mm bullae containing white fluid of the volar fat pads, most frequently of the hands. Involvement of the toes, however, can be seen as well. It occurs commonly in children up to 16 years of age and is relatively asymptomatic despite the impressive bullae. It is most commonly caused by GABHS, but *S. aureus* and *S. epidermidis* have also been reported as causes. Treatment involves incision and drainage, anti-staphylococcal antibiotics, and wet to dry dressings.

Scarlet Fever

Scarlet fever is caused by GABHS and is most common in children aged 4 to 8. Sources of GABHS include the pharynx, the tonsils, and less frequently the skin. Primary spread of disease is via respiratory droplets. Winter and spring outbreaks are common.

Fever, headache, sore throat, and vomiting occur 1 to 4 days following exposure. Twenty-four to 48 hours later, erythematous patches of the chest, axillae, and infra-auricular areas are seen. These then spread into blanching patches on the trunk, extremities, and face. These patches feel like sandpaper. The oropharynx becomes erythematous and the tongue becomes white with an associated erythema of the papillae. Over the next few days, the white coating resolves, leaving a "strawberry tongue." Cutaneous manifestations are more prominent in body folds and are accompanied by erythematous streaks, or Pastia's lines. Desquamation follows approximately 1 week later.

Leukocytosis with a left shift, eosinophilia, and positive oropharyngeal cultures can be seen on laboratory evaluation. Oral penicillin V or benzathine penicillin intramuscularly is the treatment of choice. Erythromycin can also be used.

Staphylococcal Scalded Skin Syndrome

Staphylococcal scalded skin syndrome (SSSS) typically occurs in children less than 5 years of age and is caused by *Staphylococcus aureus*, phage group II, subtypes 71, 3A, 3B, 3C, and 55. Children usually have signs and symptoms of preceding conjunctivitis or pharyngitis. This is followed by erythematous, tender patches, which develop flaccid bullae with a positive Nikolsky sign on the perineum, axillae, face, and neck. The ruptured bullae reveal an erythematous, moist base. Fever and malaise accompany the cutaneous findings.

This constellation of clinical findings is mediated by exfoliative toxins A and B, which are both produced by *S. aureus*, with toxin A being more prominent. Exfoliative toxin induces cleavage of desmoglein 1, which results in an intraepidermal split at the granular layer. Desmoglein 1 is also the target for related diseases like bullous impetigo, which is also caused by an exfoliative toxin, and pemphigus foliaceus. The mechanism of action for the effect that exfoliative toxin exerts on desmoglein 1 has yet to be elucidated. Some patients with SSSS have detectable anti-desmoglein 1 antibodies, suggesting that the toxin may trigger the desmosomal protein to become a self-antigen, thereby eliciting an immune response.

Treatment involves prompt diagnosis, initiation of antistaphylococcal antibiotics, wound care, and supportive measures. Potential sources of *S. aureus* infection, such as conjunctivitis, an abscess, pneumonia, omphalitis, endocarditis, septic arthritis, or pyomyositis, all of which can act as triggers, should be investigated. Childhood cases carry a mortality rate of 4%.

Toxic Shock Syndrome

This condition is discussed in Chapter 25.

Furuncles and Carbuncles

This condition is discussed in Chapter 1.

Cellulitis

This condition is discussed in Chapter 1.

Periorbital and Orbital Cellulitis

Periorbital cellulitis is an inflammatory process anterior to the orbital septum, which is the continuation of the orbital periosteum between the eyelids, characterized by painless erythema and edema of the eyelid. *S. aureus* and *S. pyogenes* are the most frequent causes, often following periorbital trauma. These are also the two most common bacteria to precede or infections with varicella or herpes simplex virus. Sinusitis and bacteremia related to *Haemophilus influenzae type b* (Hib) or *S. pneumoniae* are also etiologic agents for periorbital cellulitis. Buccal cellulitis is related to bacteremia with these organisms as well. With the advent of the *H. influenzae* type b conjugate vaccines, the incidence of disease related to *H. influenzae* has dropped approximately 90%.

Orbital cellulitis most commonly results from the contiguous spread of bacteria arising from ethmoid sinusitis. It can also occur if the orbital septum is breached by trauma. While it is difficult to isolate the pathogen in either periorbital or orbital cellulitis, *S. aureus*, *S. pyogenes*, Hib, *S. pneumoniae*, and anaerobes are the most commonly identified organisms in orbital cellulitis. Decreased visual acuity, proptosis, and pain should prompt ophthalmologic consultation and radiologic examination with computed tomography. This can be complicated by subperiosteal abscess and cavernous sinus thrombosis.

Clinicians should have a low index of suspicion for meningitis and sepsis. A lumbar puncture should be performed and blood cultures obtained in suspected cases. Treatment with ceftriaxone or cefotaxime in addition to clindamycin is excellent empiric therapy. This treatment regime can also be modified if the pathogenic organism is identified. Parenteral antibiotics and hospitalization are necessary for patients with orbital cellulitis.

Methicillin-resistant community-acquired staphylococcal infection

Skin abscesses less than five centimeters in size in immunocompetent children without systemic symptoms can be treated with incision and drainage alone. A culture of the purulent contents should be obtained. In those patients requiring antibiotic treatment, trimethoprim-sulfamethoxazole (8–12 mg/kg/day trimethoprim and 40–60 mg/kg/day sulfamethoxazole divided BID) or a tetracycline (doxycycline 2–4 mg/kg/day divided BID-QID) is first-line therapy. Treatment of colonization sites, such as the nares, with mupirocin has shown some effectiveness in reducing carriers, but resistance is increasing. Antibacterial soaps and twice weekly bleach baths have also shown improvement. Local resistance patterns should be considered when choosing antibiotic therapy as clindamycin and fluoroquinolone resistance is increasing. Caution should also be used in patients with in vitro erythromycin resistance and clindamycin susceptibility as there are reports of inducible clindamycin resistance, which produce a positive "D-zone" test. Such strains are usually reported as clindamycin resistant. Those patients with systemic symptoms, underlying medical problems, and children less than six months of age are at a higher risk for infection and hospitalization with parenteral therapy may be required. See chapter 1 for a more detailed discussion.

Necrotizing Fasciitis

Necrotizing fasciitis is a rare infection of the subcutaneous tissue and superficial fascia. It can be rapidly fatal. It is more common in adults, but can also be seen in children and neonates. It frequently presents on the trunk or extremities, or is related to omphalitis in infants. The affected area becomes exquisitely tender out of proportion to clinical findings and erythematous, with firm edema and systemic symptoms. The systemic symptoms include fever, hypotension, vomiting, and malaise. Skin lesions can then rapidly become blue-gray with necrosis, hemorrhagic with bullae, anesthetic with destruction of cutaneous nerves, and crepitant. Leukocytosis, anemia, and thrombocytopenia can be seen. Risk factors in children include varicella with GABHS as the causative organism, malnutrition, immunosuppression, surgery, and trauma. Mixed infections with anaerobes, gram-negative, and gram-positive organisms can frequently be seen. Reported risk factors in infants include fetal scalp electrode monitoring, circumcision, omphalitis, and temperature monitoring with rectal thermometers.

Necrotizing fasciitis is a medical and surgical emergency with prompt debridement necessary for confirmation of diagnosis and treatment. Liquid necrosis of the superficial fascia is the diagnostic finding. Antibiotic treatment should be promptly initiated with clindamycin and cefoperazone sodium while monitoring culture results. Multisystem organ failure, sepsis, and DIC can occur if untreated, with an average mortality in children of 20%.

Folliculitis

Folliculitis is a hair follicle infection of the follicular ostium, is common in children, and usually occurs on the extremities and buttocks. The most common infectious etiology is *S. aureus*, but streptococci, gram-negative organisms, *Demodex*, *Pityrosporum*, and dermatophytes can also be seen. Bockhart's impetigo, or superficial folliculitis, presents with small pustules with central hairs on an erythematous base. Extensive eruptions may require a systemic antibiotic, but the majority of cases will resolve with topical antibiotics and antibacterial soaps.

Erythrasma

Erythrasma is caused by *Corynebacterium minutissimum*, a gram-positive bacillus, and presents as well-demarcated, erythematous patches, most commonly in the intertriginous areas such as crural folds, inframammary areas, axillae, and gluteal creases. Interdigital involvement is characterized by fissuring, maceration, and scaling. Erythrasma is the most common bacterial infection of the foot in children. Risk factors include diabetes mellitus, obesity, immunosuppression, warm climate, hyperhidrosis, and poor hygiene. The diagnosis can be made by visualizing the porphyrins produced by the bacteria using a Wood's lamp, which elicits the characteristic coral red fluorescence. Other diagnostic options include gram staining of the tissue scrapings under oil immersion, or culture on special media.

In cases of mild disease, antibacterial soaps may be adequate for treatment. In those patients with more extensive disease, oral erythromycin is the treatment of choice. Tetracycline may also be used in children older than 8 years. Topical therapy with clindamycin or Whitfield's ointment (6% salicylic acid and 12% benzoic acid) daily for 4 weeks is recommended in addition to oral antibiotics in intertriginous areas. If oral treatment is not an option, topical clindamycin is also effective.

Trichomycosis Axillaris

Trichomycosis axillaris is caused by *Corynebacteria* and produces nodules or sheaths of axillary and pubic hair. The lesions can be black, yellow, or red and can cause red staining of the clothing from sweat. Antimicrobial soaps and shaving of the affected area are curative for axillary lesions while erythromycin, clindamycin, or mupirocin can be used for pubic hair involvement.

Pitted Keratolysis

Pitted keratolysis manifests as small, 1- to 7-mm depressed pits of stratum corneum most commonly on weight-bearing areas of the plantar foot. These pits may eventually coalesce into erosions (Fig. 16.3). It was originally proposed that the causative organism was *Corynebacterium*, but *Micrococcus (Kytococcus) sedentarius* has also been implicated. Research has shown that *Micrococcus* produces two proteolytic enzymes capable of degrading keratin and inducing the crater-like pits of pitted keratolysis. Patients frequently note an unpleasant odor and sliminess, as well as an underlying hyperhidrosis. Treatments include topical erythromycin, clindamycin, and management of hyperhidrosis. There have also been recent reports of resolution of refractory cases following injections of botulinum toxin.

Erysipeloid

Erysipeloid is caused by *Erysipelothrix rhusiopathiae*, a gram-positive rod. It is the cause of swine erysipelas, and has a clinical presentation in animals that ranges from polyarthritis and endocarditis to sepsis. It is also carried asymptomatically in the lymphoid tissue of 30% to 50% of all swine. Humans encounter the organism primarily via occupational exposure, with veterinarians, butchers, and fishermen at highest risk. The manifestations of human infection are termed erysipeloid and take three

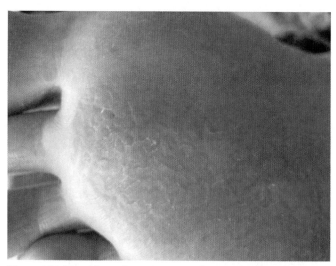

Figure 16.3. Pitted keratolysis. Honeycomb pitting on the sole in a patient with hyperhidrotic feet who presented complaining of significant foot odor. Treatment with topical agents and increased frequency of changing socks was curative.

forms: localized cutaneous (erysipeloid of Rosenbach), diffuse cutaneous, or septicemia and endocarditis.

The most common type is localized cutaneous disease, which presents as a painful, edematous, violaceous plaque of abraded or traumatized skin, 5 to 7 days after the initial injury. It frequently occurs on the fingers or hands and may spread peripherally with central clearing. When the lesions continue to progress with formation of bullae, involvement of proximal areas, and systemic symptoms of arthralgias and fever, the condition is termed *diffuse cutaneous disease*. Uncommonly, patients develop the more severe manifestations of endocarditis or sepsis, which are associated with a high mortality rate. Cardiac involvement is more common in males, and usually afflicts left-sided, native, damaged, cardiac valves with a higher propensity for the aortic valves.

Erysipelothrix can be identified on blood culture, but culture of skin lesions must be prepared on special media and may be of low yield. Organisms can be seen on a Gram stain. Both the localized and diffuse cutaneous forms may resolve spontaneously over weeks, but respond well to penicillin, ceftriaxone, or ciprofloxacin. *Erysipelothrix* is resistant to vancomycin. In patients with endocarditis, penicillin should be included as empirical antibiotic therapy for suspected cases. Preventive measures and regular cleaning of potential sources of infection with disinfectants resistant to organic matter in those persons at highest risk should be employed.

GRAM-NEGATIVE BACTERIA

Ecthyma Gangrenosum

Ecthyma gangrenosum is most commonly seen in patients with *Pseudomonas aeruginosa* bacteremia, and occurs on the buttocks, perineum, and extremities. It begins as an erythematous macule, which then becomes a hemorrhagic bulla. An ulcer with central, black eschar and inflammatory borders follows. Predisposing factors include neutropenia from an underlying immunodeficiency or chemotherapy. Cases of ecthyma gangrenosum in previously healthy children should prompt evaluation for occult immuno-deficiency. Early treatment with an antipseudomonal penicillin and an aminoglycoside is necessary.

Pseudomonal Folliculitis and Hot-Foot Syndrome

Pseudomonal folliculitis is related to improperly chlorinated swimming pools, hot tubs, or whirlpools, and results in follicular, erythematous pustules primarily in areas covered by swimsuits, but can be widespread, one to two days following exposure. Lesions usually resolve spontaneously. Some patients may complain of headache, malaise, arthralgias, and fever and can be treated with fluoroquinolones. Adequate cleaning and proper chlorination of the source will prevent re-exposure.

Children can also develop erythema and painful nodules of the weight-bearing areas of the plantar foot following exposure to Pseudomonas aeruginosa. Outbreaks have been reported following exposures at public wading pools and hot tubs. Lesions usually resolve within two weeks, but some patients can develop fever, lethargy, and significant leukocytosis requiring fluoroquinolone therapy.

Meningococcemia

See Chapter 25.

Gonorrhea

See Chapter 24.

Cat-Scratch Disease

Bartonella henselae is the cause of cat-scratch disease. It is the most common manifestation of Bartonellosis in children. Cats are the reservoir and vector, with seroprevalence being highest in young cats in warm environments. It has been proposed that the cat flea is involved in transmission between felines. Red-brown, asymptomatic papules develop over several days to 1 month following inoculation of the organism via the scratch or bite of a cat. These then become vesicular and crusted with painful enlargement of regional lymph nodes. Lymphadenopathy can last as long as 1 year, but typically resolvs within 2 months. Some patients complain of headache, malaise, anorexia, and arthralgias. Serologic evaluation is used most frequently for diagnosis. Other options include PCR testing available in some laboratories, direct observation of the organism with Warthin-Starry silver staining of affected lymph nodes, and culture(which can become positive after weeks of incubation). Treatment is not required in immunocompetent patients, as the disease is normally self-limited. However, azithromycin, trimethoprim–sulfamethoxazole, erythromycin, rifampin, doxycycline, and ciprofloxacin may offer some improvement.

Atypical cat-scratch disease can manifest as Parinaud's oculoglandular syndrome, which is characterized by a unilateral preauricular lymphadenopathy and conjunctivitis. Inoculation of the organism into the eye occurs indirectly, and infection is usually self-limited. More serious complications of atypical cat-scratch disease include encephalopathy, Leber's idiopathic stellate retinopathy and endocarditis. Immunocompromised patients can develop bacillary angiomatosis and reticuloendothelial involvement, which is known as *bacillary peliosis*.

Rocky Mountain Spotted Fever

See Chapter 25.

Ehrlichiosis

Bacteria of the family Anaplasmataceae cause the infections termed *ehrlichiosis* with three species being predominant in humans. Ehrlichiosis is a tick-borne disease, and patients present with fever, myalgias, headache, thrombocytopenia, leukopenia, and elevated liver enzyme levels. Infection occurs most commonly in the spring and summer, which directly correlates with tick activity.

Human monocytic ehrlichiosis (HME) is caused by *Ehrlichia chaffeensis* and is prevalent in the southern United States in areas where the vector *Amblyomma americanum*, or the lone star tick, is found. A rash is seen most frequently in HME and is petechial, macular, or a combination of the two in appearance. These patients are also more likely to have meningitis, encephalitis, and shock. *A. americanum* also carries *Ehrlichia ewingii*, which is the cause of human ewingii ehrlichiosis in the United States. *Anaplasma phagocytophilum* is the etiologic agent in human granulocytic anaplasmosis (HGA), which occurs internationally. *Ixodes persulcatus* ticks, including *Ixodes pacificus*, *Ixodes scapularis*, *Ixodes ricinus*, and *I. persulcatus*, are the vectors.

Diagnosis can be made with a peripheral blood smear, noting morulae in neutrophils in HGA and monocytes in HME. PCR, culture, and serologic antibody testing can also be used. Doxycycline is the treatment of choice, including seriously ill children less than 8 years of age. Treatment adversely affects diagnostic results. Rifampin has also been used in situations where doxycycline is contraindicated.

SPIROCHETES

Lyme Disease

Lyme disease in the United States is caused by *Borrelia burgdorferi* with *I. scapularis* and *I. pacificus* as the vectors of disease. Children and adults are affected by Lyme disease and clinical manifestations are consistent in each stage. Of note, children older than 8 years may be treated with doxycycline. Amoxicillin can be used in children 8 years of age and younger, with cefuroxime as an alternative for amoxicillin or doxycycline allergic patients. Refer to the discussion in the Chapter 7 on arthropod-borne infections for further review of Lyme disease.

Endemic treponematoses

Yaws, endemic syphilis (bejel), and pinta are nonvenereal treponematoses. They are commonly seen in children less than 15 years of age who also have poor hygiene and are living in rural areas of developing countries. They have characteristic stages of disease with periods of latency. Transmission is through contact of skin and mucous membranes. There is no congenital disease.

Nonvenereal and venereal treponematoses cannot be distinguished with current serologic testing. The nontreponemal tests, venereal disease research laboratory (VDRL) and rapid plasma reagin (RPR), if reactive, can identify an active infection and a treated or untreated recent infection. They can also produce a false-positive result. Nontreponemal titers can be useful for monitoring response to treatment. A four-fold decrease in titers will be seen with adequate treatment. There can also be a four-fold increase in titers with relapse or re-infection. Following treatment, the treponemal tests, enzyme-linked immunosorbent assays (ELISA), fluorescent treponemal antibody absorption test (FTA-Abs), and agglutination assays for *Treponema pallidum* (TPHA), can remain positive for many years or even for life. *T. pallidum* can also be identified on dark-field microscopy. Research is conflicting regarding the potential for cross-immunity between treponematoses. Some studies show no protection while others reflect some component of immunity related to the severity of the initial infection.

Treatment is the same for all three endemic treponematoses. Active early or late infections are treated with 1.2 million units of benzathine penicillin as a one-time dose. Children less than 10 years of age should receive 0.6 million units of benzathine penicillin. Alternative antibiotics include tetracycline, doxycycline, and erythromycin.

Treponema pallidum subspecies *pertenue* is the cause of yaws. It occurs in areas of the world with a high rainfall and temperatures greater than 80°F. The initial lesion, or "mother yaw," occurs at sites of initial infection, which are frequently on the lower extremities or buttocks. It is highly infectious, and manifests 10 days to 3 months following inoculation as an erythematous papule that enlarges into an ulcerated nodule. It may be accompanied by local lymphadenopathy. This is followed months to years later by diffuse papules and necrotic nodules with an infectious, exudative serum that is frequently on moist areas of the body. Hyperkeratotic plaques of the soles and palms, polydactylitis of the hand or foot, and osteoperiostitis of the leg or forearm are also seen. The final stage, which is characterized by destructive tissue lesions, is seen in 10% of patients. Cutaneous findings include gummas, periarticular nodules, hyperkeratosis of the palms and soles, and mottled pigmentation of the anterior lower extremities, hands, and wrists. Curvature of the tibia, termed *saber shin*, results from chronic osteitis. Perforation of the nasal septum or palate can also occur and this is referred to as gangosa.

Endemic syphilis, or bejel, is seen in hot, arid areas of the world with frequent transmission through drinking vessels in addition to skin contact. The reservoir for the *T. pallidum* subspecies *endemicum* is children between the ages of 2 and 15. The initial finding is a small papule or ulcer of the perioral area or nipple of nursing women. This is followed by second-stage periostitis, lymphadenopathy, mucous patches of the oral mucosa, and angular stomatitis of the oral commissures, which is also known as split papules. Periarticular nodules, saber shins, gangosa, and gummas can be seen in the late stage of disease.

T. carateum is the causative organism for pinta and was frequently seen in the forested areas of Central and South America. It only manifests in the skin and can occur in all age-groups, which makes it unique among the endemic treponematoses. It begins 15 to 30 days following infection as one or more papules or erythematous plaques. These lesions then slowly increase in size with central clearing and lymphadenopathy later develops. Secondary lesions, known as *pintids*, are scaly papules and plaques of a variety of colors, which include blue and grey, or hypopigmented. Two to 4 years later, symmetric, depigmented,

atrophic or hypertrophic lesions of the bony prominences characterize the late-stage. *Treponema carateum* is present in the skin from onset through the late stage.

OTHER

Pseudofolliculitis Barbae

Pseudofolliculitis barbae is a common disorder, frequently of African-Americans and patients with curly hair, characterized by erythematous, perifollicular papules and pustules of the anterior neck, chin, mandible, cheeks, and neck. It is related to a repenetration of the epidermis or hair follicle by a sharp hair shaft following close shaving. This results in a foreign-body inflammatory response. Treatments include using electric razors, depilatory creams, eflornithine, chemical peels, topical retinoids, and topical antibiotics. Current research has shown promise with Nd:YAG and diode (810 nm) laser treatment.

Eosinophilic Pustular Folliculitis

Eosinophilic pustular folliculitis (EPF) is a skin disease of unknown etiology. Three forms have been described: classic EPF, infancy-associated EPF, and immunosuppression-associated EPF. Only infancy-associated EPF, which begins within a few weeks of birth, will be discussed here. In contrast to adults, who typically present with erythematous, follicular papules and pustules in an annular or grouped configuration on the face and trunk, infants predominantly have scalp involvement, and lesions are scattered. Lesions can occasionally be found on the face and extremities. Infancy-associated EPF typically responds well to mild-to-moderate potency topical steroids.

Noma (cancrum oris)

Noma is a disease of unknown etiology seen most commonly in children ages one to four in Africa, Asia, and Latin America. It causes swelling of the gingiva or cheek followed by necrotizing stomatitis of the alveolar margin. This rapidly progresses to necrosis of the overlying cutaneous structures with eventual full thickness tissue loss, frequently exposing bony tissue. It can involve the nose, infraorbital areas, maxilla, and mandible. Systemic signs and symptoms including fever, pain, foul odor, anorexia, and excessive salivation can occur. Children often reside in unsanitary conditions and have underlying medical problems. Risk factors include malnutrition, poor oral hygiene, and preceding infection with malaria or measles. Treatment is aimed at early recognition with improvement of underlying medical issues and broad spectrum antibiotics. Reconstructive surgery is needed to correct the resulting defects.

FUNGAL INFECTIONS

Many types of fungi can lead to cutaneous infections in children, and some cutaneous fungal infections are relatively common in pediatric patients. Cutaneous fungal infections may be divided into the superficial and deep forms. There are three common causes of superficial cutaneous fungal infections: dermatophytes, tinea versicolor, and candidiasis (moniliasis).

Dermatophytes

Dermatophyte fungi are contracted from multiple sources such as animals (zoophilic such as *Microsporum canis*), humans (anthropophilic such as *Trichophyton tonsurans*), and the environment (geophilic such as *Microsporum gypseum*). These fungi are adapted to live on the skin and derive nutrients from it. Infections with these fungi are called *tinea* and they are typically classified by the body location they affect.

Tinea capitis (fungal infection of the scalp and hair) is the most common dermatophytosis of childhood. The incidence of infection in the United States is estimated at 1% to 8% in children and may be more common in urban settings.

Asymptomatic carriage (positive scalp fungal culture with no signs/symptoms of disease) is a major reservoir for disease, especially for the anthropophilic strains *Trichophyton tonsurans* and *Trichophyton violaceum*. Most carriers are African-American. Asymptomatic carriage can present as a seborrheic dermatitis-like eruption with a mild or absent inflammatory response. Dermatophyte carrier prevalence correlates with the incidence of tinea in a community. The asymptomatic carriage rate is estimated at ~15%.

There is a clear role for fomites in the spread of dermatophyte infections as well. Fungal material remains viable on fomites for months. The incubation period of dermatophyte infections can be relatively short (1–3 weeks but as fast as 2–4 days).

The type of fungus and the morphology seen in tinea capitis has changed with time. While *Microsporum audouinii* was the most common cause of tinea capitis in the United States during the mid-1900s, it is now uncommon. Infections with *T. tonsurans* increased in the 1970s, and it continues to be the most frequent agent today.

There are multiple clinical presentations of tinea capitis. As noted earlier, infection can be subtle, and can present as a mild seborrheic dermatitis-like scaling with minimal hair loss. Patients more commonly present with patches of alopecia with variable scaling of the alopecic scalp. When scale is present, it may be termed "gray type" tinea capitis. "Black dot" tinea refers to the appearance of the ends of hairs, broken at their exit from the skin surface, with minimal inflammation, that is seen especially with those dermatophytes capable of endothrix invasion of the hair shaft. Diffuse pustular forms can also occur.

Some patients develop an intensely inflammatory, boggy edematous eruption of the affected scalp with alopecia, pustules, and occasional purulence, termed a *kerion*. Aggressive therapy is indicated for these patients in order to prevent a scarring alopecia.

Favus, a form of tinea capitis rarely seen in the United States, is caused by *Trichophyton schoenleinii*. The scalp exhibits scaling, erythematous patchy lesions with striking yellow adherent crusts often with a central hair shaft (termed scutula) that form from hairs matted together by debris and hyphae. A cheesy or mouse-like odor may also be present. This condition also often leads to scarring alopecia.

Lymphadenopathy, especially cervical or postauricular, is common in patients with tinea capitis. Secondary infection of involved areas may occur, with nearly half of cases being caused by *Staphylococcus aureus*.

Dermatophytid (autoeczematization/Id) reactions occur occasionally in patients with tinea capitis especially when a kerion is present. These hypersensitivity reactions typically present with small lichenoid papules that may be pruritic. They may also occur after initiation of antifungal treatment and may raise the concern for a drug reaction. Symptomatic treatment is typically effective.

Diagnosis

Potassium hydroxide preparation can be helpful, although longer digestion times are required for detection of fungal elements within the hair shaft itself. Hairs for examination may be plucked using forceps or hemostats. However, hair extraction can be painful. The ability of dermatophytes to invade hair varies depending on the strain. Ectothrix strains exhibit fungal growth on the exterior of the hair shaft, and may fluoresce under a Wood's lamp. Whereas, endothrix fungi are able to invade the hair shaft and do not fluoresce under Wood's lamp. Favus (*T. schoenleinii*) shows infectious material with large spores interspersed with air bubbles in the hair shaft. The Wood's lamp emits filtered UV light at 365 nm, which can induce fluorescence in ectothrix strains but this is positive in only one-half of culture-positive *Microsporum canis* patients.

Fungal culture remains the gold standard diagnostic test for tinea capitis, though it can be falsely negative in up to 50% of cases. Recent reports suggest that vigorous rubbing of moistened premade bacterial culture swabs sent for fungal culture is as effective as more aggressive sampling techniques.

Treatment

Systemic treatment of tinea capitis is usually warranted as penetration of the hair follicle is necessary for cure. However, in infants topical therapies may be effective if avoidance of systemic antifungals is desired. Treatment of a kerion may require the addition of antibacterial therapy or systemic steroids.

The issue of school attendance often arises for school age children with tinea capitis. It is not practical to keep children with tinea capitis out of school as spore shedding can occur asymptomatically and such carriers may be the major source of transmission. The use of selenium sulfide or ketoconazole antifungal shampoos can suppress the carrier state and decrease potential transmission, thus alleviating anxiety for parents and teachers alike.

Systemic therapy

Griseofulvin is the only systemic antifungal medication licensed in the United States for use in children. Fungistatic in vitro, it interferes with spindle microtubule function, and leads to defective DNA synthesis and defective cell wall formation. Available as both tablets and a suspension, it is absorbed best when taken with fatty foods. Variable bioavailability and resistance among dermatophyte strains lead to some unpredictability in its ability to treat tinea capitis successfully. Thus, recent recommendations suggest higher dosing schedules than previously suggested with doses of 20 to 25 mg/kg/day divided twice daily for at least 8 weeks. A small percentage of patients exhibit headache, nausea, or rashes during treatment. While internal organ monitoring is not necessary for healthy patients on normal courses at standard doses, it may be prudent for those children on extended drug courses (>8 weeks).

Table 16.1: Antifungal Medications for Treatment of Tinea capitis in Children

Drug	Mechanism of Action	How supplied	Pediatric dose	Duration of therapy
Griseofulvin (microcrystalline)	interferes with spindle microtubule function	Tablets Suspension (125mg/5cc)	20–25mg/kg divided twice daily	Continuous: > 8 weeks
Itraconazole	inhibits lanosterol 14-demethylase	Capsule Suspension	5mg/kg/D 3mg/kg/D	Continuous: 4–6 weeks Pulse: 1 week repeat after 3 weeks
Fluconazole	inhibits lanosterol 14-demethylase	Capsule Suspension	Continuous: 6mg/kg/D Pulse: 8mg/kg/week	20 days 4–6 weeks
Terbinafine	inhibits squalene epoxidase	Tablets	<20kg–62.5mg/D 20–40 kg – 125mg/D >40kg–250mg/D or 4–5 mg/kg/D	Continuous: 4 weeks

Itraconazole, fluconazole, ketoconazole, and terbinifine have all been used to successfully treat tinea capitis in children. Table 16.1 shows recommended dosage schedules and regimens of standard antifungals in children.

Corticosteroids are rarely used in the treatment of tinea capitis but may be helpful in decreasing swelling and inflammation in extremely pronounced cases of kerion. They can also improve symptoms in diffuse Id reactions.

Concomitant use of topical antifungal shampoos may decrease the risk of transmission of the causative dermatophyte to others. Both selenium sulfide and ketoconazole shampoos (twice weekly) may be used. If pets are affected, they should be treated for dermatophytes. Dosing for affected cats is itraconazole 1.5–3 mg/kg/day for 15 days.

One difficult clinical scenario is the diagnosis of tinea capitis in children less than 1 year of age. Tinea capitis is rare in the first year of life and occurs more frequently in male infants. In this age-group it is often due to *M. canis* and *M. audouinii*. Typically, an adult caregiver is the source of the infection. Alopecia is often seen, along with scaling of the affected areas. Topical therapy may be of greater efficacy in these young patients and can be a reasonable therapeutic choice. Griseofulvin may be the systemic drug of choice, due to its long record of safety. Fluconazole, however, can also be safely used in infants.

Tinea faceii

Dermatophyte infection of the face is called *tinea faceii*. Involvement of the non–hair bearing face is relatively common in children compared to adults. These lesions may resemble the classic lesions of tinea corporis or may be more subtle.

Fungal infection of the beard is termed **tinea barbae** and typically affects adolescent and adult males.

Tinea corporis is the classic "ringworm" infection. Often presenting as annular erythematous patches, it occurs in patients of all ages but is more common in children and in the immunosuppressed. It is more frequent during warm, humid times of the year or in such climates. Patients with disorders of keratinization are more frequently affected and can present with atypical clinical findings. The causative agents include *Trichophyton sp.* and *Microsporum sp.*

Tinea corporis is frequently seen in wrestlers, transmitted by skin-to-skin contact or fomites and is termed **tinea gladiatorum**.

In cases of frequent infections, prophylactic antifungals have been used. Pets are a common source of *M. canis* infections and such zoophilic tinea infections tend to be more inflammatory than anthropophilic infections even progressing to bullae formation (Fig. 16.4).

Tinea cruris refers to infection of the genital area. Involvement of the scrotum or labia should suggest candidal infection as dermatophytes rarely affect the skin in those locations. Heat, moisture, and maceration predispose patients to dermatophyte infection in these areas. Patients with active tinea cruris often have tinea pedis as well, and this often serves as a source of infection.

Tinea pedis, or athlete's foot, is an uncommon dermatophyte infection in children with an increased incidence after puberty. It is the most common dermatophyte infection after puberty, whereas tinea capitis is the most common dermatophyte infection before puberty.

Tinea of the hand (**tinea manuum**) is rare in childhood.

Tinea incognito refers to dermatophyte infections in any location previously treated with a topical steroid or with a combination topical steroid/antifungal preparation. The use of corticosteroids can suppress the inflammatory response to dermatophytes and eliminate the erythema and scale. This makes diagnosis of tinea clinically difficult since erythema and scaling are the hallmarks of tinea infection. Immunosuppresion by topical corticosteroids may also promote the growth of the dermatophyte. Such lesions may show little to no clinical findings; yet potassium hydroxide preparation reveals numerous fungal hyphae on the skin surface. Directed treatment of the dermatophyte without corticosteroids is recommended.

Tinea unguium or **onychomycosis** is rare in children compared to adults, with an estimated incidence of ~0.6% in children in Europe (vs. 10%–20% of European adults). It has been proposed that the smaller surface area of children's nails, the decreased frequency of nail trauma, and the less frequent exposure to areas with a high prevalence of dermatophytes account for this low prevalence among children. Trauma is an important causative factor as onychomycosis is ~1.5 times more common in sports-active children compared to those who are not sports active. In ~50% of children with onychomycosis, a first-degree relative also has tinea. Often there is a positive family history or active infection in first-degree family members. In

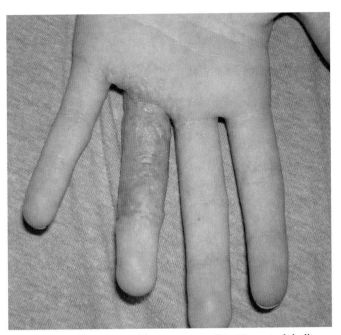

Figure 16.4. Bullous tinea – Tinea manuum. Pruritic vesiculobullous scaling eruption of the palmar aspects of the fourth digit and hand. While some of the vesicles appear herpetic in nature, the patient was a veterinarian and KOH examination of lesional scale revealed florid fungal hyphae. Antifungal therapy was rapidly curative.

addition to trauma, other predisposing factors include contact with animals, swimming, and immunosuppression. There is also a higher incidence in patients with Down's syndrome.

The most common pathogen in children is *Trichophyton rubrum. T. mentagrophytes* var. *interdigitale, Epidermophyton floccosum,* and *Candida albicans* are also reported. One report also noted *Epidermophyton floccosum* and *T. violaceum* as causative agents. Scopulariopsis brevicaulis is the most common mold responsible. Males are more commonly affected, and most manifest a distal and distolateral subungual hyperkeratosis. Onychomycosis in neonates is often due to Candida, which may be congenital.

Clinically the distal subungual type is most common. It presents with distal onycholysis and subungual thickening with occasional discoloration. It is more frequent on the toes. The proximal subungual form is more often seen in patients with HIV.

Diagnosis

The diagnosis can be confirmed by potassium hydroxide examination or periodic acid-Schiff (PAS) staining of clippings from the affected nail. Fungal culture can be definitive and allows identification of the specific dermatophyte, but false negatives are common.

Treatment

Onychomycosis can present a therapeutic dilemma when present in young patients. The necessity of treating onychomycosis in children has been debated. The risks and duration of systemic antifungal therapy must be weighed with the severity of infection, the likelihood of permanent sequelae, and the age of the child. Parents should be given as much information as possible to make an informed decision.

Topical therapy for onychomycosis exhibits greater potential than in adult patients. The thinner nail plates of children may enhance drug penetration and the more rapid growth of the nail may increase the efficacy of topical therapy.

Several reports describe the use of topical antifungals alone or in combination with chemical nail debridement such as urea with good results. The following treatments have been used successfully to treat onychomycosis in extremely young infants: Ciclopirox and Amorolfine nail lacquers, Tolnaftate solution, clotrimazole 1% solution and Bifonazole (1%) combined with urea (40%) creams applied for 15 days until the affected nail was removed, followed by bifonazole 1% cream daily for 4 weeks. Systemic therapies are listed in Table 16.2.

Tinea imbricata (Tokelau)

Tinea imbricata (TI) is a chronic dermatophyte infection of glabrous skin caused by *Trichophyton concentricum,* an anthropophilic dermatophyte belonging to the same fungal group as *T. schoenleinii.*

TI is seen in three main areas: southern Asia (China/India), the South Pacific islands, and South and Central America. The South Pacific, Polynesia, and Melanesia are the most important endemic zones in the world, with 9% to 18% of the population being infected. All are rural regions with high humidity. TI is found in both sexes and all ages from infants to the elderly. Farmers and land workers are more frequently infected. The susceptibility to infection is possibly inherited with studies favoring autosomal recessive inheritance even though there are some cases of autosomal dominance. *T. concentricum* spreads via close contact, especially from mother to child.

TI begins in childhood, often on the face, then spreads to other body areas. Patients exhibit erythematous scaly concentric and overlapping plaques mainly involving the thorax and limbs including the palms and soles. Onychomycosis, most commonly of the distal subungual type, can occur. TI can involve the scalp, creating seborrheic-like lesions, but does not infect the hair or follicle. With time the areas become lamellar and develop abundant thick scale with adherence to one side (overlapping or "imbrex"), which can lead to an ichthyosiform appearance. Pruritus is the most frequent symptom.

Treatment

Griseofulvin has been the traditional therapy for TI for many years but has a high recurrence rate, and azoles do not show good effectiveness. Terbinafine appears to be the best therapeutic option, when used at standard doses. Topical treatments include keratolytic creams such as Whitfield's ointment or the combination of systemic and topical agents. Maintenance of good skin hygiene is also helpful in treating TI.

Tinea versicolor (Pityriasis versicolor)

Multiple treatments are effective including selenium sulfide 2.5% shampoo applied in a thin layer for 10 minutes prior to rinsing, daily for 1–2 weeks. Less frequent applications (every other week or less) may maintain clearance. Ketoconazole 2% shampoo is also effective using a similar regimen. Terbinafine spray appears effective when used once to twice daily for 1–2 weeks. Severe

Table 16.2: Antifungal Medications for Treatment of Onychomycosis in Children

Drug	Mechanism of Action	How supplied	Pediatric dose	Duration
Griseofulvin (microcrystalline) [not recommended]	interferes with spindle microtubule function	Tablets Suspension (125mg/5cc)	5–10 mg/kg divided twice daily	9–18 months
Itraconazole	inhibits lanosterol 14-demethylase	Capsule Suspension	Pulse: (1 wk. on/ 3 wks. Off) 5mg/kg/D 3–5mg/kg/D	FN: 2 pulses TN: 3 pulses
Fluconazole	inhibits lanosterol 14-demethylase	Capsule Suspension	Pulse: 3–6 mg/kg/week	FN: 12 wks. TN: 26 wks.
Terbinafine	inhibits squalene epoxidase	Tablets	<20kg – 62.5mg/D 20–40 kg – 125mg/D >40kg – 250mg/D OR 4–5 mg/kg/D	FN: 6 wks. TN: 12 wks.

Abbreviations: FN: fingernail; TN: toenails
Source: Sethi A and Antaya R. Systemic antifungal therapy for cutaneous infections in children. *Pediatr Infect Dis J.* 2006;25(7):643–644. Gupta AK and Skinner AR. Onychomycosis in Children: A brief Overview with Treatment Strategies. *Pediatr Dermatol.* 2004;21(1):74–79.

or recurrent disease or follicular involvement may mandate oral therapy with ketoconazole (400mg with exercise afterward and allowing sweat to remain on skin for approximately 12 hours prior to rinsing and repeated in 1 week), itraconazole 400mg for one dose, or a single dose of 400mg fluconazole. See chapter 3 for a more detailed discussion.

Tinea nigra

Tinea nigra is a superficial cutaneous infection with the pigmented fungus *Phaeoannellomyces werneckii*. This infection is seen in warm humid areas such as the Caribbean as well as in Central and South America. It produces an asymptomatic light to dark brown or black macule, typically involving palmar skin. Scaling is rare but potassium hydroxide preparation reveals pigmented hyphae and yeast cells. Culture is confirmative and topical antifungals are curative.

Piedra

This fungal infection of the hair shaft has two clinical types. Black piedra is caused by *Piedraia hortae* and is seen in Asia, Africa, and Central America. The hair shafts of affected patients exhibit small, hard, dark nodules. Fungal culture can confirm the infection and traditionally the head was shaved to eradicate the infection. Terbinafine, however, appears to be as effective a treatment without taking such drastic measures. White piedra is caused by infection of the hair shaft with *Trichosporon beigelii*, and occurs in more temperate zones including the United States, where infections in recent immigrants are occasionally seen. Soft, white-to-tan nodules on the hair shafts can mimic hair casts or nits. Pubic hair may be involved. Fungal culture will confirm the infecting agent. Traditional treatment involved shaving of the head but itraconazole may have efficacy against *T. beigelii*. *T. beigelii* may cause disseminated infections in low birth weight infants or immunocompromised patients. Skin lesions in such disseminated infections are similar to those seen with other

disseminated fungal infections such as candida and take the form of purpuric papules and nodules with areas of necrosis. Treatment may be difficult as *T. beigelii* often exhibits resistance to amphotericin B.

Candidiasis

There are nearly 200 species of Candida and approximately 20 cause infections in humans and animals, with *C. albicans* being the main pathogen. Recently non–albicans candida (C. glabrata, krusei, parapsilosis, tropicalis, guilliermondii) infections have increased in incidence, likely because of the use of azole antifungals. Now they represent 35% to 65% of all candidemias.

Drug resistance to azoles is increasingly being reported. It was first noted in chronic mucocutaneous candidiasis patients on long-term suppressive ketoconazole therapy and now is also seen in patients with HIV. Some forms of candida are inherently resistant to antifungals, such as *C. krusei* and *C. glabrata* (both resistant to fluconazole) and *C. tropicalis* (resistant to ketoconazole). Some strains of *C. albicans* also exhibit increasing azole resistance. Cross-resistance (resistance to one azole implying resistance to alternative azoles) has also been noted but is variable.

C. parapsilosis has caused bloodstream infections, especially in neonates and those in NICUs (neonatal intensive care units), possibly from parenteral nutrition. One NICU survey found nearly 30% of Candida blood stream infections to be due to *C. parapsilosis*, which easily attaches to inert polymer surfaces and forms biofilms.

The oral, vaginal, and gastrointestinal tracts are sources of Candida. Candida carriage in the vagina increases with pregnancy with 20% to 40% of women being culture positive at the time of delivery. Approximately 30% of health care workers will be Candida culture positive on one or more occasions.

Predisposing factors for Candida infection include infancy, pregnancy, old age, occlusion of epithelial surfaces, immunodeficiency (primary or secondary), chemotherapy, immunosuppression, antibiotic use, carcinoma, and primary epithelial disease leading to a defective barrier.

Clinical

Mucocutaneous candidiasis refers to infections of the skin, nails, and mucosa. Deep-seated candidosis includes infections of internal organs. Disseminated candidal disease has markedly risen in incidence over the last few decades. It carries a significant mortality rate (~30% even with treatment). Preexisting granulocytopenia is a risk factor for the development of systemic candidiasis.

Oropharyngeal candida (thrush) is common in infants, the elderly, immunosuppressed patients, and following antibiotic therapy. Oropharyngeal candida (thrush) appears as lacy white to whitish gray patches or plaques on the oral mucosa. The mucosa may be skin colored or quite erythematous.

The plaques may be difficult to remove and doing so may reveal oozing of blood at the base. Infected infants may be irritable or asymptomatic. Oral colonization with Candida occurs rapidly in the first weeks of life, most frequently at 4 weeks of age. Candida appears to better adhere to cells from young patients. It is usually acquired either from maternal genital tract or from the hands of caregivers. Thrush is increased eight-fold in infants whose mothers had active infection and can also be acquired during breastfeeding.

The pseudomembranous form presents as solitary or confluent white plaques on the oral mucosa that are easily removed with scraping. Some patients exhibit erythematous oral lesions with loss of papillae, which is termed the *erythematous form*. Esophageal infection often occurs in patients with AIDS who have oropharyngeal infection.

Persistent or recurrent oropharyngeal lesions can develop due to asymptomatic maternal infection with contamination of nipples, pacifiers, or other frequently mouthed objects. Oral antifungals, especially fluconazole, are rapidly effective in such cases. Topical treatment for mucocutaneous candidiasis in the past utilized gentian violet, but presently nystatin is typically prescribed at one dropper full in each cheek four times a day for 7 to 14 days, along with massage of the medication onto the mucosa.

Skin infection with candida includes intertrigo, which often presents as a beefy red erythema in flexural areas. Staphylococcal overgrowth can also contribute to lesion development. Treatment considerations include drying of the skin to decrease maceration as well as antifungal therapy aimed at reducing Candida. Interdigital infections can occur if the areas are very moist. Paronychia and candidal onychomycosis are seen most often with CMC (chronic mucocutaneous candidiasis), Raynaud's, Cushing's, or with steroid therapy. CMC patients are also prone to dermatophyte and HPV infections. In such patients, attempts to avoid maintenance therapy whenever possible is reasonable because of the development of azole resistance.

Diaper dermatitis (monilial diaper dermatitis) caused by Candida is common and affected infants are usually colonized in the gastrointestinal tract. They may exhibit concomitant oral thrush. Clinically, beefy red erosions are noted, often with scattered surrounding satellite pustules. Candidiasis of the diaper area should be considered if a diaper rash does not respond to normal treatment. Candidiasis can also develop after treatment with systemic antibiotics.

Often considered a disease of adults, candidal vulvovaginitis accounts for roughly 60% of childhood/adolescent gynecologic examinations.

Angular cheilitis (perleche) is common with fissuring and inflammation at the commissures of the mouth. Childhood cases may be caused by dental malocclusion, orthodontics, or lip licking. Correction of the underlying predisposition is key to achieving resolution. Low-strength topical steroids may help, occasionally combined with topical antifungals if necessary.

Chronic paronychia is usually caused by *C. albicans*. Loss of the cuticle is typically seen. In children, it can be caused by finger/thumb sucking. Topical antifungals are usually helpful, but oral therapies may be needed.

Congenital candidiasis is a rare, congenital form of candidal infection with skin lesions developing between birth and 6 days. Contrastingly, lesions of neonatal candidiasis begin after the first week of life. Neonatal candidiasis is acquired from infection during passage through the birth canal.

Congenital candidiasis can be associated with premature labor. It is relatively benign in term infants but can cause invasive fungal dermatitis in ultra-premature infants. It presents with a maculopapular, vesicular or pustular eruption. Typically self-limited, it resolves in 1 to 2 weeks. Palmoplantar pustules are common and are a helpful diagnostic finding. Occasionally, nail changes are noted and they can be the only finding in some patients. Potassium hydroxide preparation or fungal culture allows a definitive diagnosis.

Systemic candidiasis usually occurs in low birth weight infants with an onset around 2 to 6 weeks of life. It exhibits a high mortality rate and requires aggressive therapy.

Invasive fungal dermatitis

Premature infants have a weakened cutaneous barrier with barrier function not maturing until the second week of life. Extremely low birth weight infants are at risk for Candida during the first 2 weeks of life. Candida may present as erosive lesions with significant crusting that was not present at birth. Biopsy shows invasion of fungal elements throughout the epidermis and into the dermis. Blood cultures are typically positive. In one series the mean gestation of affected neonates was 24 weeks and mean weights were <700 g. Significant associations included vaginal birth, postnatal steroid use, and hyperglycemia. In experimental studies *C. albicans* can penetrate an animal epidermis in 24 to 48 hours. Other fungi can cause invasive fungal dermatitis. The treatment of invasive fungal dermatitis is with systemic antifungals, usually amphotericin B. Prevention involves monitoring skin integrity and prevention of local trauma. It is unclear if occlusive topical ointment use plays a role.

Chronic mucocutaneous candidiasis

Chronic mucocutaneous candidiasis (CMC) represents a spectrum of disorders with persistent/recurrent candidal infections of the skin, nails, and mucous membranes. Some are genetic but all have a common immunologic defect in the production of cytokines needed to induce cell-mediated immunity to Candida, typically *C. albicans*. Despite their chronic infections, it is rare that CMC patients develop candidal sepsis or parenchymal organ infections. A familial variant of CMC occurs in consanguineous families, and consists of chronic and recurrent oral candidiasis. Onset of this variant is by the age of 2.

Chronic oral candidiasis is characterized by recurrent oropharyngeal Candida without esophageal Candida or skin/nail lesions. It is more common in middle-aged and elderly women and may occur along with iron deficiency and/or HIV infection. The presence of oral candidiasis has prognostic value for HIV-infected subjects, with affected patients more likely to progress to AIDS.

Autoimmune polyendocrinopathy-candidiasis-ectodermal dystrophy (APECED) syndrome patients exhibit recurrent oral candidiasis and diaper rashes from candida. Lesions spread to the scalp, extremities, nails, and other sites. Keratitis may be present in approximately one-third of patients. The polyendocrinopathy may manifest as hypothyroidism, adrenal failure, gonadal failure, insulin-dependent diabetes mellitus, gastric parietal cell failure, autoimmune hepatitis, or intestinal malabsorption. Hypoparathyroidism occurs in approximately 79% of patients, hypoadrenalism in 72%, and ovarian failure in 60%. About 60% of APECED patients have two or more conditions, and nearly 50% have four or five of these disorders. The endocrinopathies may have an onset later than childhood or adolescence and these patients require annual evaluation of endocrine function. The disorder is caused by autosomal recessive defects in the AIRE (autoimmune regulator) gene.

Lesions of chronic localized candidiasis are also known as *candidal granulomas*. Affected patients present with skin lesions characterized by hypertrophic, adherent crusts on the scalp and face, with some patients developing striking lesions similar to cutaneous horns. Most also have oral Candida. Lesion onset is in early childhood (before age 5) with an equal sex distribution. There is no clear genetic cause.

The hyper-IgE syndrome, an autosomal dominant syndrome characterized by high serum IgE levels as well as impaired cell-mediated immune responses can exhibit chronic candidal infections of the skin and nails in 83% of patients. Importantly, one report noted a 50% incidence of additional non-candidal infections in CMC patients.

Treatment of CMC may be topical or systemic. Patients frequently relapse upon discontinuation of therapy. The timing of response to treatments is variable and if long-term therapies are employed appropriate monitoring should be performed.

CONGENITAL INFECTIONS

Congenital infections may be caused by multiple infectious agents including viruses, bacteria, or parasites. Most important are the so-called TORCH infections: Toxoplasmosis, Others (such as syphilis, varicella, and HIV), Rubella, Cytomegalovirus, and Herpes.

Congenital toxoplasmosis

Toxoplasmosis is caused by infection with the parasite *Toxoplasma gondii*, an intracellular protozoan that can invade multiple tissues including the heart, liver, spleen, CNS, and lymph nodes.

In normal hosts most infections are asymptomatic and limited. Pregnant women are more susceptible and can have poor fetal outcomes if fetal infection occurs, including seizures, mental retardation, and blindness. The greatest risk for transplacental transmission occurs from primary maternal infection during the third trimester, however, the severity of fetal infections is worse with first-trimester infections. *T. gondii* is acquired through the consumption of raw or poorly cooked meat such as pork, mutton, and wild game or via ingestion of oocysts from feline fecal matter.

Fetal toxoplasmosis can cause stillbirth or prematurity with signs and symptoms occurring at birth or developing in the first weeks of life. The classic clinical triad of toxoplasmosis includes chorioretinitis, hydrocephalus, and intracranial calcifications. Clinical findings include fever, vomiting, diarrhea, and malaise. Lymphadenopathy, microphthalmia, hepatosplenomegaly, cataracts, microcephaly, pneumonitis, a bleeding diathesis, and seizures can also occur. Up to 80% of patients will have visual or learning disabilities later in life.

Skin lesions associated with toxoplasmosis include the classic "blueberry muffin"-like lesions and a rubella-like maculopapular eruption that typically spares the face, palms, and soles. Skin lesions occur during the first week of illness and may last up to 1 week with postinflammatory desquamation or hyperpigmentation. Patients may exhibit anemia, thrombocytopenia, eosinophilia, and occasionally severe leukopenia. Diagnostic testing includes *T. gondii*-specific IgG and IgM antibodies. A diagnostic quandary is the persistence of *T. gondii*-specific IgM, even though the presence of these antibodies does not necessarily indicate an acute infection. In addition, the presence of IgG only in the first 6 months may be due to maternal transplacental transmission. In questionable cases, more elegant testing methods can usually resolve such dilemmas.

Most infected infants show few to no symptoms. However, because of the high frequency of later neurologic sequelae all patients should be treated regardless of symptoms. Treatments for both mother and child include sulfadiazine, pyrimethamine, folinic acid, and spiramycin.

Congenital syphilis

While rare in most developed countries, worldwide, congenital syphilis is a major health problem. In recent years, the incidence of syphilis in the United States and some European countries has increased. The rate of syphilis in pregnant women in some Asian and African countries varies between 3% and 10%.

Syphilis is caused by *Treponema pallidum* with transplacental infection occurring after 14 weeks of gestation. It is estimated that up to 40% of infected pregnancies result in fetal loss and that two-thirds of affected live born infants are symptom free at birth. The risk of vertical transmission from an untreated infected mother to her fetus decreases as maternal disease progresses. This finding is termed *Kassowitz's law*. The risk of transmission during primary syphilis is 70% to 100% but is approximately 40% for early latent syphilis and only 10% for late latent disease.

Clinical findings of congenital syphilis are divided into early (onset <2 years of age) and late (onset >2 years of age).

The earliest sign of congenital syphilis is frequently a nasal discharge, termed *snuffles* which occurs 1 to 2 weeks before the onset of a syphilitic maculopapular eruption. The discharge results from ulceration of the nasal mucosa, which, if deep enough, can later lead to saddle nose deformity. It is teeming with spirochetes and provides a medium for diagnostic testing.

Additional early findings include hepatosplenomagaly, jaundice, lymphadenopathy (epitrochlear is considered characteristic), and a rash. The more pronounced the early manifestations, the poorer the outcome for the patient.

The eruption of congenital syphilis is seen in one-third to one-half of infants and exhibits variable appearances. It most typically resembles the eruption of secondary syphilis seen in adults, including palmoplantar involvement. Palmoplantar vesiculobullous lesions are rare but are proposed to be highly suggestive of congenital syphilis. Either can be followed by desquamation. Condyloma lata-like lesions may be seen in warm, moist areas such as the anogenital region, around the nares, and at the angles of the mouth. Mucous patches are present in approximately one-third of infants. Both forms of these lesions are teeming with spirochetes and are highly infectious. Fissures may develop at mucocutaneous junctions, which can later lead to deep wounds that heal with characteristic radiating, ragged scars, known as *rhagades*.

The umbilical cord may exhibit a necrotizing funisitis, leading to spiral areas of red and blue discoloration with internal white streaks, termed a *barber pole umbilical cord*. This occurs in premature neonates and is associated with a high mortality.

Bony lesions are not common at birth but are present by the second month in 90% of patients. Although any bone can be involved, involvement of the long bones of the extremities is most common. Osteochondritis, the most common and earliest lesion, is often asymptomatic but severe lesions can cause subepiphyseal fractures leading to dislocation and "pseudoparalysis of Parrot." Periosteal inflammation of the frontal bones can lead to the flattened forehead described in congenital syphilis and frontal bossing is noted in 30% to 60% of patients. The periosteal inflammation is diffuse, in contrast to the osteochondritis, and can lead to thickening of the external portions of the bony cortex. When this occurs on the tibia it can cause anterior bowing, the so-called "saber shins."

Late stigmata of congenital syphilis are also well described. Most pronounced are dental changes such as Hutchinson's incisors, which show central notching and tapering toward the free edge of the tooth. When seen along with interstitial keratitis and eighth nerve deafness (a rare complication, typically of sudden onset around 8–10 years of age). These findings are classically referred to as Hutchinson's triad. Mulberry molars are lower first molars malformed because of crowded, poorly developed crusts on the crown. These decay early in life and are often lost by puberty, but are considered pathognomonic for congenital syphilis when present.

Unilateral thickening of the inner third of the clavicle has been termed *Higoumenakis sign* and is considered a finding of congenital syphilis. However, similar lesions can be produced from clavicular fractures at birth, thus this sign is not considered pathognomonic. Focal erosion of the inner proximal tibia leads to metaphyseal destruction. The radiologic changes associated are termed *Wimberger's lines*. Clutton's joints, of hydrarthrosis, typically involve the knees and elbows with an onset between 8 and 15 years of age. Late skin changes are typically nodules or gummas.

Diagnosis and Treatment

Routine screening of maternal serology for syphilis is performed for most women seeking prenatal care. While there are inadequacies in the testing methods, currently recommendations are for newborns of seropositive mothers to be tested using the same nontreponemal test (VDRL/RPR) as their mother. A four-fold higher titer in the infant is considered a probable infection. Confirmation using a treponemal test (FTA-Abs/ MHA-TP) is reasonable. Additionally, examination of the placenta in suspected cases (including dark-field microscopy of the umbilical vein or moist lesions) may be positive.

Treatment of congenital syphilis is with parenteral penicillin G 100,000 to 150,000 IU/kg/day IV for 10 days. Both the World Health Organization and Centers for Disease Control and Prevention recommend that asymptomatic infants born to seropositive mothers be treated with a single dose of benzathine benzylpenicillin at 50,000 IU/kg. Close follow-up with appropriate laboratory studies are strongly recommended.

Congenital rubella

Rubella is also known as German measles as it was first described in the German literature. It is typically a mild disease but its effects on the developing fetus have led to widespread vaccination. If acquired in the first 12 weeks of pregnancy, more than 80% of fetuses will exhibit congenital defects.

Rubella is a togavirus, an RNA virus with a surrounding capsid and envelope. Congenital rubella is quite rare, with most recent cases occurring in unvaccinated immigrants. In the United States, young Hispanic women may represent an at-risk population.

Exposure of the fetus after 16 weeks gestation rarely results in any sequelae. An infection before 12 weeks gestation may result in the classic triad of abnormalities called the congenital rubella syndrome. It includes cataracts, heart defects, and sensorineural deafness.

Some manifestations of congenital rubella syndrome are transient such as low birth weight, thrombocytopenia, hepatosplenomegaly, and meningoencephalitis. These findings tend to resolve over days or weeks, but they may exhibit failure to thrive during infancy. The purpuric eruption occurs in the first few days of life and exhibits a "blueberry muffin" appearance. These lesions may represent true purpura or extramedullary hematopoiesis. Other skin findings reported include urticarial lesions, reticulate erythema, and generalized, nonpurpuric eruptions.

Permanent defects include heart defects which are found in more than 50% of children infected during the first 8 weeks of gestation. Patent ductus arteriosus is the most common finding. Pulmonary artery stenosis and hypoplasia are also seen. CNS defects include mental retardation, psychomotor retardation, microcephaly, speech, and language delay. Eye defects, such as cataracts, which occur in one-third of cases and are bilateral in 50%, micropthalmia, and "salt and pepper" retinopathy are also noted. Deafness (sensorineural or central auditory) is the single most common defect and may be the only finding when infection has occurred after 12 weeks gestation.

Late onset defects may not show themselves until after several years of life, especially defects in development, hearing, or ocular function.

Diagnosis

The virus may be isolated from nasopharyngeal swabs, urine, or other bodily fluids. Congenital rubella is most easily diagnosed by the detection of rubella-specific IgM in the serum or oral fluid before 3 months of age. A negative result at this time indicates that the diagnosis of congenital rubella is highly unlikely.

Treatment

Nursing patients in isolation can avoid spreading the infection because of high excretion of rubella virus for up to 1 year. Close long-term follow-up including ophthalmology is warranted.

Congenital Cytomegalovirus

CMV is an enveloped DNA virus of the herpes virus family. Following primary infection, it establishes lifelong latency. It is spread via contact with contaminated body fluids. It is one of the most common viral congenital infections in developed countries and is a major cause of hearing loss and neurodevelopmental disabilities in children. It affects 0.15% to 2% of newborns. Primary CMV infections occur in 1% to 4% of seronegative mothers during pregnancy, with a risk of fetal transmission of 30% to 40%. CMV reactivation during pregnancy occurs in 10% to 30% of seropositive females with a 1% to 3% transmission risk. Only approximately 5% to 15% of infants with congenital CMV will be symptomatic.

There is a wide range in clinical sequelae. While most infections are vertical with transplacental spread or during birth, breast milk is also a source of CMV, and infants with low birthweight and early postnatal virus transmission are at the greatest risk for symptomatic infection.

Up to one-third of symptomatic infants are delivered prematurely. Various findings such as fetal hydrops, intrauterine growth retardation, microcephaly, ventriculomegaly, and periventricular calcifications may be detected during prenatal ultrasounds and suggest the diagnosis.

Skin lesions may be petechial or purpuric, creating a blueberry muffin–like eruption similar to rubella and toxoplasmosis. However, nonspecific maculopapular exanthems may also be seen.

Additionally, hepatosplenomegaly, jaundice, anemia, thrombocytopenia, and interstitial pneumonia can occur.

Most symptomatic cases are fatal in months, with survivors exhibiting severe deficits. In contrast, asymptomatic infants rarely (5%–15%) show any future findings. Diagnosis can be made with viral culture or strongly positive IgM anti-CMV antibody testing. No consistent pharmacologic drug exists for CMV. The efficacy of ganciclovir in this setting is unclear.

Children with congenital CMV will shed the virus for years. Overall, 80% to 90% of children with congenital CMV have a normal outcome and one-third of children with symptomatic congenital CMV will have a normal outcome.

Congenital and neonatal herpes simplex virus (HSV)

Congenital HSV due to intrauterine infection is rare, representing only about 5% of neonatal HSV cases. Such infections may be acquired in an ascending manner or possibly after maternal viremia via the placenta. Up to 70% of cases are caused by HSV type 2. Most infants (85%) acquire infection during birth and 10% acquire it postnatally. Transmission of infection is influenced by type of maternal infection (primary vs. secondary), maternal immunity, duration of membrane rupture, mucocutaneous barrier integrity, and method of delivery. Infants born to mothers during a primary episode of genital HSV are at a much higher risk (57%) than those with recurrent disease (2%) for the development of neonatal HSV. The incidence of neonatal HSV is estimated at 1:3200 live births. Most infants with neonatal HSV are born to mothers who are asymptomatic.

Clinically, infants with congenital HSV may have chorioretinitis, microphthalmia, abnormal brain imaging, and microcephaly. Cutaneous lesions may be active vesicles or simply scars from intrauterine vesiculation. The range in severity of clinical lesions is broad.

Neonatal HSV may have a variety of presentations including disseminated disease involving multiple organs, central nervous system disease in the presence or absence of skin lesions, and finally only superficial lesions limited to the skin, eyes, and mouth. Those infants with primary CNS disease tend to present later (16–19 days) than infants with disseminated or superficial disease (10–12 days). Most infants become ill within the first month of life.

The incidence of disseminated disease has decreased with the introduction of effective antiviral therapies. Over 20% of infants with disseminated disease do not exhibit cutaneous vesicles during their infection. These infants may clinically appear septic and present around 10 to 12 days of age and often exhibit hepatitis and pneumonitis. Consider HSV if bacterial cultures are negative after 2 to 3 days and the infant is not responding to antimicrobial therapy. Disseminated disease has an overall mortality approaching 60%.

Nearly one-third of all infants with HSV infection have some form of CNS involvement. Approximately two-thirds of infants with CNS involvement will have cutaneous vesicular lesions at some point in the course of infection. The localized superficial form of neonatal HSV infection is typically seen in about 20% of cases although this frequency has increased with the more frequent early institution of antiviral therapies. Cutaneous lesions may exhibit a variety of appearances from erythematous macules to vesicles. Vesicles often become pustular in 1 to 2 days followed by crusting and ulceration. Occasionally, patients will have large bullae reminiscent of epidermolysis bullosa. Others may appear purpuric, petechial or even zosteriform. Often, the presenting aspect of the infant is the area most severely involved. Ocular lesions are less common.

Diagnosis

Viral culture remains the definitive modality for diagnosis. Serology is not greatly helpful in diagnosing neonatal HSV. PCR-based assays may prove helpful in the future. Direct fluorescent antibody–based assays are rapid and allow differentiation between viral types. Their sensitivity, however, is lower.

Known risk factors for fatal outcomes include CNS and disseminated disease, impaired consciousness at presentation/onset of treatment, and prematurity. For infants with disseminated disease the presence of pneumonitis and disseminated intravascular coagulation are poor prognostic indicators.

Mothers with active HSV lesions should be delivered by Caesarean section. The role of acyclovir is unclear. Avoidance of fetal scalp electrode monitoring in such cases may also be helpful.

A newborn with suspected HSV lesions should be isolated using contact precautions, treated with empiric antiviral therapy, and aggressively evaluated. Ophthalmologic evaluation and prophylactic topical antivirals are critical. Within 1 month after discharge, 5% to 10% of infants with neonatal HSV will present with a flare of lesions requiring treatment.

The recommended treatment of suspected neonatal HSV is acyclovir 60 mg/kg/day divided every 8 hours for 21 days unless limited only to superficial lesions, where 14 days will suffice. Neutrophil counts should be monitored during therapy. Additionally, all patients should have lumbar puncture at completion of therapy to allow confirmation of PCR negativity. If the patent is PCR positive, therapy is continued until a negative result is obtained.

Congenital varicella

The group of developmental abnormalities associated with congenital varicella infection, termed *congenital varicella syndrome*, occur after maternal infection and in the first 13 to 20 weeks of gestation. The incidence following maternal infection is 0.5% to 1.5% above the background risk for major malformations. Thus, most women who acquire varicella during pregnancy deliver unaffected infants. Maternal zoster is almost never associated with any untoward sequelae for the fetus unless it is disseminated.

Clinical findings of congenital varicella infection include ophthalmologic defects such as microphthalmia, cataracts, and chorioretinitis, low birth weight, limb hypoplasia, neurologic defects, and gastrointestinal and genitourinary defects. Some infants exhibit scars or even vesicles in a dermatomal distribution. The erosions in some cases resemble cutis aplasia.

Neonatal varicella is most severe if maternal rash occurs between 5 days before to 2 days after delivery. These infants must be treated immediately with Varicella-zoster immune globulin (VZIG) and intravenous acyclovir as mortality approaches 30%. Maternal eruptions before or after these periods are typically associated with mild infections, if any.

Congenital parvovirus B19

Parvovirus B19, the only parvovirus to infect humans, is one of the smallest viruses, nonenveloped and made up of single-stranded DNA. Maternal infection during pregnancy can cause fetal infection due to the high viral loads during the 6 to 8 days of most significant infection. Nearly two-thirds of pregnant females are immune to parvovirus and most infants born to mothers who are infected during pregnancy are normal. Viral targeting of erythroid precursor cells and possibly fetal cardiac tissues leads to severe anemia, edema, heart failure, and fetal hydrops, which

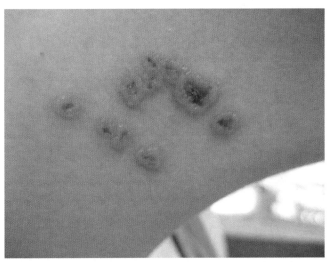

Figure 16.5. Herpes simplex virus type 1. Grouped umbilicated vesicles on an erythematous base on the neck.

can lead to death in some cases. The greatest risk occurs in pregnancies with infection before 20 weeks gestation with fetal loss occurring in 2% to 9% of patients.

VIRAL DISEASES OF THE SKIN

Herpes simplex virus

Outside the neonatal period, most primary HSV infections in children and infants are asymptomatic. HSV-1 is typically transmitted through contact with lesions or oral secretions, whereas HSV-2 is transmitted through sexual activity or contact with genital secretions. Typical cutaneous HSV lesions are shown in Figure 16.5.

Primary HSV gingivostomatitis is likely the most common clinical manifestation, which is usually caused by HSV-1 and occurs in children between 1 and 5 years of age. An ulcerative painful enanthem of the gingival and oral mucous membranes, it often leads to decreased oral intake with dehydration as an occasional complication. Affected areas may exhibit swelling with friability and easy bleeding. Vesicles rapidly progress to erosions and ulcers. Affected children may exhibit fever as well as localized lymphadenopathy. Spread of lesions to the lips, cheeks, and chin will occur in a majority of patients to some degree. Resolution within 10 to 14 days is typical and acyclovir may be helpful if therapy is initiated early enough. Children with a history of eczema should be monitored closely for dissemination and may require antiviral therapy outside of this time range to suppress the infection. A similar eruption due to HSV-2 is described in sexually active adolescents/young adults.

Eczema herpeticum is a widespread eruption of HSV occurring in patients with preexisting skin diseases such as atopic dermatitis, Darier's disease, pemphigus, or burns. Patients become febrile and ill with the sudden outbreak of widespread vesicles. Viral lesions are often worse or more concentrated in areas of active skin disease. Multiple complications can occur, including keratoconjunctivitis, secondary bacterial infections, dehydration, and systemic viremia. Early systemic therapy is mandatory and typically parenteral. Ophthalmogic evaluation is important. Skin care utilizes bland emollients early to aid healing followed by topical anti-inflammatory agents to control dermatitis.

Herpetic whitlow involves single or multiple, painful, deep-seated HSV vesicles, typically on the distal aspects of a digit. It can arise via autoinoculation from oral or genital HSV or as an occupational dermatosis in those who come into contact with such secretions. Resolution in 2 to 3 weeks is typical.

Herpes gladiatorum occurs in wrestlers or rugby players, where repeated skin trauma along with skin-to-skin contact and skin-to-fomite contact predisposes to transmission of HSV. Approximately one-third of wrestlers develop herpes gladiatorum at some point. Lesions typically involve areas of skin contact and may not have a typical vesicular appearance. Occasionally, patients exhibit systemic symptoms. Treatment is indicated and athletes are allowed to return to play once lesions have crusted. Episodic or prophylactic therapy may also be indicated.

HSV keratoconjunctivitis occurs with primary HSV infection of the eye, leading to severe inflammation with superficial corneal erosions or ulcers. HSV is the leading cause of recurrent kerato-conjunctivitis with eventual corneal opacification and blindness. Viral culture and HSV PCR on tear film can confirm the infection, although corneal scrapings may be better sources of the virus. Topical and/or oral antivirals are the mainstays of therapy.

Herpes genitalis may be caused by HSV-1 or HSV-2. While the cause of infection is typically HSV-2, the frequency of genital HSV-1 infection is increasing among young adults/college students. Frequency of HSV-2 infection directly correlates with the number of sexual partners, and transmission is dramatically reduced with condom use, offering another reason for the strong promotion of condom use among sexually active adolescents. The diagnosis of genital HSV in a child should prompt concern regarding sexual abuse. Recurrence rates of HSV tend to be higher in the first years after initial infection.

HSV is the most common cause of erythema multiforme (EM) minor in both children and adults. Recurrences of HSV are followed by the eruption of tender, inflammatory, targetoid lesions, often acral and especially on the palms and soles (Figs. 16.6 and 16.7). Control of the HSV infection often prevents recurrence of the EM.

HSV lesions in immunosuppressed patients may present with a variety of atypical skin manifestations including verrucous, pustular, crusted, necrotic, or exophytic presentations. A high index of suspicion with a low threshold for appropriate testing allows earlier diagnosis of such outbreaks. HSV may cause persistent or recurrent ulcers in immunosuppressed patients such as those with AIDS. Widespread or large lesions may be seen (Figs. 16.8 and 16.9).

Primary varicella zoster virus (VZV) infection has become infrequent in the USA with the advent and widespread administration of the live attenuated varicella vaccine. It is highly contagious with a 14–16 day incubation period; traditionally it was most common in the colder months of the year. Spread occurs from person to person via respiratory droplets and children are no longer contagious within 7–8 days of rash onset. Affected patients often exhibit a low grade fever early in the illness with the generalized eruption beginning on the scalp or trunk. Lesions

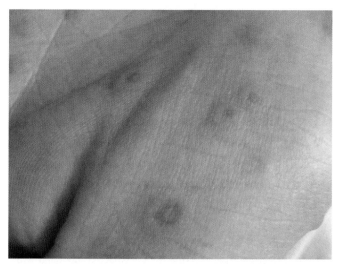

Figure 16.6. Erythema multiforme simplex due to HSV. Tender targetoid lesions on palms in a patient with a recent outbreak of orolabial HSV.

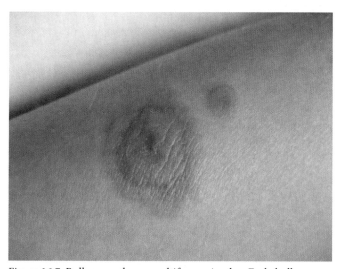

Figure 16.7. Bullous erythema multiforme simplex. Early bullous lesion from the lateral distal upper extremity. Note targetoid appearance of lesion and early central bullae.

begin as erythematous macules but rapidly become vesicular, crust and begin to heal (see Figure 16.10). Mucous membrane lesions are common and the pruritus from skin lesions is often intense. Varicella often exhibits a more severe course in older patients and very young infants. The most common complication of primary varicella is secondary infection of the skin lesions, usually caused by Staphylococcus and group A streptococcal infections. Serious infections such as necrotizing fasciitis and purpura fulminans can occur. Tzanck preparations, direct fluorescent antibody testing, and viral culture from vesicular fluid can aid diagnosis. The differential includes some forms of enteroviral exanthems which can produce clinical lesions mimicking varicella. Children with primary varicella are no longer contagious once all the lesions have crusted.

Herpes zoster is more common in children who are immunosuppressed or who had their primary varicella infection in the first year of life. With implementation of the varicella vaccine, cases have occurred due to apparent reactivation of the

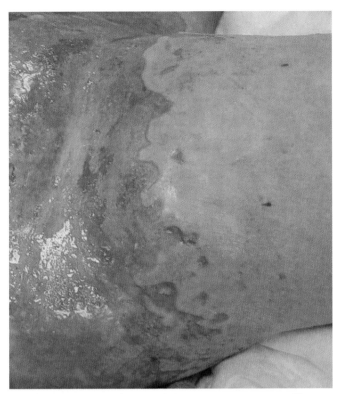

Figure 16.8. Recurrent chronic HSV in an immunosuppressed host. Note widespread angulated ulcers with punched out lesions on periphery.

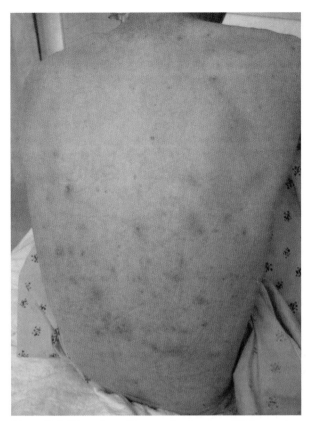

Figure 16.9. Disseminated herpes simplex virus. Widespread vesicular lesions arising on erythematous bases in an immunosuppressed patient. Tzanck preparation was positive for multinucleated giant cells and viral culture revealed herpes simplex virus type 1.

viral VZV strain. Hutchinson's sign refers to varicella lesions of the nasal tip, which can reflect involvement of the nasociliary branch and signal a risk of corneal lesions. Such patients require prompt initiation of antiviral therapy and ophthalmologic consultation. Treatment is with high-dose antivirals, and severe or disseminated infections should be treated parenterally.

Treatment of both primary and secondary VZV infections is supportive in uncomplicated cases, mainly focused on control of pruritus and prevention of excoriation which could increase the chance of secondary skin infections. If systemic therapy is necessary acyclovir is the treatment of choice. Immunosuppressed or other high risk patients may require passive immunization with varicella zoster hyperimmune globulin (VZIG).

Verruca

Human papillomavirus (HPV) is a double-stranded DNA virus that causes various clinical lesions. Infection of squamous cells leads to the formation of benign tumors called warts, verruca, or papillomas. Lesions on acral surfaces are most common and children are the most common hosts, with an incidence estimated at 10%.

Condylomas are HPV-induced lesions of the genital tract and are one of the most common sexually transmitted diseases. Multiple modes of transmission exist: vertical spread (perinatal); benign (nonsexual) inoculation from a parent or caregiver; autoinoculation; fomite spread; and sexual contact. Clinically they appear as soft, verrucous, occasionally pedunculated, skin colored papules. Although commonly located in the perianal region they can be located anywhere in the genital area. Typically, they are asymptomatic although some lesions may exhibit bleeding and pain if irritation occurs. An important consideration in

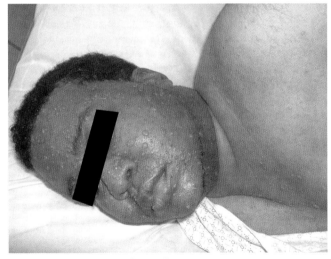

Figure 16.10. Disseminated varicella. Immunocompetent patient; note umbilication creating resemblance to pox virus infections. Image courtesy of Mike Swann, MD.

the differential of condyloma in young children is the perianal pyrimidiform protrusion, a flesh colored to pink soft tissue swelling along the median raphe more commonly seen in females. The lesions may be mistaken for condylomas but often appear in association with a history of diarrhea or constipation. They often resolve with normalization of the gastrointestinal function.

Diagnosis of condyloma in children should raise the possibility of sexual abuse as the mode of HPV acquisition. While HPV typing is often considered in the work-up of such patients, it does not allow differentiation between the forms of viral transmission. A directed history is necessary, screening for timing of onset, as well as maternal history of HPV infection or abnormal PAP smears and the personal or family history of verruca. An appreciation of the child's social environment is helpful. The risk of sexual abuse as a cause of condyloma in children is higher for those patients older than 3 to 4 years. Infections are believed to be acquired in a nonsexual manner in the following instances; children <3 years of age (especially with lesions that began in the first year of life), the presence of other nongenital warts verrucae in close contacts, a positive maternal history and no physical findings for abuse. Any suspicion of abuse should prompt referral to a child protective services team and consideration of a SAFE exam.

Treatment of verrucae is challenging, as there is no one perfect effective therapy. Spontaneous resolution may occur in at least 54% of patients within 5 years from their diagnosis. Because of this observation, minimal intervention can be a reasonable therapeutic choice. Overly painful or aggressive therapies or those that could scar are usually avoided. The choice of therapy is variable, depending on the individual child and the parents' input. Though parents may occasionally press for aggressive (and thus painful) therapies for their children, always consider the risk–benefit ratio for the child and recommend therapy accordingly.

Topical therapies such as salicylic acid may be used with or without occlusive dressings. Resolution of the verruca may require 2 to 12 weeks.

Cryotherapy, ideally using liquid nitrogen, is effective but painful. Use of a cotton-tipped applicator to apply the liquid nitrogen may be less frightening for small children rather than using a cryogen spray gun. When using cryotherapy, care must be taken not to freeze the skin too deeply, or hypopigmentation and/or scarring can result. In addition, debriding the hyperkeratotic material from the surface of the verruca before cryotherapy can speed improvement. Treatments are then continued every 3 to 4 weeks.

Additional treatments for verruca involve modulation of the immune response, such as cimetidine (30 mg/kg/day divided into three doses for 6 to 8 weeks of therapy), topical imiquimod applied with varying frequency (three times per week on thin or genital skin – more frequently, up to twice daily on more keratinized surfaces), and stimulation of allergic contact dermatitis using squaric acid dibutylester or diphenylcyclopropenone (DPCP). Use of these agents is painless and is well tolerated even by the youngest patients. Pulsed dye laser therapy has been used with reasonable efficacy but the cost of this modality limits its use to those verruca resistant to other therapies.

Care must be taken when treating verruca plana with destructive therapies so as not to induce undue scarring or hypopigmentation. For this reason and because large areas are often involved by these lesions, topical agents such as imiquimod and/or topical retinoids may be preferred.

The high rate of spontaneous involution for condyloma makes observation a reasonable option for therapy. Topical destructive agents such as podophyllin or trichloracetic acid may be used. Imiquimod is also highly effective. Surgical debulking of large lesions may be necessary. Destructive modalities such as cryotherapy and pulsed dye laser may be used but may require sedation in children or adolescents.

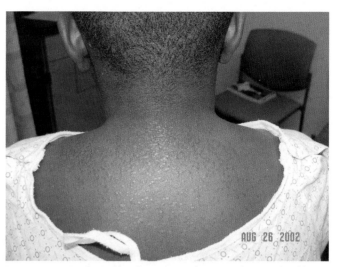

Figure 16.11. Epidermodysplasia verruciformis. Otherwise healthy patient with widespread flat-topped lesions. Histopathology was consistent with human papillomavirus infection. Improved greatly on isotretinoin.
Image courtesy of Karen Edison, MD.

Oral HPV infection is associated with respiratory papillomatosis as well as cervical and genital lesions. Respiratory papillomatosis, the most common laryngeal neoplasm of children, is caused by HPV types 6 and 11, usually acquired via vertical transmission and is not considered a marker of sexual abuse. Recent work suggests that oral HPV acquisition before 1 year is typically via vertical transmission. Heck's disease is one form of oral verruca characterized by unique HPV subtypes 13, 24, and 32. In the absence of Heck's disease, mucosal strains of HPV such as types 6 and 11 are often detected. In these patients, the epidemiology of HPV acquisition likely mimics that of condyloma. Younger children are more likely to have been infected with HPV via innocuous transmission, while older children are more likely to have had sexual transmission.

Epidermodysplasia verruciformis is a genetically mediated disease. Affected patients have an increased susceptibility to wart infections. The disease is caused by mutations in two novel genes EVER1 and EVER2. It is estimated that ~50% of affected patients will undergo malignant degeneration of lesions in adulthood. The onset of skin lesions is in early childhood and patients often present with widespread hypopigmented macules that can mimic tinea versicolor in addition to verruca plana–like lesions. More verrucous lesions may be found on the face and extremities (Fig. 16.11). Cutaneous malignancies typically occur in sun-exposed areas, and strict aggressive sun protection measures are necessary.

An autosomal dominant syndrome has been described with patients exhibiting hypogammaglobulinemia, infections, and myelokathexis (retention of white blood cells in the bone marrow), in addition to widespread verrucae. This has been termed the *WHIM syndrome*.

Molluscum and poxviridae

Molluscum contagiosum is now a common viral skin infection of childhood caused by the molluscum contagiosum virus (MCV). Recent decades have seen a significant increase in MCV infection frequency and MCV is now the main disease causing

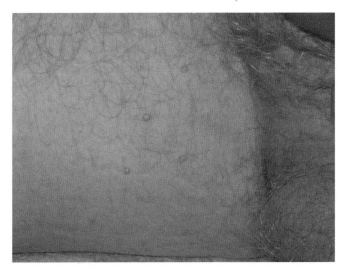

Figure 16.12. Molluscum. Umbilicated, pearly papules located on the inner thigh.

poxvirus in humans. While in adults MCV infection is associated with immunodeficiency or sexual transmission, in children it is typically acquired innocuously. Several forms of MCV have been identified with the MCV-1 form typically causing MC in children and the MCV-2 form being more often sexually transmitted. MCV is easily spread via skin-to-skin contact or via fomites. Swimming pools are thought to be a major source of transmission. Autoinoculation and koebnerization are common modes of spread once infected. Patients with underlying skin disorders, especially children with atopic dermatitis, are particularly susceptible to disseminated MC lesions.

Clinically MC appears as pearly, pink-to-flesh colored papules of variable size. Often a central umbilication is present (Fig. 16.12). The immune response to these lesions is variable but when severe, the deep-seated inflammation can lead to tenderness and drainage similar to what is seen in a furuncle.

Molluscum dermatitis is an eczematous reaction occurring around MC lesions or clusters of lesions that may represent virally induced modulation of the local immune system. Pruritus from the dermatitis may lead to scratching and further spread of the virus. Eyelid lesions can be problematic as conjunctivitis or superficial punctate keratitis can occur if an inflammatory response develops.

Course

Most patients with MC will undergo spontaneous remission between 6 months and 2 years after the onset of infection. For this reason, watchful waiting is a reasonable mode of management although pruritus, pain, concerns over spread to other children or classmates, and the cosmetic impact of lesions may prompt parental requests for more aggressive treatments.

Treatment

Modalities employed in the treatment of MC in adults such as curettage and cryotherapy may not be tolerated by small children. Application of cantharidin, an extract from the blister beetle, is a painless alternative and produces a superficial blistering reaction that can result in removal of MC lesions. This treatment is usually well tolerated without any resultant discomfort and thesmall

vesicles typically resolve within a few days. Postinflammatory hyperpigmentation may occur and parents should be cautioned about this temporary side effect. Parents should also be counseled that, as a poxvirus, MC infections can leave a residual "pock mark" that, while small and often innocuous, represents a scar caused by the infection. These marks, which develop from ~7% of lesions, often fade with time as the child grows but can be disturbing to parents when first noticed.

Other treatments used for MC include topical imiquimod, topical retinoids, tape stripping, keratolytic agents, pulsed dye laser, and oral cimetidine.

Other poxviruses may infect pediatric patients. **Orf** (ecthyma contagiosum) and **milker's nodules** are caused by exposure to infected goats and sheep (orf) or cattle (milker's nodules). Both are caused by parapox viruses and after onset, the clinical infection progresses through several typical clinical stages. The first stage begins as macules that develop into papules and then into vesicles. These vesicles then erode to become weeping nodules, which then evolve into verrucous lesions, eventually develop a dry crust and then shed with wound healing. Occasionally, erythema multiforme may occur. Lesions typically heal without scarring over 4 to 8 weeks. No other treatment is needed. These lesions are rarely seen in a dermatology clinic as most patients involved in the husbandry of susceptible animals recognize the infection and realize it will resolve with no therapy.

Monkeypox

In the spring of 2003, an outbreak of febrile illness with associated vesiculopustular lesions led to the identification of the first outbreak of monkeypox in the Western Hemisphere. Several of the patients including the index case were children, infected via bites from or exposures to ill pet prairie dogs, which had acquired the illness from an infected Gambian giant rat. While several patients became quite ill, all recovered. Cutaneous lesions were variable in appearance and often made up of deep-seated vesiculopustules, some with pronounced surrounding erythema. In most patients, a variable number of satellite and disseminated lesions developed over several days. Larger lesions often resolve with scars.

Vaccinia and Variola

Concern over weaponization of smallpox, or variola major, though eradicated from the planet since 1977, has been on the rise due to recent terrorist events. This has led to resumption of smallpox vaccination using vaccinia virus in at-risk persons such as military personnel and certain workers in the medical community. Thus, familiarity with both smallpox and the complications associated with vaccination against smallpox is now much more important.

Acquisition of variola occurs via the respiratory tract with viral replication in regional nodes followed by viremia. Onset of symptoms typically occurs after an incubation period of 7 to 17 days. An enanthem of erythematous macules on the oral mucosa (palate, tongue, and pharynx) begins 1 to 2 days before the exanthem. The exanthem is characterized by erythematous macules progressing to vesicles and then pustules over a 4 to 7 day period with most lesions at the same developmental stage in each area of the body. The pustules are deep seated and firm (in contrast to varicella) due to their dermal location. Lesions typically begin on the face and spread downward. Crusting of lesions begins at 8 to 9 days, and healing leaves significant scarring. The mortality is ~30%. Variant presentations such as the hemorrhagic and malignant forms are almost universally fatal. Variola minor (alastrim) occurs when individuals with some preexisting immunity are infected with variola and has a much lower mortality rate. Once infection occurs, patients are infectious for ~10 days from the onset of the rash. Suspected cases must be isolated. Cidofovir may help in treatment.

Another major concern with resumption of smallpox vaccination is risks from the vaccine. Most importantly, **eczema vaccinatum** can occur when a person with active or a past history of certain skin diseases, such as atopic dermatitis or Darier's disease, is exposed to vaccinia. Worsening of the eruption can happen quickly with rapid viral dissemination. While no cases of eczema vaccinatum had been reported since the late 1980s, recently eczema vaccinatum has occurred in a male child with severe eczema and a history of failure to thrive. After exposure to his father, who had recently been vaccinated for smallpox in preparation for deployment, the child became febrile and then began to develop vesicular skin lesions. Dissemination of the infection led to a clinical presentation similar to smallpox. Aggressive treatment was necessary, the child required intubation and administration of vaccinia immune globulin as well as cidofovir and an investigational drug.

Complications can include secondary infection, shock, and even death. Vaccinia immune globulin has been approved since 2005 for treatment of eczema vaccinatum. People that are vaccinated for smallpox should avoid contact with people who have a history of generalized dermatoses. At present, smallpox vaccination is not recommended for those under 18 years of age.

INFESTATIONS

Pediculosis

Pediculosis humanus capitis infestation is usually seen in children aged 3 to 12 and has no socioeconomic barriers. The oval hair shafts of African-Americans are somewhat resistant to infestation. Lice are transmitted via direct contact or via fomites that have a less than 24-hour survival off the scalp of the human host. Eggs, or nits, are firmly attached to the base of the hair shaft by the female louse at a rate of approximately ten per day. They hatch in 10 to 14 days. The life cycle from nit to adult louse is approximately 3 weeks. Nits are often found in the posterior auricular area and occipital scalp. Pruritus begins 3 to 4 weeks after the first infestation, allowing for the development of a delayed hypersensitivity response to the louse saliva.

Treatment with pediculicides is the first line of treatment. Many over-the-counter products exist and are effective in the treatment of head lice. Pyrethrins, in addition to piperonyl butoxide, are found in a shampoo form, which is neurotoxic to the lice. A 10-minute incubation period on dry hair is recommended, followed by rinsing with cool water to minimize cutaneous absorption. This treatment is partially ovicidal as well, but approximately 30% may persist. Therefore, a second treatment is recommended in 7 to 10 days. Resistance does occur, and patients with ragweed or chrysanthemum sensitivity should avoid this product, as there is potential for allergic reaction.

The treatment of choice is permethrin 1%, a synthetic pyrethroid, which can be found over-the-counter as a cream rinse. It should be applied to damp hair following shampooing and the hair should be allowed to dry for ten minutes before rinsing. This is pediculocidal and partially ovicidal and repeat treatment in 7 to 10 days is recommended.

Lindane should be used cautiously as CNS toxicity can produce seizures in children. It is available as a prescription shampoo, has low ovicidal activity, and resistance has been noted. Malathion carries a risk of flammability and respiratory depression with ingestion, but does have ovicidal activity. Permethrin 5% and crotamiton 10% have had some effectiveness in patients with pediculosis, but have not been studied extensively. Oral treatment with sulfamethoxazole–trimethoprim in combination with pediculocidal agents has been effective but carries the potential for serious side effects including Stevens–Johnson syndrome. Ivermectin is not recommended in children weighing less than 15 kg as they are at higher risk for penetration of the blood–brain barrier.

Studies in children have shown that only 20% to 30% of children with nits develop infestation with adult lice, which should encourage schools to eliminate the "no nit" policy seen in some school districts. Treatment should be advised for children and close contacts with evidence of live lice, or nits within 1 cm of the scalp as these are more likely to be viable. Following treatment, removal of nits from wet hair with a fine-toothed comb can be done but may not be necessary. Bedding, clothing, and personal care items should be cleaned. Objects, which cannot be washed, may be vacuumed or placed in a closed plastic bag for 2 weeks.

The body louse, *Pediculus humanus humanus*, infests individuals in crowded, unsanitary conditions. The louse resides in the clothing of affected individuals and can be found along the seams. It also has a preference for warmer areas of the body. The louse is larger than *Pediculus humanus capitis* and has a life span of 18 days. Approximately 3 weeks are required for a nit to develop into a mature louse. The body louse can live for 3 days without feeding. Treatment involves cleaning affected clothing and improving personal hygiene.

Pthirus pubis, or the crab louse, is transmitted via sexual contact, and can be visualized with the naked eye attached to the hairs of the pubic and adjacent body areas. The body of the louse is wide with clawed legs, which allow it to grasp the hairs. Adult lice live approximately 2 weeks and require 3 weeks to progress from nits to the mature adult. Blue-gray macules on the trunk and thighs, known as maculae ceruleae, can be seen in chronic infections. Nits may also be noted on the eyelashes, and scalp involvement can occur as well. Patients should be screened for other sexually transmitted diseases as there is a 30% rate of concurrence between the two infections. Permethrin 5% cream is recommended for the treatment of pubic lice, with petrolatum for eyelash involvement. Patients should also be advised to abstain from sexual intercourse and to thoroughly cleanse all linens and garments.

Mites

Sarcoptes scabiei var. *hominis* is the mite responsible for the manifestations of scabies and is transmitted by human-to-human contact. A worldwide distribution is seen, but is very common in areas of poverty, in persons with dementia, in persons with nutritional deficiencies, in persons with poor hygiene, and in the homeless. It also occurs frequently in children.

Skin manifestations include burrows, which are usually found in the digital web spaces, or at the elbows, wrists, umbilicus, nipples, and genital areas. Erythematous, sometimes excoriated papules can also be seen. Bullous lesions can be seen in the elderly or immunosuppressed, but cases have been reported in children as well. Generalized pruritus occurs 3 to 4 weeks following initial infection, as it is a delayed hypersensitivity response to the eggs, scybala, or saliva of the mite. In reinfested patients, pruritus occurs within a few days of infection.

Lesions in children may become secondarily infected with *S. aureus* or *S. pyogenes*. Infants normally develop nodules, vesicles, and pustules of the face, head, axillae, and genital area. Palmoplantar involvement can also be seen. Red-brown, pruritic nodules of the male genitalia and axillae, described as nodular scabies, are seen in 7% of patients. These are hypothesized to be manifestations of an exuberant hypersensitivity reaction. Immunosuppressed patients may develop Norwegian, or crusted scabies, which is characterized by acral, hyperkeratotic plaques and subungual involvement.

Female mites lay one to three eggs in burrows created in the stratum granulosum. The larval forms hatch in 2 to 4 days and undergo a molting process, with mature mites being produced in 10 to 14 days. The average patient carries 10 to 15 adult female mites, while patients with crusted scabies may be infested with more than one million organisms. The life cycle then repeats, with male mites dying after mating.

Diagnosis can be made by microscopic visualization of mites, eggs, or scybala after scraping a burrow with a blade coated in oil. Dermatoscopy can be useful in some cases, but histologic exam is only consistent with an arthropod bite reaction unless the organism or eggs are noted.

Permethrin 5% cream, a synthetic pyrethroid, is the most effective topical treatment and is safe to use in children older than 3 months. It can cause irritant cutaneous reactions and rarely dystonic reactions. There is no potential for allergic reaction in patients with chrysanthemum sensitivity. Lindane should be used with caution in children and avoided in infants as neurologic symptoms including seizures and irritability can occur. Infants can be treated with crotamiton 10% cream, which has been shown to be more effective than permethrin in infants and children. Potential side effects include conjunctivitis and erythema. Systemic treatment with ivermectin is not recommended in children less than 5 years of age as safety has not yet been established, and permeability of the blood–brain barrier has been seen in some patients. Pruritus can persist for weeks following treatment. Patients should be advised to use sensitive skin care measures and given topical steroids and antihistamines for symptom control.

Harvest mites, or chiggers, are in the family *Trombiculidae* and frequently cause skin lesions in the summer and fall. The larval form is found on the ground and painlessly feeds on the lower extremities or waistline. Pruritic papules appear within 24 hours and resolve over weeks.

Cheyletiella blakei, *Cheyletiella yasguri*, and *Cheyletiella parasitvorax* are mites of cats, dogs, and rabbits, respectively. They are the cause of pruritic papules, which may become vesicular, pustular, and crusted in areas of the body where pets are frequently in contact with the patient. The animals are asymptomatically infected, and microscopic examination of fur scrapings will identify the organisms as they are rarely found on the affected human. Eradication of the mites is curative and skin lesions can be treated symptomatically.

Spiders

Brown recluse spiders, *Loxosceles reclusa*, can be seen in the southern United States from Nebraska to Ohio with the Gulf of Mexico as the southernmost border. The tan spider can be identified by the characteristic violin marking of the head and thorax, and its three pairs of eyes. The brown recluse does not bite unless provoked and can be found under rocks, in basements, and in boxes. Bites may initially cause slight discomfort followed by increasing pain and erythema. Subsequent necrosis occurs in 48 to 72 hours. Systemic symptoms of fever, chills, arthralgias, nausea, and serious complications of hemolytic anemia mediated by the sphingomyelinase D toxin, renal failure, and pulmonary edema are more common in children. Treatment involves rest and elevation with antibiotic coverage in cases where secondary infection is a concern. Supportive measures are indicated in patients with systemic effects.

Lactrodectus mactans is the most common species of black widow spiders in the United States and can be identified by the red hourglass located on the abdomen of the black spider. It lives on webs in the protected areas of buildings. Bites can be painful and are incurred after disruption of the spider's habitat. Neuronal depolarization occurs following inoculation of the α-latrotoxin resulting in erythema and piloerection at the site, with systemic symptoms of abdominal pain, nausea, vomiting, paresthesias, hypertension, and headache. Antivenin can be used in severe cases. Benzodiazepines and calcium gluconate are also helpful.

Scorpions

Scorpions are found predominantly in the southwestern United States and stings cause burning pain followed by anesthesia. Scorpions retaliate if they are disturbed or trapped. Stings related to *Centruroides exilicauda* are of particular concern in children as they are potentially fatal. Children should be monitored in an intensive care unit as the scorpion's neurotoxin can cause respiratory distress, vision changes, muscles spasms, and slurred speech. Antivenin and supportive measures are the treatments of choice. *Centruroides* scorpions can be identified by a spine at the base of their stinger.

Papular urticaria

Papular urticaria is caused by an arthropod bite-induced hypersensitivity reaction. The most common pathogens are *Cimex lectularius*, *Ctenocephalides canis*, *C. felix*, and *Pulex irritans*, which are bedbugs and the cat, dog, and human fleas, respectively. Children require prior exposure to these arthropods to mount the hypersensitivity response. This allows infants to be relatively spared, and teens often develop hyposensitization with chronic exposure. Cutaneous lesions are commonly seen on the arms and legs and manifest as urticarial, sometimes vesicular, papules that are extremely pruritic. Symptomatic treatment of pruritus with antihistamines and mild topical steroids is helpful, but the primary focus should be on elimination of the source of infection.

Fleas

Fleas can cause a papular, pruritic dermatitis, which results from the injection of antigenic saliva into the skin. Treatment is symptomatic and eradication of the organism is key, as some species of *Xenopsylla* are vectors for typhus and bubonic plague. The sand flea, or *Tunga penetrans*, can also cause tender, pruritic nodules of the feet secondary to burrowing of the flea into the skin. This infection is known as *tungiasis* with potentially serious complications of secondary infection and occasionally digital amputation.

Bedbugs

Cimex lenticularis is seen in developing countries and lives in cracks in paint, wallpaper, and furniture. They feed nocturnally and typically bite painlessly. Bites tend to be grouped or linear, and pruritic papular lesions with a central punctum are the result. Treatment should focus on symptomatic management and prevention of secondary infection.

Stinging Insects

The order *Hymenoptera* contains three families of stinging insects. Honeybees are in the family *Apidae*. They commonly live in buildings or hollow trees and sting only when provoked, leaving the stinger and venom sack in the skin. Phospholipase A_2 is the primary allergen in honeybee venom.

Wasps, hornets, and yellow jackets are members of the *Vespidae* family. Hornets are aggressive and commonly make nests in trees and shrubs. Honeycomb nests in shrubbery and protected areas of buildings are the homes of wasps. Yellow jackets reside in walls, hollow spaces, and the ground. They are attracted to food and garbage and tend to be very aggressive. The major allergen in yellow jackets and hornets is antigen 5, which has significant cross-reactivity. Wasps, however, show only a moderate cross-reactivity.

Reactions to insect stings can be categorized as normal, large local, anaphylactic, and toxic. Most components of the reaction are mediated by the vasoactive amines, peptides, and proteins found in the venom. Tenderness, swelling, and erythema, that resolves within a few hours are considered normal reactions. Patients with 24 to 48 hours of increasing local symptoms followed by slow resolution have large local reactions. These carries a slightly higher but less than 10% risk of more severe reactions to future stings for these patients. Toxic reactions can occur following inoculation of significant quantities of venom. These are manifested physiologically as reactions to the venom components. Urticaria, angioedema, hypotension, bronchospasm, and shock can be seen in 0.5% to 1.5% of stings and are classified as anaphylactic reactions. Children are more likely to have an anaphylactic reaction, but atopy only minimally increases this risk.

Care should be taken in the removal of residual stingers, as additional venom can be inoculated if the venom sac is compressed. The recommendation is to scrape the stingers from the skin. Treatment for local reactions is primarily symptom driven. Patients with large local reactions may consider carrying self-injectible epinephrine, which is mandatory in patients with anaphylactic reactions. Immunotherapy following skin testing by an allergist can reduce the risk of severe reactions to less than 5% in patients with a history of anaphylaxis. Avoidance measures should also be utilized.

Stinging ants are in the family *Formicidae* with *Solenopsis invicta* as the most common fire ant species in the United States. They live in large groups in nests or mounds and are aggressive, resulting in multiple stings per insect. Their venom is primarily alkaloid and produces a pustule within 24 hours at the site of stings. Reactions are categorized in the same manner as the flying insects and immunotherapy can be used to treat severe reactions as well.

Blister beetles

Blister beetles of multiple species produce a characteristic dermatitis when crushed. Vesicles and bullae occur after cantharidin, which is produced by the beetles, comes in contact with the skin. This phenomenon is used therapeutically in controlled settings to treat other infectious disease in children such as verrucae and molluscum contagiosum. Treatment involves cleansing the area to remove the chemical and wound care for bullous lesions.

Caterpillars and Moths

Lepidopterism is the term used to describe the cutaneous and systemic effects related to moths, caterpillars, and butterflies of the order *Lepidoptera*. The fine hairs, or setae, of these organisms are responsible for the manifestations of disease, which may be mediated via toxins, hypersensitivity reaction, or mechanical irritation. Tape stripping of the setae following exposure is helpful in treatment. Outbreaks can occur in areas of high concentration, such as those reported at Boy Scout camps. Linear, erythematous, pruritic papules are most commonly seen, but urticaria and exacerbation of underlying respiratory problems can occur as well. Some *Lepidoptera* produce a distinct cutaneous manifestation, such as the painful, tram-track lesions that are seen following the sting of *Megalopyge opercularis*, or the puss caterpillar.

PITFALLS AND MYTHS

Cutaneous infections in children are common. While many diagnoses are straightforward, many common infections may present with atypical clinical features, which can delay the diagnosis or lead to an initial misdiagnosis. Additionally, some skin diseases common to childhood may mimic infectious processes, such as the frequent misdiagnosis of granuloma annulare as tinea corporis. Familiarity with the timing, presentation, and course of these typical cutaneous infections of childhood is important and can allow for more rapid testing, diagnosis, and treatment.

SUGGESTED READINGS

Paller, Amy S, and Mancini, Anthony J. *Hurwitz Clinical Pediatric Dermatology*, 3rd edition. Saunders: Elsevier, 2006.
Schachner, Lawrence A and Hansen, Ronald C. *Pediatric Dermatology*, 3rd edition. Mosby, London, 2003.

SKIN INFECTIONS IN THE ELDERLY

Noah S. Scheinfeld

INTRODUCTION

"All things collapse the center can not hold," wrote W.H. Auden. While he was likely speaking of politics in Western Europe before World War II, he might well have been speaking of the skin in old age. The skin of old age is the product of a gradual loss of skin structures and a decrease in skin integrity that occurs through adulthood and middle age.

Skin infections of all types are more common in the elderly than in the young. The reasons for this are multifold and include the following:

(1) Decreased skin integrity due to
   (a) the decreased function and number of sweat glands
   (b) the decline in the ambient moisture content of the skin
   (c) thinning of the epidermis and dermis and
   (d) decreases in fascial function, which facilitates the ingress of fungi into the skin and nails
(2) Cardiovascular impairment, which
   (a) decreases skin integrity
   (b) hinders immune cell deployment and
   (c) sometimes leaves parts of the skin and nails as virtual cul-de-sacs outside regulation of the body's various homeostatic systems
(3) Decreased immune function, which manifests with
   (a) inability to mount fevers
   (b) a tilt toward the TH2 arms of immune function at the expense of the TH1 arm
   (c) fewer and less functional immune cells
(4) Physical factors such as pressure effects on weakened skin, leading to breakdown secondary to a sedentary life style, immobility, or neuropathy
(5) malnutrition and
(6) hormonal alterations that include decreased estrogen and testosterone levels and insulin resistance.

I will expend on these points further.

The symptoms that surround infections in the elderly are less florid. The elderly are less able to mount a fever or increase their white blood cell count in response to infection. Acute disorientation, anorexia and weakness, and simple erythema of the skin are all nonspecific signs that can be the presenting signs of infection, making the diagnosis of infection difficult.

Diseases that provide the foundation for infection increase in incidence in the elderly. Specifically, diabetes and cancers decrease the function of the immune system. Diseases that undermine the cardiovascular system such as coronary artery disease, peripheral vascular disease, hyperlipidemia, and hypertension decrease blood flow to the skin decreasing the capacity of the elderly to defeat infection. Decreased blood flow slows healing, increases xerosis, and decreases epidermal integrity. This decrease in epidermal integrity permits bacteria and fungi to enter broken skin, such as cuts, sores, abrasions, erosions, ulcers, and fissures. Ulcers can occur on the feet as a result of neuropathy secondary to diabetes in many cases and get infected (Fig. 17.1).

As the implications for missing a diagnosis are high and the potential for a confusing clinical picture is great, elderly patients who are examined should be approached with a high index of clinical suspicion. Initiation of treatment should be considered as soon as an infection is suspected. Apposite diagnostic testing should be performed promptly. Culturing pus, fluids, blood, and scale should be considered before treatment is started.

When assessing the results of laboratory tests, some results may be suggestive of a diagnosis rather than diagnostic. Some positive culture results represent colonization rather than infection of the skin. Inflammatory skin diseases and systemic diseases can mimic skin infection. To achieve a definitive diagnosis, tests such as a Gram stain, blood chemistry tests, urine analysis, and skin biopsy can be helpful.

HISTORY

The sixth age shifts
Into the lean and slipper'd pantaloon,

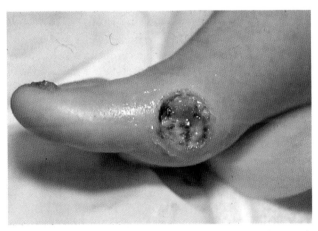

Figure 17.1. Malperforans ulcer in an elderly diabetic with secondary infection.

With spectacles on nose and pouch on side,
His youthful hose, well saved, a world too wide
For his shrunk shank; and his big manly voice,
urning again toward childish treble, pipes
And whistles in his sound. Last scene of all,
That ends this strange eventful history,
Is second childishness and mere oblivion,
Sans teeth, sans eyes, sans taste, sans everything.
Shakespeare's *As You Like It*

The burden of skin disease has always weighed on the elderly. Before the middle of the 20th century, relative to today, few persons reached age 65. The atrophy of skin and waning immune function affected people before 1950, particularly and intensely. This was due in part to the fact that effective antibiotic and antifungal agents were not available. Few classical authors attributed skin disease to old age although they did note the wrinkles and sagging skin of old age. As people lived better and longer, starting in the 20th century skin diseases could be separated more readily between those of the adult and those of the elderly.

BACTERIAL INFECTIONS

The most common pathogens associated with infections of the skin are *Staphylococcus aureus* and Streptoccocal species. Rarely, gram-negative organisms can be involved, and this should be remembered when starting empirical treatment. These pathogens result in a variety of infections that include cellulitis (in particular of the lower legs), erysipelas, necrotizing fasciitis, folliculitis, impetigo, folliculitis, and furunculosis.

Cellulitis and Erysipelas

In the elderly, cellulitis and erysipelas are common infections. Cellulitis should be clinically distinguished from erysipelas. Erysipelas involves the dermis, most commonly involves the legs, and tends to be sharply demarcated. Cellulitis also most commonly occurs on the lower legs, but also involves the subcutaneous fat. It is deeper andless demarcated. A classic sign of both cellulitis and erysipelas is the orange-peel (peau d'orange) texture of affected skin. Vesicles and bullae may be present in areas affected by cellulitis and erysipelas. Streptoccocal species are the most common cause of cellulitis and erysipelas. *S. aureus* and gram-negative organisms can cause cellulitis and are more serious than cellulitis caused by *Streptococcus*.

Prompt treatment of cellulitis and erysipelas is necessary as cellulitis and erysipelas can evolve into septicemia, thrombophlebitis, septic arthritis, osteomyelitis, and endocarditis.

Cellulitis and erysipelas require antibiotic treatment. In most cases, these infections should be treated with intravenous antibiotics if complicated, if of significant extent or if present with coincident disease. The most common antibiotics used to treat cellulitis and erysipelas are penicillins and cephalosporins. Other therapeutic options include clindamycin, quinolones, and macrolides. With the increase of methicillin-resistant pathogens, the use of glycopeptides (particularly vancomycin) has increased. And vancomycin is now first-line therapy until a pathogen and its susceptibilities are identified. The typical duration of therapy is 10 to 14 days for simple skin and skin structure infections.

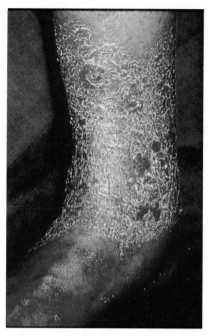

Figure 17.2. Stasis Dermatitis with secondary infection.

Complicated skin and skin structure infections such as cellulitis associated with leg ulcers usually requires longer courses of intravenous treatment. These courses can last up to 3 to 4 weeks.

The entity most often confused with cellulitis/erysipelas is stasis dermatitis. The former is usually warm to the touch, unilateral rather than bilateral, and sometimes painful. The latter is of the same temperature as the surrounding skin, is more often brown than red, is bilateral rather than unilateral, and is not painful. While stasis dermatitis can be colonized or impetiginized, even in such cases, it is not an interchangeable entity with cellulitis/erysipelas (Fig. 17.2). Other entities that can mimic cellulitis/erysipelas include allergic contact dermatitis and deep venous thrombosis. If cellulitis and deep venous thrombosis are confused when a leg is red and painful, a Doppler ultrasound or related imaging test should be carried out to rule out thrombophlebitis and clotting.

Impetigo, folliculitis, and furunculosis

Staphylococcus aureus and β-hemolytic streptococci are the most common organisms that cause impetigo, folliculitis, and the more serious infections of cellulitis and erysipelas.

Impetigo appears as honey-colored crusted erosions. Care givers should obtain a sample of fluid or pus for a Gram stain and culture it to define the causative organism. However, the diagnosis of impetigo can usually be made clinically. Methicillin-resistant *S. aureus* is the cause of a higher and higher percentage of hospital- and community-acquired skin infections. A nasal culture of the patient and other family members is often helpful in assessing if nasal carriage of *S. aureus* is the source of the infection (up to 20%–25 % of persons carry *S. aureus* in their noses).

Folliculitis refers to a bacterial infection of the pilosebaceous unit. Folliculitis occurs on body surfaces with hair such as the scalp, neck, beard area, axillae, buttocks, and limbs. A fungal folliculitis (Majocci granuloma) can occur if a superficial fungal infection is treated with topical steroids. A furuncle or boil is the manifestation of a deeper infection of the hair follicle generally with *S. aureus*. It results in a red, hot, tender inflammatory nodule (a boil) from which pus can be expressed. Carbuncles are multiloculated or multiple furuncles. The differential diagnosis for a furuncle is an inflamed epidermal or pilar cyst. Although antibiotics may help treat an inflamed cyst because it is secondarily infected or because antibiotics may have anti-inflammatory effects, the definitive treatment of an epidermal cyst is surgical.

A variety of conditions may increase the likelihood of infections of the superficial skin and hair follicle. These factors include bacterial carriage in the nostrils, scabies, vigorous scratching of the skin, diabetes mellitus, obesity, lymphoproliferative neoplasms, malnutrition, and the administration of glucocorticosteroids and other immunosuppressive drugs.

The optimal treatment begins with culture of eruptions that are suspected of having infectious etiologies. Empiric treatment should be started if an infection is suspected. While resistance and atypical organisms can be the cause of a skin infection, treatment should be directed toward gram-positive organisms with the expectation that some response will be seen in 2 to 3 days. If the patient has systemic symptoms (fever, malaise, nausea, vomiting) or the infection occurs on a sensitive area (e.g., genital or ocular sites), the patient should be admitted to the hospital and treated with intravenous antibiotics. If the culture of fluid of a folliculitis or furunculosis reveals that the infection is resistant to the initial therapy, treatment should be altered. Alternatives for organisms resistant to penicillins include intravenous vancomycin and oral linezolid. Typical courses of therapy are 7 to 10 days.

Necrotizing fasciitis

Necrotizing fasciitis describes a destructive, usually polymicrobial, infection causing rapidly advancing deep tissue necrosis, which can result in significant morbidity and mortality. The etiologies of necrotizing fasciitis are diverse and include prior injury, surgery, irradiation, cancer, diabetes mellitus, alcoholism, and malnutrition.

Treatment for necrotizing fasciitis requires surgical intervention in combination with multiantibiotic therapy using drugs effective against gram-positive and gram-negative pathogens as well as pathogens that are aerobes and anaerobes. Proper nutrition, hydration, close monitoring, and supportive care are essential if the patient is to recover from necrotizing fasciitis.

HERPES ZOSTER

Herpes zoster involves the recrudescence of infection with varicella-zoster virus whose source is a quiescent virus residing in a nerve, which usually spreads along a single dermatome (Fig. 17.3). Herpes zoster has a different profile in the elderly than it does in the young. Herpes zoster is a disease of old age and is best considered an exception in the young. The incidence of herpes zoster increases constantly with age so while it is rare in the young, it is not uncommon in those older than 65. Zoster rates are highest among individuals over age 80 (10.9 per 1,000 person-years, i.e., 1% of persons are suffering from it at any time). Secondly, disseminated zoster, while rare, is a disease

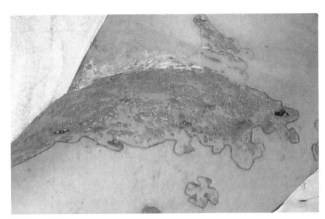

Figure 17.3. Herpes Zoster in an 81-year-old male patient in his groin area.

associated with non–Hodgkin's lymphoma, which is a disease that is most common in the old and very old. Finally, postherpetic neuralgia (PHN) is most common and most severe in the elderly.

In recent years, the approach toward the treatment and prevention of zoster has changed with the approval of a vaccine for zoster. This vaccine is significant in that it prevents the recrudescence of disease rather than its genesis. The vaccine is identical in content to the childhood vaccine for the prevention of chickenpox except the herpes zoster vaccine provides a higher dose of the active ingredient. The use of the zoster vaccine diminished the burden of illness due to herpes zoster by 61.1%, diminished the incidence of PHN by 66.5%, and diminished the incidence of herpes zoster by 51.3% ($P<0.001$). Patients who develop herpes zoster have a milder clinical course if they have been vaccinated. Reactions at the injection site when present were generally mild and were more frequent among vaccine recipients.. Tricyclic antidepressants, topical lidocaine, gabapentin, nerve root injections with steroids or aneshetics, acupuncture, and opiates may all be used as treatments for PHN.

FUNGAL INFECTIONS

The incidence of all fungal infections, with the exception of tinea versicolor, increases with age. This is true of onychmycosis, tinea pedis, cutaneous candiadias, perléche, and intertrigo.

Candidiasis

Candidiasis is a yeast infection most commonly due to *Candida albicans* that increases in incidence in diabetic or obese patients. These patient groups have a higher prevalence in the elderly. It is also more common for elderly patients to be on chronic antibiotics, chronic oral and topical corticosteroids, immunosuppressive drugs, and have poor nutrition. These factors lead to an increased incidence of candidal infections. Obese elderly patients are more apt to be poorly mobile and this increases prolonged occlusion, moisture, and warmth in skin flexures. Once again these are conditions that lead to candida.

Oral candidiasis, termed *thrush,* occurs commonly in elderly persons. Poor dentition, immunosupression, systemic and oral corticosteroid use are all predisposing factors. Thrush manifests as white plaques that can be easily removed, and overly erosions or ulcerations on the buccal, palatal, or oropharyngeal mucosa. These plaques overly areas of mucosal erythema. Candida infection or superinfection of erosions and inflammation occurring at the mouth's lateral angles is termed *angular cheilitis* or *perléche*. Denture stomatitis presents as chronic mucosal erythema typically beneath the site of a denture and is a related condition.

Maceration of the finger web spaces (most commonly seen in the third web space between the middle and ring fingers) is caused by candida and gram-negative bacteria and is termed *erosio interdigitalis blastomycetica* (interdigital candidiasis). Liquid exposure played out against a background of a weakened epidermis, obesity, diabetes and immunosuppression seems to be the basis for erosio interditalis blastomycetica. Erosio interdigitalis blastomycetica responds to drying agents and topical antiyeast agents.

Onychomycosis

Onychomyocosis is an infection of nails by fungi and is more difficult to treat than fungal infections of the skin. The prevalence of onychomyocosis increases constantly with age. The prevalence of fungal nail infections is about 20% in the 60 to 79 years age-group compared to ~1% in patients younger than 21 years. Onychomycosis is a common disease affecting as much as 8% of the general population. A greater prevalence of onychomycosis is associated with greater age, male gender, diabetes mellitus, family history of onychomycosis, psoriasis, concurrent intake of immunosuppressive drugs, and cardiovascular and peripheral vascular disease. Onychomycosis can cause pain or limited mobility impairing quality of life. Difficulty walking and wearing shoes and embarrassment are common complaints. Moreover, in patients with recurrent cellulitis, onchomycosis and tinea pedis are thought to provide portals of entry for bacteria and are thus a predisposing factor for cellulitis.

Dermatophytes are the most commonly cultured organisms, appearing in ~75% to 91% of nails with fungal involvement. *Tinea rubrum* is the most common dermatophyte to cause onychomycosis or tinea unguium. Other species of tinea including *T. mentagrophyte* can cause onychomycosis. *Candida* (*Candida Parapsilosis, Candida guilliermondii, Candida albicans*) and nondermatophyte molds and related pathogens (e.g. *Scopulariopsis brevicaulis, Aspergillus spp., Alternaria spp., Curvularia spp., and Fusarium spp.*) can also cause onychomycosis. Periodic acid–Schiff (PAS) stain of the nails is the best test for diagnosing onychomycosis but it will not distinguish between species of tinea. As terbinafine will cover all dermatophytes (but not *Candida* or nondermatophyte molds) speciation of tinea is not important. A PAS is useful because nail dystrophy from psoriasis, lichen planus, and eczema can result in an onychodystrophy that may resemble onychomycosis.

Onychomycosis is divided into four types: distal subungual onychomycosis, proximal subungual onychomycosis, white superficial onychomycosis, and candidal onychomycosis. Distal subungual onychomycosis, which manifests with thickened and friable nails with associated discoloration and subungual hyperkeratosis, is the most prevalent type and accounts for 75% to 85% of cases.

Treatments exist for onychomycosis. Treatment is not uniformly effective as elderly patients possess special risk factors for poor response to therapy for onychomycosis, including frequent nail dystrophy, slow growth of nails, and increased prevalence of cardiovascular and peripheral vascular disease and diabetes mellitus. Onychomycosis can be treated with oral terbinafine (250 mg daily for 3 months) oral itraconazole, topical amorolfine or ciclopirox nail lacquer. Terbinafine is the most effective agent with the fewest drug interactions. Terbinafine is only effective against dermatophytes while itraconazole is effective against yeasts and molds. Topical application of urea 20% to 50% gel or cream, breaks down keratin and softens the nail plate. It may enhance penetration of topical antifungal drugs when used in tandem. After therapy is initiated, it can take up to 6 months to assess therapeutic effect. Combinations of treatments (e.g. oral and topical or oral/topical and surgical) seem to enhance cure rates.

Tinea Pedis and Manuum

Tinea pedis (athlete's foot) and manuum commonly occur in the elderly. Tinea commonly occurs on both feet and one hand for unknown reasons. Tinea pedis manifests as maceration in the interdigital toe web folds and as scaly plaques on the feet, often in a moccasin distribution. Treatment involves the use of topical antifungal (e.g. ketoconazole, ciclopirox) gels, creams, foams, or solutions with or without a keratolytic agent (e.g., lactic acid, urea or salicylic acid). The examination of a KOH preparation can establish the diagnosis for tinea pedis. Tinea pedis and manuum must be distinguished from xerosis, allergic contact dermatitis, and dyshydrotic eczema, which can be accomplished by examination of a KOH preparation.

Tinea corporis commonly occurs on the torso of elderly persons. Tinea corporis has a variety of presentations that include nummular patches, annular plaques with a rim of scaly erythema, and polycyclic annuli (Fig. 17.4). Examination using a KOH preparation can establish the diagnosis of tinea corporis. Tinea corporis can be treated effectively with a topical antifungal agent.

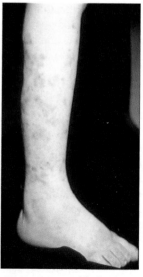

Figure 17.4. Tinea Corporis in an elderly patient under a leg brace.

Elderly people with diabetes should be treated for onychomycosis to prevent secondary bacterial infections and subsequent complications. Terbinafine is the drug of choice for dermatophyte onychomycosis, with greater mycological cure rates, less serious and fewer drug interactions, and a lower cost than continuous itraconazole therapy. Adjunct debridement may improve the clinical and complete cure rates compared with terbinafine alone. Common adverse effects of terbinafine in the elderly include nausea, sinusitis, arthralgia, and hypercholesterolemia. For onychomycosis caused by Candida or nondermatophyte molds, there is no superior systemic therapy. In general, topical nail lacquers, amorolfine and ciclopirox, are not practical for elderly patients because of the recommended frequency of application, periodic routine debridement of affected nails, and long duration of therapy. However, nail lacquers may be a good option as monotherapy or in combination with systemic antifungal therapy.

PITFALLS AND MYTHS

A key pitfall in diagnosing skin infections in the elderly is that they do not present in the same manner as infections in adulthood. That is, "atypical presentations" occur commonly. The host response of the elderly can be less vigorous and thus the hallmarks of infection – i.e. rubor, calor, and dolor can be less pronounced. Thus, those who examine the elderly must have a high index of clinical suspicion. Another pitfall is clinically not appreciating the role that the impaired integrity of the integument plays in the facilitation of infection and that for infection to be dealt with, breaks in the skin from xerosis and poor circulation must be dealt with. Finally, it is important to understand that florid stasis dermatitis is not the same thing as cellulitis.

SUGGESTED READING

Insinga RP, Itzler RF, Pellissier JM Saddier P, Nikas AA. The incidence of herpes zoster in a United States administrative database. *J Gen Intern Med* 2005;20(8):748–753.

Scheinfeld N, Mones J. Seasonal variation of transient acantholytic dyskeratosis (Grover's disease). *J Am Acad Dermatol* 2006;55(2): 263–268.

Scheinfeld N. Infections in the elderly. *Dermatol Online J* 2005; 11(3):8.

Brian B. Adams

INTRODUCTION

Cutaneous infections afflict athletes sometimes in epidemic proportions. Several aspects of sporting activities place the athlete at a greater risk of developing and transmitting these infections. First, many athletic endeavors involve intense, close skin-to-skin contact, which facilitates the spread of infectious microorganisms between athletes and among teams. Second, sweating, inherent to athletics, results in a macerated epidermis that easily facilitates the penetration of microorganisms. Third, many athletes wear occlusive equipment, which provides an ideal environment for the growth of microorganism (warm, dark, and moist). Finally, trauma (gross or micro) related to athletic activities further impairs the stratum corneum's barrier.

The microorganisms that plague athletes of all skill levels include bacteria, viruses, fungi, atypical mycobacteria, and parasites. Knowledge of these infections in the context of athletics permits the clinician to treat the athletic patient more effectively. Through this focused approach, the clinician can minimize disruption to an individual's athletic activities and prevent team and league epidemics.

HISTORY

Sports dermatology began with several isolated case reports of unusual skin conditions in athletes. Interest in the field blossomed with the identification of epidemics of viral, fungal, and bacterial skin infections among those involved in sports of all kinds. The transmission of herpes virus among athletes with close skin-to-skin contact (primarily among wrestlers) has predominated in the sports dermatology literature. Research and close observation in the 1990s and early 2000s also documented epidemics of tinea corporis gladiatorum. With the advent of epidemics of community-acquired methicillin-resistant *Staphylococcus aureus* (MRSA), attention has turned to the role of athletic participation and the transmission of MRSA. Considerable practice time and competition is lost to skin infections and our attempts at adequately preventing the transmission of these skin infections in athletes remains at its infancy.

BACTERIAL INFECTIONS

Clinical Features

Impetigo

While impetigo routinely affects athletes of all sorts, only one epidemiologic study exists that noted an epidemic at a national

AAU wrestling championship. *S. aureus, MRSA, Streptococcus pyogens, and Streptococcus agalactiae* can all cause impetigo. Athletes with close skin-to-skin contact (wrestlers; rugby ["Scrum strep"], football, and basketball players) and others wearing occlusive equipment (fencers; hockey and soccer players) seem particularly susceptible. The lesions are distributed over areas of skin-to-skin contact or areas occluded by equipment. Well-defined erythematous, yellow-crusted papules or plaques develop in these exposed athletes (Fig. 18.1). Mature lesions demonstrating these clinical features make the diagnosis straightforward. However, early lesions may lack characteristic findings. As such, clinicians may mistake beginning lesions of impetigo for acne, papular dermatitis, or other infectious conditions related to sports such as herpes gladiatorum or tinea corporis gladiatorum. Termed "scrum kidney," poststreptococcal nephritis has developed as a complication of impetigo in rugby players.

Furunculosis

A significant body of work exists regarding the epidemiology of furunculosis in athletes. Epidemics ranging from 9% to 56% have plagued football and basketball teams at the high school, collegiate, and professional levels. Caused by *S. aureus* and increasingly by *MRSA*, athletically related furunculosis occurs on areas of skin-to-skin contact. Not infrequently, however, athletes (such

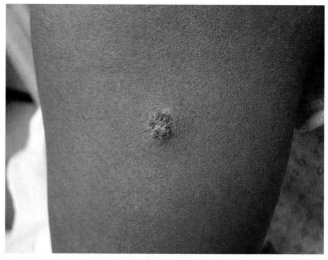

Figure 18.1. This is a typical lesion of impetigo in an athlete. Reprinted from *Sports Dermatology* © 2006, Brian B. Adams, MD, MPH Chapter 1, Figure 1 with permission from Springer Science and Business Media LLC.

as soccer and field hockey players) develop furunculosis beneath protective equipment on the lower legs. Tight-fitting garments also predispose athletes to furunculosis.

Several studies have highlighted important risk factors that place athletes at a high risk for infection. Athletes with turf burns (caused by frictional trauma with the playing field) or who practice body shaving demonstrate a six to seven times higher prevalence of furunculosis compared to athletes without those characteristics. Increasing weight among football players appears to increase the risk of infection. A player's position on the field also tends to play a role. Cornerbacks experience a 17.5 times higher risk of Staphylococcal infection, and in another study, lineman had a 10 times higher risk.

Well-defined, tender, erythematous nodules develop in locations of skin-to-skin contact and/or beneath occlusive equipment. Very early lesions may mimic acne, papular dermatitis, herpes gladiatorum, or tinea corporis gladiatorum.

Folliculitis

Unlike impetigo and furunculosis, no epidemiology of folliculitis in athletes exists. Caused by *S. aureus* and increasingly by *MRSA*, folliculitis in athletes occurs in areas of skin-to-skin contact. Not infrequently, however, athletes develop an infectious folliculitis beneath protective equipment on the lower legs (such as soccer and field hockey players). Tight-fitting garments also tend to predispose athletes to staphylococcal folliculitis. Erythematous papules and follicular pustules occur at these sites but can be easily confused with other infections such as molluscum contagiosum and noninfectious entities such as acne mechanica.

Diagnosis

Culture confirms the diagnosis of these bacterial infections. Occasionally, biopsies are required, especially early in the course of the infection and with very small lesions. During epidemics or in cases of recurrent disease, clinicians should culture the nares of the infected individuals and consider cultures of asymptomatic teammates. Fomites play an unknown role in the transmission of these infections. Multiple studies have failed to document the presence of these bacteria on mats or equipment.

Therapy and Prevention

Treatment varies with the severity of disease. First and foremost, athletes should apply warm moist washcloths to the affected area for 10 minutes three times per day. Oral (dicloxacillin or cephalexin) and topical (mupirocin) antibacterial agents for 7 to 10 days clear the eruption. Folliculitis, furunculosis, or impetigo caused by *MRSA* clears with sulfamethoxazole–trimethoprim. Athletes with positive *S. aureus* or *MRSA* nasal cultures require twice daily application of mupirocin ointment or cream to both nares for 10 days; this regimen can be repeated every 6 months or more frequently depending on the rapidity of recurrence of colonization. Clinicians should also consider applying mupirocin (ointment or cream) to the perianal region and the axilla.

Prevention is paramount. In one highly publicized epidemic among professional football players, rampant towel sharing (three athletes to one towel), improper cleaning of weight room equipment, and inadequate access to hand sanitizer for training

Table 18.1: Prevention Techniques That May Help Avoid Skin Infection Epidemics

Frequent, if not daily, skin checks by athletes and trainers

Daily showers immediately after practices or competition

Routine antibacterial soap use in the showers

Frequent hand washing by trainers and affected athletes

Universal availability of alcohol-based, waterless, soap cleansers

Regular laundering of equipment and clothing

Mandatory no-sharing policy for equipment and personal items

Required personal towels

Meticulous covering of all wounds

Periodic formal education for the athletes, coaches, and trainers

Reprinted from *Sports Dermatology* © 2006, Brian B. Adams, MD, MPH Chapter 1, Table 1–1 with permission from Springer Science and Business Media LLC.

staff were identified as the major risk factors. Athletes should practice impeccable hygiene that includes showering immediately after practice and competitions, washing with antibacterial soaps or Hibiclens, and not sharing equipment or towels. While no evidence exists that these approaches decrease the incidence or transmission of folliculitis, furunculosis, or impetigo, these hygienic measures only seem reasonable. Athletes with recurrent disease should also minimize the amount of skin exposed during skin-to-skin contact. Long-sleeved moisture-wicking synthetic clothing allows the athlete's skin to stay dry and helps prevent the transmission of infectious organisms among other athletes (Table 18.1).

Disqualification of athletes from competition remains quite a controversial issue. At the high school athletic level, regulations vary among states while the National Collegiate Athletic Association (NCAA) has uniform regulations regarding disqualification of infected athletes from competition. For example, skin checks, starting with the lowest weight categories and proceeding up, occur at all wrestling competitions. Certified athletic trainers or physicians make the final determination at the venue. At high school competitions, the referee, who may or may not have any medical training, makes the disqualification determination.

NCAA guidelines note that in order for these athletes with bacterial infections to be eligible to compete, they must not have any new lesions less than 48 hours before competition, must have taken oral antibiotics for at least 72 hours before competition, and must also have covered the area with a bandage that cannot be dislodged (Table 18.2).

Pitted Keratolysis

Caused by micrococcus or cornybacteria species, pitted keratolysis occurs in athletes even though its epidemiology is not yet well documented. Runners and tennis and basketball players seem particularly prone. The warm, dark, and moist environment of the athletic shoe provides an ideal climate for these two organisms. Well-defined, pitted lesions particularly

Table 18.2: Guidelines for Return to Competition for Impetigo/Furunculosis (Based on NCAA Guidelines)

1) Take 72 hours of oral antibiotics

2) Lack new lesion for at least 48 hours

3) Cover lesion with non-permeable bandage

NCAA 2006 Wrestling Rules and Interpretations. Appendix D Skin Infections.

distributed on the weight-bearing aspects of the sole typify pitted keratolysis. The soaking of the sole enhances the prominence of the pits. Treatment includes topical antibiotics (clindamycin or erythromycin) or topical benzoyl peroxide or both. To prevent pitted keratolysis, athletes can apply aluminum chloride solution to decrease exertional hyperhidrosis. Synthetic moisture-wicking socks, available at most athletic specialty stores, can keep the sole dry and cool.

Gram-Negative Infections (Hot tub folliculitis, green foot, tropical ulcers, hot foot syndrome)

Hot Tub Folliculitis

Hundreds of epidemics of hot tub folliculitis have occurred involving both athletes and nonathletes. Athletes are at risk this infection, caused by *Pseudomonas aeruginosa,* due to exposure to hot tubs after practice or during rehabilitation. Inadequate chlorination allows the organism to proliferate. The hot, turbid water and heavy usage by athletes dissipates the chlorine. On any submerged skin surface, but often concentrated on areas covered with clothing, and sparing the palms and soles, follicular erythematous papules and pustules develop. In rare case reports the presence of green pustules has been documented. Systemic manifestations often occur and include pharyngitis, lymphadenopathy, and malaise. The differential diagnosis includes other types of folliculitis including those resulting from *Staphylococcus, pityrosporum*, acne, and anabolic steroid use.

No treatment for the immunocompetent athlete is necessary as hot tub folliculitis resolves spontaneously in 7 to 10 days and those athletes treated with antibiotics risk recurrence. Proper cleaning and chlorination of the hot tubs prevent hot tub folliculitis. Heavily used hot tubs in the training room need more frequent cleaning and chlorination than a typical hot tub.

Green Foot

Athletes may acquire a green discoloration on their feet and toenails as a result of contact with *Pseudomonas* growing in their shoes. The discoloration does not wipe away and takes about 1 month to resolve. By making the link between athletic participation and subsequent culture of the organism from the insole, the clinician can best reassure the athlete and prevent future recurrences.

Tropical Ulcers

Seven members of one rugby team who competed in an international competition developed painless ulcers on their knees, hands, and wrist caused by *Fusobacterium ulcerans.* In areas of traumatic abrasions, resulting from their sport, the rugby players demonstrated many well-defined, shallow ulcers with indurated borders. Cultures confirm the diagnosis.

Hot Foot Syndrome

One case series studied 40 children swimmers who developed this condition caused most likely by *Pseudomonas aeruginosa.* Their median age was 6 years. The pathogenesis of this condition is not well understood. Ten to 40 hours after pool exposure, these mostly young swimmers developed intensely painful, erythematous, and violaceous nodules on the soles. Some swimmers in this study also had fever, nausea, and fatigue. The lesions may persist for 2 weeks but resolve spontaneously. The differential diagnosis includes athletically related neutrophilic eccrine plantar hidradenitis and plantar urticaria. Neutrophilic eccrine plantar hidradenitis, however, typically develops after repeated pounding trauma on the soles, while sports-related plantar urticaria resolves rather quickly (few minutes to few hours). No effective therapy exists except for symptomatic relief.

VIRAL INFECTIONS

Herpes Simplex Virus

Reactivation

Outdoor athletes exposed to excessive ultraviolet radiation risk reactivating their herpes labialis. Snow-related sports place the athlete at even greater risk because of chapping of the skin and reflection of sunlight off the snow. At high altitudes, the atmosphere absorbs less ultraviolet radiation and the snow reflects up to 100% of the ultraviolet radiation. About 12% of skiers (with a history of herpes labialis) will develop herpes labialis during a 1-week stay at the slopes. The median time to development of lesions after arriving at the ski slopes is 3.5 days. Athletes should take 2 grams of valacyclovir twice in one day at the first sign of the prodrome.

To prevent reactivation of herpes labialis, outdoor athletes with a history of HSV should take daily suppressive dosing of valacyclovir or famcyclovir. These athletes also need to apply sunscreen. One study documented herpes labialis lesions in 71% of skiers not wearing lip sunscreen and in 0% of individuals wearing lip sunscreen.

Skin-to-skin transmission

Researchers have extensively delineated the epidemiology of HSV-1 infection primarily in wrestlers and rugby players. The median prevalence was 20%. Of all skin infections in athletes, herpes gladiatorum (wrestlers) and herpes rugbeiorum (rugby players) can cause the most individual morbidity and team disruption. Wrestlers transmit their skin infections as a result of intense and repeated skin-to-skin contact (such as the "lock-up" position), while, rugby players experience close contact during the scrum. An unaffected wrestler competing with an infected wrestler has a one-third probability of obtaining the infection. When the nonaffected wrestler develops herpes gladiatorum, the lesion develops between 4 to 11 days after exposure.

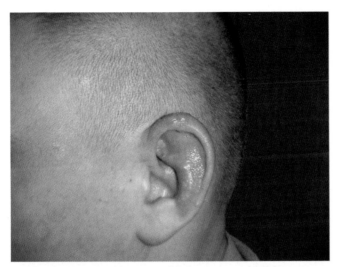

Figure 18.2. Herpes gladiatorum of the ear.
Reprinted from Sports Dermatology © 2006, Brian B. Adams, MD, MPH Chapter 2, Figure 2 with permission from Springer Science and Business Media LLC.

Table 18.3: Clinical Appearance of Lesions of Herpes Gladiatorum or Herpes Rugbeiorum Based on Duration

Clinical Appearance	Age of Lesion
Red papule	Very early, 1–2 days
Grouped blisters	2–6 days
Crusted papule	5–14 days

Reprinted from *Sports Dermatology* © 2006, Brian B. Adams, MD, MPH Chapter 2, Table 2–3 with permission from Springer Science and Business Media LLC.

Mature lesions of herpes gladiatorum demonstrate well-defined, grouped vesicles on an erythematous base (Fig. 18.2), whereas crusted lesions typify late lesions. Very early-detected lesions may not have vesicles or the grouped morphology, which makes prompt diagnosis challenging (Table 18.3). These lesions predominantly develop on the upper extremities, head, and neck regions. Headache, fever, and chills occur in one-quarter of infected wrestlers. The differential diagnosis includes impetigo, tinea corporis gladiatorum, acne, and subacute dermatitis. Tzanck preparation represents the quickest method to confirm herpes gladiatorum but it is technically difficult. Viral cultures take 24 hours but direct immunofluorescence yields results in hours. Early detection allows rapid institution of therapy and proper athlete isolation to prevent epidemics. One state's high school wrestling program suffered an epidemic after many competitors were incorrectly diagnosed and subsequently returned to competition. Of the misdiagnosed wrestlers (90% of wrestlers with herpes gladiatorum), 70% were initially diagnosed with impetigo, while 20% were thought to have either dermatitis (10%) or tinea corporis gladiatorum (10%).

First and foremost, athletes should apply warm moist washcloths to the affected area for 10 minutes three times per day. Infected athletes should at the first sign of the prodrome

Table 18.4: Guidelines for Return to Competition for Herpes Gladiatorum (Based on NCAA Guidelines)

1) All lesions must be dried with an adherent crust and

2) The wrestler must have been on oral antiviral therapy for 120 hours and
   * Evidence-based data suggest 96 hours is sufficient
   ** Valacyclovir's one time dosing would allow competition 96 hours later

3) No systemic symptoms of herpes gladiatorum and

4) No new blisters within 72 hours of precompetition skin check-in

Reprinted from *Sports Dermatology* © 2006, Brian B. Adams, MD, MPH Chapter 2, Table 2–6 with permission from Springer Science and Business Media LLC.

take 4 g total of valacyclovir in one day (in two separate doses of 2 g each). After 96 hours, no viral shedding exists and the wrestler can safely return to wrestling. Current NCAA regulations, however, allow for safe return to wrestling after 120 hours from the initiation of oral antiviral agents. The competitor must also be free from systemic symptoms, have no new lesions in the past 72 hours, and possess at most only crusted lesions (Table 18.4).

Clinicians caring for these athletes should recognize the complications associated with herpes gladiatorum. Secondary bacterial infections can occur as well as monoarticular arthritis, keratitis, and conjunctivitis. Cognizant athletes (typically at the high school level), in an attempt to escape detection and possible disqualification, may modify the grouped vesicle morphology by using sandpaper or bleach. These maneuvers can cause significant disruption to the epidermal barrier.

To prevent the transmission of herpes gladiatorum, clinicians must identify, treat, and potentially isolate athletes as early as possible in the course of their disease. Athletes should practice impeccable hygiene that includes showering immediately after practice and competitions, washing with antibacterial soaps or Hibiclens, and not sharing equipment or towels. While no evidence exists that fomites transfer the viral organism, it seems only reasonable to avoid sharing equipment (such as pads and headgear) and towels. Athletes with recurrent disease should also minimize the amount of skin exposed during skin-to-skin contact. Long-sleeved moisture-wicking synthetic clothing allows the athlete's skin to stay dry and helps prevent the transmission of HSV among other athletes (Table 18.1). Pharmacologically, high-risk athletes should take 1 g of valacyclovir daily during the entire season. One study documented a decrease in herpes gladiatorum prevalence from 33% to 8% using this season-long prophylaxis.

Molluscum

Caused by the Poxvirus, molluscum contagiosum infects athletes that come into contact with swimming pools and other infected athletes' skin. Athletes who share protective equipment such as pads, gloves, and helmets are also at risk for infection. One study of over 7,000 individuals demonstrated that swimmers

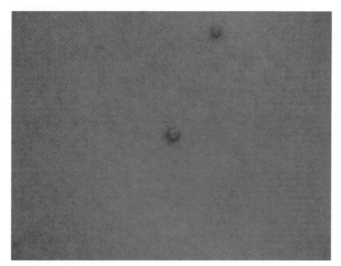

Figure 18.3. Molluscum contagiosum (especially small lesions) can be confused with folliculitis).
Reprinted from *Sports Dermatology* © 2006, Brian B. Adams, MD, MPH Chapter 2, Figure 5 with permission from Springer Science and Business Media LLC.

Table 18.5: Guidelines for Return to Competition for Molluscum (Based on NCAA guidelines)

1) Curette all lesions

2) Cover solitary lesions with op-site or bioclusive

3) Cover with stretch tape

NCAA 2006 Wrestling Rules and Interpretations. Appendix D Skin Infections.

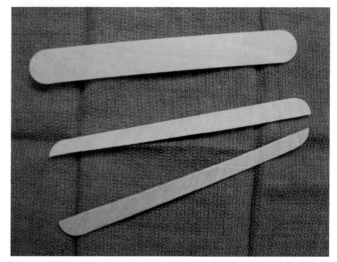

Figure 18.4. A tongue depressor split longitudinally provides a readily available curette to remove molluscum. The curved end can scoop out the lesions quickly.
Reprinted from *Sports Dermatology* © 2006, Brian B. Adams, MD, MPH Chapter 2, Figure 7 with permission from Springer Science and Business Media LLC.

experienced two times the risk of infection with molluscum compared to nonswimmers. Another interesting report highlighted an epidemic wherein 8% of 1,400 cross-country runners developed molluscum. The researchers theorized that the runners transmitted the organism through their use of shared courses through the woods or shared towels.

Most athletes develop small, white, occasionally slightly erythematous papules on their skin under protective equipment or on the head, neck, and extremities (sites of close skin-to-skin contact). The cross-country runners, in the previously mentioned epidemic, demonstrated lesions on the anterior knees and thighs. Mature lesions present with central umbilication, but early lesions often lack this characteristic finding (Fig. 18.3). The differential diagnosis includes infectious folliculitis and acne mechanica. Curettement of the lesions cures the athlete. Athletes should return for follow-up as microscopic lesions may exist and grow within several weeks after removal. Without an easily accessible curette, clinicians in the training room can fabricate one by splitting a tongue depressor longitudinally (Fig. 18.4). NCAA regulations mandate the removal of molluscum before competition. Solitary lesions may be covered with bioclusive or op-site and then subsequently covered with stretch tape (Table 18.5).

Athletes should practice impeccable hygiene that includes showering immediately after practice and competitions, washing with antibacterial soaps or Hibiclens, and not sharing equipment or towels. While no evidence exists that fomites transfer the viral organism, it seems only reasonable to avoid sharing equipment (such as pads and headgear) and towels. Athletes with recurrent disease should also minimize the amount of skin exposed during skin-to-skin contact. Long-sleeved moisture-wicking synthetic clothing should be recommended since it allows the athlete's skin to stay dry and helps prevent the transmission of molluscum among fellow athletes (Table 18.1).

Verruca

Caused by the human papilloma virus, verrucae of all varieties plague the athlete. Several studies have implicated swimming pool decks and locker room showers in the transmission of these infections. One study demonstrated that crewmembers developed verruca 2.5 times more frequently than cross-country runners. The use of gloves and weight rooms seems to be associated with this increased prevalence. Athletes may harbor these viruses in calluses that are intrinsic to several different sporting activities.

Clinicians need to differentiate among calluses, warts, and corns. Paring the well-defined hyperkeratotic lesion will demonstrate pericapillary hemorrhages in verrucae, a central core in corns, and no loss of skin ridges in calluses. While destructive methods seem to best remove verruca, athletes often require therapies that minimize loss of practice or competition. The blisters and pain induced by liquid nitrogen or cantharidin may detrimentally affect (in some cases dangerously so) an athlete's grip or gait. Topical medications such as salicylic acid, 5-fluorouracil, and imiquimod under occlusion (duct tape or coban) provide often a more gradual destruction. However, on occasion, this chemical approach can induce pain as well. Athletes should never walk barefoot in the locker room.

Table 18.6: Epidemiology of Tinea Pedis among Various Sports in One Study

Sport	Prevalence (%)	Relative Risk (compared to nonathletes)
Basketball	39	2
Judo	23	1
Running	56	4
Soccer	44	2.6
Swimming	55	4
Water polo	53	3.7

FUNGAL INFECTIONS

The three main cutaneous fungal infections that afflict athletes include tinea pedis, tinea corporis gladiatorum, and tinea cruris. Tinea cruris, as it pertains to athletes, does not vary significantly from that in nonathletes. Details of tinea cruris are described elsewhere in this book (see Chapter 3).

Tinea Pedis

All three varieties of tinea pedis (namely moccasin, interdigital, and vesicular) affect athletes. *Trichophyton rubrum* predominantly causes the moccasin and interdigital variants, whereas *Trichophyton mentagrophytes* mainly causes the vesicular or inflammatory variety. *Trichophyton mentagrophytes* dominates as the primary organism causing occult disease. The dark, moist, warm nature of sports' shoes places the athletes at an increased risk of developing tinea pedis. Several studies have documented a higher prevalence of tinea pedis among athletes compared to the nonathletic population. In a study of over 100,000 individuals, those people involved in sports experienced a 1.6- to 2.3-fold increase in tinea pedis compared to nonathletes.

Different sports were also studied together in one large study (Table 18.6). A recent study identified an unknown epidemic wherein 61% of soccer players (69% of professional players and 57% of collegiate players) had tinea pedis. No difference in prevalence existed between genders or between professional and collegiate athletes. Interestingly, clinical examination of the professional soccer players' toenails slightly overestimated the prevalence of tinea pedis. The duration and intensity of activity experienced by the professional players may cause a skin trauma that mimics tinea pedis (especially the interdigital variant).

Another study examined poolside areas along walkways and discovered 54 dermatophytes/mm². Other researchers found that 77% of their cultures taken from the pool deck, locker rooms, and springboard grew dermatophytes. The springboard area accounted for nearly 50% of all positive cultures.

Athletes with interdigital tinea pedis demonstrate scaling plaques between the toes, whereas the inflammatory variant presents with pruritus, scaling, vesicular papules, and plaques that are located most often on the instep. Close inspection excludes other diagnoses that occur on athletes' soles such as pitted keratolysis and allergic contact dermatitis. Sports clinicians

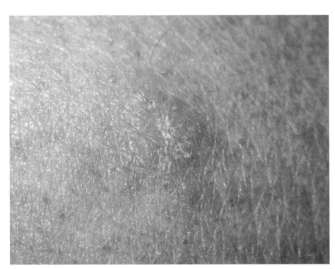

Figure 18.5. A well-defined, erythematous scaling round papule typifies tinea corporis gladiatorum.

and athletes themselves most often confuse the moccasin variety with dry skin. However, potassium hydroxide examination will reveal hyphae among the scale.

Therapy for tinea pedis is discussed elsewhere in this book (see Chapter 3). However, athletes can employ specific preventative measures. Athletes should wear synthetic moisture-wicking socks that can be found in most cities at local sports specialty stores or on the Internet. Athletes should change socks frequently, dry their feet completely before putting on their socks, and alternate their athletic shoes every other day to allow them to dry. By wearing sandals in the locker room and showers as well as using antifungal powders, athletes can prevent tinea pedis. Prompt diagnosis and therapy by the clinician will also help stop epidemics. Most athletes with tinea pedis fail to recognize the condition and do not bring it to the attention of proper medical personnel.

Tinea Corporis Gladiatorum

Multiples names exist for tinea corporis in athletes (most often occurring in wrestlers). These terms include tinea gladiatorum and trichophytosis gladiatorum. Studies have shown that 20% to 75% of individuals on any given team can be affected at any given time. The large difference in prevalence relates to study methodology. Some teams had known epidemics whereas other teams were studied without previous knowledge of an epidemic. Unlike typical tinea corporis, in which *Trichophyton rubrum* dominates as the leading organism, both *T. rubrum* and *Trichophyton tonsurans* share the top spot in tinea corporis gladiatorum. The high prevalence of *T. tonsurans* in lesions of tinea corporis gladiatorum suggests a possible link to asymptomatic scalp shedding by some athletes. The mats play little role in transmission of these infectious organisms. Only very rarely have investigators demonstrated dermatophytes on the wrestling mats. If mats did play a role, lesions on the legs would not be as uncommon as they are.

Well-defined, round, erythematous, scaling papules and plaques typify tinea corporis gladiatorum (Fig. 18.5). The annular morphology, typical of tinea corporis, is often not found. Lesions of tinea corporis gladiatorum occur most commonly on

Table 18.7: Guidelines for Return to Competition for Tinea Corporis Gladiatorum (Based on NCAA Guidelines)

1) Use a topical fungicidal agent for at least 72 hours

2) Wash with ketoconazole shampoo

3) Cover with naftifine or terbinafine

4) Cover with op-site or bioclusive

5) Cover with tape

NCAA 2006 Wrestling Rules and Interpretations. Appendix D Skin Infections.

the head and neck (32%), upper extremities (38%), and trunk (24%). The differential diagnosis, especially early in the course of the disease, includes herpes gladiatorum, impetigo, subacute dermatitis, and acne.

First and foremost, athletes should apply warm moist washcloths to the affected area for 10 minutes three times per day. Several studies have documented pharmacologic options for tinea corporis gladiatorum. No studies have investigated either the oral or the topical form of the allylamines. Not surprisingly, oral antifungal agents clear tinea corporis gladiatorum much more quickly. Half of the wrestlers, in one study, had negative cultures after 23 days while using topical clotrimazole twice daily. However, the same number of wrestlers had negative cultures after only 11 days while taking once-weekly fluconazole. No clear evidence-based data exists for appropriate return to competition after experiencing tinea corporis gladiatorum. The current recommendations for return to NCAA competition include the use of topical fungicidal agents for at least 72 hours. In addition, to compete, the athlete must wash with ketoconazole shampoo and cover the lesion with naftifine or terbinafine, followed by op-site or bioclusive and then tape (Table 18.7).

While little evidence supports the transmission of tinea corporis gladiatorum via mats, headgear, or pads, sharing of equipment should be discouraged. Athletes should practice impeccable hygiene that includes showering immediately after practice and competitions, washing with antibacterial soaps or Hibiclens, and not sharing equipment or towels. Athletes with recurrent disease should also minimize the amount of skin exposed during skin-to-skin contact. Long-sleeved moisture-wicking synthetic clothing also should be used since it allows the athlete's skin to stay dry and helps prevent the transmission of tinea corporis gladiatorum among other athletes (Table 18.1).

At-risk athletes should take season-long pharmacological prevention, which consists of weekly fluconazole (100 mg) or every other week itraconazole (400 mg in divided doses). Studies have demonstrated a decrease in prevalence compared to placebo with both regimens. Clinicians should consider obtaining baseline liver function tests before subjecting the athlete to these therapies since they last several months.

ATYPICAL MYCOBACTERIA (*SWIMMING POOL GRANULOMA*)

Caused by *Mycobacterium marinum*, swimming pool granuloma once caused an epidemic in 290 swimmers from a single pool. The clinical morphology presents with a myriad of morphologies including papules, nodules, and ulcers distributed on skin surfaces exposed to the microorganism (most often the extremities in swimmers). Biopsy and culture of fresh tissue confirms the diagnosis, since the clinical differential diagnosis is vast. The cultures may take several weeks to grow. Various treatments exist and include combinations of minocycline, clarithromycin, or rifampin. Aquatic athletes need to attend carefully to abrasions to prevent this swimming pool granuloma.

PARASITES (*CUTANEOUS LARVA MIGRANS*)

Ancyclostoma has caused cutaneous larva migrans in sand volleyball players. Infected animals' feces contain the organisms' eggs. The larvae that hatch from these eggs penetrate athletes' skin especially if the stratum corneum possesses any disruption related to the individual's sporting activity. The larvae migrate within the skin and create a linear erythematous plaque that in athletes happens to occur most often on the lower extremities. This hookworm may migrate several centimeters per day within the epidermis. Treatment includes topical thiabendazole for limited disease or oral thiabendazole for diffuse or recalcitrant conditions.

PITFALLS AND MYTHS

The most common pitfall in sports dermatology is to misdiagnose cutaneous infections. Athletic trainers, coaches, and athletes, with heightened awareness, are often concerned about very small lesions early in the course of disease. As a result, clinicians are called upon to make accurate diagnoses based on fairly nonspecific morphologic features. Early lesions of tinea corporis, herpes simplex, and impetigo can easily be confused. Cultures and direct examination are invaluable tools in making a correct diagnosis.

Additionally, very small lesions of molluscum contagiosum (often found beneath protective clothing or tight-fitting uniforms or undergarments) can easily be confused with noninfectious folliculitis or acne. Appropriate therapy, may therefore be delayed, which results in the spread of the causative organism to other areas of the athlete's skin or among teammates or competitors.

Athletes and clinicians often fail to recognize the presence of verruca in lesions they believe to be calluses. Calluses are common to sporting activities and there is some evidence to suggest that viruses that cause warts find refuge in these sports-related calluses. Not all thick areas of skin on the hands or feet of an athlete are calluses; if careful sharp paring of the thick skin reveals pinpoint black hemorrhages, the callus is or contains a wart.

Lastly, athletes and those entrusted to care for their medical needs frequently ignore "dry skin" on their feet. This "dry skin" is frequently KOH positive. Most of the 70% of collegiate and professional athletes who had KOH positive tinea pedis did not identify that they had "athlete's foot."

SUGGESTED READING

Adams BB. Tinea corporis gladiatorum. A cross-sectional study. *J Am Acad Dermatol* 2000;43:1039–1041.

Adams BB. Sports dermatology. *Adolesc Med* 2001;2:305–322.

Adams BB. Dermatologic disorders of the athlete. *Sports Med* 2002;32:309–321.

Adams BB. Tinea corporis gladiatorum. *J Am Acad Dermatol* 2002; 47:286–390.

Adams BB. *Sports Dermatology*. New York, New York: Springer Science and Business Media LLC, 2006.

Anderson BJ. The effectiveness of valacyclovir in preventing reactivation of herpes gladiatorum in wrestlers. *Clin J Sport Med* 1999;9:86–90.

Belongia EA, Goodman JL, Holland EJ et al. An outbreak of herpes gladiatorum at a high-school wrestling camp. *New Engl J Med* 1991;325:906–910.

Biolcati G, Alabiso A. Creeping eruption of larva migrans – A case report in a beach volley athlete. *Int J Sports Med* 1997;18: 612–613.

Chandrasekar PH, Rolston KVI, Kannangara W et al. Hot tub associated dermatitis due to Pseudomonas aeruginosa. *Arch Dermatol* 1984;120:1337–1340.

Detandt M, Nolard N. Fungal contamination of the floors of swimming pools particularly subtropical swimming paradises. *Mycoses* 1995;38:509–513.

Hazen PG, Weil ML. Itraconazole in the prevention and management of dermatophytosis in competitive wrestlers. *J Am Acad Dematol* 1997;36:481–482.

Kamihama T, Kimura T, Hosokawa JI et al. Tinea pedis outbreak in swimming pools in Japan. *Pub Health* 1997;111:249–253.

Kohl TD, Martin DC, Berger MS. Comparison of topical and oral treatments for tinea gladiatorum. *Clin J Sport Med* 1999;9:161–166.

Kohl TD, Martin DC, Nemeth R, Hill T, Evans D. Fluconazole for the prevention and treatment of tinea gladiatorum. *Pediatr Infect Dis J* 2000;19:717–722.

Lindenmayer JM, Schoenfeld S, O'Grady P et al. Methicillin-resistant Staphylococcus aureus in a high school wrestling team and the surrounding community. *Arch Intern Med* 1998;158:895–899.

Philpott JA, Woodburne AR, Philpott OS et al. Swimming pool granuloma. A study of 290 cases. *Arch Dermatol* 1963;88: 158–161.

Selling B, Kibrick S. An outbreak of herpes simplex among wrestlers (herpes gladiatorum). *N Engl J Med* 1964;270:979–982.

Sosin DM, Gunn RA, Ford WL, et al. An outbreak of furunculosis among high school athletes. *Am J Sports Med* 1989;17:828–832.

19 | SKIN INFECTIONS IN DIABETES MELLITUS

Nawaf Al-Mutairi

Skin infections are common in diabetic patients. They can even be the presenting feature of diabetes mellitus. A high index of suspicion in patients suffering from recurrent common skin infections, or with severe uncommon or rare infections, sometimes helps in detecting diabetes in a person previously not known to have this common condition. There can be many factors underlying increased susceptibility to skin infections in diabetics including poor microcirculation, hypohidrosis, peripheral vascular disease, peripheral neuropathy, and the decreased immune response seen in diabetics. Some of these factors may result in poor wound healing for these patients.

Decreased neutrophil chemotaxis and phagocytosis predisposes diabetic patients to an increased susceptibility of infections. The incidence of colonization as well as infections of the skin with bacteria such as *Staphylococcus, Streptococcus,* and *yeast (Candida albicans)* in patients with poor control of diabetes is increased. Dermatophyte infections are not more frequent in diabetic than in nondiabetic individuals. Some of the rare but serious and life-threatening infections of skin such as necrotizing fasciitis, malignant otitis externa, and mucormycosis are more common in diabetics and require special mention.

HISTORY

Before the advent of insulin and antibiotics, bacteria causing severe or extensive furuncles, carbuncles, ecthyma, cellulitis, and styes were frequent among diabetic patients. These infections are still commonly encountered among diabetic patients especially in developing countries where the lifelong management of underlying diabetes in many patients may not be optimum because of the cost involved or ignorance.

EPIDEMIOLOGY

Poor glycemic control is often associated with an increased incidence of skin infections in diabetics. At least one-third of persons with diabetes have some cutaneous involvement during the course of this chronic disease. Cutaneous infections are among the more common skin manifestations of diabetes. The incidence of skin infections in diabetics shows a close correlation to the patients' mean blood glucose levels. Skin infections occur in 20% to 50% of diabetics, but more often in type 2 diabetic patients.

DIAGNOSIS

Any person presenting with frequent, unusually severe or extensive common bacterial skin infections such as furuncles, carbuncles, cellulitis, ecthyma, erythrasma, or rare but life-threatening infections such as necrotizing fasciitis, malignant otitis externa, and mucormycosis should be investigated to rule out diabetes. Skin signs and symptoms may sometimes be surprisingly misleading even in the presence of serious infections in diabetics. Bacteriologic culture and sensitivity evaluation of the properly collected material in common infections, and blood in severe infections, is of paramount importance in management of these infections. A simple investigation such as Gram's stain of the purulent material may provide an early clue to the etiology. Gram's stain is better than KOH examination in demonstrating corynebacteria causing erythrasma. Material for culture may be collected via swabbing, injecting saline into the affected area and then aspirating the material, aspiration of blister fluid, or biopsy. However, even with all these procedures bacterial culture may not yield positive results in conditions such as erysipelas and cellulitis. Streptococcal serology may be helpful retrospectively. At onset of disease, high titers indicate infection. Serology at days 1 and 14 are also helpful but early institution of antibiotics can alter the antibody response. Immunofluorescence identifies streptococcal group antigens on biopsy specimens. Recurrent balanitis (infection of the prepuce) or balanoposthitis (infection of the foreskin and glans penis) in males and vaginal discharge (moniliasis) in females due to *Candida albicans* should also prompt laboratory investigation for diabetes. Simple KOH examination of swabs from genitalia will reveal the yeast which should be budding in active infection.

Cellulitis, erysipelas, and necrotizing fasciitis are primarily streptococcal diseases. Sometimes pure staphylococcal infection can cause cellulitis, and mixed infection with both may be present in many cases. Other bacteria such as pseudomonas can also rarely cause these infections.

CUTANEOUS INFECTIONS THAT MAY BE INDICATIVE OF UNDERLYING DIABETES MELLITUS

Candida infections

Infections of the mouth (oral thrush, angular cheilitis), nail folds (paronychia), and genitalia (balanitis/balanoposthitis in males, and moniliasis/vaginal thrush in females) due to the commonly present commensal yeast *Candida albicans* are frequent in diabetics. Candidiasis may be the first presenting clinical feature

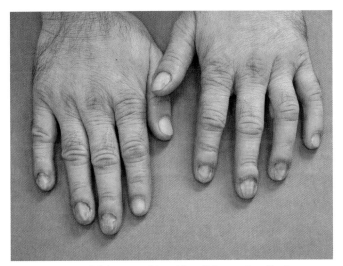

Figure 19.1. Candidal paronychia with nail dystrophy affecting multiple fingers.

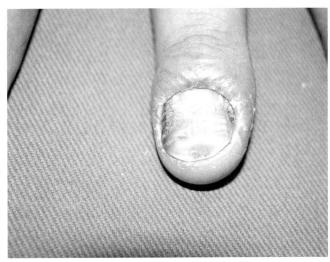

Figure 19.2. Paronychia with nail dystrophy.

of diabetes, and it is frequently seen in patients whose diabetes is not well controlled. A crucial factor is the amount of available glucose in the oral cavity and if this is markedly elevated, as in diabetes, the normal bacterial flora will not inhibit the yeast. In the mouth, carbohydrate levels are important. Food debris, likely to be present in the mouth of the severely ill patient with inadequate oral hygiene, should not be ignored. High glucose levels in urine, general tissue fluids, and sweat may make diabetics more susceptible to candidal infections. Phagocytosis is also impaired in diabetics. Any form of local tissue damage may be important in the pathogenesis of candidiasis. Increased levels of glucose in the saliva seem to be responsible for oral candidiasis in diabetics.

Dermatophyte Fungal Infections

It is traditionally mentioned in most textbooks that the incidence of superficial dermatophytic fungal infection of the skin is not increased in diabetic patients. Some of the recent studies, however, have contradicted this. The incidence of superficial dermatophyte fungal infections, especially the moccasin-type tinea pedis and some other clinical types, has been reported to be underreported among diabetics.

Angular stomatitis/cheilitis is characterized by redness, erosions, or fissures at the angles of the mouth. Paronychia (Figs. 19.1 and 19. 2) produces redness, swelling, pain of proximal and lateral nail folds, and sometimes loss of the cuticle. It is a very chronic and resistant condition, especially in persons involved in jobs involving frequent or prolonged contact with water such as housewives, cooks, chefs, and others. Secondary bacterial infection with *Pseudomonas* can result in severe pain and pus discharge from under the nail fold. Persistent paronychia invariably results in nail dystrophy (Fig. 19.2).

Candida infections of the female genitalia producing curd white vaginal discharge, soreness, redness, and itching in the vulva is fairly common in women with diabetes. Intertrigo (erythema and/or maceration of the skin) over inframammary area in obese female diabetic patients (Fig. 19.3) and web space skin between the toes (Fig. 19.4) and fingers (Fig. 19.5) (especially the middle and fourth toes) is also a common occurrence in both

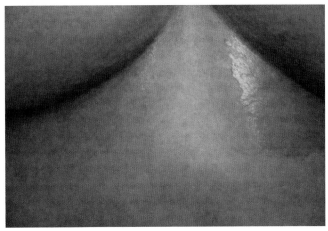

Figure 19.3. Candidal intertrigo of the inframammary area in an obese diabetic female.

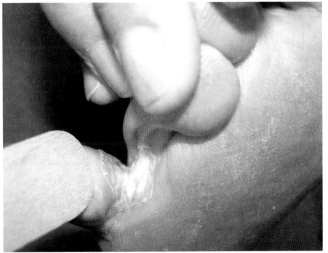

Figure 19.4. Intertrigo of a toe web: a potential source of cellulitis of the lower limbs.

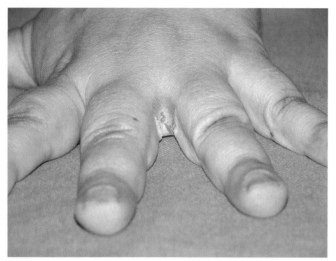

Figure 19.5. Candidal intertrigo of finger webs.

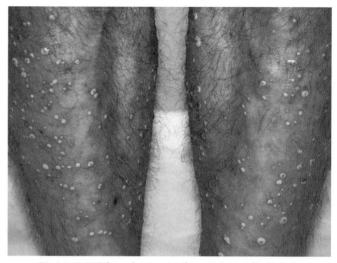

Figure 19.7. Bilateral extensive furunculosis of both legs.

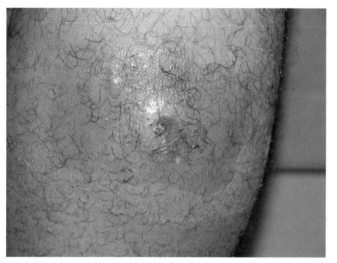

Figure 19.6. Large furuncle affecting the lower limb.

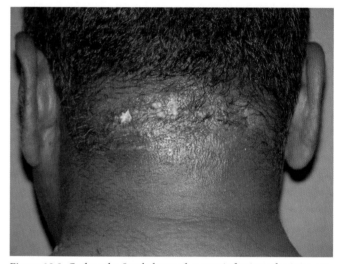

Figure 19.8. Carbuncle: *Staphylococcal aureus* infection of contiguous hair follicles in the nape of the neck.

male and female diabetics. Redness, superficial white scaling, and linear erosions of the foreskin (balanoposthitis) and glans penis (balanitis), which can cause some discomfort, pain, or itching in some patients can be the presenting feature of diabetes in males. Phimosis is a common complication in these patients. Control of blood sugar and treatment with topical antifungals usually clears these infections. However, oral ketoconazole is sometimes required, especially for cases of paronychia. Single-dose oral fluconazole 150 mg is an effective and convenient treatment for vaginal candidiasis in women.

Cutaneous Bacterial Infections in Diabetics

Common bacterial infections of the skin in diabetics are usually caused by *Staphylococcus aureus* and β-hemolytic streptococci. They include clinical presentations such as recurrent furuncles, carbuncles, ecthyma, cellulitis, and erysipelas.

A furuncle (Fig. 19.6) is an acute, usually necrotic, infection of the hair follicle with *S. aureus*, which results in an abscess of the hair follicle. The perifollicular abscess then necroses and destroys the hair follicle. Clinically this produces an erythematous, warm,

tender, painful nodule centered around a hair follicle, which forms a pus point on top of the lesions. It is a common infection in normal people but recurrent and extensive furuncles (Fig. 19.7) in a patient should prompt work-up for the presence of diabetes. The main defence against staphylococci is ingestion and killing by phagocytes, a function which may be deficient in diabetics. Resistance to staphylococcal infection is reduced in patients with poorly controlled diabetes.

A carbuncle (Fig. 19.8) is a deep infection of a group of contiguous hair follicles with *S. aureus*, accompanied by intense inflammatory changes in the surrounding and underlying connective tissues and subcutaneous fat. Carbuncles occur mainly in men, and usually in middle or old age. They may be seen in the apparently healthy but are more common in diabetics. The term "carbuncle" in Latin means "a small, fiery coal". It aptly describes the painful, hard, red lump that is the initial stage of infection. The carbuncle is smooth, dome-shaped, and acutely tender. It increases in size for a few days, to reach a diameter of 3 to 10 cm or occasionally more. Suppuration begins after some 5 to 7 days, and pus is discharged from the multiple adjacent follicular orifices. Most lesions occur on the back of the neck (Fig. 19.8), the shoulders or the hips and thighs. Although usually solitary, these lesions can be multiple or associated with one or more furuncles. Constitutional symptoms may accompany, or even precede the development of skin lesions. Fever may be high, and malaise and prostration may be extreme if the carbuncle is large or if the patient's general condition is poor. The lesion heals slowly to leave a scar. However, in patients with poor general health, death may occur from toxemia or from metastatic infection.

A swab of the pus must be taken for culture and sensitivity. Treatment, however, should not be postponed until bacteriological confirmation is available. Cloxacillin or another penicillinase-resistant antibiotic should be given.

Erysipelas is a bacterial infection of the lower dermis and the superficial part of subcutaneous tissue resulting in the sudden appearance of a bright red, edematous, warm, tender swelling with a well-defined edge, usually on the face or legs. Blistering and hemorrhage in the superficial skin may result. The patient can look ill and toxic with constitutional symptoms. Group A streptococci are usually implicated. Pus and blood cultures are essential parts of management. Swabs taken from intact overlying skin, saline injection followed by needle aspiration, biopsy, and even blister fluid may not yield any results. Some organisms are present in very small numbers.

Blood cultures and swabs from possible entry sites, like wounds or inflammatory lesions situated distal to the infection occasionally yield relevant organisms. Streptococcal serology may be helpful retrospectively. Poor glycemic control predisposes to erysipelas, however, at the same time the infection can result in hyperglycemia.

Cellulitis refers to the acute, subacute, or chronic inflammation of subcutaneous tissue. The infectious agent is usually bacterial. Minor injuries or scratches can introduce the infection. A firm, red, tender, diffuse swelling without a well-demarcated edge of the involved part, usually a limb or the face, is produced. It has been observed many times that features of both **cellulitis** and erysipelas can coexist. In such cases, a well-defined edge is present in one part, and there is diffuse involvement in the other part of the lesion. Moreover, erysipelas can extend deeper into the subcutaneous tissue, and cellulitis may spread upward into the superficial skin, making clinical distinction between the two conditions impossible. Currently, erysipelas is accepted as a form of superficial cellulitis by many. Streptococci are usually the pathogens responsible for both conditions. However, *S. aureus* alone can also cause cellulitis. Constitutional symptoms are invariably present in both erysipelas and cellulitis. Exceptions to this rule can be found in some milder cases. Severe cellulitis can result in bullae (Fig. 19.9), dermal necrosis, myositis, and fasciitis. In one study, cultures of biopsy specimens, needle aspirates, and samples from probable sites of entry in 50 patients with cellulitis gave a positive result in only 26% of the cases.

Erythrasma

Erythrasma is a mild, chronic, localized superficial infection of the skin caused by the aerobic coryneform bacterium, *Corynebacterium minutissimum*. It is frequently present as normal flora, especially in the toe clefts. A warm, humid climate is a predisposing factor. A Wood's lamp examination shows a coral

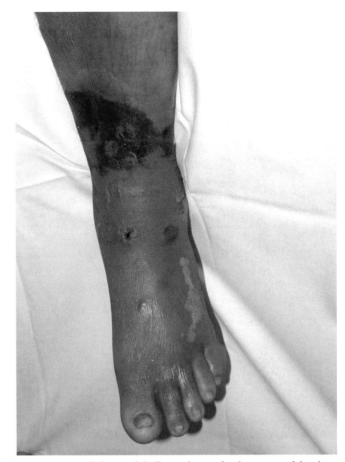

Figure 19.9. Cellulitis with bullae and superficial necrosis of the skin.

red fluorescence. Erythrasma is a common infection in diabetics. Erythrasma that is extensive and persistent and involves the axillae, inframammary folds, and large areas of the trunk and groins, is particularly common in obese, middle-aged women. Gram's staining of the scales reveals gram-positive rods and filaments (Figs. 19.10 and 19.11).

Irregular, sharply demarcated, initially red, but later brown patches with fine branny scaling are produced (Fig. 19.12). In colder regions, erythrasma is asymptomatic. In the warmer areas, however, irritation of lesions in the groins may lead to scratching and lichenification. Pruritus ani can be a symptom in lesions involving perianal skin. Clinical differential diagnosis includes tinea versicolor, dermatophytosis, psoriasis, and candidiasis. Wood's light examination and bacterial and fungal cultures help in diagnosis. Topical azole antifungal creams such as clotrimazole or miconazole are helpful in treating this condition. The antibiotic cream fucidin applied twice a day for 2 weeks is also effective. Rarely, systemic treatment with erythromycin 500 mg QID for 2 weeks is required.

LIFE-THREATENING INFECTIONS IN DIABETICS

Certain skin and soft tissue infections that are potentially lethal are more common in diabetics than in normal healthy individuals. Two of these are necrotizing fasciitis and malignant external otitis. Both of these conditions deserve special mention.

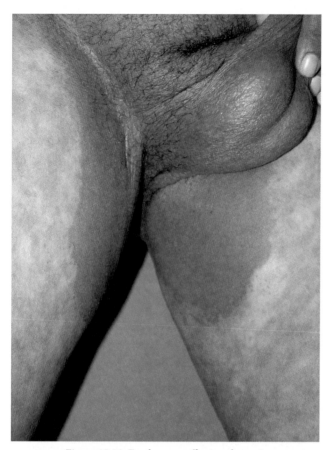

Figure 19.10. Erythrasma affecting the groins.

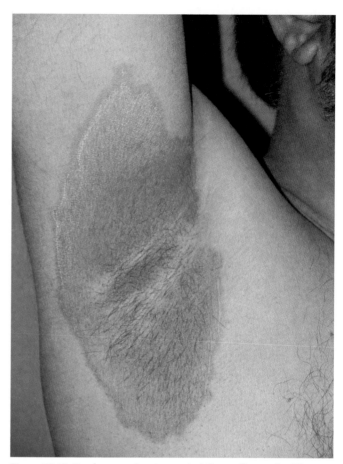

Figure 19.12. Erythrasma showing typical fine scaling and mild erythema.

Necrotizing fasciitis

This is a serious, life-threatening infection of the subcutaneous tissue associated with severe necrosis of underlying tissues (subcutaneous adipose tissue, muscle, fascia, and sometimes, even bone). The hallmark of this infection is an extensive necrosis accompanying cellulitis. There are two types. One is pure streptococcal (β-hemolytic Group A streptococci) and mixed infections type which consists of multiple organisms, and one is usually an anaerobe. The infections of mixed bacterial origin are common in diabetics, and include *Streptococcus pyogenes,* *S. aureus,* anaerobic streptococci and Bacteroides. The patient is usually severely ill and toxic, and mortality of over 45% has been reported in some case studies. Trauma, infection, diabetes mellitus, and previous surgery are the predisposing factors. Clinical features appear to be part of a spectrum ranging from cellulitis to myonecrosis. Erythema, which may become dusky red, appears within 24 to 48 hours. Bullae that are initially clear can develop. These later on become hemorrhagic or maroon. Bullae indicate an already extensive deep soft tissue destruction such as necrosis of the fascia or muscle. The extent of infection is variable. In some cases, pathology is restricted to a zone bound by fascia while in others infection extends to involve muscle and deep vessels. Swabs from the skin surface are usually negative. The most important step in diagnosis and management is surgical exploration in which subcutaneous tissues down to the fascia are found to be necrotic and may contain chains of

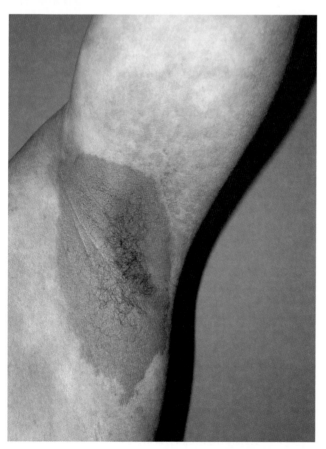

Figure 19.11. Erythrasma affecting the axilla.

gram-positive bacilli. A high index of suspicion and meticulous physical examination is required to make an early diagnosis. The diagnosis can be life saving because progression from an indolent presentation starting as a benign infectious process such as a furuncle to the one resulting in extensive tissue damage, toxicity, loss of limb, or even death can take place fairly rapidly among diabetics. Institution of high-dose IV penicillin therapy with metronidazole and supportive care while awaiting results of microbiologic work-up is crucial. Surgical debridement of infected devitalized tissue and surrounding areas is essential and should not be delayed. High-dose IV antibiotics should be started empirically, before awaiting the results of culture and sensitivity. Antibiotics alone, without surgical debridement, are rarely successful in saving the patient or the affected limb. Even with optimal care involving surgery and antibiotics, mortality rate is as high as 20% to 45%. It must be emphasized that 80% of cases of necrotizing fasciitis begin as a trivial skin lesion such as a boil, insect bite, or injection site infection. Decubitus ulcers along with the skin of the perineum and extremities are often sites where the condition first starts.

Fournier's Gangrene

These patients are usually diabetic. It is a suddenly erupting and rapidly progressing infection that involves the fascial planes of the lower abdominal wall, and extends to the scrotum and perineum. It can be caused by group A streptococci or multiple organisms. More commonly, however, it is caused by the latter. The condition carries a high mortality rate of around 40% despite surgical intervention or antibiotic use. It has been regarded as a synergistic necrotizing cellulitis or a subtype of necrotizing fasciitis. The management is similar to that of necrotizing fasciitis.

Malignant otitis externa

It is an invasive infection of the external auditory canal that typically occurs in immunocompromised individuals. The patients are usually elderly diabetics. Diabetic microangiopathy of the ear canal causing poor perfusion of the pinna or an increase in the pH of ear canal cerumen may be responsible. However, no correlation has been found with poor glycemic control. *Pseudomonas aeroginosa* is the causative organism in more than 95% of the cases. The patient presents with a purulent ear discharge and severe pain. The condition begins as cellulitis in the preaural area and surrounding skin. It can then progress to chondritis, osteomyelitis of the skull base, cerebritis, and thrombosis of the intracranial vessels. A tender pinna and preauricular area, a swollen external auditory canal, purulent discharge, and granulation tissue at the junction of the cartilaginous and bony parts are all clinical signs. A high level of clinical suspicion along with laboratory investigations showing leukocytosis and a markedly raised ESR are suggestive. CT, MRI, bone scan, and thallium scan can reveal the extent of bony involvement. Treatment consists of ear canal irrigation, drainage, debridement of devitalized tissue if needed, along with parenteral or oral quinolones for 6 to 8 weeks, especially if osteomyelitis is present. Resistant pseudomonas infection requires prolonged treatment with IV antipseudomonal β-lactam with or without an aminoglycoside. Correction of acid–base imbalances is also necessary.

Rhinocerebral mucormycosis

Hyperglycemia may permit nonpathogenic organisms to establish an infection in traumatized skin. Patients with uncontrolled diabetes are predisposed to deep fungal infections. Rhinocerebral mucormycosis is a rare life-threatening complication of diabetes. It may be a presenting feature of diabetes in the elderly. Diabetic ketoacidosis is present in most patients at the time of diagnosis. The causative organism is the fungus belonging to the class Zygomycetes, which is ubiquitous in nature, and can be found on decaying vegetation and in the soil. Hyperglycemia, acidosis, and the increased serum iron levels in diabetic patients provide favorable growth conditions for these fungi.

The clinical features include fever, facial cellulitis, periorbital edema, proptosis, blindness, and black eschars in the nasal mucosa or the palate due to ischemic necrosis of the tissue. The infection can spread throughout the sinuses and cause cranial nerve palsies, and it can also cause the patient to become obtunded. Facial numbness from infarction of the fifth cranial nerve can also be seen.

The diagnosis should be suspected in any poorly controlled diabetic presenting with sinusitis and purulent nasal discharge, metabolic acidosis, altered mentation, and/or nasal or palatal infarction. Endoscopy of the sinuses to look for infarction and to obtain specimens for culture is recommended. Characteristic broad nonseptate hyphae with right angle branching are seen using calcoflour white or methanamine silver stains. CT and MRI imaging is required to assess sinus involvement and to evaluate contiguous ocular and intracranial structures. Surgical debridement and parenteral amphotericin B are the treatments of choice.

PITFALLS AND MYTHS

In diabetic patients signs of inflammation may be missing even in the presence of severe, life-threatening cutaneous infections like necrotizing fasciitis. Pain may be absent because of peripheral neuropathy. Contrastingly, some diabetic patients with an underlying bacterial infection can present only with severe pain and no obvious cutaneous signs. In these cases, bacteria are present in affected tissues in low numbers. Even with multiple techniques of collecting samples for microbiologic studies the diagnosis can be difficult. The culture positivity is low in erysipelas and cellulitis. Swab from fissures, erosions, ulcers or injury sites distal to the site of these infections may yield relevant organism in some cases. Surface swabs from intact skin are unhelpful. In the case of facial infections, the pathogen should be sought in the nose, throat, conjunctiva, and sinuses. Toe webs must always be examined to look for evidence of intertrigo (maceration of the skin between toewebs) as that may be the portal of entry or source of bacteria for cellulitis on the legs. Deep vein thrombosis of the lower limbs can mimick cellulitis to a great extent. Phlebography, plethysmography, and Doppler ultrasound helps to decipher between the two. A simple and inexpensive test is to determine the protein concentration of the edema fluid; levels more than 10g/L indicate cellulitis whereas levels are usually around 5 g/L in deep vein thromboses.

PRINCIPLES OF THERAPY IN DIABETIC PATIENTS WITH CUTANEOUS INFECTIONS

1. Any patient suffering from recurrent or extensive furuncles, cellulitis, erysipelas, ecthyma, candidal balanitis/balanoposthitis, vaginal candidiasis, paronychia, and intertrigo should be investigated for diabetes.

2. Cutaneous signs and symptoms of infection may be absent even in presence of severe infection due to peripheral neuropathy. A high index of suspicion is required especially in elderly diabetics.

3. Therapy should not be delayed until the results of culture studies are available in cases presenting with clinical features suggestive of erysipelas/cellulitis, necrotizing fasciitis, malignant otitis externa, or Fourniers' gangrene as these are all possibly life threatening conditions. IV antibiotics should be started promptly. High-dose parenteral IV penicillin along with metronidazole in suspected mixed infection origin cases of necrotizing fasciitis and Fournier's gangrene should be started immediately, pending availability of culture results.

4. Surgical debridement is life saving in necrotizing fasciitis and should not be postponed unnecessarily.

5. Samples for microbiology should be collected from blister fluid, erosions, ulcers, injury, or inflammatory lesions distal to the site of cellulitis/erysipelas, necrotizing fasciitis, malignant otitis externa, and Fourniers'. Blood cultures should also be part of the work-up.

6. In facial infections, samples should be taken from the throat, nose, conjunctiva, and sinuses. Needle aspiration for collecting samples on the face should be avoided.

7. Measures to control hyperglycemia, management of fluid, and acid–base balance should be an integral part of the management, especially in severe infections.

8. Diabetic foot care to prevent detect and treat toe web intertrigo early can reduce the incidence of cellulitis and necrotizing fasciitis.

SUGGESTED READING

Ahmed I, Goldstein B. Diabetes mellitus. *Clin Dermatol* 2006;24(4):237–246.

Al-Mutairi N, Zaki A, Sharma AK, Al-Sheltawi M. Cutaneous manifestations of diabetes mellitus. Study from Farwaniya hospital, Kuwait. *Med Princ Pract* 2006;15(6):427–430.

Al-Mutairi N. Skin diseases seen in diabetes mellitus. *Bulletin Kuwait Institute of Medical Specialization* 2006;5:30–39.

Ferringer T, Miller F 3rd. Cutaneous manifestations of diabetes mellitus. *Dermatol Clin* 2002;20(3):483–492.

Mayser P, Hensel J, Thoma W, Podobinska M, Geiger M, Ulbricht H, Haak T. Prevalence of fungal foot infections in patients with diabetes mellitus type 1 – underestimation of moccasin-type tinea. *Exp Clin Endocrinol Diabetes* 2004;112(5):264–268.

Muller LM, Gorter KJ, Hak E, Goudzwaard WL, Schellevis FG, Hoepelman IM, Rutten GE. Increased risk of infection in patients with diabetes mellitus type 1 or 2. *Clin Infect Dis* 2005;41(3):281–8.

Rajagopalan S. Serious infections in elderly patients with diabetes mellitus. *Clin Infect Dise* 2005;40(7):990–996.

Rich P. Treatment of uncomplicated skin and skin structure infections in the diabetic patient. *J Drugs Dermatol* 2005;4(6 Suppl): s26–29.

Saw A, Kwan MK, Sengupta S. Necrotizing fasciitis: a life-threatening complication of acupuncture in a patient with diabetes mellitus. *Singapore Med J* 2004;45(4):180–182.

Tabor CA, Parlette EC. Cutaneous manifestations of diabetes. *Signs of poor glycemic control. Postgrad Med* 2006;119(3):38–44.

Tan JS, Joseph WS. Common fungal infections of the feet in patients with diabetes mellitus. *Drugs Aging* 2004;21(2):101–112.

Yoga R, Khairul A, Sunita K Suresh C. Bacteriology of diabetic foot lesions. *Med J Malaysia* 2006;61 Suppl A:14–16.

PART V: INFECTIONS OF SPECIFIC SKIN-ASSOCIATED BODY SITES

INFECTIONS OF THE SCALP

Shannon Harrison, Haydee Knott, and Wilma F. Bergfeld

INTRODUCTION

As an important component of skin, the hair-bearing scalp represents a unique microenvironment, which is afflicted by unique infections caused by many organisms such as fungi, viruses, parasites, and bacteria. Scalp infections affect all ages, both males and females and all races. This chapter describes the distinctive features of the hair-bearing scalp and its associated infections with highlights of current treatment regimes.

HISTORY

Scalp symptoms and conditions are common. Given the significance of scalp hair in today's society, visible changes in the hair and scalp such as erythema, scaling, and hair loss can cause considerable psychological distress and affect self-esteem. Although there are many causes of hair loss not associated with infections, infections of the scalp can lead to alopecia. Scalp infections are caused by various pathogenic organisms and were described years ago in Ancient Egypt.

SCALP ANATOMY

The scalp is comprised of five distinct layers: the skin, the subcutaneous layer, the galea aponeurosis, the loose areolar layer, and the periosteum. The frontalis and occipitalis muscles merge with the galea anteriorly and posteriorly respectively, and the temporalis muscle lies deeper under the loose areolar layer laterally. Important for scalp infections is the density of hair follicles and sebaceous glands (pilosebaceous units). In individuals without alopecia, the hair-bearing scalp contains approximately one hundred thousand (100, 000) hair follicles, which provide not only UV protection, but also considerable thermal insulation, creating an environment, which is warmer, darker, and more moist than in the non–hair-bearing parts of the body. The follicular environment supports the growth of microorganisms.

The pilosebaceous unit consists of the hair shaft, the hair follicle, the sebaceous gland, the sensory end organ, and the arrector pili muscle. The hair follicle can be structurally divided into three components. The inferior component is located below the insertion of the arrector pili muscle and includes the hair bulb. The middle component is called the *isthmus* and corresponds to

Dr. Harrison was funded by the F.C. Florance Bequest through the Australasian College of Dermatologists in 2008.

the insertion of the arrector pili muscle to the infundibulum and includes the bulge. The topmost component, or infundibulum, extends from the skin surface to the opening of the sebaceous gland. The hair shaft arises from the hair bulb, a rounded structure that contains the hair matrix, or cells, which give rise to the hair. The infundibulum hosts many normal organisms such as *Malassezia* species, *Staphylococcus epidermidis*, and occasionally *Demodex*. When the follicle is overwhelmed with the overgrowth of organisms, a folliculitis is frequently observed.

The sebaceous glands are unilobular or multilobular structures, which empty into the hair follicle via a short duct. The sebaceous glands produce an oily substance (sebum) which supplies emollients for the hair and skin. Sebum production peaks in late adolescence and thereafter declines with age. Sebum production is linked to androgen production, signaling the increase in circulating androgen levels in puberty and the decrease in androgen production with increasing age.

The unique anatomical and structural elements of the scalp reflect the characteristic diseases seen on the scalp. The dense covering of hair follicles on the scalp provides a warm, dark environment for microorganisms to flourish. Furthermore, due to the density of hair follicles on the scalp, increased absorption of topical agents occurs via the hair root sheaths. The scalp is associated usually with a high rate of sebum production, which provides a rich source of nutrition for microorganisms, particularly when combined with desquamated skin. The integrity of the scalp epidermis can be disrupted by friction and physical trauma from the use of combs, brushes, and other grooming tools, as well as chemicals used during the hair dying, perming, and straightening processes. These processes may create portals for infection on the scalp. In addition, shared hats, scarves, and hair accessories can introduce infection. The use of some hair products and occlusive emollients on the scalp can also predispose the hair follicle to infection. Therefore, the scalp is susceptible to a variety of infections, including superficial mycoses, parasitic and bacterial infections, and infective scarring processes.

FUNGAL INFECTIONS

Seborrheic dermatitis and pityriasis capitis

Seborrheic dermatitis and pityriasis capitis (dandruff) are recognized as two manifestations of a single disease process, although differing in severity (Table 20.1). Caused by *Malassezia* species, previously known as *Pityrosporum* species, these lipophilic, putative yeasts feed off of the lipids in sebum in patients with high levels of sebaceous gland activity. Global lifetime prevalence rates of Malassezia verge on 50%. Seborrheic dermatitis most commonly occurs in adults, between the ages of 15 and 50 years, in susceptible individuals with the postpubertal increase in androgen levels and the following rise in sebum production. Seborrheic dermatitis can persist into senescence. Seborrheic dermatitis, commonly known as "cradle cap" is also seen in the infant, likely still under the influence of circulating maternal androgens.

Immunocompetence is important in limiting the disease incidence, with approximately 30% to 35% prevalence in immunocompromised adults. Seborrheic dermatitis is associated with HIV infection where it may cause a generalized dermatitis requiring therapy with oral ketaconazole. Seborrheic dermatitis is also increased in patients with neurological conditions such as Parkinson's disease, cerebrovascular accidents, and head trauma.

The etiology of these diseases has recently been elucidated in greater detail. While colonization with *Malassezia globosa* and *Malassezia restricta* (yeasts) occurs in normal scalps, increased activity of these organisms has been linked to the development of the disease state. The lipophilic yeast is believed to digest sebaceous triglycerides, producing free fatty acids. These free fatty acids then penetrate the stratum corneum, disrupting the skin's barrier function, leading to inflammatory changes, pruritus, and dryness. It remains unknown why patients develop one clinical manifestation versus another, but it is believed to be due to the severity of the disease, the immune response, and the yeast burden.

Patients with pityriasis capitis (a variant of seborrheic dermatitis) classically experience loosely adherent, small white or grey flakes, while patients with the more severe seborrheic dermatitis, experience inflammatory changes of erythema, associated with yellow, greasy scales that collect to form crusts. Telogen effluvium can also occur in response to scalp inflammation such as severe seborrheic dermatitis. Occasionally, due to the pruritus and scratching, secondary bacterial infection can occur (Table 20.1). Frequently, seborrheic dermatitis not only occurs on the scalp, but also involves other areas of high sebum production including the face, posterior auricular area, posterior neck, and the body. A Wood's lamp can be helpful in confirming the presence of the *Malassezia* organisms, which fluoresce orange in active infections. Seborrheic dermatitis will often demonstrate repeated exacerbations and remissions over decades, and the treatment protocol needs to be relatively straightforward to ensure high levels of patient compliance.

Treatment consists of mono- or combined topical therapy using antifungal, keratolytic, or antiproliferative agents (Table 20.1). Management involves treating the acute exacerbation as well as continued therapies for prevention and control. Antifungal shampoos (ketoconazole, sulfur, selenium sulfide, pyrithione zinc, ciclopirox) are widely available and have been shown to be effective. Daily shampooing with an antifungal agent until the condition is under control is helpful. Tar shampoos are antiproliferative and useful in reducing scale, but are not user friendly, given their tendency to stain lighter colored hair and be odiferous. If the scale is thick or severe, the use of keratolytic agents such as salicylic acid in formulary preparations overnight to the scalp for a short period will be required to dislodge and remove scale. Tar formulary preparations can also be used as an antiproliferative agent in more severe cases. Patients with more severe presentations also require topical corticosteroid to the scalp for a short period to reduce inflammation and itch. The use of hair conditioners then can be considered if the topical therapies are drying.

If a secondary bacterial infection is suspected, culture and appropriate antibiotics should be started. Once the exacerbation is controlled, regular maintenance of therapies includes use of an antifungal shampoo every second day or three times per week. Alternating with another shampoo or another medicated shampoo should be continued to ensure levels of yeast on the scalp remain under control.

Pityriasis Amiantacea

Pityriasis amiantacea is characterized by thick, closely adherent overlapping scales on the scalp surrounding the hair shafts. It can be associated with temporary alopecia, or rarely a scarring alopecia. The etiology is unknown; however, it is believed to possibly involve multiple pathologies including seborrheic dermatitis, tinea capitis, pyogenic infection, and poor hygiene in addition to other inflammatory conditions of the scalp such as lichen planus and psoriasis. It may even be idiopathic.

Management involves removal of the scale with a salicyclic acid and/or tar preparations left on the scalp overnight or at least 4 to 5 hours before shampooing the hair. This needs to be continued daily until the scale is removed. Antifungal or tar shampoo needs to be continued daily. The underlying condition then needs to be treated appropriately.

Tinea Capitis

Tinea capitis is a dermatophytosis of the hair follicles of the scalp and while it is most common in childhood, it may present at any age. Tinea capitis can spread by exposure to infectious contacts or fomites. There are three genera of dermatophytes: *Microsporum, Trichophyton,* and *Epidermophyton* (Table 20.1). *Epidermophyton* does not invade the hair shaft. Both *Microsporum* and *Trichophyton* can infect the hair follicle. *Trichophyton tonsurans,* an anthrophilic agent, is the most common agent in North America, Western Europe, and Australia and is increasing in incidence. Infections in African-American and Latino children are also more likely to be caused by *T. tonsurans.* In Eastern Europe, *Trichophyton violaceum* is the most common etiologic agent. It should always be remembered that immigrants can be infected by the organisms endemic to their country of origin.

Tinea capitis infections may be classified according to the microscopic pattern of fungal invasion: endothrix, ectothrix, and favus. Ectothrix infection is defined by sporulation around of the hair shaft, weakening the cuticle and the shaft fractures several millimeters from the scalp, leading to patchy alopecia with grayish-white broken hair ends. This is most commonly associated with *Microsporum spp.,* including *Microsporum canis, Microsporum audouinii, Microsporum distortum,* and also *Trichophyton ferrugineum.* In the United States, *M. canis* is the most commonly encountered ectothrix pathogen. Endothrix infection grows within the hair shaft and the hair breaks at the scalp surface, leading to "black dot" alopecia. Both *T. tonsurans* and *T. violaceum* are endothrix infections (Table 20.1). Favus infections are usually caused by *Trichophyton schoenleinii.* Favus is recognizable by firm yellow crusts of hyphae and skin debris at the follicular orifices. This type of infection can lead to a scarring alopecia. It is most common in rural Africa and rural central Asia.

Symptoms of tinea capitis include well-demarcated or irregular alopecia, scaling, pruritus, and broken hair shafts (Table 20.1) (Fig. 20.1). Clinically, tinea capitis can be inflammatory and noninflammatory. The noninflammatory variant usually presents

Table 20.1: Fungal Infections of the Scalp

Condition	Organism	Clinical Presentation	Investigations	Treatment
Seborrheic dermatitis/ Pityriasis capitis	*Malassezia globosa, Malassezia restricta*	Pruritus, grayish white-to-yellow greasy scales with erythema and crusting ± telogen effluvium	Wood's light positive; orange fluorescence Bacterial cultures if secondary infection suspected	Antifungal shampoo (selenium sulfide, zinc pyrithione, ketoconazole, ciclopirox), tar shampoo Topical keratolytics (salicylic acid) Topical antiproliferatives (tar) Topical corticosteroids
Tinea capitis	*Microsporum canis, M. audouinii, M. distortum, T. ferrugineum*	Ectothrix infections causing white scaling patchy alopecia Pruritus	Small spore ectothrix infections may fluorescence green under Wood's light	Antifungal shampoo (selenium sulfide, zinc pyrithione, ketoconazole, ciclopirox) Systemic antifungal agent (griseofulvin, terbinafine-see text for further details) Systemic antibiotic if secondary bacterial infection Cleaning of combs, brushes, hair accessories and fomites
	Trichophyton tonsurans, T. violaceum, T. mentagrophytes, T. verrucosum	Pruritus Endothrix infection causing "black dot" tinea or inflammatory kerion ±lymphadenopathy	(Endothrix infections do not) Scrapings and hair clippings for culture and microscopy Bacterial swab if secondary infection suspected	
Piedra (Black and white variants)	*Piedra hortae Trichosporon asahii, T. asteroides, T. cutaneum, T. inkin, T. mucoides, T. ovoides*	Gritty adherent black or beige annular nodules encircling the hair shaft	Direct hair microcopy with KOH preparation and culture	Antifungal shampoo (selenium sulfide, zinc pyrithione, ketoconazole, ciclopirox) Cutting/shaving hair Systemic azole antifungal agent (see text)

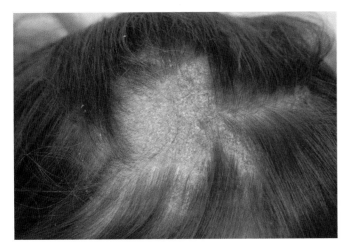

Figure 20.1. Scaling dermatitis on the scalp of a child with hair loss of tinea capitis.
"Photo courtesy of the Cleveland Clinic Department of Dermatology."

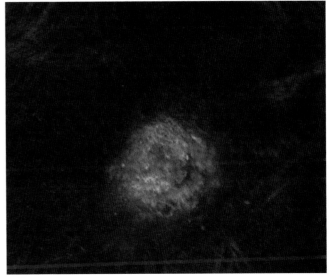

Figure 20.2. A boggy mass on the scalp of a child with hair loss is typical of a kerion.
"Photo courtesy of the Cleveland Clinic Department of Dermatology."

with oval patches of fine scaling with or without associated alopecia. Black-dot tinea capitis presents as areas of alopecia with black dots on the scalp surface. Inflammatory tinea capitis is characterized by a more aggressive presentation, ranging from pustules to abscess formation and even the development of kerions. Associated lymphadenopathy can be found in the primary nodal basins (Table 20.1). Kerions are boggy, inflammatory scalp masses (Fig. 20.2) often associated with infection by zoophilic fungi such as *T. mentagrophytes* or *T. verrucosum*, but can also be seen with the anthrophilic *T.tonsurans* infection. If untreated or inadequately treated, scarring alopecia may result.

Some scalp fungal infections fluoresce under Wood's light. Endothrix infections like *T. tonsurans* do not fluoresce (Table 20.1). Light-green fluorescence is seen with small spore ectothrix infections with *Microsporum*, while *Trichophyton schoenleinii* causing favus can also show a duller green fluorescence under Wood's light. Other ectothrix infections do not fluoresce. Wood's light examination may help confirm suspected infection, but never rules out infection.

The diagnosis of tinea capitis is often clinical. However, direct microscopy with 20% KOH (potassium hydroxide) of scalp skin scrapings and infected hair shafts allows the fungal infection to be visualized. Differentiation between ectothrix and endothrix infections can also be made. The scale and broken-off hairs can be obtained by scraping or rubbing the scalp with a disposable toothbrush or moist gauze. These samples can then be sent for culture in Sabouraud's agar to identify the causative species (Table 20.1). Once tinea capitis is confirmed, the family members of the patient should also undergo scalp microscopy and culture to rule out any infected family members or carriers.

Treatment of tinea capitis is currently undergoing extensive innovation. Griseofulvin has long been the treatment of choice; however, itraconazole, fluconazole, and terbinafine are also available (Table 20.1). Only griseofulvin is approved by the U.S. Food and Drug Administration (FDA) for the treatment of tinea capitis. Griseofulvin is fungistatic and griseofulvin-resistant organisms have developed. Doses are 20 to 25 mg/kg daily or 10 to 15 mg/kg daily of the ultra-microsize form for 6 to 8 weeks. Griseofulvin should be taken with a fatty meal to increase bioavailability and is usually well tolerated. Griseofulvin may cause gastrointestinal effects including nausea, diarrhea and vomiting, as well as skin rashes, headache, antabuse-like effect, and photosensitivity. Griseofulvin is a P450 enzyme inducer in the liver, and results in multiple drug interactions. Given the side effects and duration of therapy, noncompliance can become an issue. *T.tonsurans* appears to be less sensitive to griseofulvin compared to other species like *M. canis*.

Terbinafine is an allylamine fungicide, which inhibits synthesis of ergosterol in fungal cells. Terbinafine accumulates in hair follicles and stratum corneum rapidly. It has less drug interactions than griseofulvin with a shorter course of therapy. However, it is not FDA-approved for the treatment of tinea capitis. Treatment with oral terbinafine using a weight-based protocol (62.5 mg for patients weighing less than 20 kg, 125 mg for 20–40 kg patients, and 250 mg for patients greater than 40 kg) for 2 to 4 weeks is effective if the causative agent is *T. tonsurans*. Usually longer therapy is required to eradicate *Microsporum* species. Side effects of terbinafine include mild gastrointestinal upset, skin rashes, abnormal taste, and rarely, abnormal liver function. Reports of Stevens–Johnson syndrome and toxic epidermal necrolysis also exist for terbinafine.

In another recent study, itraconazole given in suspension or capsule form at 5 mg/kg/day for 6 weeks achieved a cure of 88% in children with tinea capitis caused by *M. canis*, and the cure rates were maintained in all subjects when evaluated 12 weeks following the cure. Adverse effects were noted in 6.7% of the children in the study, with only one child discontinuing the medication as a result. Itraconazole is an azole antifungal agent and side effects include gastrointestinal symptoms such as dyspepsia, nausea and vomiting, skin rashes, dizziness, and headache. It can also rarely cause abnormal liver function and Stevens–Johnson syndrome, and has multiple drug interactions.

Fluconazole is another azole antifungal that has been studied in the treatment of tinea capitis. It also has multiple drug interactions. A study showed in children with tinea capitis using once weekly fluconazole 8 mg/kg showed that 60 out of 61 children obtained a mycologic cure. The course duration ranged from 8 to 16 weeks. Side effects of fluconazole include headache, dizziness, nausea, and abnormal taste. Rare cases of Stevens–Johnson syndrome have been reported. Ketoconazole is associated with the rare but serious side effect of hepatotoxicity, and is therefore rarely selected for tinea capitis. Any systemic treatment should be continued until mycological cure is confirmed by negative mycological cultures.

In addition to a systemic antifungal agent, an antifungal shampoo such as ketoconazole or selenium sulfide shampoo should be used on the scalp 2 to 3 times per week to reduce the period of infectivity. Children should not share brushes, combs, hats, or scarves. Combs, brushes, and other fomites should be cleaned. Unaffected family members should also use an antifungal shampoo.

The treatment of a kerion has previously involved oral griseofulvin, an oral antibiotic, and usually oral corticosteroid. This regimen has been shown to improve itching and scaling more rapidly than griseofulvin alone. Recently, terbinafine has also been reported for kerion treatment. Currently, an oral antifungal agent as well as an antifungal shampoo is the treatment of choice for kerion. Any secondary bacterial infection should be cultured and treated appropriately.

Piedra

Meaning "stone" in Spanish, piedra represents a group of fungal infections that present as gritty nodules adherent to the hair shaft. Piedra can present as white or black variants, depending on the causative agents. Black piedra is caused by *Piedra hortae*, an ascomycete fungus. White piedra is caused by different *Trichosporon* species: *Trichosporon asahii*, *Trichosporon asteroides*, *Trichosporon cutaneum*, *Trichosporon inkin*, *Trichosporon mucoides*, or *Trichosporon ovoides*. Each species tends to occupy specific corporeal niches; while *T. inkin* infects the genitals, *T. asteroides*, *T. cutaneum*, and *T. ovoides* have been reported to cause scalp infections (Table 20.1). White piedra is less common and occurs in temperate climates. Black piedra occurs more frequently in the tropics and subtropics, and mainly affects the scalp. While rare in the United States, the infection appears to be increasing. This is largely attributed to the immigrantion of populations of a lower socioeconomic status. Transmission in humans is uncertain, although it is believed that close contact is responsible.

Diagnosis of piedra is based on clinical findings and supported by laboratory testing. The nodules are easily seen, encircling the hair shaft, and may be black, white, or tan. The shafts may become weakened by the infection and break at the level of the nodules. Direct microscopy and KOH mounting demonstrates focal, bulbous concretions on the hair shafts composed of hyphae, asci, and ascospores in black piedra. White piedra nodules contain hyphae, blastoconidia, and arthroconidia. Fungal stains and cultures may further confirm the diagnosis (Table 20.1).

Traditional treatment focused on complete removal or shaving of the affected hair, and treatment with topical antifungal agents

Table 20.2: Parasitic Infections of the Scalp

Condition	Organism	Clinical Presentation	Investigations	Treatment
Pediculosis capitis (Head Lice)	*Pediculosis humanis capitis*	Pruritus and live lice within 2 and 1/2" from the scalp Nits firmly attached to hair shafts	Clinical diagnosis Head lice can be visualized by dermoscopy and on microscopy Bacterial cultures if secondary infection suspected	Permethrin 1% cream rinse (See text for alternatives) Screen family and close contacts Cleaning of combs, brushes, hair accessories and fomites Antihistamines and topical corticosteroids may be needed for pruritus
Demodecidosis	*Demodex follicularum, D. brevis*	Erythema and pustular folliculitis	Clinical diagnosis Mites can be seen on skin biopsy histology	Topical permethrin or topical metronidazole (see text for alternatives)
Scabies	*Sarcoptes scabiei var. hominis*	Pruritus Erythematous papules, burrows, and vesicles in web spaces, volar wrists, waist, genitals and axillae Scalp and face involvement in children ± Secondary bacterial infection with crusting	Clinical diagnosis Mites can be visualized under direct microscopy Bacterial cultures if secondary infection suspected	Permethrin 5% cream (See text for alternatives) Screen and treat family and close contacts Cleaning of clothes, towels, linens and fomites Antihistamines and topical corticosteroids may be needed for pruritus

such as ciclopirox, imidazoles, and selenium sulfide. Black piedra has been treated with terbinafine with good effect, if shaving is not appropriate. Use of oral azole antifungals for 3 to 4 weeks combined with an antifungal shampoo for 2 to 3 months has recently been shown to be an effective treatment and avoids the need for shaving of the affected hair in white piedra in children (Table 20.1).

PARASITIC INFECTIONS

Pediculosis capitis

Pediculosis capitis is caused by the obligate human parasite *Pediculosis humanus capitis* or the human head louse (Table 20.2). The female head louse lives for 30 days and feeds off the host every 4 to 6 hours. She lays approximately 10 eggs per day, which hatch 10 to 14 days later. Head lice rarely can survive without their host; however, in certain climates nits may survive for 10 days away from the host. This infection is particularly common among children and occurs in all socioeconomic strata. *P. capitis* is much more commonly seen among White or Latino children, due to the difficulty of the lice adhering to the tightly curled hair of children of African heritage. Girls are more commonly infected than boys, likely due to their favoring of long hair and sharing of hair accessories. Transmission is common through direct contact with fomites that are found on shared combs, brushes, hats, helmets, bed linens, and clothing.

P. capitis is confined to scalp hair, and pruritus is the most common symptom. The severity of the pruritus varies among individuals, depending on the immune hypersensitivity response to the lice's salivary antigens. The lice load usually is heavier in the occipital and post-auricular regions of the scalp. Secondary effects are due to itch and scratching, causing crusting, secondary bacterial infection, and cervical adenitis (Table 20.2).

The diagnosis is made with clinical recognition of active lice in the hair. The nits (eggs) are usually more easily seen as white particles firmly attached to the hair shafts near the scalp skin, but unlike the concretions of piedra, nits are not completely circumferential. The eggs can sometimes be mistaken for hair casts, however, hair casts easily slide along the hair and are annular. The adults measure 3 to 4 mm in size and can therefore be seen with the naked eye; however, the lice load varies among individuals. In active infection, the lice are attached to the hairs within 2½ inches from the scalp surface. Wet combing with a fine-tooth comb can assist in visualizing the nits. Dermoscopy can aid in visualizing the lice or nits. Lice and nits can be identified under direct microscopy (Table 20.2).

Treatment of *P. capitis* is almost universally topical (Table 20.2). A variety of therapies are available, including permethrin, pyrethrin extracts, lindane, malathion, and carbaryl, which are typically applied twice. The second treatment follows the first treatment by 7 to 10 days to eliminate any active lice/nits that survived the initial therapy. Permethrin is a synthetic pyrethroid with a good safety profile. Permethrin 1% cream rinse is applied to clean and partially dry hair and is left for 10 minutes. It is then rinsed off and should be repeated in 7 to 10 days time. Resistance to permethrin has been reported. Pyrethrins plus piperonyl butoxide have also been used to treat head lice. They are less effective than permethrin and should not be used in patients with chrysanthemum allergy. Malathion 0.5% lotion is applied to hair for 8 to 12 hours and is thought to be safe if used as directed. Malathion is flammable and accidental ingestion can cause respiratory depression. It is recommended that malathion only be used in treatment-resistant cases. Lindane 1% shampoo can cause neurotoxicity and seizures in children and should be avoided if possible. After topical treatment, the nits need to be removed physically using a fine-tooth comb daily until the nits and lice are removed.

Alternate therapies include essential oils as well as petroleum jelly, mayonnaise (avoid reduced fat varieties), and conditioner, which are believed to suffocate the lice and nits. These alternative therapies do not appear to be effective and require further study. Any secondary bacterial infection should be cultured and treated with the appropriate antibiotics. Antihistamines and topical steroids are occasionally needed for itch relief. Family members may also be affected, and should be screened to prevent reinfection. All clothes and bed linens should also be washed in hot water and machine dried. Toys should be washed and dried in a clothes dryer or sealed in plastic bags for 2 weeks. Carpets and upholstery should be thoroughly vacuumed. Topical drug-resistant strains are emerging, and oral courses of ivermectin or cotrimoxazole are effective in eradicating these strains. Systemic treatment may also need to be considered in treatment failures.

Demodecidosis

Demodecidosis is a cutaneous infection caused by an infestation with demodex mites (Table 20.2). Two species have been implicated in active disease: *Demodex folliculorum* and *Demodex brevis*. Demodecidosis is not limited to the scalp, but may be encountered on the forehead, nose, cheeks, eyelids, as well as more distant locations such as the upper chest and genitals. Demodex colonization is directly related to areas of high sebum production. As such, there are low rates of colonization in children and adolescents, with an increasing prevalence among adults.

The demodex mite measures approximately 0.3 to 0.4 mm, and has a life span of 2 weeks. A strong distinction must be made between colonization by *Demodex spp* and active infection, since colonization rates approach 100% in adults. Therefore, biopsy specimens containing occasional demodex mites is of no significance, but the finding of more than 5 mites per low power field or more than 5 per cm^2 is believed to be correlated with disease development. Nevertheless, the ubiquity of the mites among normal hosts makes pathogenicity controversial. In some conditions, multiplication of the follicle mites and mites in an intradermal location may contribute to disease. Immunocompetent adults and children can rarely develop infections, but active disease is more common among immunocompromised adults and children. Case reports have associated demodecidosis with HIV and leukemia. Demodex mites have been implicated in rosacea and pustular folliculitis of the scalp. Rarely, severe scalp demodicidosis in children can resemble favus.

A variety of oral and topical agents have demonstrated effectiveness against demodex mites. Lindane, permethrin, metronidazole, crotamiton, benzyl benzoate, and ivermectin have all shown efficacy (Table 20.2).

Scabies

Scabies is an intensely pruritic skin infestation caused by the mite, *Sarcoptes scabiei var. hominis* (Table 20.2). Scabies may afflict patients of any background, ethnic group, or age. While scabies usually spares the scalp and face among adults, in children it often involves the scalp. The severe crusted variant known as *Norwegian scabies*, commonly involves the scalp, and is encountered among patients who are immunocompromised or debilitated.

The scabies mite can survive up to 3 days without a host, so while direct human contact is the most common mode of transmission, infested bedding or clothing may serve as a reservoir of infection. The mite moves through the epidermis by secreting proteases that degrade the stratum corneum on which they feed, leaving scybala (feces) behind.

Clinically, nocturnal pruritus is characteristic. Scabies is characterized by small papules, vesicles, and burrows over the flexor aspects of the wrists, the interdigital web spaces of the hands and feet, axillae, elbows, waist, and genitalia. In children, vesicles and papules can be seen on the hands and feet, but the scalp and face can also be involved (Table 20.2). Secondary impetiginization and eczematization can occur. Patients with Norwegian scabies typically have crusting on the hands and feet with associated nail dystrophy, as well as crusting of the head and face. Hair loss can also be associated with Norwegian scabies.

BACTERIAL INFECTIONS

Folliculitis

Folliculitis can occur in any hair-bearing area of the skin, including the scalp. Folliculitis is inflammation of the hair follicle and is usually caused by infection. Occlusion, friction, and some topical agents also predispose to folliculitis. Folliculitis can be superficial or deep. Superficial folliculitis involves the superior portion of the hair follicle, and deep folliculitis, the entire follicle or inferior portion of the hair follicle is involved. Superficial folliculitis is seen as small tender or nontender pustules that can have associated pruritus and usually heal without scarring. The clinical presentation of deep folliculitis is different with erythematosus, tender papules, pustules, and nodules, which may heal with scarring. Folliculitis can be caused by many different organisms.

Staphylococcal folliculitis

Staphylococcal folliculitis is the most common type of folliculitis (Table 20.3) (Fig. 20.3). It can be superficial or present as furuncles and carbuncles. A furuncle is a single infective perifollicular abscess, and is less common on the scalp, but can affect the face and neck. A carbuncle is a deeper infection of a group of hair follicles and can occur in the scalp and posterior neck. It can be associated with constitutional symptoms and diabetes mellitus, obesity, chronic renal impairment, and malnutrition. Corticosteroid treatment can predispose to infection. Pustules should be swabbed and sent for culture.

The mainstay of treatment is appropriate oral antistaphylococcal antibiotics and avoidance of overheating, friction, and occlusion (Table 20.3). In superficial folliculitis, topical antibiotics and compresses may only be needed. Antibacterial washes with chlorhexidine or betadine can reduce the bacterial skin load. Surgical incision and drainage may be required for furuncles and carbuncles. Carrier status of *Staphylococcus aureus* in the anterior nares, perineum, and axillae can also occur in patients with *Staphylococcal* infections or close family members. Swabs and cultures should be done. Physicians should always remember that the incidence of methicillin-resistant *Staphylococcal aureus* (MRSA) is increasing in the community.

Table 20.3: Bacterial Infections of the Scalp

Condition	Organisms	Clinical Presentation	Investigations	Treatment
Folliculitis	*Staphylococcus aureus*, *Staphylococcal spp.* MRSA *Pseudomonas*, *Klebsiella, Aermonas, Proteus spp*	Superficial folliculitis with erythema and folliculocentric pustules Furuncles and carbuncles	Bacterial swab for microscopy, culture and sensitivities MRSA carrier swabs and cultures	Systemic antibiotics Anti-bacterial wash Incision & drainage if needed for furuncles & carbuncles
Impetigo	*Staphylococcus aureus*, *Streptococcal spp.*	Erythematous blisters, crusting and erosions	Bacterial swab for microscopy, culture and sensitivities	Systemic antibiotics Anti bacterial wash
Erysipelas	*Streptococcal spp.* Group A	Well demarcated erythematous painful plaque ± fever and lymphadenopathy	Bacterial swab for microscopy, culture and sensitivities CBC for leukocytosis.	Systemic antibiotics
Scalp cellulitis	*Staphylococcus aureus*, *Staphylococcal spp. Streptococcal spp.* Group A	Poorly demarcated erythematous, swollen painful plaque ± fever and lymphadenopathy	Bacterial swab for microscopy, culture and sensitivities CBC for leukocytosis	Systemic antibiotics
Postoperative infection	*Staphylococcus aureus*, *Staphylococcal spp.*, MRSA, *CA-MRSA, Streptococcal spp.* Group A	Erythematous, swollen painful wound ± crusting ± fever and lymphadenopathy	Bacterial swab for microscopy, culture and sensitivities CBC for leukocytosis	Systemic antibiotics
Infections secondary to intrauterine fetal monitoring devices	*Staphylococcal spp., MRSA. Streptococcal spp.*, mixed anaerobes and aerobes	Abscess, cellulitis or osteomyelitis Rarely meningitis and sepsis	Bacterial swab for microscopy, culture and sensitivities	Systemic antibiotics

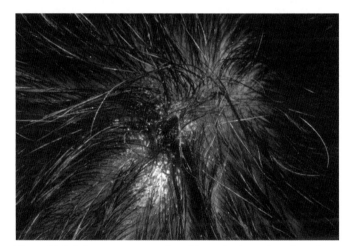

Figure 20.3. Inflammatory pustules of the scalp that cultured staphylococcus aureus making the diagnosis of staphylococcal folliculitis. "Photo courtesy of the Cleveland Clinic Department of Dermatology."

It should be remembered that folliculitis can involve not only the hair follicles of the scalp but other areas of the body as well. Dermatophyte, *Pityrosporum*, and candidial infections can mimic a bacterial folliculitis. Gram-negative bacteria such as *Pseudomonas, Klebsiella*, and *Proteus* can also cause folliculitis. *Pseudomonas* folliculitis occurs after using a hot tub or contaminated pool. The folliculocentric lesions occur typically under the bathing suit, but do not affect scalp hair follicles. *Aeromonas hydrophilia* may also be responsible for a case of hot tub folliculitis.

Eosinophilic pustular folliculitis

Eosinophilic pustular folliculitis (EPF) is a noninfectious folliculitis presenting as red papulopustules. The cause is unknown, but may be associated with immune dysfunction to certain infectious pathogens. Infancy-associated eosinophilic pustular folliculitis usually starts within the first few weeks of life and affects particularly the scalp, as well as the face and extremities. Classic EPF presents as sterile annular papulopustules with peripheral extension and commonly affects the face, while immunosuppression-associated EPF is mostly HIV-related and also involves the face, showing more discrete pruritic, erythematous papules. Histology shows infiltration with eosinophils and lymphocytes at the follicular isthmus and minimally surrounding the outer root sheath and sebaceous glands. In infancy-associated EPF, flame figures may be present in the scalp. Topical corticosteroids are the first-line treatment and immunosuppression-associated EPF may require narrow-band UV light therapy.

Impetigo

Impetigo can be primary or secondary and is a superficial skin infection caused by *Staphylococci, Streptococci*, or both (Table 20.3). Primary impetigo presents as erythematous crusting or blisters, particularly on the face, scalp, and extremities. Secondary impetigo or impetiginization with *Staphylococci* presents in skin with impaired barrier function or in traumatized skin. Secondary infection can occur in the scalp affected by seborrheic dermatitis, psoriasis, eczema, pediculosis capitis, or insect bites. Swabs and cultures should be taken and appropriate oral antibiotic therapy commenced. Antibacterial washes with chlorhexidine or betadine can reduce the bacterial skin load. Soaks of aluminum acetate (Burow's solution) or saline are useful to remove crusting, and the underlying condition in secondary impetigo should also be treated.

Erysipelas and Scalp Cellulitis

Erysipelas is an infection of the upper dermis usually caused by Group A Streptococci (Table 20.3). The scalp can be involved due to extension from the face or pinna or due to a scalp wound or chronic skin condition. Clinically, a well-demarcated erythematous plaque with associated fever is seen. Lymphadenopathy can be associated. An acute telogen effluvium can follow this infection. Lymphedema predisposes to this infection.

Cellulitis or infection involving the deep dermis and subcutaneous fat can be caused by *Streptococcus pyogenes* and/or *Staphylcoccus aureus or* MRSA (Table 20.3). Entry for the bacteria can be a scalp wound, scalp surgery, or a chronic skin condition. Diffuse, poorly demarcated erythema, heat, swelling, and pain are the hallmarks of cellulitis. Systemic symptoms and lymphadenopathy can also be associated. Laboratory investigations of cellulitis rarely identify a specific causative organism. Diagnosis is clinical, with possible identification of the infecting agent on skin swabs and cultures. Blood cultures are recommended in elderly patients with fever and leukocytosis as well as in immunocompromised patients. For both erysipelas and cellulitis, treatment with systemic antibiotics is required.

Postoperative Scalp Infections

Scalp infection post hair transplant is a surgical risk. Scalp infection following neurosurgery must also be considered. A recent study highlighted risk factors for the development of any infection. The following conditions were found to be risk factors having a scalp infection following neurosurgery, being >70 years in age, being male, and having a postoperative cerebrospinal fluid (CSF) leak.

Methicillin-resistant *Staphylococcus aureus* (MRSA) is a well-known nosocomial pathogen that can cause soft tissue infections such as abscesses and cellulitis and should always be considered as a potential pathogen in scalp infections (Table 20.3). The rate of community-acquired MRSA (CA-MRSA) infections is on the rise and should also be kept in mind as a potential pathogen in cutaneous infections. Culture and antimicrobial sensitivities should be obtained and appropriate antibiotic therapy should be instituted. Intravenous vancomycin, or linezolid if vancomycin is contraindicated, is a highly effective treatment option for MRSA-positive wounds.

Intrauterine fetal monitoring devices

Bacterial infections of the scalp following the placement of intrauterine fetal monitoring (IFM) devices, which are used to monitor fetal circulation and oxygenation, are also increasing. Cutaneous infection following placement of IFM devices is between 0.1% and 5.2%. Sensitive culture techniques have revealed a diverse microbiology including aerobic, anaerobic, and mixed aerobic and anaerobic organisms. Use of multiple IFM devices, cephalohematoma, amnionitis, endometritis, and a long duration of monitoring have all been implicated in these infections.

The infection may present as cellulitis, abscess, osteomyelitis or bacteremia. In the case of cellulitis or abscess, the infection is usually centered over the area where the electrode had been placed. Aspiration or placement of a drain may be required if the abscess does not drain spontaneously. Effective treatment depends on culture-directed antibiotic therapy. Patients with minimal infection may improve spontaneously, but most cases need parenteral antibiotic therapy. If insufficiently treated, osteomyelitis of the occipital bone, meningitis, and sepsis may all occur as sequelae.

SCALP CONDITIONS WITH PRESUMED BACTERIAL ETIOLOGY:

Acne miliaris necrotica

The etiology of acne miliaris necrotica is unknown. However, bacterial infection with *Propionibacterium acnes* has been suggested. Acne necrotica miliaris is the milder form of the disease, and acne necrotica varioliformis is the deeper form of the condition, which can cause varicella-like scars. Clinically, tender, itchy, erythematous papules, which then ulcerate and crust centrally, occur along the scalp hairline. Biopsy and bacterial swabs and cultures should be taken. Histology shows a lymphocytic perifollicular infiltrate with plasma cells and lymphocytes invading the outer root sheath. The outer root sheath also demonstrates keratinocyte cell necrosis.

Treatment involves topical antibiotics such as 1% clindamycin lotion for the mild form of the disease and an oral antibiotic such as tetracycline or doxycycline for the more severe condition. Topical and oral steroids are occasionally needed as an adjunctive therapy.

Folliculitis keloidalis (Acne keloidalis)

Folliculitis keloidalis is a form of scarring alopecia, in which staphylococcal infection is a postulated etiology. Clinically, it presents as grouped follicular papules, pustules, and hypertrophic scars at the nape of the neck and occipital scalp. Occasionally, it can also occur at the vertex and overlap with folliculitis decalvans. African-American men are commonly affected. Scalp biopsy and bacterial swabs and cultures should be taken. Biopsy shows hair follicles with a mixed acute or chronic granulomatous inflammation and hypertrophic scarring with loss of the sebaceous glands. Treatment is difficult. Antibiotic therapy with cephalosporins, penicillins or tetracyclines in conjunction with topical and intralesional corticosteroids is usually required. Carbon dioxide laser and surgery may be needed in some cases.

Folliculitis Decalvans and Dissecting Cellulitis of the Scalp

Folliculitis decalvans and dissecting cellulitis of the scalp are neutrophilic-predominant cicatricial alopecias (Fig. 20.4). Inflammatory follicular nodules, pustules, and papules precede areas of scarring hair loss. Activity is intermittent, but slowly progressive. In folliculitis decalvans, any area of the scalp can be involved.

Table 20.4: Unusual Infections of the Scalp

Condition	Organism	Clinical Presentation	Investigations	Treatment
Syphilis	*Treponema pallidum*	Diffuse alopecia or moth-eaten patchy hair loss Less commonly, gumma, papulopustular or noduloulcerative lesions	Skin biopsy with Warthin-Starry staining and PCR	Recommended CDC syphilis therapeutic regime (see text for website details)
Mycobacterial infection	*Mycobacterium neoaurum.* *Mycobacterium spp.*	Erythematous indurated plaque of scarring alopecia Skin ulcers and soft tissue infections	Skin biopsy with Ziehl-Nelson staining, culture and PCR	Antimycobacterial treatment according to species identified on culture or PCR Certain mycobacterial species infections require surgery as treatment (Management can be reviewed.)

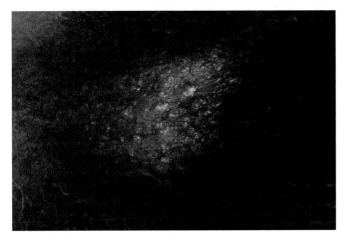

Figure 20.4. Alopecia of the nuchal scalp with inflammatory papules and scarring of folliculitis decalvans.
"Photo courtesy of the Cleveland Clinic Department of Dermatology."

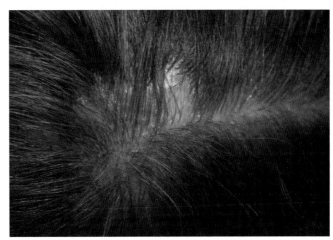

Figure 20.5. Grouped pustules on a person with fair skin that already shows significant alopecia of the scalp. This is early erosive pustular dermatosis.
"Photo courtesy of the Cleveland Clinic Department of Dermatology."

In dissecting cellulitis of the scalp, inflammatory nodules are accompanied by abscesses and sinus formation. The etiology for folliculitis decalvans and dissecting cellulitis of the scalp is not clear, but is believed to be an abnormal host response to Staphylococcal antigens. They occur more commonly in African-American men. Scalp biopsy can confirm the diagnosis and bacterial swabs and cultures should be taken. Histology shows keratin plugging of the follicle orifice and many intraluminal neutrophils, the follicles rupture and there is an interstitial and perifollicular inflammatory infiltrate with dermal abscess formation. Over time, fibrosis and a chronic inflammatory infiltrate with granulomas are seen, followed by scarring. In dissecting cellulitis of the scalp, sinus formation is also seen on histology, with a deep mixed inflammatory cell infiltrate and foreign body granulomas.

Treatment consists of prolonged courses of systemic anti-staphylococcal antibiotics. Combination treatment with rifampicin and clindamycin can be effective in resistant cases. Fusidic acid and zinc have also been used. Topical and intralesional corticosteroids are frequently needed. Isotretinoin is now an effective choice for dissecting cellulitis of the scalp. Surgery and hair removal lasers have also been used for dissecting cellulitis of the scalp.

Erosive Pustular Dermatosis of the Scalp

The etiology of erosive pustular dermatosis of the scalp is unknown. However, abnormal immune responses to infectious organisms such as *Staphylococcus aureus* have been suggested. It is usually seen in chronically sun-damaged scalps of older, balding individuals. Sterile pustules coalescing into lakes with crusting and erosions on the scalp are seen. Scarring alopecia can be an end result (Fig. 20.5). Histology shows a suppurative folliculitis with adnexal involvement and later, fibrosis and a chronic inflammatory infiltrate. Treatment involves potent topical steroids, and topical or oral antibiotics with a medicated shampoo. Isotretinoin has also been used. Topical tacrolimus 0.1% has also been reported to be effective in erosive pustular dermatosis of the scalp.

UNUSUAL INFECTIONS

Syphilis Infection

Hair loss can occur in secondary and tertiary syphilis. Syphilis is caused by the spirochete, *Treponema pallidum* (Table 20.4).

Primary syphilis does not cause hair loss unless the primary chancre involves the scalp. Hair loss in syphilis can present as a diffuse alopecia mimicking telogen effluvium, but more classically presents as a "moth-eaten" pattern of hair loss with irregular patches of scalp hair loss. Other lesions of syphilis can occur in the scalp including gummata in tertiary syphilis and a papulopustular or noduloulcerative eruption in secondary syphilis.

Diagnosis of syphilis is based on serological testing. Dark-field microscopy of lesions or tissue identifying the spirochetes can assist in diagnosis. Scalp biopsy is also helpful for active scalp lesions, and in the noduloulcerative form spirochetes may be seen with the Warthin-Starry stain. In cases of diffuse and moth-eaten alopecia, spirochetes had not been seen previously and histology showed a sparse perifollicular lymphocytic infiltrate with plasma cells. However, recently *Treponema pallidum* has been identified in the peribulbar region in a patient with patchy nonscarring alopecia due to syphilis infection. The recommended treatment schedule for syphilis from the Centers for Disease Control and Prevention (CDC) should be followed (www.cdc.gov/std/syphilis).

Mycobacterial infection

Cutaneous mycobacterial infection can cause scalp hair loss. *Mycobacterium neoaurum* has been shown to cause an indurated plaque of scarring alopecia in an immunocompetent host (Table 20.4). Histology showed granulomatous inflammation and PCR was positive on scalp biopsy for *Mycobacterium neoaurum;* however, culture was negative. Supportive of the causative origin of this alopecia, antimycobacterial treatment was instigated and the plaque improved and flattened; however, no hair growth returned. Other nontuberculosis mycobacteria species could also infect the scalp, causing soft tissue infections and skin ulcers. Biopsy, culture, and PCR should be done on any suspected atypical infection. Treatment is guided by the mycobacterium species identified on culture or PCR.

VIRAL INFECTIONS

Warts

Rarely, viral infections can affect the scalp (Table 20.5). Warts can occur on the scalp, usually via direct inoculation of the human papilloma virus (HPV). The peak incidence of warts is in childhood and warts can occur in immunosuppressed individuals. Warts typically appear as firm hyperkeratotic papules. They can resolve spontaneously, and treatment depends on the size and location of the warts. Topical keratolytics and topical immunotherapy can be used. Curettage under local anesthetic and cryotherapy are also possible treatment options.

Molluscum contagiosum

Molluscum contagiosum caused by a DNA poxvirus can occur on the face and scalp. Typically, umbilicated skin-colored-to-pink papules can be identified and rarely can mimic folliculitis in hair-bearing areas. Giant molluscum has been reported in the scalp, and diagnosis is through histology on biopsy. Treatment involves irritant strategies with tape stripping, topical retinoids, topical imiquimod, or physical therapies of cryotherapy or curettage for large lesions. The lesions normally resolve spontaneously, so treatment is not always necessary.

Herpes viral infections

Herpes zoster can involve the scalp. It is caused by a DNA herpes virus (VZV) involving the ophthalmic branch of the trigeminal nerve, and grouped, painful vesicopustules occur in the distribution of the unilateral ophthalmic branch. Crusting, ulceration, secondary bacterial infection, and hair loss can sometimes occur. Herpes simplex virus (HSV) can also affect hair follicles and can mimic bacterial folliculitis. Primary and secondary lesions of HSV present as grouped, painful vesicopustules on an erythematous base. A Tzank smear of the lesions can clinically corroborate the diagnosis. Viral culture and/or PCR can confirm the infection. Valacyclovir, acyclovir or famciclovir is the treatment of choice in herpes zoster. Postherpetic neuralgia is an important consequence of herpes zoster infection and prompt treatment is essential. Herpes simplex infection can also be treated with systemic antivirals. Any secondary bacterial infection should be treated with appropriate antibiotics.

INFECTIONS IN TRANSPLANT PATIENTS

Transplant patients are at risk for infection from their transplanted organ, from the surgery itself, from reactivation of latent infections, and from opportunistic infections during the iatrogenic immunosuppression following their transplant. Success rates of transplants have improved with increased patient and graft survival in heart and lung transplant recipients. As a reflection, clinicians are diagnosing more opportunistic and atypical infections secondary to immunosuppression. These infections frequently involve the skin and scalp.

In transplant patients, the scalp can be affected by all the organisms that can affect immune competent individuals. Conditions such as tinea capitis, which are more commonly seen in children, can be seen in transplant adult patients because of immunosuppression. Primary invasive cutaneous *Microsporum canis* infections have been reported in a transplant recipient and an HIV-positive patient. Norwegian scabies, which can involve the scalp, is also more commonly seen in debilitated or immune-compromised patients. In addition, skin cancers on sun-damaged scalp can occur in the setting of immunosuppression post transplant. Infections in transplant patients are often more severe and life threatening. Prophylactic regimens have been developed to reduce posttransplant infective complications. Any infection in a transplant patient must be diagnosed and treated early.

PITFALLS AND MYTHS

Itchy scalp is a very frequent presenting complaint, and although it is commonly believed to be a sign of infection, there are noninfective scalp disorders that can produce pruritus. Allergic contact dermatitis to certain hair dyes and products can occur and cause pruritus. Pruritus is also an important symptom of inflammatory scalp conditions such as eczema, seborrhea, irritant dermatitis,

Table 20.5: Viral Infections of the Scalp

Condition	Organism	Clinical Presentation	Investigations	Treatment
Warts	*Human papilloma virus*	Firm, hyperkeratotic papules	Clinical diagnosis. Rarely histological confirmation needed	Observation, topical keratolytics, immunotherapy, cryotherapy, curettage
Molluscum	*Molluscum contagiosum DNA pox virus*	Umbilicated skin-colored to pink papules	Clinical diagnosis. Rarely, histological confirmation needed	Observation, tape stripping, topical retinoids, cantharidin, imiquimod, cryotherapy, curettage
Herpes Zoster	*Varicella-Zoster virus*	Unilateral grouped painful erythematous vesicopustules	Viral swab for microscopy, culture and PCR. Tzanck smear	Oral valacyclovir or famciclovir or acyclovir
Herpes Simplex	*Herpes simplex virus*	Grouped painful erythematous vesicopustules	Viral swab for microscopy, culture and PCR. Tzanck smear	Oral valacyclovir or famciclovir or acyclovir

and psoriasis. Certain forms of cicatricial alopecia such as lichen planopilaris and discoid lupus erythematosus can also lead to scalp pruritus. Pruritus of the scalp invariably leads to scratching and possible secondary bacterial infection. When examining a scalp for possible infection, it should be remembered that more than one may be present. It should also be remembered that the scalp is an area of skin that can easily be forgotten when examining the skin of a patient, and complete skin examination includes a thorough examination of the scalp.

Importantly, the scalp and its hair follicles can only react to infectious and/or other pathological processes in a finite number of patterns. These include flaking, erythema, and hair loss. As such, there can be similarities among the clinical presentations of different conditions and diseases of the scalp, which can occasionally make accurate diagnosis difficult. Swabs for culture, hair and skin microscopy, as well as histology can sometimes be needed to confirm the diagnosis.

A common myth is that only people with poor hygiene habits develop scalp infections. Another myth is that sleeping with wet hair can cause fungal scalp infections. These are false beliefs as infection is usually transmitted through direct head contact with an infected individual or through sharing of infected fomites such as brushes, hats, and hair accessories and not through poor hygiene or sleeping with a wet scalp. Dandruff and seborrheic dermatitis are also incorrectly believed by some to be from inadequate scalp hygiene or a build up of pollutants or residues from hair products and the atmosphere. Dandruff and seborrheic dermatitis are caused by resident *Malassezia* yeasts present in small numbers on all adult scalps, which under certain influences, such as hormonal variations and not poor hygiene, can multiply and cause the clinical picture of itch and scaling. Cradle cap seen on the scalp of babies was falsely believed to reflect poor parental care or a serious illness. However, it is caused by the same yeasts that cause dandruff in adults, which multiply under the influence of the maternal circulating androgens. Once these hormonal influences have resolved, the cradle cap often improves.

Normally, scalps are protected by the hair follicles; however, with aging, the hair follicle density can decrease and can be affected by androgenetic alopecia (patterned hair loss). Balding scalps are exposed to UV light, predisposing them to skin cancer.

A skin cancer can either be mimicked by a primary skin infection or it can be a primary skin cancer that is secondarily infected. Therefore, an isolated crusted or itchy papule or nodule on a balding scalp should always be regarded with suspicion and may require a biopsy as well as bacterial swab and culture to exclude malignancy.

Hair loss is a common symptom, and usually is not associated with scalp infection. However, infections can cause different types of hair loss including telogen effluvium, and diffuse or patchy alopecia, and scarring alopecia. Severe inflammatory conditions of the scalp including seborrheic dermatitis can trigger a telogen effluvium. Inflammatory tinea capitis or kerions and nontuberculous mycobacteria can also cause scarring hair loss. Syphilis can cause both a diffuse alopecia and a patchy alopecia, while tinea capitis can cause a patchy or localized nonscarring alopecia. In some cases of hair loss, scalp biopsy and culture, in addition to microbiological swabs, may be needed to exclude a possible infective cause of hair loss.

There are many home remedies and natural therapies postulated to cure dry hair, dandruff, head lice, tinea capitis, and hair loss. Tea-tree oil has been used as a natural antiseptic and antifungal. Apple cider vinegar has been used as a remedy for dandruff. There are many natural products and herbal concoctions that claim to help hair loss such as aloe vera and saw palmetto, as well as hair care products containing natural ingredients. Although natural ingredients such as plant extracts may provide possible therapeutic activities, there is a lack of clinical trials for these products. There is a need to understand these chemicals and possible contaminants, as well as their safety for the community, before they become accepted therapies. In this chapter, current recommended treatments for scalp infections have been discussed.

CONCLUSION

The structural and anatomic features of the scalp predispose it to a variety of infections from fungal, parasitic, bacterial, and viral organisms. Unusual infections such as syphilitic and mycobacterial infections can also involve the scalp. Interestingly, the scalp can also be affected by a set of unique conditions that can mimick a bacterial infection but are not. These conditions are unique to the scalp and can result in cicatricial alopecia. Clinically, many of these conditions are recognizable; however, microscopy, culture, and biopsy can assist in diagnosis. Antimicrobial resistance, newly emerging agents, and the increasing number of immunosuppressed patients require that clinicians update their knowledge regarding etiologic agents and treatment protocols.

SUGGESTED READINGS

Apache PG. *Eczematous dermatitis of the Scalp*. In: Zviak, C, ed. The Science of Hair Care. New York, Marcel Dekker, 1986: 513–521.

Ashack RJ, Frost ML, Nornins AL. Papular pruritic eruption of Demodex folliculitis in patients with acquired immunodeficiency syndrome. *J Am Acad Dermatol* 1989;21:306–307.

Aste N, Pau M, Biggio P et al. Kerion Celsi: A clinical epidemiological study. *Mycoses* 1998;41:169–173.

Aylesworth R, Vance JC. *Demodex folliculorum* and *Demodex brevis* in cutaneous biopsies. *J Am Acad Dermatol* 1982;7(5):583–589.

Baima B, Sticherling M. Demodicidosis revisited. *Acta Derm Venereol* 2002;82:3–6.

Bayeral C, Feller G, Goerdt S. Experience in treating molluscum contagiosum in children with imiquimod 5% cream. *Br J Dermatol* 2003;149(Suppl 66):25–29.

Bennett RG: Anatomy and physiology of the skin. In: Papel, ID, ed. *Facial Plastic and Reconstructive Surgery*. 2nd edition. New York, New York: Thieme, 2002.

Bergfeld WF & Elson DM. Cicatricial Alopecias. Olsen EA. *Disorders of Hair Growth: Diagnosis and Treatment*. 2nd edition. McGraw-Hill 2003.

Bettencourt M, Olsen E. Pityriasis amiantacea : A report of two cases in adults. *Cutis* 1999;64:187–189.

Brook T. Cutaneous and subcutaneous infections in newborns due to anaerobic bacteria. *J Perinat Med* 2002; 30:197–208.

Burgess IF. Cutaneous parasites. *Curr Opin Infect Dis* 1998;11:107–111.

Burkhart CG & Burkhart CN. Asphyxiation of lice with topical agents, not a reality…yet. *J Am Acad Dermatol* 2006;54:721–722.

Burkhart CN, Burkhart CG. Fomite transmission in head lice. *J Am Acad Dermatol* 2007; 56(6):1044–1047.

Burns DA. Follicle mites and their role in disease. *Clin Exp Dermatol* 1992;17:152–155.

Carroll KC. Cases and clinical correlation. In: Brooks GF, Carroll KC, Butel JS, Morse SA. eds. *Jawetz, Melnick, & Adelberg's Lange Medical Microbiology*, 24th edition. The McGraw-Hill Companies Inc. USA 2007.

Cenkowski MJ & Silver S. Topical tacrolimus in the treatment of erosive pustular dermatosis of the scalp. *J Cutan Med Surg* 2007; 11(6):222–225.

Cotsarelis G, Millar S, Chan EF. Embryology and anatomy of the hair follicle. In: Olsen EA, ed. *Disorders of Hair Growth: Diagnosis and Treatment*, 2nd edition. McGraw-Hill Publishing, 2003.

Dawson TL Jr: *Malassezia globosa and restricta*: Breakthrough understanding of the etiology and treatment of dandruff and seborrheic dermatitis through whole-genome analysis. *J Investig Dermatol Symposium Proceed* 2007;12:15–19.

De Maeseneer J, Blokland I, Willems S et al. Wet combing vs. traditional scalp inspection to detect head lice in school children. An observational study. *Br Med J* 2000;231:1187–1188.

Dragos V, Lunder M. Lack of efficacy of 6-week treatment with oral terbinafine for tinea capitis due to *Microsporum canis* in children. *Pediatr Dermatol* 1997;14(1):46–48.

Elewski BA. Clinical diagnosis of common scalp disorders. *J Investig Dermatol Symp Proc* 2005;10:190–193.

Elewski BE. Tinea capitis. A current perspective. *J Am Acad Dermatol* 2000;42:21–24.

Fisher DA. Acne necroticans (varioliformis) and *Staphlococcus aureus*. *J Am Acad Dermatol* 1987;16:1007–1014.

Fishman JA. Infection in solid-organ transplant recipients. *N Engl J Med*. 2007;357(25):2601–2614.

Forton F, Song M. Limitations of standardized skin surface biopsy in the measurement of the density of *Demodex folliculorum*. A case report. *Br J Dermatol* 1998;139:697–700.

Garcia-Vargus A, Mayorga-Rodriguez JA, Sandoval-tress C. Scalp demodicosis mimicking favus in a 6 year old boy. *J Am Acad Dermatol* 2007;57:S19–21.

Garrity ER, Moore J, Mulligan MS et al. Heart and lung transplantation in the United States, 1996–2005. *Am J Transpl* 2007;7 (Part 2):1390–1403.

Ginarte M, Pereiro M, Fernandez-Redondo V et al. Case reports: Pityriasis amiantacea as a manifestation of tinea capitis due to *Microsporum canis*. *Mycoses* 2000;43:93–96.

Ginter-Hanselmayer G, Smolle J, Gupta A: Itraconazole in the treatment of tinea capitis caused by *Microsporum canis*, experience in a large cohort. *Pediatr Derm* 2004;21(4):499–502.

Gip L. Black piedra: the first case treated with terbinafine. *Br J Dermatol* 1994;130 (Suppl 43):26–28.

Griffith DE, Aksamit T, Brown-Elliott BA et al. An official ATS/IDSA statement: Diagnosis, treatment and prevention of nontuberculous mycobacterial diseases. *Am J Respir Crit Care Med* 2007;175:367–416.

Grimalt R. A practical guide to scalp disorders. *J Investig Dermatol Symp Proc* 2007;12(2):10–14.

Gupta AK, Dlova N, Taborda P et al. Once weekly fluconazole is effective in children in the treatment of tinea capitis: a prospective multicentre study. *B J Dermatol* 2000;142:965–968.

Habif TP. Infestations and bites. In: Habif TP, ed. *Clinical Dermatology* 4th edition, Edinburgh: Mosby Inc. 2004; Chapter 15: pages 497–546.

Habif TP. Bacterial Infections. In: Habif TP, ed. *Clinical Dermatology* 4th edition, Edinburgh: Mosby Inc. 2004; Chapter 9: pages 267–306.

Hengge UR, Currie BJ, Jager G, Lupi O, Scwartz RA. Scabies: a ubiquitous neglected skin disease. *Lancet* 2006;6:769–779.

Honig PJ, Caputo GL, Leyden JJ et al. Treatment of Kerions. *Pediatr Dermatol* 1994;11: 69–71.

Ivy SP, Mackall CL, Gore L, Gress RE, Hartley AH. Demodicidosis in childhood acute lymphoblastic leukemia: an opportunistic infection occurring with immunosuppression. *J Pedriatr* 1995; 127:751–754.

Jordaan HF & Louw M. The moth-eaten alopecia of secondary syphilis. A histopathological study of 12 patients. *Am J Dermatopathol* 1995;17:158–162.

Katoch VM. Infections due to non-tuberculous mycobacteria (NTM). *Indian J Med Res* 2004;120:290–304.

Kiken DA, Sekaran A, Antaya RJ, et al: White piedra in children. *J Am Acad Dermatol* 2006;55:956–61.

King D, Cheever LW, Hood A et al. Primary invasive cutaneous *Microsporum canis* infections in immunocompromised individuals. *J Clin Microbiol* 1996;34(2):460–462.

Langtry JAA, Ive IA. Pityriasis amiantacea, an unrecognized cause of scarring hair alopecia described in four patients. *Acta Derm Venereol* 1991;71:352–353.

Lopez FA & Lartchenko S. Skin and soft tissue infections. *Infect Dis Clin N Amer* 2006;20:759–772.

Martigoni E, Paccheti C, Berardesca E et al. Is seborrhea a sign of autonomic impairment in Parkinson's diseases? *J Neural Transm* 1997;104:1295–1304.

Martin LK, Lawrence R, Kossard S et al. Cutaneous *Mycobacterium neoaurum* infection causing scarring alopecia in an immunocompetent host. *Br J Dermatol* 2007;157: 204–205.

Miskjian HG. Demodicosis (Demodex infestation of the scalp). *Arch Dermatol* 1951;63:282–283.

Moon CM, Schissel DJ. Pityriasis amiantacea. *Cutis* 1999;63:169–170.

Mulholland A & Yong-Gee S. A possible new case of spa bath folliculitis: *Aeromonas Hydrophila*. *Aus J Dermatol* 2008; 49:39–41.

Nam-Cha SH, Guhl G, Fernandez-Pena P, Fraga J. Alopecia syphilitica with detection of *Treponema pallidum* in the hair follicle. *J Cut Pathol* 2007; 34 (Suppl. 1):37–40.

Nervi SJ, Schwartz RA, Dmochowski M. Eosinophilic pustular folliculitis: A 40 year retrospect. *J Am Acad Dermatol* 2006;55:285–289.

Ogiso T, Shiraki T, Okajima K et al. Transfollicular drug delivery: penetration of drugs through human scalp skin and comparison of penetration between scalp and abdominal skins in vitro. *J Drug target* 2002;10(5):369–378.

Olsen EA, Bergfeld WF, Cotsarelius G et al. Summary of North American Hair Research Society (NAHRS) sponsored workshop on cicatricial alopecia, Duke University Medical Center, February 10 and 11, 2001. *J Am Acad Dermatol* 2003;48:103–110.

Peter RU, Barthauer U. Successful treatment and prophylaxis of scalp seborrheoic dermatitis and dandruff with 2% ketoconazole shampoo. *Br J Dermatol* 1995;132:441–445.

Plewig G, Jansen T. Acniform dermatoses. *Dermatology* 1998;196:102–107.

Ressel GW. AAP Releases clinical report on head lice. *Am Fam Phys* 2003;67(6):1391–1392.

Roberts JL & DeVillez RL. Infectious, physical and inflammatory causes of hair and scalp abnormalities. In: Olsen EA. ed. *Disorders of Hair Growth: Diagnosis and Treatment* 2nd edition. USA: McGraw-Hill Publishing, 2003.

Rogers RL, Perkins J. Skin and Soft Tissue Infections. *Prim Care Clin Office Pract* 2006;33:697–710.

Rook A & Dawber R. The comparative physiology, embryology and physiology of human hair. In: Rook A & Dawber R, eds. *Diseases of the Hair and Scalp*. Oxford: Blackwell Science, 1982;1–17.

Rook A & Dawber R. Infection and Infestations Pp: 367–408. In: Rook A & Dawber R eds. *Diseases of the Hair and Scalp*. Oxford: Blackwell Science Publications, 1982.

Schaller M, Sander CA, Plewig G. Demodex abscesses: clinical and therapeutic challenges. *J Am Acad Dermatol* 2003;49:S272–274.

Schwartz RA. Superficial fungal infections. *Lancet* 2004;364:1173–1182.

Shinoura N, Yamada R, Okamoto K, Nakamura O: Early prediction of infection after craniotomy for brain tumors. *Brit J Neurosurg* 2004;18(6):598–603.

Sinclair R, Banfield C, Dawber R, eds. Inflammatory dermatoses of the scalp. In: Malden, MA. *Handbook of Diseases of the Hair and Scalp*. Blackwell Science 1999; 201–208.

Sinclair R, Banfield C, Dawber R, eds. Infections and Infestations of the hair. In: Malden MA. *Handbook of Diseases of the Hair and Scalp*. Blackwell Science 1999; pp: 191–200.

Skinner RB, Zanolli MD, Noah PW, et al. Seborrhoeic dermatitis and AIDS. *J Am Acad Dermatol* 1986;14:147–148.

Sperling LC, Homoky C, Pratt L, et al. Acne keloidalis is a form of primary scarring alopecia. *Arch Dermatol* 2000;136:479–484.

Sullivan JR & Kossard S. Acquired scalp alopecia. Part II. A Review. *Austral J Dermatol* 1999;40:61–72.

Taplin D, Meinking TL, Chen JA, Sanchez R. Comparison of crotamiton 10% cream (Eurax) and permethrin 5% cream (Elimite) for the treatment of scabies in children. *Pediatr Dermatol* 1990;7:67–73.

Virgili A, Zampino MR. Relapsing tinea capitis by *Microsporum canis* in an adult female renal transplant recipient. *Nephron* 1998;80:61–62.

Zhang AY, Camp WL, Elewski BE. Advances in topical and systemic anti-fungals. *Dermatol Clin* 2007;25:165–183.

21 | INFECTIONS OF THE NAIL UNIT

Gérald E. Piérard, Claudine Piérard-Franchimont, and Pascale Quatresooz

HISTORY

The nail unit has probably been the target of infectious processes since the origin of humanity. However, the causative agents have changed over time. No information is available on bacterial infections, but it is likely that few changes have occurred over the past centuries. By contrast, the nature of onychomycoses has considerably changed during the 20th century with the progressive spread of *Trichophyton rubrum* to many parts of the world. The history of nail infections is also geographically influenced by geoclimatic conditions as well as by occupational activities, and cultural habits, and lifestyle habits.

NAIL UNIT STRUCTURE

The nail unit has a unique structure consisting of four distinct components, namely, the matrix, the nail bed, the nail plate, and the nailfolds. The matrix is mostly located under the proximal nailfold and its distal portion, which corresponds to the whitish lunula.

The nail plate is composed of approximately 25 layers of flattened, cornified onychocytes that are tightly bound together. This structure is organized as three superimposed layers corresponding to the dorsal and intermediate layers originating from the matrix and the ventral layer which are both derived from the nail bed (Fig. 21.1). The dorsal part is a few cell layers thick containing hard keratin. This structure represents the main barrier to drug and xenobiotic penetration into the nail plate and

beyond. The intermediate layer, which contains soft keratin, represents almost three quarters of the whole nail thickness. Below this structure, the ventral layer rich in soft keratin is a few cells thick and is located firmly at the interface between the nail plate and the underlying nail bed.

The proximal nailfold consists of a crescentic sheet of tissue covered with epidermis on its dorsal and undersurface. Its sharp and angled free margin produces the cuticle. The hyponychium between the nail underface and pulp epidermis corresponds to the distal end of the nail structure.

It is also important to distinguish microbial paronychial infections from onychomycoses.

MICROBIAL PARONYCHIAL INFECTIONS

The proximal nailfold with its cuticle attached to the nail plate, the lateral nailfolds, and the ventral hyponychium normally forms tight closures. They normally prevent infections and xenobiotics from entering the subungual area. Microbial paronychia is an infectious and inflammatory condition of these periungual soft tissues. The disorder may correspond to an acute or chronic infection. Conceptually paronychia is therefore not a primary disease, but follows some physical or chemical damages. This evidence does not apply to superficial infections, such as impetigo or herpes simplex affecting the dorsum of the proximal nailfold.

Acute Paronychia

Most often, a minor physical trauma under the distal edge of the nail or in a lateral groove is the cause of acute paronychia. It may consist of a break in the skin, the inclusion of a splinter, a prick from a thorn, or a subungual infection following a hematoma. The bacteria most commonly responsible for acute paronychia are staphylococci and less commonly β-hemolytic streptococci and gram-negative enteric bacteria. Paronychia presents as local erythema, swelling, and throbbing pain. The purulent reaction often takes several days to localize. A bead of pus is often visible underneath the nail or in the periungual folds. At this stage, a topical antibiotic treatment is indicated, combined or not, with appropriate oral antibiotic therapy. Clinicians should be weary of response to topical and systemic antibiotics because it may mask an underlying yeast infection or tumor.

The collected pus tends to create a cleft between the nail and its underlying proximal attachment. The firmer attachment of the nail at the site of the lunula often temporarily limits the spread of the pus. However, the nail matrix is particularly fragile in early childhood and can be destroyed within a couple of days

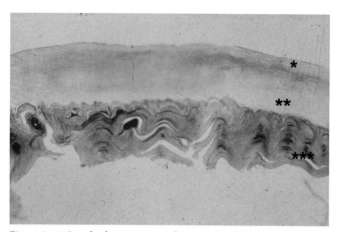

Figure 21.1. Standard microscopy of a normal nail plate showing 3 superimposed structures: the thin dorsal layer (*), the thicker intermediate layer (**) and the ventral layer (***).

by an acute bacterial infection. Distal subungual pyogenic infections may accompany periungual involvement. In some cases, extension of the infection can involve the finger pulp or the matrix. In other instances, evacuation of a paronychial abscess can uncover a narrow sinus. This sinus suggests the presence of a "collar-stud" abscess communicating with a deep-seated necrotic zone.

In general, acute paronychia involves only a single nail. The differential diagnosis should include several conditions including eczema, herpes simplex, psoriasis, Reiter's disease, and acute vascular impairment. Bacterial culture and allergy screening are often indicated.

Chronic Paronychia

Chronic paronychia is a common inflammatory disorder of the proximal nailfold typically affecting hands that are frequently exposed to both wet environments and repeated minor traumas altering the cuticle. The index and middle fingers of the dominant hand are most often affected. In addition, the periungual skin can be quite vulnerable to harsher surfactants. If the epidermal cover of the cuticle or any other parts of the nailfold is impaired, these structures will be exposed to an ingress of a variety of xenobiotics including irritants and allergens.

The periungual erythema and swelling form a cushion at the proximal and lateral nailfolds. With time, the adherence of the cuticle is weakened and the proximal nailfold retracts and becomes thicker and rounded. This condition is further prolonged as molecular xenobiotics, foreign particles, and microorganisms lodge beneath the nailfold, and further contribute to the inflammation and infection. In some cases, pus will arise from the nailfold. The histological presentation of chronic paronychia commonly reveals spongiotic dermatitis on the ventral portion of the proximal nailfold.

The course of chronic paronychia is occasionally accompanied by paroxysmal exacerbations of painful inflammation. In some instances, episodes can be due to secondary *Candida* spp. and bacterial infections or even superinfections, where small pustules develop between the proximal nailfold and the nail plate. These microbial abscesses often drain spontaneously and heal without any treatment in a couple of days. Acute exacerbations of chronic paronychia are not only due to microbes but also to irritant or allergen xenobiotics penetrating deep into the proximal nailfold. Contact allergies to foodstuffs, latex, and topical drugs are not uncommon. In addition, fragments of foreign particles such as hair, foodstuffs, and various other debris can collect in the proximal nailfold. This multifaceted process often causes retraction of the nailfold and a persistence of the paronychial process.

In the early stages of paronychia the nail plate is preserved, but one or both lateral edges may develop surface roughness as well as yellowish, brownish, or blackish discoloration. This discoloration may further extend over a large portion or even the totality of the nail plate. This type of chromonychia is believed to be caused by dihydroxyacetone produced by the microorganisms in the nailfold. By contrast, *Pseudomonas* spp. tend to produce a greenish hue caused by a pigment called pyocyanin. The lateral edges of the nail plate become cross-ridged when the disease affects the lateral nailfold. The surface of the nail commonly becomes rough and friable, and numerous irregular transverse ridges and grooves appear, due to repeated acute exacerbations. Eventually, the nail becomes considerably reduced in size because of swelling in the surrounding soft tissues.

There is some disagreement as to the importance of *Candida* spp. colonization or infection in chronic paronychia because these organisms can behave as commensals or pathogens. Various factors can damage the area and allow *Staphylococcus aureus* and *Candida* spp. under the cuticle of the nail plate. In children, the habit of thumb or finger sucking represents the most common predisposing factor. This condition is potentially more harmful than occupational hand immersion, as saliva is more irritating than tap water. Chronic paronychia can also develop in patients with eczema or psoriasis involving the nailfolds. Chronic paronychia may also develop in association with ingrown toenails or, more rarely with diabetes or peripheral vascular impairments. Chronic paronychia can be related to nail infections caused by *Scytalidium* spp. In such instances, brown chromonychia can start at the lateral edges of the nail plate and spread centrally into the nail. *Fusarium* spp. can also produce chronic paronychia.

Syphilitic paronychia can represent a painful chancre. Pemphigus can alter the nailfold, mimicking chronic paronychia. Psoriasis, Reiter's disease, and eczema can also involve the proximal nailfold.

FUNGAL INFECTIONS OF THE NAIL

Onychomycosis is defined as a fungal infection of the nail. It is not a clinical diagnosis and the presence of the fungus must be confirmed by laboratory procedures. The common clinical signs include thickening, discoloration, and splitting of the nail plate, as well as lifting of the nail plate from the nail bed. The disease has a high incidence in the general population. The main predisposing factors for onychomycosis include old age, diabetes, HIV infection, psoriasis, peripheral vascular impairment, peripheral neuropathies, podiatric abnormalities, certain sporting activities, and traumatic nail disorders.

This condition represents about 50% of all nail disorders. It has a high occurrence throughout the world and recent epidemiological data indicates a prevalence ranging from 2% to 15%. Thus, onychomycosis is the most common progressive nail disease by fungi. Some clinicians claim to be able to predict the presence of a fungus in a dystrophic nail. However, it is very difficult. Dermatophytes are the pathogens most commonly responsible for primary onychomycoses. Yeasts and nondermatophyte molds both account for about 5% to 15% of cases. Onychomycosis more frequently affects the toenails than the fingernails. This is probably explained in part by the fact that the toenail growth rate is 3 times slower than that of fingernails. Different clinical patterns of onychomycosis due to the way by which fungi invade the nail have been described. The type of nail invasion depends on both the nature of the fungus, the host susceptibility and the site at which the nail is invaded.

Five main categories of onychomycosis have been established. They are the distal and lateral subungual type, the proximal subungual type, the white or black superficial type, the midplate type, and the total dystrophic type. There are also mixed variants of onychomycosis, as well as unusual patterns seen in onychomycosis relapses.

It is not within the scope of this chapter to detail laboratory procedures, but it is important to stress the necessity of sending suitable specimens to the laboratory. Clippings taken from affected areas are best, however, this is not always possible. It may be necessary to scrape or slice off areas of dystrophic nail with a scalpel blade.

Traditional methods used for the diagnosis of onychomycosis are fungal nail culture on Sabouraud's dextrose agar and KOH preparation of nail samples. Although these have been the standard methods used in clinics, the diagnostic accuracy range for these tests is as low as 50% to 70%, depending on the methods used to collect and prepare the samples. There is evidence that histomycology when compared to culture shows higher discriminatory ability and a higher accuracy rate.

Distal and Lateral Subungual Onychomycosis

Distal and lateral subungual onychomycosis (DLSO) represents the most common type of onychomycosis. This condition is frequently caused by *Trichophyton rubrum*, which reaches the nail through the hyponychium or the lateral nailfolds and invades the nail bed spreading proximally. The skin of the palms and soles is the primary site of infection.

In DLSO, the distal and lateral free edges of the nail exhibit subungual hyperkeratosis and eventual onycholysis (Fig. 21.2a, b & c). In early evolving DLSO, the fungi are confined to the deeper portion of the nail plate (Fig. 21.3). The onycholytic area appears as opaque, yellow-white areas spreading proximally. Yellow streaks along the lateral margin of the nail and/or presence of yellow onycholytic areas in the central portion of the nail represent air-filled tunnels or clumps of dermatophytes named *dermatophytomas* (Fig. 21.4). As the disease progresses, the nail plate usually becomes more friable and grossly hyperkeratotic. Various color changes can also be present in DLSO.

Aspergillus spp., *Fusarium* spp. and *Scopulariopsis brevicaulis* may produce DLSO that involves a single toenail, creating the diffuse nail invasion associated with paronychia. DLSO due to *Acremonium* spp. usually presents as one or a few longitudinal white streaks extending proximally from the distal margin. In DLSO due to *S. brevicaulis*, *Alternaria* spp. and *Scytalidium* spp., the periungual tissues and the nail plate often show a brown to black pigmentation.

Sometimes DLSO occurs secondary to posttraumatic onycholysis. The initial space created becomes the potential site for colonization and infection.

Proximal Subungual Onychomycosis

Proximal subungual onychomycosis (PSO) is one of the least common variants of onychomycosis in the general population, but it does represent the most common type of onychomycosis among immunocompromised patients (particularly those infected by HIV where T. rubrum is most likely the etiology). Fungi most likely target the nail plate through the underface of the proximal nailfold and the area under the cuticle. The infection typically spreads to the ventral portion of the nail plate. PSO presents with or without paronychia. Clinically, PSO presents as a focal leukonychia appearing from beneath the proximal nailfold. The affected nail shows a deep, milky-

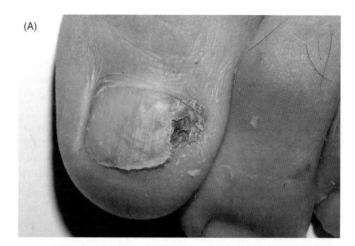

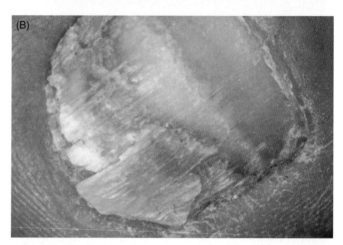

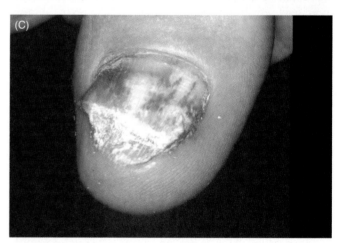

Figure 21.2. A,B&C. Distal and lateral subungual onychomycosis. (A) Lateral type; (B) distal onycholytic type; (C) hyperkeratotic type.

white or yellowish discoloration that overtakes the lunula (Fig. 21.5a & b). It then spreads to involve the whole nail plate very rapidly.

Secondary PSO is much more common than the primary variety, and chronic paronychia is usually the predisposing factor. In chronic paronychia mixed flora of microorganisms can

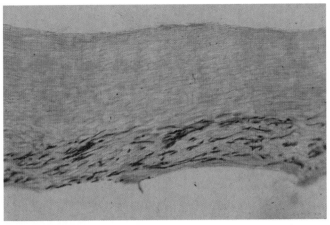

Figure 21.3. Deep invasion of the nail plate. Fungi are oriented in parallel arrays (PAS stain).

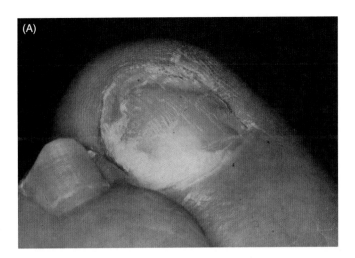

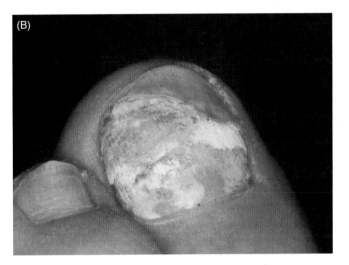

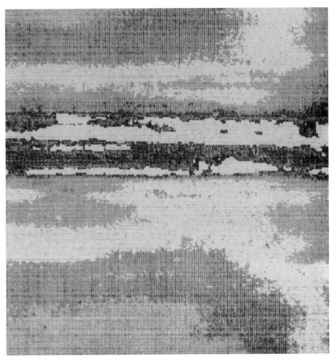

Figure 21.4. Streaky pocket of fungi (black) inside a nail plate as revealed by image analysis of a histological section.

Figure 21.5. A&B. Proximal subungual onychomycosis. (A) Native aspect of the nail; (B) Aspect of the nail involvement after scraping the upper portion of the nail plate. The distinction between this PSO type and a "deep white superficial onychomycosis" is difficult to establish.

be isolated from the nailfold area. *Candida* species, especially *Candida albicans* and *Candida parapsilosis*, are most consistently found. They are also likely to be the main pathogens. In secondary PSO, the nail plate can be affected centrally or at one or both lateral edges. The resulting dystrophy then gradually spreads up the nail. Apart from the cosmetic appearances, the nail bed is often painful, and sometimes pus can be expressed by applying pressure to the proximal nailfold.

PSO caused by *Aspergillus* spp., *Fusarium* spp. and *Scopulariopsis brevicaulis* are typically associated with marked, painful paronychia. Some patients complain of inflammatory flares with purulent discharge, especially when *Aspergillus* is the cause.

White or Black Superficial Onychomycosis

White superficial onychomycosis (WSO) and black superficial onychomycosis (BSO) affect the dorsal surface of the nail plate. The common type of WSO is usually caused by *T. interdigitale* that possesses keratolytic enzymes able to metabolize the hard keratin of the superficial nail plate (Fig. 21.6). Clinically, the nail shows one or more small white opaque chalky spots that can easily be scraped off. They may coalesce gradually to cover the whole nail plate.

In HIV-infected patients, WSO is usually due to *T. rubrum*. In these patients, it is not only seen in the toenails but also in the fingernails. Clinically, the affected nails appears diffusely opaque and white, with leukonychia often reaching the proximal portion of the nail. A similar clinical picture of "deep WSO" is seen in children who present with infections due to *T. rubrum* and nondermatophyte molds.

The most common species of nondermatophyte molds that are able to invade the superficial nail plate include *Fusarium* spp.,

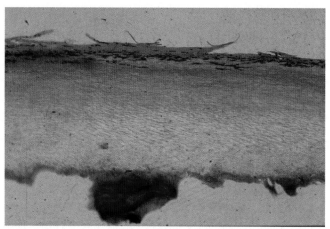

Figure 21.6. White superficial onychomycosis with fungal cells confined to the upper portion of the nail plate.

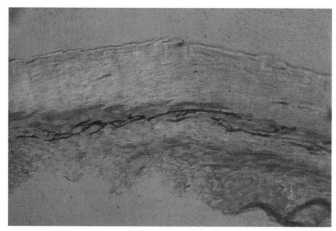

Figure 21.7. Midplate onychomycosis with a parallel pattern of fungal infiltration.

Aspergillus spp., and *Acremonium* spp. Mold WSO usually affects a single toenail (mainly the big toe). In some instances, WSO is complicated by a deeper pattern of nail invasion. This diffuse and deep nail plate involvement makes it difficult to distinguish a "deep WSO" from PSO progressing superficially. As seen in the other types of onychomycosis due to nondermatophyte molds, paronychia may be associated. However, it usually presents without a pustular discharge.

The uncommon "WSO zebra type" (WSOZ), or superficial white transverse onychomycosis is characterized by alternating transversal bands of white and native nail colors. This clinical presentation is probably due to a primary paroxysmal alteration in the structure of the dorsal aspects of the nail plate. The focal transversal defect in keratinization allows *T. rubrum* invasion at these places.

In rare instances, *Scytalydium dimidiatum* causes BSO with superficial black patches on the nail plate.

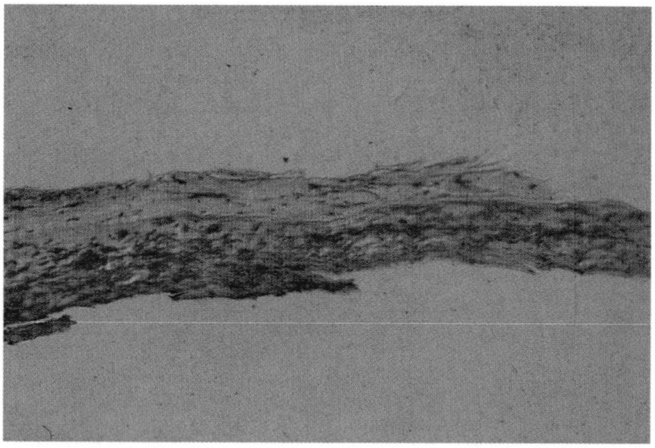

Midplate onychomycosis

In midplate onychomycosis (MPO), also called endonyx onychomycosis, fungi invade the nail via the free margin of the nail-plate. Instead of infecting the nail bed, the fungus penetrates the mid part of the nail plate where it remains confined (Fig. 21.7). This rare type of onychomycosis is predominantly caused by *Trichophyton soudanense* and *Trichophyton violaceum*. In midplate onychomycosis the nail plate appears diffusely opaque and white in the absence of onycholysis and subungual hyperkeratosis. Plantar infection can also be associated.

Total Dystrophic Onychomycosis

Total dystrophic onychomycosis (TDO) rarely occurs as a primary condition. Most commonly, it represents the endpoint of severely evolving DSO, PSO, "deep" WSO, and MPO. TDO occurs when the entire nail plate and nail bed are invaded and dissociated from the fungal pathogen (Fig. 21.8). Eventually, the nail crumbles away, leaving a hyperkeratotic bed. The common acquired TDO type is the expression of a dermatophyte infection.

By contrast, the rare primary type of TDO is usually due to *Candida*, and typically affects immunocompromised patients, such as those suffering from chronic mucocutaneous candidiasis,

Figure 21.8. Total dystrophic onychomycosis with fungi present at all levels of the nail plate.

iatrogenic immunosuppression, or HIV infection. In the chronic mucocutaneous type, TDO is associated with paronychia of the proximal nailfold, and it involves the nail matrix, the nail bed, and the hyponychium. The nail bed is hyperkeratotic and the nail plate is considerably thickened and dystrophic in TDO. Several nails are generally affected, including both fingernails and toenails. In these patients, oral candidiasis is often associated.

In HIV-positive patients and iatrogenic immunocompromised individuals the clinical presentation of *Candida* onychomycosis is less severe, and only one or a few fingernails are affected.

Candida albicans is frequently isolated from the subungual area of onycholytic nails and from the proximal nailfold in chronic paronychia. In both of these conditions, however, *Candida* colonization may not represent true infection.

COMBINED VARIANTS OF ONYCHOMYCOSIS

The histological examination of onychomycoses discloses combined variants of onychomycosis associating different patterns

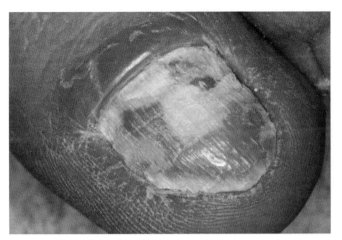

Figure 21.9. Combined variant of onychomycosis.

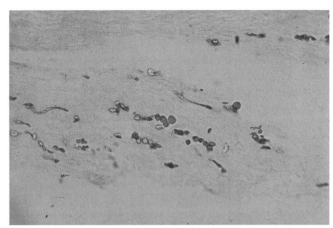

Figure 21.11. Mixed type onychomycosis due to a dermatophyte (hyphae) and large spores of *Scopulariopsis brevicaulis*.

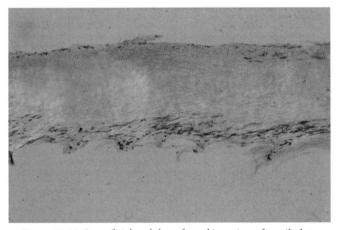

Figure 21.10. Superficial and deep fungal invasion of a nail plate.

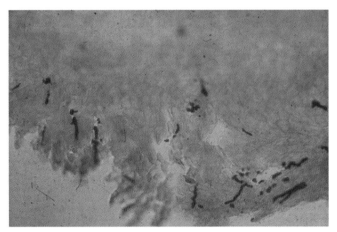

Figure 21.12. Fungal conidia and small hyphae trapped in a nail plate and surviving after antifungal treatment.

of fungal invasions. PSO, WSO, deep WSO, and MPO can be variably associated in any given nail (Figs. 21.9 and 21.10). These combined patterns of fungal invasion should not be confused with mixed onychomycosis, which indicates the presence of differing species of fungi in a single nail (Fig. 21.11).

ONYCHOMYCOSIS RELAPSE

Onychomycosis is a challenging infection to treat, with treatment failures and relapses being very common occurrences. The recurrent onychomycosis clinically is not always the same as in the primary phase of the disease. The sites of early recurrence can be inside the nail plate where fungal conidia have survived the antifungal treatment (Fig. 21.12). In other instances, sites of recurrence correspond to a site of recontamination from shoes, fomites, or other environmental structures. In the latter instance, fungal propagules are found inside cracks in the nail (Fig. 21.13). A sporodochium can develop in rare instances.

PITFALLS AND MYTHS

Clinical confusion between noninfectious onychodystrophies and infections of the nail unit is the main pitfall. Another

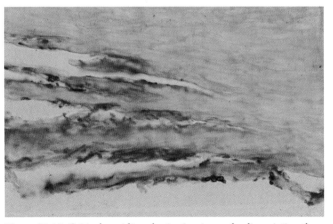

Figure 21.13. Critical conidia colonization in cracks dissociating the distal edge of a nail plate.

important pitfall deals with the identification of the causative fungus in onychomycosis. Retrieving a fungus at culture does not mean that it is a pathogen. A myth concerns the extrapolation that in vitro antimicrobial testing correlates with clinical diseases (such as psoriasis, lichen planus and eczema).

CONCLUSION

The nail unit can be infected by a variety of microorganisms. The unique anatomy of the nail is responsible for specific patterns of microbial colonization and infection. All conditions merit medical attention because each diagnosis is different, and merits a specific treatment. In these disorders, clinical assessment must be combined with culture and histomycology to obtain the correct diagnosis.

SUGGESTED READINGS

Arrese JE, Piérard-Franchimont C, Piérard GE. Fatal hyalohyphomycosis following Fusarium onychomycosis in an immuno-compromised patient. *Am J Dermatopathol* 1996;18:196–198.

Arrese JE, Piérard-Franchimont C, Piérard GE. Facing up to the diagnostic uncertainty and management of onychomycoses. *Int J Dermatol* 1999;38: 1–6.

Arrese JE, Piérard GE. Treatment failures and relapses in onychomycosis: a stubborn clinical problem. *Dermatology* 2003;207: 255–260.

Baran R, hay R, Perrin C. Superficial white onychomycosis revisited. *J Eur Acad Dermatol Vener* 2004;18:569–571.

Effendy I, Lecha M, Feuilhade de Chauvin M, Di Chiacchio N, Baran R. Epidemiology and clinical classification of onychomycosis. *J Eur Acad Dermatol Vener* 2005;19:S8-S12.

Ghannoum MA, Hajjeh RA, Scher R, et al. A large-scale North American study of fungal isolates from nails: the frequency of onychomycosis, fungal distribution, and antifungal susceptibility patterns. *J Am Acad Dermatol* 2000;43:641–648.

Gupta AK, Jain HC, Lynde CW, et al. Prevalence and epidemiology of onychomycosis in patients visiting physicians's offices: a multicenter Canadian survey of 15,000 patients. *J Am Acad Dermatol* 2000;43:244–248.

Gupta AK, Lynch LE. Onychomycosis: review of recurrence rates, poor prognostic factors, and strategies to prevent disease recurrence. *Cutis* 2004;74:S10–S15.

Gupta AK, Ricci MJ. Diagnosing onychomycosis. *Dermatol Clin* 2006;24: 365–369.

Haneke E. Surgical anatomy of the nail apparatus. *Dermatol Clin* 2006;24: 291–296.

Piérard GE, Arrese JE, Pierre S, Bertrand C, Corcuff P, Lévêque JL, Piérard-Franchimont C. Diagnostic microscopique des onychomycoses. *Ann Dermatol Venereol* 1994;121:25–29.

Piérard GE, Arrese JE, De Doncker P, et al. Present and potential diagnostic techniques in onychomycosis. *J Am Acad Dermatol* 1996;4:273–277.

Piérard GE, Piérard-Franchimont C, Quatresooz P. Fungal thigmotropism in onychomycosis and in a clear hydrogel pad model. *Dermatology*, in press.

Piérard GE, Quatresooz P, Arrese JE. Spottlight on nail histomycology. *Dermatol Clin* 2006;24: 371–374.

Piérard GE. Spores, sporodochia and fomites in onychomycosis. *Dermatology* 2006;213:169–172.

Scher RK, Baran R. Onychomycosis in clinical practice: factors contributing to recurrence. *Br J Dermatol* 2003;149:S5–S9.

Weinberg JM, Koestenblatt EK, Tutrone WD, Tishler HR, Najarian L. Comparison of diagnostic methods in the evaluation of onychomycosis. *J Am Acad Dermatol* 2003;49:103–107.

INFECTIONS OF THE MUCOUS MEMBRANES

Julia S. Lehman, Alison J. Bruce, and Roy S. Rogers, III

HISTORY

Infections involving the mucous membranes have been documented since antiquity. For example, Hippocrates (460–377 B.C.) referred to condyloma and leprosy in his writings. Genital ulcers were first proposed to be transmitted sexually in the 1100s A.D. by Roger of Palermo. Syphilis, one of the most historically significant mucosal infections, was initially described during the late fifteenth century. Understanding of the pathogenesis of and recognizing the organisms implicated in these diseases blossomed during the latter half of the 1800s with the development of new microbiology and histopathology techniques, as well as the introduction of the Germ Theory paradigm.

The clinical presentation of certain diseases has evolved over time as a consequence of changing cultural norms. For example, whereas HSV-1 infection historically was limited to the oral mucosa and HSV-2 to the genitalia, both viral strains are identified frequently in both anatomic locations in recent times due to changing sexual practices. Moreover, disease epidemiology is continually changing as a result of medical advances. For example, syphilis has become much less common in the developed world after the development of penicillin. However, the recent increase in iatrogenic immunosuppression and other acquired immunodeficiency states has given rise to a modified set of diseases and disease presentations involving the mucosa. Finally, the ease of world travel has removed geographic boundaries that previously limited the spread of many infections, making it necessary for all practitioners – particularly primary care physicians, dermatologists, dentists, infectious disease specialists, gynecologists, and urologists – to be familiar with the spectrum of infectious diseases affecting the mucosa.

Mucosal epithelium, the biologic lining of all orifices of the human body, is continuously exposed to potentially pathogenic endogenous and exogenous organisms. Multiple local regulatory factors contribute to defense against infection of the mucosal membranes. First, the stratified squamous epithelium of mucosal membranes offers a physical barrier against invading microbes. Additional protection is provided by epithelial keratinization at some sites, such as the gingiva, hard palate, and filiform papillae of the tongue. Susceptibility to infection increases when mucosal membranes are disrupted, as is seen with radiation or chemotherapy-related oral mucositis, for example. Second, mucosal surfaces are colonized by a myriad of native microorganisms that inhibit invading organisms. The normal flora regulates the growth of pathogenic organisms by providing competition for available nutrients, limiting the number of sites to which exotic organisms may adhere, and releasing antimicrobial substances (described below). When the normal pattern of flora is altered, as occurs with antibiotic or corticosteroid usage, mucosal membranes are rendered more vulnerable to infection. Third, in many sites, mucous membranes harbor cilia that clear pathogens mechanically. Patients with disturbed ciliary function, such as those with primary ciliary dyskinesis, for example, are more likely to develop certain infections. Fourth, salivary and vaginal secretions not only flush organisms but also alter regional pH and oxidation–reduction potential, thus selecting which organisms can thrive in the mucosal environment. For example, conditions causing xerostomia, such as Sjögren's disease, head and neck irradiation, and medication side effects, predispose the host to a higher incidence of oral infection. Fifth, mucous epithelial cells intrinsically produce antimicrobial peptides, such as defensins, histatins, and bacteriocins, which comprise part of the innate immune system and function as a chemical shield. Moreover, host epithelial cells secrete cytokines and other mediators that recruit and activate complement, cellular immunity, and humoral immunity. Thus, host defense of the mucous membranes is achieved by an intricate, multi-tiered system comprised of locally protective factors and selective activation of innate, cellular, and humoral immunity.

Although mucosal membranes line much of the gastrointestinal, respiratory, and genitourinary tracts, this chapter will focus on infections that cause disease in the oral cavity and lower genital tract. Diagnosis of mucosal membrane infections can be challenging, particularly as mucosal response to insult is often nonspecific. Optimally, therapeutic decisions are guided by an accurate diagnosis. In serious or systemic disease, however, treatment may need to be started empirically. Airway management is another important consideration in infections of the oropharyngeal mucosa. In addition to treating the underlying disease and predisposing factors, a variety of therapeutic modalities may be used to alleviate the symptoms of oral infection. For example, pain may be relieved with the use of topical therapies, such as topical viscous lidocaine, benzocaine-containing preparations (e.g. Anbesol, Orajel), or analgesic mouthwashes, such as diphenhydramine elixir. Systemic agents, such as nonsteroidal anti-inflammatory drugs, acetaminophen, and opioid medications, may be required to achieve adequate analgesia in select cases.

VIRAL INFECTIONS: DNA VIRUSES

Human herpesviruses

Human herpesvirus (HHV) is a double-stranded DNA virus with multiple serotypes that have been implicated in the development of mucosal disease in humans (Table 22.1). Pathogenesis

Table 22.1: Human Herpesviruses and Associated Disease or Syndrome Potentially Involving Mucous Membranes

Human Herpesvirus Serotype	Virus Name	Associated Disease or Syndrome Potentially Affecting Mucous Membranes
1	Herpes simplex virus type 1	*Primary disease:* Acute herpetic gingivostomatitis; ulcerative pharyngotonsillitis; mononucleosis-like syndrome *Recurrent:* Herpes labialis; recurrent HSV stomatitis
2	Herpes simplex virus type 2	*Primary disease:* Genital herpes *Recurrent:* Genital herpes
3	Varicella-zoster virus	*Primary:* Varicella (*chicken pox*) *Recurrent:* Herpes zoster (*shingles*); Ramsay Hunt Syndrome
4	Epstein-Barr virus	Mononucleosis (*glandular fever*); oral hairy leukoplakia; Burkitt lymphoma; nasopharyngeal lymphoma; posttransplantation lymphoproliferative disorder
5	Cytomegalovirus virus	Mononucleosis (*glandular fever*)
6	Roseola virus	Exanthema subitum (*roseola infantum*)
7	Human herpesvirus 7	Unclear (possible link to *roseola infantum*)
8	Human herpesvirus 8	Kaposi sarcoma

results from virus-mediated cytopathic change and host immune-mediated cell damage.

Human herpesvirus 1 and human herpesvirus 2

Herpes simplex virus (HSV)-1 and HSV-2 cause primary and recurrent mucosal lesions. Seropositivity for HSV-1 ranges from 58% to 90%, while seropositivity for HSV-2 is less frequent in the general population. HSV-1 is usually isolated from oral herpes lesions, whereas HSV-2 is found more commonly in genital herpes lesions. Both serotypes may be responsible for either oral or genital disease, however. HSV is transmitted to oral, nasal, genital, or conjunctival mucosa via contact with an infected individual. Infection can also result from autoinoculation, dental work, and contact with fomites. Moreover, HSV can be transmitted vertically from mother to newborn via passage through an infected birth canal.

After primary infection, HSV travels to the sensory ganglion innervating the site of inoculation via retrograde intra-axonal transport. Following a latency period, HSV can undergo antegrade axonal transport, leading to recurrent infection. Recurrent infection can arise spontaneously or can be precipitated by emotional stress, fatigue, fracture of the facial bones, neurosurgical axonal injury, or ultraviolet light exposure. Recurrent infection is seen in 40% of patients infected with HSV-1 but is less common with HSV-2 infection.

CLINICAL PRESENTATION

Primary HSV infection often occurs during childhood and is asymptomatic or unrecognized in the vast majority of infected patients. When symptomatic in children, primary oral HSV infection most frequently appears as painful, fragile vesicles on the gingiva and other oral surfaces (acute herpetic gingivostomatitis). In adolescents, primary HSV infection often presents as ulcerative pharyngotonsillitis. In adults, primary oral HSV infection results in painful vesicles and erosions of the keratinized and nonkeratinized oral mucosa. Pharyngitis, tonsillitis, dysphagia and associated dehydration, or a mononucleosis-like syndrome may accompany oral herpetic lesions. Differential diagnosis of primary oral HSV infection is broad and includes hand-foot-and-mouth disease, herpangina, infectious

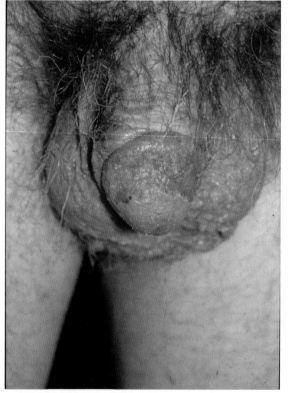

Figure 22.1. Primary herpes simplex virus infection of the genitalia.

mononucleosis, streptococcal stomatitis, acute necrotizing ulcerative gingivitis, and immunobullous diseases, such as pemphigus vulgaris and paraneoplastic pemphigus.

Primary genital HSV infection is associated with vesicles and ulcers on the external genitalia (i.e., labia majora, labia minora, vaginal vestibule, and introitus in women, and the glans penis, prepuce, shaft of the penis, and scrotum in men) (Fig. 22.1). Tender regional lymphadenopathy may accompany mucosal findings. Because partial immunity develops during primary infection, recurrent HSV is not usually associated

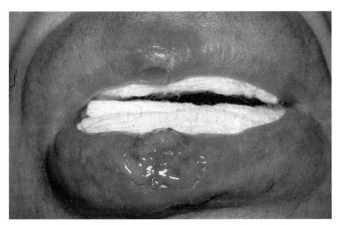

Figure 22.2. Herpes labialis (*herpes simplex virus*).

with significant constitutional symptoms. Urethritis and associated dysuria or urinary retention may occur in either sex but are more commonly seen in women. Herpetic proctitis can also result from receptive anal intercourse with an infected individual. The differential diagnosis of HSV infection of the genitalia includes chancroid, lymphogranuloma venereum, granuloma inguinale, Behçet's disease, and immunobullous disorders.

Lesions of primary herpes simplex develop 5 to 10 days following exposure, persist for 10 to 14 days, and heal without scarring. Despite the absence of signs or symptoms of HSV infection, asymptomatic carriers are contagious, because they shed infectious viral particles in mucosal secretions.

In most patients, recurrent HSV presents initially with a prodrome of tingling, burning, or itching sensation. Recurrent oral herpes arises commonly at the cutaneous lip and vermilion border (herpes labialis; Fig. 22.2) but only rarely presents intraorally. Unlike lesions of primary oral herpes, those of recurrent oral herpes lesions are typically confined to the keratinized mucosa. In the immunocompetent host, recurrences occur up to 3 to 4 times each year and last 7 to 10 days. In immunocompromised patients, however, recurrences are more frequent, last for a longer period, and may disseminate widely. Recurrent intraoral HSV infection is frequently confused with recurrent aphthous stomatitis. The clinical features of the two conditions differ in several respects, however. Specifically, lesions of recurrent intraoral HSV infection appear as grouped, punched-out ulcers found exclusively on keratinized mucosa and are reasonably mild in intensity. The lesions of recurrent aphthous stomatitis, however, are found on nonkeratinized mucosa, and although they may appear similar morphologically to those of recurrent intraoral HSV infection, they often are solitary and can be exquisitely tender.

Epidemiologic and molecular studies have consistently demonstrated an association between HSV seropositivity and erythema multiforme (EM), with approximately 36% to 75% of patients with EM having evidence of previous infection with HSV. EM is thought to arise as a result of an exuberant host cytopathic response to circulating immune complexes. EM is characterized by the appearance of targetoid, erythematous lesions with a dusky center. Mucosal manifestations of EM are present in 40% of cases and present as a desquamative stomatitis. Frequently involved sites include the buccal mucosa, palate, and lips. Other nonmucosal sequelae of HSV

infection include aseptic meningitis, encephalitis, ganglionitis, and myelitis.

DIAGNOSIS

Primary and recurrent HSV infections are usually diagnosed clinically, based on the appearance of characteristic lesions. The gold standard for detection of all herpesviruses is culture, which is most useful early in the disease course during the replicative phase. Once the lesion has crusted over or regressed, however, viral culture becomes less sensitive because of reduced viral shedding. Histopathology with hematoxylin and eosin stain shows ballooning and reticular epidermal degeneration with characteristic multinucleated keratinocytes. These findings are nonspecific, as they are also seen with varicella-zoster virus infection. Tzanck smear is a rapid, inexpensive test that demonstrates multinucleated giant cells with viral inclusions. Even with optimal technique, however, test sensitivity is about 50% to 65% and cannot differentiate among various human herpesviruses.

Polymerase chain reaction for the detection of HSV DNA is being used increasingly because of its high sensitivity. However, it is significantly more costly than traditional diagnostic modalities. Also, detection of serum antibodies to HSV-1 and HSV-2 with direct immunofluorescence testing or in situ hybridization is another diagnostic strategy but may be insensitive in early disease.

TREATMENT

In immunocompetent hosts, initial management of HSV infection is supportive. As intraoral herpetic infection can lead to dysphagia, adequate oral intake of fluids should be stressed. Symptomatic relief can be achieved with mouth rinses containing topical anesthetic agents, such as viscous lidocaine, benzocaine preparations, dental pastes, or a diphenhydramine elixir with Maalox (1:1). Salicylates, nonsteroidal anti-inflammatory drugs, and acetaminophen can be used for additional analgesia. In children, however, salicylates should be avoided because of the potential to develop Reye's syndrome. Secondary bacterial infections, which are uncommon, should be treated with appropriate antibiotics.

When antiviral therapy is indicated in primary HSV infection, acyclovir is the drug of choice. Valacyclovir may be preferred for its more convenient dosing schedule, however. A randomized controlled trial demonstrated efficacy of oral acyclovir in childhood acute herpetic gingivostomatitis. Topical acyclovir is not particularly effective, likely because of poor intraoral drug absorption. In addition, this medication may contribute to antiviral resistance.

For recurrent herpes simplex, oral antiviral therapy has been shown to be effective as preventive and suppressive therapy in immunocompetent patients. Acyclovir, valacyclovir, or famciclovir may be used. Topical use of sunscreen on the lips may prevent herpes labialis by blocking ultraviolet light, and docosanol 10% cream (Abreva) and topical penciclovir (Denavir) have been shown to decrease duration of symptoms in herpes labialis.

In immunocompromised hosts, disease can be severe or disseminated and is more likely to be associated with complications. Therefore, aggressive antiviral therapy is recommended. Oral acyclovir can be used as suppressive therapy for HSV infection. Though not approved by the U.S. Food and Drug Administration (FDA) for this indication, famciclovir is as effective as high-dose acyclovir in the treatment of recurrent herpes labialis in patients with HIV infection. Intravenous foscarnet may be used in acyclovir-resistant HSV infection.

Human herpesvirus 3 (varicella-zoster virus)

CLINICAL PRESENTATION

Varicella infection can cause painful, shallow vesicles and ulcerations on the palate, buccal mucosa, and pharyngeal mucosa. These oral lesions are accompanied by the characteristically pruritic eruption of varicella, as well as fever, malaise, and myalgias. Incubation period is usually 14 to 16 days. Although generally self-limited in children younger than 10 years, primary varicella infection in adolescents, adults, and immunocompromised individuals can be severe. Complications include secondary bacterial infection, otitis media, pneumonia, arthritis, uveitis, Reye's syndrome (particularly with administration of salicylates in children), nephritis, and encephalitis. Congenital varicella syndrome (CVS), acquired during the first half of pregnancy, is rare, because most women of childbearing age have viral immunity.

Recurrent VZV infection (herpes zoster, *shingles*) is heralded by the onset of pain, tingling, or pruritus in a dermatomal distribution. One to 2 days later, clustered herpetic lesions arise in a unilateral dermatomal segment. Oral lesions develop when the second and third divisions of the trigeminal nerve are involved and typically affect the palate, buccal mucosa, tongue, and oropharynx. Usually, lesions resolve within 2 to 3 weeks but can impart residual chronic pain, known as postherpetic neuralgia. Other oral complications are rare but include tooth exfoliation and mandibular necrosis. Ramsay Hunt Syndrome (herpes zoster of cranial nerves VII and VIII) may involve herpetic lesions on the anterior two-thirds of the tongue, soft palate, external auditory canal, and pinna. Associated symptoms include facial palsy, nystagmus, tinnitus, otalgia, ageusia, vertigo, and hearing loss. Other diseases that mimic oral VZV infection or herpes zoster include recurrent aphthous stomatitis, acute herpetic gingivostomatitis, erythema multiforme, oral pemphigoid, and pemphigus vulgaris. Unilaterality and dermatomal distribution of lesions may be helpful in distinguishing herpes zoster from other conditions.

DIAGNOSIS

Both primary and recurrent VZV infection can be diagnosed based on clinical findings alone. When the diagnosis is in question, VZV can be differentiated from HSV by culture, PCR, direct immunofluorescence, or *in situ* hybridization. Culture and PCR are insensitive for the presence of varicella-zoster virus, however, because the organism does not persist in the oropharynx following incubation. As with HSV infection, histopathology of VZV-infected tissue demonstrates ballooning epidermal degeneration and multinucleated giant cells. Tzanck smear is 75% to 80% sensitive in herpes zoster.

TREATMENT

Topical and systemic analgesics are used for symptomatic relief. Antiviral therapy is used rarely for primary varicella in otherwise healthy children, as the disease course is generally uncomplicated. Also, antiviral therapy is discouraged because of concerns regarding the development of resistant viral strains and the cost incurred with therapy. In patients older than 13 years and immunocompromised individuals, however, oral acyclovir is indicated because it decreases duration and severity of the disease.

In the treatment of herpes zoster, narcotic analgesics are often necessary for pain management. Antiviral drugs of choice are oral acyclovir or valacyclovir, with the greatest efficacy achieved when started early in disease course. Antiviral therapy can shorten disease duration but has not been shown to prevent postherpetic neuralgia. For disseminated or severe local disease, systemic acyclovir, famciclovir, and valacyclovir have similar efficacy and safety profiles. In acyclovir-resistant herpes zoster, foscarnet or cidofovir are recommended, although these are both associated with significant toxicity.

Previously a common disease of childhood, varicella is becoming much less common since the development and distribution of an effective vaccine. Varivax vaccine, the live, attenuated Oka/Merck vaccine, is FDA-approved for children older than 12 months and immunocompromised persons. It is thought to be 70% to 90% effective in preventing infection, and those patients who do develop varicella following vaccination generally have a milder course. The ProQuad vaccine, a new quadrivalent vaccine for measles, mumps, rubella, and varicella, has similar efficacy to the separate administration of MMR and Varivax vaccines. When used in adults aged 60 or older, the varicella vaccination (Zostavax) is effective in reducing the incidence of herpes zoster and postherpetic neuralgia.

Human herpesvirus 4 (Epstein-Barr virus)

Epstein-Barr virus (EBV) is a ubiquitous organism that is transmitted via oral contact.

CLINICAL PRESENTATION

Oral findings of EBV-related infectious mononucleosis include palatal petechiae, oropharyngeal ulceration, erythema of the posterior oropharynx, exudative tonsillitis, and, in severe cases, necrotizing gingivitis. These signs are accompanied by fever, profound malaise, and neck lymphadenopathy. A diffuse morbilliform exanthem develops in a minority of cases, particularly in children treated with amoxicillin for presumed or concurrent streptococcal pharyngitis. The incubation period ranges from 5 to 50 days. Differential diagnosis includes streptococcal pharyngitis, leukemia, syphilis, diphtheria, primary HIV infection, and drug reaction.

Oral hairy leukoplakia presents as an asymptomatic white patch or hyperkeratotic plaque on the lateral aspect of the tongue. It can also extend to the dorsal and ventral tongue, buccal mucosa, palate, and tonsils. While usually bilateral in distribution, lesions can also be unilateral. Hypertrophy of the surface contributes to the development of hair-like projections. Lesions of oral hairy leukoplakia are fixed and cannot be scraped away with a tongue depressor. Though intrinsically benign, oral hairy leukoplakia is only seen in the presence of underlying immunocompromise, as with HIV infection or renal transplantation. In patients with HIV infection, the presence of oral hairy leukoplakia portends a greater likelihood of developing *Pneumocystis jiroveci* (*P. carinii*) pneumonia.

EBV has been linked to a variety of different cancers, including Burkitt lymphoma, nasopharyngeal cancer, and post-transplantation lymphoproliferative disorder. In one series of immunosuppression-related oral lymphomas, EBV was present universally. Burkitt lymphoma, a form of non–Hodgkin's lymphoma, has endemic (African) and non-endemic (sporadic) forms. While EBV infection is strongly linked to endemic Burkitt lymphoma (particularly in African children with concurrent malarial infection), EBV infection is also identified in about 20% of nonendemic cases. Burkitt lymphoma is associated with pharyngitis, cervical lymphadenopathy, jaw masses, loosened teeth, and odontalgia. EBV-related nasopharyngeal cancer, a poorly differentiated anaplastic carcinoma, is seen predominantly in Southern China and Northern Africa. A case of posttransplantation EBV-related diffuse, large B-cell lymphoma initially presenting with an oral lesion has been described.

DIAGNOSIS

Diagnosis of EBV-related infectious mononucleosis is clinical but is supported by the presence of the virus-specific IgM heterophile antibody, detected by the monospot test. Test positivity occurs within 1 to 2 weeks of primary illness. Infectious mononucleosis is also associated with the presence of large numbers of atypical lymphocytes on differential cell count. Diagnosis may be confirmed by the presence of other serum viral antigens, such as those of the viral capsid and membrane.

Oral hairy leukoplakia is diagnosed when EBV is detected in biopsy specimens of typical oral lesions using *in situ* hybridization, Southern blotting, direct immunofluorescence testing, or electron microscopy. EBV-associated lymphomas are diagnosed by biopsy. The presence of EBV in association with lymphoma development is demonstrated with serologic tests or in situ hybridization.

TREATMENT

Infectious mononucleosis typically resolves spontaneously after approximately 4 weeks and is treated symptomatically. Bed rest and avoidance of activities that could predispose the patient to splenic rupture (e.g. contact sports) are recommended. Acyclovir has not been shown to be effective in limiting duration or severity of disease, although it reduces subclinical viral shedding. Although co-infection with *Streptococcus pyogenes* should be investigated and treated, amoxicillin or ampicillin should be avoided because of the risk of associated skin eruption.

Oral hairy leukoplakia responds to a 10- to 14-day course of high-dose acyclovir. Efficacy of topical 0.1% vitamin A acid and topical podophyllum resin in 25% solution has been reported. With all therapies, however, recurrence is common upon discontinuation of the medication if the underlying immunosuppression persists. In patients with HIV infection, lesions of hairy leukoplakia usually regress with antiretroviral therapy.

Burkitt lymphoma may respond initially to chemotherapy but usually recurs. Nasopharyngeal carcinoma is often diagnosed after it has metastasized. Treatment is irradiation, although prognosis is poor.

Human herpesvirus 5 (cytomegalovirus)

Although cytomegalovirus (CMV) is ubiquitous, it rarely causes illness in immunocompetent people. CMV is present in mucosal secretions and is transmitted via exposure to bodily fluids of an infected individual. Risk factors for illness from CMV infection include transplantation, iatrogenic immunosuppression, and concurrent HIV infection.

CLINICAL PRESENTATION

Oral manifestations of CMV are rare in immunocompetent hosts. Enlargement of the salivary glands with an accompanying mononucleosis-like syndrome may develop, although infection is commonly asymptomatic. In immunocompromised individuals, oral findings include oropharyngeal ulcerations, gingival hyperplasia, sialadenitis, and necrotizing gingivitis. Oral lesions may be accompanied by mild hepatitis, thrombocytopenia, or hemolytic anemia. In this patient population, CMV infection is associated with increased morbidity and mortality. The incubation period is approximately 4 to 8 weeks. Primary infection with or reactivation of CMV during the first two trimesters of pregnancy can confer significant teratogenicity to the developing fetus, including chorioretinitis, intracerebral calcifications, and hepatosplenomegaly. Differential diagnosis for oral CMV manifestations includes EBV-related mononucleosis, primary HIV infection, acute herpetic gingivostomatitis, recurrent aphthous stomatitis, mumps, and immunobullous disorders such as pemphigus vulgaris.

DIAGNOSIS

In otherwise healthy patients, diagnosis is usually based on clinical findings. In cases in which diagnosis must be established, enzyme-linked immunosorbent assay (ELISA) can be used to detect CMV IgM antibodies. Other diagnostic tests include culture with fibroblast media, in situ hybridization, or PCR. On histopathology, the presence of basophilic intranuclear inclusions and granular cytoplasmic inclusions ("owl eyes") is specific for CMV. CMV particles may also be seen on electron microscopy.

TREATMENT

In immunocompetent patients, treatment is limited to supportive measures. In immunocompromised patients, ganciclovir is the treatment of choice. Foscarnet should be reserved for resistant disease. Prolonged therapy is often required, as current antiviral therapies suppress but cannot cure viral disease. Although acyclovir is generally not effective against CMV, resolution of CMV-induced oral lesions with high-dose acyclovir has been reported. In bone marrow transplant recipients, CMV prophylaxis with ganciclovir or valganciclovir may be indicated.

Human herpesvirus 6

HHV-6 causes exanthem subitum (*roseola infantum*) in children and is transmitted via salivary secretions. HHV-6 infection is very common during the first 2 years of life, and almost all children are seropositive for HHV-6 by age 4. Following primary infection, the virus remains latent in salivary glands.

CLINICAL PRESENTATION

The first signs of exanthema subitum include high fever and malaise, followed by the eruption of erythematous macules on the soft palate and uvula (*Nagayama spots*). A generalized eruption of small, rose-colored macules on the chest, back, and abdomen follows. Lymphadenopathy, diarrhea, and cough may be associated. Complications are rare but include febrile seizures, pneumonitis, encephalitis, diarrhea, meningitis, hepatitis, and bone marrow failure. Co-infection of HHV-6 with HIV is synergistic and can accelerate cytopathic effects. The incubation period is approximately 7 to 10 days. Differential diagnosis of exanthema subitum includes measles, rubella, and drug eruption. Some molecular evidence implicates HHV-6 in the development of recurrent aphthous stomatitis, although this remains to be confirmed.

DIAGNOSIS

In otherwise healthy individuals, diagnosis is usually based on the presence of classic clinical findings. When the identity of the etiologic agent is required, immunofluorescence testing

Table 22.2: Mucosal Manifestations of Human Papillomavirus Infection with Commonly Associated HPV Serotypes

Disease	Typical Area of Mucosal Involvement	Most Commonly Associated HPV Serotypes
Squamous papilloma	Palatine, buccal, gingival, or labial mucosa	6, 11
Oral verruca vulgaris	Palatine, buccal, gingival, or labial mucosa	2, 4, 6, 11, 16
Condyloma acuminatum	Anogenital mucosa	6, 10, 11, 16, 18, 33
Focal epithelial hyperplasia	Buccal mucosa; lower lip	11, 13, 32
Cervical intraepithelial neoplasia; cervical cancer	Uterine cervix	16, 18

demonstrates the presence of HHV-6 IgM antibodies or a fourfold increase in IgG with serial testing in acute disease. A rapid shell vial assay is sensitive and specific for HHV-6. While specific, viral culture is insensitive and impractical in clinical practice.

TREATMENT

As exanthema subitum is generally benign and self-limited, treatment is supportive. In disease complicated by CNS involvement, pneumonia, or hepatitis, ganciclovir and foscarnet are used but have not been proven effective.

Human herpesvirus 7

First isolated from salivary secretions in 1989, HHV-7 has not been definitively linked to disease. Some evidence links HHV-7 to an exanthem subitum-like syndrome, although this has not been confirmed.

Human herpesvirus 8

HHV-8 is a B-cell lymphotropic human herpesvirus that, unlike other human herpesviruses, is not present ubiquitously in the general population. However, HHV-8 is associated with virtually all lesions of Kaposi sarcoma (KS), a low-grade, multicentric vascular neoplasm. The mechanism of pathogenesis has not been well established, although HHV-8 infection has been associated with changes in the host response to cytokines and angiogenesis. The development of KS in HHV-8-positive individuals is more frequent in men than in women, thus suggesting a possible role of hormones in the development of KS. HHV-8 has also been associated with multiple myeloma, Waldenström's macroglobulinemia, angiolymphoid hyperplasia with eosinophilia, multicentric Castleman's disease and primary effusion lymphoma, a condition characterized by malignant effusions without an identifiable contiguous solid tumor mass.

CLINICAL PRESENTATION

Initial lesions of KS are usually found intraorally and appear as asymptomatic erythematous, violaceous or blue macules, patches, plaques, ulcers, or nodules. In individuals with darker skin, lesions may appear brown or black. The hard palate, soft palate, tongue, and gingiva are involved frequently. In a minority of cases, intraoral KS is associated with pain, bleeding, or ulceration. Differential diagnosis includes ecchymosis, hemangioma, lymphangioma, granular cell tumor, and plaques of discoid lupus erythematosus.

DIAGNOSIS

Diagnosis can be confirmed by typical findings on biopsy. Early lesions are characterized by the presence of atypical vascular channels and lymphocytes, while later lesions demonstrate numerous mitotic figures, erythrocytes, eosinophilic bodies, and a prominent spindle cell component. PCR or serologic testing can also identify evidence of an HHV-8 infection. An HIV test should be performed, and a chest radiograph should be obtained to screen for pulmonary KS.

TREATMENT

The following treatments for isolated lesions of Kaposi sarcoma have been reported to be efficacous: surgical excision, cryotherapy, injection of a sclerosing agent, intralesional interferon, intralesional vinblastine, topical retinoids, and local radiotherapy. For widespread or aggressive disease, systemic agents, such as liposomal anthracyclines, paclitaxel, antiangiogenic medications, and oral retinoids, may be indicated. Treatment of underlying immunosuppression is also necessary to prevent recurrence.

Human papillomavirus

Human papillomavirus (HPV) is a small, double-stranded DNA virus and has been associated with several mucosal manifestations, including squamous papilloma, oral verruca vulgaris, condyloma acuminatum, focal epithelial hyperplasia, cervical dysplasia and cancer (Table 22.2).

CLINICAL PRESENTATION

Commonly described as oral warts, squamous papillomas (associated with HPV types 6 and 11) and oral verruca vulgaris (associated with HPV types 2, 4, 6, 11, and 16) are soft, pink, exophytic papules that arise on the lips, tongue, hard and soft palates, and uvula. Papillomas are pedunculated and persistent, whereas verrucae are sessile and more likely to resolve spontaneously. Although usually painless, lesions may be tender at the base.

Condyloma acuminatum (linked to HPV types 6, 10, 11, 16, 18, and 33) appears as multiple soft, sessile, pink or grey papules on the anogenital mucosa (Fig. 22.3). Rarely, palatal and tongue lesions arise from autoinoculation, hematogenous spread, or sexual transmission. Oral lesions are small, white, exophytic papules, though they can coalesce to form nodules.

Focal epithelial hyperplasia (Heck disease) is seen most commonly in native Americans, residents of Greenland, Alaska, South America, and in patients with HIV infection. This disease presents with multiple tender, pink, soft papules commonly arising on the lower lip and buccal mucosa. HPV types 11, 13 and 32 have been implicated.

Some evidence links oral HPV infection with an increased risk for oral squamous cell carcinoma. Differential diagnosis for oral HPV lesions includes traumatic fibromas, oral

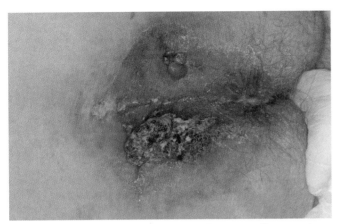

Figure 22.3. Condyloma acuminatum (*human papillomavirus*).

lesions of Cowden disease, fibrous hyperplasia, verruciform xanthoma, focal dermal hypoplasia syndrome, and squamous cell carcinoma.

In women, genital infection with high-risk HPV serotypes (e.g., 16 and 18) confers a higher chance for the development of squamous intraepithelial lesions of the cervix and, ultimately, cervical cancer.

DIAGNOSIS

Diagnosis of oral infection by HPV is generally made on the basis of clinical findings and is confirmed when lesions turn white with the application of acetic acid (aceto-whitening). Papanicolaou-stained (Pap) smear is used to screen for high-risk HPV infection of the cervix. When Pap smear results are abnormal, colposcopy and colposcopy-guided biopsy are performed. Excisional biopsy may be required in some cases, and HPV serotype can be determined with PCR or in situ hybridization.

TREATMENT

As with cutaneous verrucae, oral HPV lesions can resolve spontaneously or may require ablative therapy with podophyllum, topical 5-fluorouracil, cryotherapy, laser therapy, electrodessication, or excision. Therapeutic interventions are most effective if the entire base of the lesion is destroyed, although recurrences are common regardless of the therapeutic modality used. To avoid autoinoculation, all lesions should be targeted in a treated patient. Patients with periungual HPV lesions should be counseled to avoid nail biting.

In focal epithelial hyperplasia, topical interferon-β and carbon dioxide laser have been used, although lesions may resolve spontaneously.

For primary prevention of cervical dysplasia and cancer, highly effective recombinant HPV vaccines containing virus-like particles from high-risk HPV genotypes have been developed. The American Cancer Society recommends routine vaccination among all females between the ages of 11 and 12 and all females between the ages of 13 and 18 who have not previously received all three doses of the vaccination. For secondary prevention, the American Cancer Society recommends regular cervical cancer screening for vaccinated and unvaccinated women starting 3 years after onset of vaginal intercourse and no later than age 21. Treatment of cervical intraepithelial neoplasms and cervical cancer is based on particular histopathologic findings and may involve surgical resection, chemotherapy, or radiotherapy.

Parvovirus B19

A member of the *Parvoviridae* family, parvovirus B19 is a single-stranded DNA virus that is transmitted via inhalation of aerosolized respiratory droplets or via receipt of contaminated blood products. Frequently, parvovirus B19 infection is asymptomatic. However, it may be associated with several syndromes, including erythema infectiosum (*slapped cheek syndrome; Fifth Disease*), Henoch-Schönlein purpura, vasculitis, glomerulonephritis, aplastic crisis, myocarditis, arthritis, and papular-purpuric "gloves and socks" syndrome. When transmitted vertically from mother to developing fetus, hydrops fetalis may result.

CLINICAL PRESENTATION

In the majority of parvovirus B19-associated syndromes, mucosal findings are absent. However, oral lesions may develop in the rare condition, papular-purpuric "gloves and socks" syndrome. These are usually multiple painful, erythematous macules, erosions, or papules on the hard palate. Intraoral petechiae may also be seen. Rarely, parvovirus B19 infection has been associated with erythema multiforme and erythema nodosum.

DIAGNOSIS

Diagnosis is usually based on the presence of classic clinical findings. PCR is a useful tool in detecting parvovirus B19 DNA. ELISA testing can demonstrate IgM antibodies in acute infection.

THERAPY

Mucosal involvement is self-limited, so supportive measures are adequate. No specific antiviral therapy is currently available for treatment of parvovirus B19. Blood and platelet transfusions and intravenous immunoglobulin (IVIG) may be required for hematologic complications.

Molluscum contagiosum

In children, MC lesions in the anogenital region may be a sign of sexual abuse or may occur from autoinoculation.

CLINICAL PRESENTATION

Typically a cutaneous pathogen, it rarely causes conjunctival or oral disease (Fig. 22.4).

RNA Viruses

RNA viral syndromes with frequently implicated viruses and associated mucosal findings are listed in Table 22.3.

Hand-foot-and-mouth disease

Hand-foot-and-mouth disease is caused by coxsackieviruses such as coxsackievirus A16 or less commonly, A4, A5, A9, and A10. Other enteroviruses, such as enterovirus 71, have also been implicated. Transmitted via saliva and feces, hand-foot-and-mouth disease is highly contagious and occurs in outbreaks among children and young adults.

CLINICAL PRESENTATION

Oral lesions of hand-foot-and-mouth disease include painful, fragile vesicles, erosions, or ulcerations of the palate, buccal mucosa, or tongue (Fig. 22.5). Lesions typically arise after 1 to 2 days of flu-like symptoms. Oral lesions are accompanied or followed by the development of papules, vesicles, or ulcers on the dorsal and ventral surfaces of the hands and feet. Complications

Table 22.3: RNA Viral Syndromes with Frequently Implicated Viruses and Associated Mucosal Findings

Syndrome	Most Commonly Implicated Viruses	Mucosal Findings
Hand-foot-and-mouth disease	Coxsackieviruses (A16) Enteroviruses (71)	Vesicles, erosions, ulcerations on the palate, buccal mucosa, and tongue
Herpangina	Coxsackieviruses (group A, types 1–6, 8, 10, and 22; group B) Echovirus	Small vesicles with an erythematous base on the soft palate and posterior oropharynx
Measles	Paramyxovirus	Small erythematous macules with white necrotic core (*Koplik spots*)
Mumps	Paramyxovirus	Swelling of the parotid, submandibular, submental salivary glands; edema at the opening of Stensen's duct
Rubella	Togavirus	Petechiae and pinpoint erythematous macules (*Forschheimer spots*) on the palate and uvula

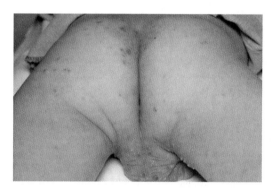
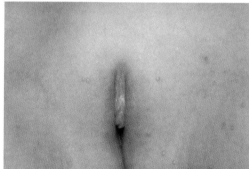

Figure 22.4. Molluscum contagiosum.

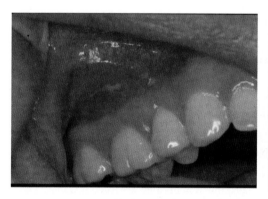
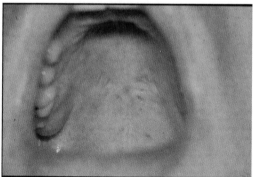

Figure 22.5. Oral manifestations of hand-foot-and-mouth disease.

are rare but may include meningitis, encephalitis, myocarditis, or pneumonia. The incubation period is 3 to 5 days, and clinical disease persists for 5 to 10 days. Differential diagnosis includes herpangina, erythema multiforme, syphilis, Epstein-Barr virus infection, cytomegalovirus infection, varicella, acute herpetic gingivostomatitis, and recurrent aphthous stomatitis. Infection during pregnancy may lead to spontaneous abortion or intrauterine growth retardation.

DIAGNOSIS

Diagnosis is made clinically. In atypical cases, serologic testing may be used. Moreover, virus can be cultured from the saliva or feces, although this is rarely followed in clinical practice.

TREATMENT

As hand-foot-and-mouth disease is self-limited, symptomatic treatment is usually adequate. In complicated cases, oral acyclovir may have some efficacy. Low-level laser therapy may shorten duration of oral lesions.

Herpangina

Herpangina is caused by coxsackievirus group A, types 1–6, 8, 10, and 22 and, less commonly, by coxsackievirus group B and echovirus. Disease is usually transmitted via the fecal–oral route, although infection can be acquired via inhalation of respiratory droplets. Herpangina is common in children under the age of 5 years and among school-aged children, particularly during epidemics in the summer and fall.

CLINICAL PRESENTATION

Herpangina is associated with the development of small vesicles on an erythematous base that may be covered with exudate. Lesions are confined to the soft palate and posterior oropharynx and usually develop after the abrupt onset of fever. The incubation period lasts for 1 to 2 weeks, and symptoms persist for 4 to 6 days. Differential diagnosis includes acute herpetic gingivostomatitis, recurrent aphthous stomatitis, streptococcal pharyngitis, hand-foot-and-mouth disease, and erythema multiforme. Unlike the intraoral lesions of hand-foot-and-mouth disease, those of herpangina do not involve the anterior oral cavity and can be covered by a pseudomembrane.

DIAGNOSIS

Diagnosis is usually based on clinical findings. Although virus can be isolated from oral or fecal culture, laboratory testing is often not indicated. Serologic testing can be used to confirm diagnosis when necessary.

TREATMENT

Disease course is usually mild. Conservative therapy is recommended.

Measles

Measles (rubeola) is caused by a paramyxovirus of the *Morbillivirus* genus and is rare in the United States because of widespread vaccination. Measles is transmitted via airborne respiratory droplets and is highly contagious in unimmunized populations.

CLINICAL PRESENTATION

Pathognomonic for measles, Koplik spots are the primary oral manifestation of this disease. Koplik spots are small, bluish macules with an erythematous background and a white necrotic core. They generally arise on the buccal mucosa apposing the first and second molars. This finding precedes the development of the classic, caudally progressive, maculopapular exanthem of measles by 1 to 2 days. Other gingival and oral manifestations of measles include necrotizing stomatitis, ulcerative gingivitis, and superinfection with candida. Some evidence suggests that measles virus is associated with recurrent aphthous ulcers, but this remains to be confirmed. The incubation period ranges from 10 to 12 days. Complications include otitis media, pneumonia, diarrhea, blindness, croup, acute encephalitis, and subacute sclerosing panencephalitis. Differential diagnosis of oral manifestations of measles includes recurrent aphthous ulcers, acute herpetic gingivostomatitis, varicella, exanthem infantum, and infectious mononucleosis.

DIAGNOSIS

Diagnosis is made based on typical clinical findings or by the presence of virus-specific IgM antibodies on serologic testing. Alternatively, measles virus RNA may be detected in respiratory secretions of acutely infected individuals using molecular methods.

TREATMENT

In uncomplicated measles, treatment involves supportive measures, such as hydration and local analgesia. The disease is prevented by administration of the live-attenuated MMR (Measles, Mumps and Rubella) vaccination series.

Unimmunized individuals are protected via herd immunity in regions of the world in which vaccination is widespread. Unimmunized pregnant women should be advised to wait until after delivery and hospital discharge before receiving the MMR vaccine.

Mumps

Mumps is caused by a paramyxovirus of the *Rubulavirus* genus that, like measles, is transmitted via aerosolized respiratory droplets. Although rare in the United States, an outbreak of cases was seen as recently as 2006. Mumps most often affects children aged 5 to 15 during winter and spring.

CLINICAL PRESENTATION

The primary intraoral sign of mumps is localized erythema and edema at the opening of Stensen's duct, opposite from the upper molars on the buccal mucosa. Mumps is characterized by a 3–5-day prodrome of low-grade fever, chills, and malaise, swelling of the parotid, submandibular, and submental salivary glands, and development of a morbilliform eruption. Incubation period is 2 to 3 weeks. Complications are uncommon but include myocarditis, pancreatitis, orchitis, meningitis, encephalitis, and unilateral deafness. Differential diagnosis includes acute suppurative parotitis, parotid enlargement from medications, buccal cellulitis, sialolithiasis, angioedema, Sjögren syndrome, Mikulicz syndrome, tuberculosis, syphilis, systemic lupus erythematosus, Heerfordt syndrome, and salivary gland neoplasms. When contracted in the first trimester of pregnancy, mumps may lead to spontaneous abortion.

DIAGNOSIS

Mumps is usually a clinical diagnosis. The presence of mumps-specific IgM antibodies on serologic testing is diagnostic. Moreover, the virus may be isolated with saliva culture. Elevated serum amylase or lymphocyte percentage in the cell count differential corroborates the diagnosis.

TREATMENT

Supportive therapy is recommended. Mumps is prevented by the MMR vaccination, as described earlier.

Rubella

Rubella (German measles) is caused by a togavirus of the *Rubivirus* genus and is transmitted via respiratory droplets and saliva. In the United States, rubella is usually only seen in unimmunized adults and immigrants because of widespread immunization with the MMR vaccine.

CLINICAL PRESENTATION

The presence of *Forschheimer spots*, dark red macules on the palate and uvula, is a nonspecific intraoral sign of rubella present in 20% of cases. A macular eruption develops on the face and later involves the neck, trunk, and extremities. Lymphadenopathy of the head and neck, particularly in the suboccipital region, is frequent. In adults, the eruption is usually preceded by constitutional symptoms. Incubation period is approximately 14 to 21 days. Complications are rare but may include arthralgias, arthritis, thrombocytopenia, hemolytic anemia, Guillain-Barré syndrome, and postinfectious encephalopathy. Differential diagnosis includes erythema infectiosum (*Fifth Disease*), mucocutaneous lymph node syndrome (Kawasaki Disease), measles, roseola infantum, scarlet fever, streptococcal pharyngitis, infectious mononucleosis, and juvenile rheumatoid arthritis. When contracted within the first 20 weeks of pregnancy, rubella may lead to congenital rubella syndrome.

DIAGNOSIS

Diagnosis is usually made based on classic physical findings, although serologic testing may demonstrate the presence of virus-specific IgM immunoglobulin.

TREATMENT

As rubella is usually benign and self-limited, symptomatic treatment is appropriate. Isolation precautions should be taken while the patient is infectious to prevent transmission, particularly to pregnant women. Disease prevention is achieved with widespread administration of the MMR vaccination.

RNA Retroviruses

Human immunodeficiency virus

Human immunodeficiency virus (HIV) is an RNA retrovirus that is transmitted by direct exchange of bodily fluids, as with sexual transmission, transfusion of contaminated blood products, intravenous drug use, vertical transmission from mother to fetus during pregnancy, or horizontal transmission from mother to newborn via lactation. Progression from HIV infection to acquired immunodeficiency syndrome (AIDS) occurs a median of 11 years after initial infection and predisposes the patient to opportunistic pathogens.

CLINICAL PRESENTATION

Oral findings are present in about 55% to 60% of patients with HIV infection worldwide, and their frequency is inversely proportional to the patient's CD4+ T-lymphocyte count. Nonspecific oral erythema and ulceration may be present at the time of seroconversion. The most common oral disease among patients with HIV infection is oropharyngeal candidiasis, which ultimately develops in up to 90% of patients. Other frequent intraoral findings include KS, disseminated herpes zoster, oral hairy leukoplakia, perioral or intraoral molluscum contagiosum, recurrent aphthous ulcers, local or generalized ulcerative periodontitis, and acute necrotizing ulcerative gingivostomatitis. In the developing world, oral tuberculosis also has a high prevalence in this patient population. Azidothymidine (AZT), a thymidine analog used to delay progression of HIV infection, can cause oral hyperpigmentation. HIV infection is also associated with an increased prevalence of genital candidiasis. Co-infection with other sexually transmitted infections with manifestations of the mucosa, such as chlamydia, gonorrhea, chancroid, syphilis, and HPV, is common. In fact, the ulcerated lesions of chancroid and other causes of genital ulceration are thought to facilitate the acquisition of HIV in exposed individuals.

DIAGNOSIS

Since ELISA is very sensitive for the presence of HIV-specific antibodies, it is used for screening. Reactive tests are repeated. If two ELISA tests are reactive, then Western blot is utilized, as it has a very high specificity. A positive Western blot test confirms diagnosis.

TREATMENT

Treatment of mucosal manifestations of HIV infection should be tailored to the particular disease process. Moreover, pharmacotherapy of the underlying HIV infection is necessary to avoid recurrence.

Table 22.4: Viral Organisms That Do Not Usually Cause Disease of the Oral or Genital Mucous Membranes

Adenovirus	Ebola Virus	Orthomyxovirus
Arbovirus	Hantavirus	Papovavirus
Calcivirus	Viral hepatidides (A, B, C, D, E)	Parainfluenza virus
Coronavirus	Influenza virus	Poliovirus
Dengue virus	Norwalk virus	Respiratory syncytial virus

Human T-lymphotropic virus

Associated with adult T-cell leukemia and lymphoma, the RNA retrovirus human T-cell lymphotropic virus type 1 is not typically associated with intraoral manifestations. However, two cases of HTLV-1-associated acute T-cell leukemia/lymphoma presenting with oral findings have been reported. One patient had a painful, ulcerated lesion on the hard palate, and the other developed lymphoproliferative disease at the posterior tongue.

Viral organisms that do not usually cause disease of the oral or genital mucous membranes include (Table 22.4) adenovirus, arbovirus, calicivirus, coronavirus, Dengue virus, Ebola virus, hantavirus, hepatitis A, B, C, D, and E, influenza virus, Norwalk virus, orthomyxovirus, papovavirus, parainfluenza virus, paramyxovirus, poliovirus, and respiratory syncytial virus.

FUNGAL INFECTIONS

Superficial Mycoses

Candida spp.

Candida spp., saprophytic dimorphic yeast, are the most frequent colonizing fungal organisms of the oral and genital mucosa and can function as opportunistic pathogens. Risk factors for candidal infection are numerous and include previous infection of the mucosa, antibiotic use, diabetes mellitus, and other endocrine disorders, malnutrition, various primary immune deficiencies, neutropenia, denture usage, usage of immunosuppressive medications (such as topical corticosteroids, corticosteroid inhalers, systemic corticosteroids, chemotherapy agents, and others), xerostomia, certain nutritional deficiencies, and malignancy.

Candida spp. bind to mucosal surfaces and degrade epidermal keratin, which permits invasion. Although both the yeast and mold forms of Candida albicans may be present in infection, branching mycelia predominate. Engulfment of these large mycelia by host phagocytes is difficult. Moreover, Candida spp. are capable of undergoing phenotype switching, a phenomenon that can contribute to increased organism virulence and to the development of drug resistance. Candida spp. are responsible for a range of mucosal disease syndromes, which are described subsequently (Table 22.5).

CLINICAL FEATURES

Acute pseudomembranous candidiasis (thrush) from Candida is common in neonates, young children, chronically ill adults, and the elderly. Thrush presents with thick, creamy white,

Table 22.5: Syndromes and Physical Findings Associated with Infection with *Candida* Spp

Syndrome	Physical Findings
Acute pseudomembranous candidiasis	White patches and plaques with an erythematous base
Denture stomatitis	Erythema and edema of the hard palate
Acute atrophic candidiasis (candidal glossitis)	Tender erythematous atrophy of dorsal tongue and palate
Angular cheilitis	Linear erythema and fissures at the commissures
Oral leukoplakia (candida leukoplakia, hyperplastic candidiasis)	Persistent, tender oral lesions
Median rhomboid glossitis	Rhomboid-shaped region of atrophy on the dorsal tongue
Candidal infection of the tongue and nonspecific inflammation of the palate (CIT-NIP)	Findings of median rhomboid glossitis with tender erythema of the hard palate
Chronic mucocutaneous candidiasis	Chronic candidal infection of skin, mucous membranes, and nails
Systemic candidiasis	Candidemia, fever, myalgias

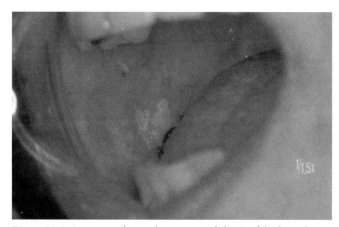

Figure 22.6. Acute pseudomembranous candidiasis of the buccal mucosa.

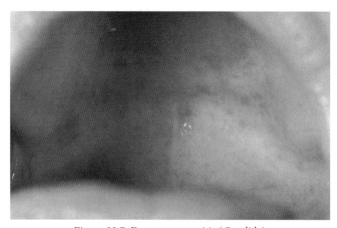

Figure 22.7. Denture stomatitis (*Candida*).

cheese-like patches and plaques on the mucosa, which often have an erythematous or ulcerated base (Fig. 22.6). A pseudomembrane may develop in severe cases. These plaques can be removed with scraping, but a bleeding surface often remains. In most otherwise healthy patients, infection remains confined to the mucosa.

Denture stomatitis results from contact between the palate and a dental appliance that has been colonized by *Candida* (usually *C. albicans*). Denture stomatitis is characterized by asymptomatic or painful erythema and edema of the hard palate (Fig. 22.7). The combination of appliance colonization, local tissue trauma, and presence of a moist, occluded local environment contributes to pathogenesis.

Acute atrophic candidiasis (candidal glossitis) presents with tender, smooth, erythematous lesions of the dorsal tongue and palate. Atrophy results from the loss of filiform papillae, a feature that distinguishes lesions of acute atrophic candidiasis from those of local trauma or nonspecific inflammation. Use of inhaled corticosteroids predisposes the patient to this condition in a dose-dependent fashion.

Candidal infection can cause angular cheilitis (*perlèche*), a condition associated with linear erythema and commissural fissuring. Risk factors for this condition include situations in which the oral commissures are chronically moist, as with denture usage and the edentulous state. Nutrient deficiencies and hematologic dyscrasias may also be associated with angular cheilitis. These predisposing factors must be addressed before antifungal therapy can be maximally effective. Infection may be polymicrobial and bacterial pathogens such as *Staphylococcus aureus* often coexist. Therefore, synchronous antibacterial therapy may be necessary.

Candida has been found to be a risk factor for oral leukoplakia, also known as candida leukoplakia or hyperplastic candidiasis. Oral leukoplakia is characterized by the presence of persistent, tender, speckled, white oral lesions that are not removed easily with mechanical scraping. Histopathology reveals epithelial hyperplasia, which is associated with cytologic atypia or malignant conversion in 3% to 6% of patients.

Median rhomboid glossitis appears as painless atrophy in a distinctive rhomboid pattern at the central portion of the tongue. This condition was previously attributed to the congenital persistence of the tuberculum impar. However, it is now thought that chronic oral candidiasis contributes to pathogenesis, because candidal hyphae are often seen in intralesional focal neutrophilic microabscesses, and antifungal therapy frequently leads to cure. Although median rhomboid glossitis intrinsically is benign, the concern for HIV infection or AIDS arises when the condition is accompanied by erythema and pain at the hard palate. This phenomenon is seen in a condition known as CIT-NIP (candidal infection of the tongue and nonspecific inflammation of the palate). Although occasionally confused with the presence of a lingual thyroid, median rhomboid glossitis differs morphologically in several respects. Specifically, median rhomboid glossitis is located anterior to the foramen cecum and is generally macular, whereas lingual thyroid is present posterior to the foramen cecum and is raised.

Genital candidiasis is typically seen in people during their sexually active years. Vulvovaginal candidiasis is a common cause of vaginitis and presents with thick, white vaginal discharge, localized pruritus, and dysuria. *C. albicans* causes 93% to 98% of vulvovaginal candidiasis in healthy women, although *Candida glabrata* and other non-albicans species are causative more frequently in patients with recurrent disease. In men, candida may infect the coronal sulcus, prepuce, or perimeatal area and is characterized by localized pruritus, pain, and erythema. Disease may also be asymptomatic in either sex.

Differential diagnosis of mucosal candidiasis includes chronic cheek bite keratosis, morsicatio buccarum, chemical and thermal burns, oral hairy leukoplakia, lichen planus, syphilis, hereditary benign intraepithelial dyskeratosis, and white sponge nevus.

DIAGNOSIS

In most uncomplicated cases, diagnosis is made clinically. Round or oval yeast forms, hyphae, or pseudohyphae are seen on KOH preparation and culture. Isolation of candida alone cannot confirm candidiasis, however, since candida is often part of the normal mucosal flora. Colposcopy may have a role in the diagnosis of chronic vulvar candidiasis.

TREATMENT

Treatment of localized *Candida* typically involves the use of topical nystatin, topical imidazoles (such as clotrimazole in an oral troche or cream), or oral imidazoles. For candidiasis confined to the mouth, duration of treatment should be at least twice as long as it takes for the signs and symptoms to resolve. In immunocompromised patients, early treatment is crucial to avoid dissemination. Moreover, management of underlying predisposing factors is necessary to avoid recurrence.

Subcutaneous Mycoses

Chronic mucocutaneous candidiasis

Chronic mucocutaneous candidiasis (CMC) results from a diverse group of congenital or acquired conditions that render patients unable to clear *Candida* spp. Recent research revealed that CMC is associated with deficits in the production of type 1 cytokines (such as IL-2 and IL-12) and overproduction of type 2 cytokines (IL-6 and IL-10) in response to *Candida*. These alterations in cytokine response to infection appear to be specific to *Candida* and are due to upstream immune defects.

Primary CMC results from a variety of primary immunodeficiencies, all of which disrupt host response to candidal infection. Primary CMC may arise as a spontaneous mutation or through autosomal dominant or autosomal recessive inheritance. Secondary CMC is associated with HIV infection, corticosteroid usage, and denture usage.

CLINICAL PRESENTATION

CMC is characterized by chronic candidal infection of the skin, mucous membranes, and nails. Painful, hyperkeratotic vegetating lesions that are exacerbated by the consumption of acidic or spicy foods develop in the mouth. When the esophagus is involved, dysphagia may result. Infections tend to remain superficial, although deep or disseminated disease may follow. When inherited in an autosomal recessive manner, primary CMC has been associated with endocrine and inflammatory disorders. In cases of adult-onset CMC, concomitant presence of thymoma has been reported.

DIAGNOSIS

CMC is diagnosed clinically in patients with recurrent or persistent candidal infections. Reversible causes for cell-mediated immune deficiency should be sought.

TREATMENT

Acute flares are treated with topical or systemic antifungal agents, depending on the severity of the infection. Long-term prophylaxis with antifungal therapy is also indicated, as most patients with CMC experience recurrent infection upon discontinuation of antifungal medications. Immunomodulatory therapy is being investigated.

Deep Mycoses (Table 22.6)

Deep mycotic infections with frequently implicated fungal organisms and associated mucosal findings are listed in Table 22.6.

Non-Endemic Mycoses

Disseminated candidiasis

Disseminated candidiasis, or candidemia, is seen exclusively in immunocompromised individuals and can arise from proliferation or migration of *Candida* from colonized gastrointestinal or urinary tracts, oral mucosa, heart valves or central venous catheters. Although *Candida albicans* is the most common nosocomial fungal infection, other *Candida* species are common in some immunocompromised populations. Systemic candidiasis causes significant morbidity and mortality and, in patients with HIV, its presence is a strong predictor of HIV progression rate.

CLINICAL PRESENTATION

Disseminated candidiasis may be associated with nonspecific oral lesions and classically presents with the triad of fever, skin eruption, and myalgias. Potentially life-threatening complications include esophageal rupture, *Candida* pneumonia, and widespread dissemination.

DIAGNOSIS

The consistent presence of *C. albicans* or other *Candida* spp. in blood cultures in the immunocompromised patient is suggestive of systemic infection. Histologic examination of skin lesions is relatively sensitive and may offer identification of the offending organism before blood culture results are available.

TREATMENT

Although amphotericin B used to be the drug of choice in disseminated candidiasis, fluconazole and other systemic azoles are now preferred because of their more favorable side effect profile. However, azole-resistant *Candida* has emerged in HIV patients. Underlying immunosuppression should be addressed.

Mucormycosis (zygomycosis)

Mucormycosis is a rare condition caused by *Rhizopus* and *Mucor* spp., which are found commonly in the soil and on moldy bread. Application of contaminated medical tape and bandages over facial wounds has also been implicated in disease transmission. Mucormycosis is seen in patients with diabetes mellitus (particularly those in diabetic ketoacidosis), burns, uremia, malnutrition, neutropenia, iatrogenic immunosuppression, or liver cirrhosis. Since iron is a growth stimulant for the causative

Table 22.6: Deep Mycoses with Mucosal Manifestations and the Appearance of Pathogenic Organism upon Histopathologic Examination

Systemic Mycosis	Mucosal Findings	Appearance of Organism on Histopathology
Disseminated candidiasis	Nonspecific oral lesions	Round or oval yeast cells; hyphae; pseudohyphae
Mucormycosis	Ulcer with black, necrotic eschar; hard palate perforation	Broad, nonseptate, right-angled hyphae
Aspergillosis	Single ulcer with grey exudate or surrounding eschar; hard palate perforation	Hyphae with septae branching at 45 degrees
Histoplasmosis	Tender, nonhealing ulcers; granulomatous lesions	Yeast within monocytes, histocytes, or neutrophils
Blastomycosis	Ulcer with verrucous surface vegetating plaque; granulomatous edema	Broad-based budding yeast
Cryptococcosis	Ulcer with vegetating surface; granulomatous nodule	Encapsulated narrow-based budding yeast
Paracoccidioidomycosis	Painful, destructive, granulomatous lesions (*mulberry lesions*); hard palate perforation	Budding yeast in "ship's steering wheel" or "Mickey Mouse" forms
Coccidioidomycosis	Ulcerative tongue lesion resembling squamous cell carcinoma (very rare)	Spherules and loose endospores

agents of mucormycosis, this condition can also arise in patients with iron overload states, such as hemochromatosis.

CLINICAL PRESENTATION

Mucormycosis is a highly destructive infection that erodes arteries of the nasal membranes, upper and lower respiratory tracts, gastrointestinal system, and central nervous system, leading to thrombosis, ischemia, and necrosis. Tissue necrosis appears as an ulcer surrounded by a black, necrotic eschar. Resultant perforation of the palate has also been reported. Disseminated disease typically starts with orbital cellulitis with or without proptosis and may result in cranial nerve palsy. Other associated symptoms include low-grade fever, malaise, epistaxis, sinus pressure, and retro-orbital headache. Associated mortality is high. Differential diagnosis includes lethal midline granuloma, tuberculosis, squamous cell carcinoma, anthrax, aspergillosis, nasopharyngeal carcinoma, syphilis, Wegener's granulomatosis, and systemic mycoses.

DIAGNOSIS

Histopathology and smear examination demonstrate the presence of broad, right-angled hyphae (Fig. 22.8) and tissue necrosis. Culture is necessary to identify the involved species. Serum ferritin, total iron-binding capacity, and glucose and electrolyte levels should also be checked. Computed tomography can aid in diagnostic confirmation, delineation of disease extent, and surgical planning.

THERAPY

Effective treatment of mucormycosis often requires surgical debridement and systemic antibiotic therapy with amphotericin B. Because of the nephrotoxicity associated with amphotericin B, particular caution must be used in patients with poorly controlled diabetes mellitus. Although most azoles and echinocandins are not effective in this disease, posaconazole, a new azole, has been shown to have in vitro and in vivo efficacy. Predisposing factors must also be controlled.

Cryptococcosis

Cryptococcosis, caused by the encapsulated yeast *Cryptococcus neoformans,* generally is acquired via the respiratory tract and

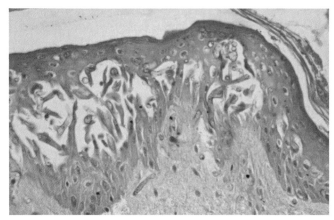

Figure 22.8. Broad, sharply-angled hyphae of *Mucor* spp.

classically occurs by inhalation of aerosolized bird feces. While *C. neoformans* var *neoformans* affects immunocompromised patients, *C. neoformans* var *gattii* may cause disease in healthy individuals.

CLINICAL PRESENTATION

Oral findings in cryptococcosis are uncommon and typically represent manifestations of disseminated disease. Mucosal cryptococcosis appears as erythematous papules that evolve into ulcerative lesions. Reported sites of intraoral involvement include the tongue, palate, gingiva, and sites of previous tooth extraction. Diseases mimicking mucosal manifestations of cryptococcosis include squamous cell carcinoma, chancroid, lethal midline granuloma, tuberculosis, syphilis, traumatic ulcer, and other systemic fungal infections.

DIAGNOSIS

The diagnosis of cryptococcosis is supported by the presence of encapsulated, narrow-budding yeast on histopathology (Fig. 22.9). Special stains, such as methenamine silver periodic acid-Schiff, Mayer mucicarmine or Masson-Fontan silver stains, often are required to visualize the organism and its distinctive capsule. Diagnosis may be confirmed by in situ hybridization or isolation of the organism on fungal culture.

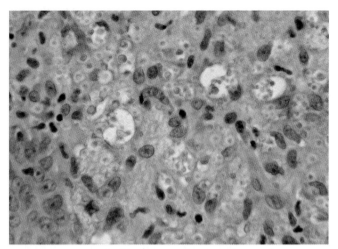

Figure 22.9. Narrow-budding, encapsulated organisms of *Cryptococcus* spp. (*mucin stain*).

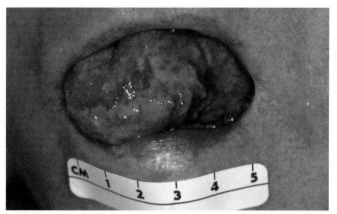

Figure 22.10. Oral histoplasmosis.

THERAPY

In symptomatic cryptococcosis, fluconazole is considered the first-line therapy. In severe disease, amphotericin B may be required. Patients with HIV infection may require lifelong suppressive therapy.

Aspergillosis

Aspergillis spp. are ubiquitous airborne fungi that can spread on the hands of health-care providers and via ventilation systems, particularly in hospitals during times of renovation. The most common cause of invasive aspergillosis is *Aspergillus fumigatus.* Risk factors include leukopenia, lymphoma, iatrogenic immunosuppression, and HIV infection.

CLINICAL PRESENTATION

Primary intraoral aspergillosis is extremely rare but has been reported. When present intraorally, primary aspergillosis appears as an isolated ulcer covered with a grayish exudate on the gingiva, hard palate, soft palate, and dorsum of the tongue. In disseminated aspergillosis, mucosal lesions are present in about 10% of cases. Intraoral lesions of disseminated aspergillosis develop as a result of hemorrhagic necrosis and appear as ulcerated eschars on the palate and posterior tongue. Hard palate perforation from invasive aspergillosis has been reported in several patients with acute leukemia. Disseminated aspergillosis can be life threatening. Differential diagnosis of mucosal lesions includes mucormycosis, lethal midline granuloma, nasopharyngeal carcinoma, Wegener's granulomatosis, tuberculosis, syphilis, and other systemic mycoses.

DIAGNOSIS

On tissue histology, *Aspergillus* spp. can be visualized as hyphae with septae branching at 45 degrees with Gomori methenamine silver stain. Cultures are often negative and, when positive, might represent colonization. Other diagnostic methods, such as PCR and ELISA, have been developed.

THERAPY

Surgical debridement may be useful in primary intraoral aspergillosis. In disseminated aspergillosis, empiric treatment often must be instituted while diagnostic work-up is pending, since early treatment is required for reduction in mortality. Although amphotericin B used to be the drug of choice,

voriconazole is now preferred. Caspofungin can also be used in refractory cases or in patients who do not tolerate azoles or amphotericin. Consistent hand washing and the use of laminar airflow or high-efficiency particulate air (HEPA) filtration can limit the dissemination of airborne *Aspergillus* organisms.

Endemic Mycoses

Histoplasmosis

Histoplasma capsulatum, the causative agent in histoplasmosis, is endemic to the Mississippi and Ohio River Valleys of the United States, as well as parts of Africa and Australia. It can be found in soil contaminated by bat or bird feces. Human disease can result from the inhalation of airborne spores or more rarely, the direct inoculation of organisms into the skin or mucous membranes. The sporulated organism converts to a yeast form and replicates at body temperature.

CLINICAL PRESENTATION

Histoplasmosis can cause oral lesions as part of primary or disseminated disease. Oral histoplasmosis can present with one or multiple tender, nonhealing, friable ulcers or as nodular, verrucous, or granulomatous lesions (Fig. 22.10). These are found on the tongue, palate, and buccal mucosa. Reactivation of latent histoplasmosis of the oropharynx following radiation therapy for laryngeal squamous cell carcinoma has been documented. Histoplasmosis may also cause macroglossia via tongue infiltration. Differential diagnosis of oral findings includes squamous cell carcinoma, lethal midline granuloma, mucocutaneous leishmaniasis, CMV infection, Wegener's granulomatosis, lymphoma, tuberculosis, sarcoidosis, and other deep mycoses.

DIAGNOSIS

The diagnosis of oral histoplasmosis can be confirmed by visualizing yeast within phagocytes with the use of routine and special stains, such as periodic acid-Schiff and methenamine silver nitrate stains on histopathology. In situ hybridization is also an effective mode of diagnosis. Serologic tests can demonstrate the presence of organism-specific antibodies, although false negatives can occur in immunocompromised individuals. Serum and urine antigen tests may also be helpful. As the organism is fastidious, fungal culture is often insensitive.

THERAPY

Cutaneous lesions may be self-limited, so treatment is warranted only if disease is prolonged or systemic. Although

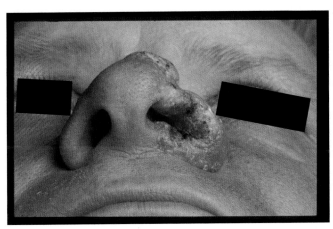

Figure 22.11. Blastomycosis.

Table 22.7. Fungal Organisms That Do Not Usually Cause Disease of the Oral and Genital Mucous Membranes

Dermatophytes	*Malassezia furfur*
Exophiala werneckii	*Piedraia hortai*
Fonsecaea pedrosoi	*Pseudallescheria boydii*
Fonsecaea compacta	*Trichosporon beigelii*
Madurella grisea	*Sporothrix schenckii*
Madurella mycetomatis	*Wangiella dermatitidis*

amphotericin B used to be the preferred agent for complicated histoplasmosis, systemic azole derivatives are now the treatment of choice.

Blastomycosis

Blastomycosis, caused by the thermal dimorphic fungus *Blastomyces dermatitidis,* occurs in parts of North America and Africa. Blastomycosis is not as closely linked as the other systemic endemic mycoses with immunocompromise.

CLINICAL PRESENTATION

As with other systemic endemic mycoses, oral lesions associated with blastomycosis can be the first clue to the presence of systemic disease. Lesions of oral blastomycosis usually take one of three morphologies: (1) painless solitary ulcers with a verrucous surface and thin, raised edges, (2) vegetating plaques, or (3) granulomatous edema. Blastomycosis can also infiltrate the nasal mucosa or the larynx (Fig. 22.11), mimicking squamous cell carcinoma or the tongue, resulting in macroglossia. Other areas of potential disease involvement include the genitourinary tract, central nervous system, skin, and bone. Diseases that mimic oral blastomycosis include tuberculosis, squamous cell carcinoma, sarcoidosis, Wegener's granulomatosis, syphilis, and other deep mycoses. One group reported a case of oral blastomycosis with secondary bacterial infection that mimicked actinomycosis because the infection eroded through from the mandible to the oral cavity.

DIAGNOSIS

Presumptive diagnosis can be made by the demonstration of broad-based budding yeasts with doubly refractile cell walls on direct examination of the sputum or histopathology. Diagnosis is confirmed by in situ hybridization and tissue culture.

THERAPY

Blastomycosis is treated with azole derivatives and amphotericin B. In immunocompromised individuals, early and aggressive treatment with amphotericin B is indicated.

Paracoccidioidomycosis

Paracoccidioidomycosis (formerly South American blastomycosis) is a systemic endemic mycosis caused by the dimorphic fungus, *Paracoccidioides brasiliensis. Paracoccidioides brasiliensis* is found in the soil in countries of Central and South

America and primarily affects men, with a male-to-female ratio of 15:1. Although inhalation is the most common route of infection, direct inoculation can occur when contaminated twigs are used to clean teeth, as is the practice in some areas of rural Brazil.

CLINICAL PRESENTATION

Oral findings are present in about half of all patients with paracoccidioidomycosis. Paracoccidioidomycosis causes painful, destructive, granulomatous lesions (*mulberry lesions*), which can be found on the tongue, lips, gingiva, hard palate, buccal mucosa, and, less commonly, nasal mucosa. These lesions can lead to dysphagia and dysphonia. Other previously documented presentations of paracoccidioidomycosis include squamous cell carcinoma–like lesions and hard palate perforation. Associated cervical lymphadenopathy is common. Differential diagnosis includes mucocutaneous leishmaniasis, actinomycosis, lymphoma, squamous cell carcinoma, Wegener's granulomatosis, necrotizing sialometaplasia, sarcoidosis, and other systemic fungal infections.

DIAGNOSIS

Tissue biopsy is the gold standard for diagnosis. Multiple budding yeast in "Mickey Mouse" or "ship's steering wheel" forms, as well as granuloma formation, can be seen with Gomori methenamine silver (GMS) stain. A small study of patients with biopsy-demonstrated oral paracoccidioidomycosis found that cytology obtained through direct smear was positive in all infected patients. A subsequent trial found that cytology from direct smear had a sensitivity of 68% and a specificity of 92%. Therefore, cytology may be a reasonable first test for oral paracoccidioidomycosis, but biopsy should be performed if cytology is unrevealing and the clinical index of suspicion remains high.

THERAPY

Slow-acting sulfonamides are the preferred treatment option in paracoccidioidomycosis. Other reasonable pharmacologic options include fluconazole, terbinafine, and amphotericin B.

Coccidioidomycosis

Coccidioidomycosis is a systemic mycosis caused by *Coccidioides immitis*, which is endemic to the southwestern United States. Although not usually associated with mucosal lesions, one case of coccidioidomycosis of the tongue has been reported. The tongue lesion resembled squamous cell carcinoma and responded to systemic antifungal medication.

Fungal organisms that do not usually cause disease of the oral or genital mucous membranes include (Table 22.7)

Table 22.8: Sexually Transmitted Bacterial Infections with the Associated Disease Syndrome and Characteristic Mucosal Lesions

Organism	Disease Syndrome	Lesions
Chlamydia trachomatis Types A-C	Trachoma (conjunctivitis)	Injection of the bulbar conjuntivae, ulceration and scarring of the cornea, ocular discharge, pre-auricular lymphadenopathy
Types D-K	Cervicitis, urethritis, epididymitis, pharyngitis	Oral mucosa: Diffuse erythema and small pustules in the tonsillar area Genital mucosa: Purulent vaginal or urethral discharge, dysuria, dyspareunia
Types L1-L3	Lymphogranuloma venereum	Phase 1: Small, painless papule or ulceration Phase 2: Lymphadenopathy, buboe formation Phase 3: Chronic ulceration and stricture
Neisseria gonorrheae	Cervicitis, urethritis, vaginitis, pharyngitis	Oral mucosa: Erythema of posterior oropharynx, painful oral ulcers with pseudomembranes, necrosis of gingivae and intradental papillae Genital mucosa: Purulent vaginal or urethral discharge, dysuria, dyspareunia Conjunctiva: Erythema of bulbar conjunctiva, profuse purulent discharge
Trichomonas vaginalis	Trichomoniasis	Mucosal petechiae, overlying exudate, dysuria, profuse vaginal discharge, urethral discharge, dysuria, dyspareunia
Haemophilis ducreyi	Chancroid	Tender ulcerated lesions with grey or purulent base, lymphadenopathy
Calymmato-bacterium granulomatis	Granuloma inguinale (Donovaniasis)	Erythematous, moist papule at site of inoculation that enlarges and spreads along body folds; no significant lymphadenopathy
Treponema pallidum	Syphilis	See Table 22.9.

dermatophytes, *Exophiala werneckii*, *Fonsecaea pedrosoi* or compacta, *Madurella grisea or mycetomatis*, *Malessezia furfur*, *Piedraia hortai*, *Pseudallescheria boydii*, *Trichosporon beigelii*, *Sporothrix schenckii*, and *Wangiella dermatitidis*.

BACTERIAL INFECTIONS

A range of bacterial species cause disease of the mucous membranes. These will be categorized as (1) sexually transmitted bacterial organisms, (2) spirochetes, (3) mycobacteria, and (4) other.

Sexually Transmitted Infections of Bacterial Origin (Table 22.8)

Sexually transmitted bacterial infections with frequently implicated bacterial organisms and associated mucosal findings are listed in Table 22.8.

Chlamydia

Chlamydia trachomatis, an obligate intracellular organism transmitted via sexual activity, has multiple immunoptypes that can impart one of three diseases to the host. Specifically, *C. trachomatis* immunotypes A-C cause trachoma (conjunctivits), D-K infect the genital tracts and other mucosal membranes and L1-L3 cause lymphogranuloma venereum (LGV). In the United States, C. trachomatis is the commonest pathogen responsible for urethritis and cervicitis in young adults and, when associated with pelvic inflammatory disease, is a leading cause of infertility in women. LGV is rare in the United States. For a more detailed discussion of Chlamydia see chapter 24.

TREATMENT

The treatment of choice for uncomplicated chlamydial infection is azithromycin or doxycycline. Sexual partners should also be treated to prevent reinfection. LGV is treated with tetracycline, doxycycline, or erythromycin. Some authors have reported azithromycin to be effective, although definitive evidence is lacking. Buboes may be aspirated for symptomatic relief. Strictures and fistulas may require operative intervention.

Gonorrhea

Gonorrhea is a sexually transmitted infection caused by the gram-negative diplococci of *Neisseria gonorrheae*. From 1981-1991, it was the most frequently reported sexually transmitted infection in the United States and is currently second in frequency only to Chlamydia. For a more detailed discussion of Gonorrhea, see chapter 24.

TREATMENT

Symptoms are often self-limited but can be transmitted to others if left untreated. Given the high prevalence of co-infection with Chlamydia, treatment strategies should cover both organisms. The drug of choice for gonorrhea is intramuscular ceftriaxone. Ciprofloxacin and levofloxacin are alternative antimicrobial agents, although resistance to fluoroquinolones is rising. The use of chlorhexidine as a vaginal lubricant was shown to prevent transmission of gonorrhea in one study.

Chancroid

Chancroid, a sexually transmitted infection caused by the small gram-negative rod, *Haemophilus ducreyi*, is the commonest cause of genital ulceration worldwide. It is only rarely seen in the developed world, where it is generally associated with prostitution, crack cocaine use, and travel to an area with high prevalence of chancroid. Chancroid may be associated with HIV infection and other sexually transmitted infections. The male to female ratio is 3:1. For a more detailed discussion of Chancroid, see chapter 24.

TREATMENT

Antimicrobial therapy consists of erythromycin, azithromycin, ciprofloxacin, ceftriaxone, or spectinomycin. Resistance is emerging against penicillins, aminoglycosides, trimethoprim-sulfamethoxazole, and tetracycline, however. When possible, in vitro antimicrobial susceptibility testing should guide therapy. Treatment failure is commonest in patients with HIV infection. Since rupture of buboes may cause chronic ulceration, aspiration or incision and drainage may be indicated.

Spirochetes

Spirochetes are long, helically coiled cells with flagella that run between the cell membrane and cell wall. These flagella permit active movement of the organism. The two phyla of spirochetes that cause disease in the mucosal membranes of humans are *Treponema* and *Borrelia*.

Syphilis

Syphilis is a systemic disease caused by the spirochete, *Treponema pallidum*. Although the incidence of syphilis decreased significantly in the mid-20th century with the introduction of penicillin, changing sexual practices, availability of crack cocaine, and increased prevalence of HIV infection have led to a resurgence in the United States and Europe. Syphilis can be acquired via maternal transmission to the fetus (i.e. congenital syphilis) or via mucosal contact with an infected individual. Syphilis is extremely infectious, with reported transmission rates ranging from 18 to 80%. Mucosal findings can be seen in almost every stage of syphilis (Table 22.9).

CLINICAL PRESENTATION

Syphilis is characterized by an early stage (involving primary, secondary, and early latent phases) and a late stage (involving late latent and tertiary phases). The patient is highly infectious in early syphilis but becomes less contagious once late syphilis has developed due to reduced spirochetemia.

Primary syphilis is marked by the development of a relatively painless solitary ulcer (*chancre*) at the site of inoculation. Classically, this primary lesion begins as a dome-shaped papule and erodes into a punched out, clean ulcer with distinct edges and a firm, granular base. Lesions are covered with a grey, serous exudate. Although primary syphilis affects the genital mucosa in the vast majority of cases, oral manifestations may be the presenting sign of primary syphilis in about 10% of cases. The most frequent anatomic sites for primary oral syphilis are the lips, tongue, and tonsillar fauces, depending on the method of disease transmission. Primary oral chancres are commonest on the upper lip in men and the lower lip in women. These lesions are associated with regional, nontender lymphadenopathy and appear approximately 3 weeks following inoculation. Ulcers of primary syphilis resolve spontaneously without residual scarring in 2 weeks. Without treatment, 25% of patients will develop secondary syphilis from persistent spirochetemia, while others develop latent syphilis, a phase characterized by the absence of physical signs of disease despite continued infectivity.

Table 22.9: Mucosal Lesions of Syphilis, by Disease Phase

Organism	Disease Syndrome	Mucosal Lesions
Treponema pallidum	Early stage	
	Primary phase	Solitary, painless ulcers (chancres)
	Secondary phase	Mucous patches, snail-track ulcers, macular and papular syphilides, oral hairy leukoplakia-like lesions, pseudomembranous lesions, condyloma lata
	Early latent phase	(No physical signs of disease)
	Late stage	
	Late latent phase	(No physical signs of disease)
	Tertiary phase	Destructive granulomas (gummas), syphilitic leukoplakia, interstitial glossitis, syphilitic sialadenitis
	Congenital	High arched palate, Hutchinson's teeth, Mulberry molars, mucous patches, rhagades at commissures

Secondary syphilis presents with constitutional symptoms and a widespread maculopapular eruption involving the palms and soles. Mucosal manifestations are common in secondary syphilis, occurring in at least 30% of patients. Mucous patches, shallow gray-white necrotic patches surrounded by erythema, are the most frequent intraoral sign of secondary syphilis. Other mucosal manifestations of secondary syphilis include macular syphilides (erythematous, oval macules), papular syphilides (painless, grayish nodules), snail-track ulcers (confluent mucous patches), oral hairy leukoplakia-like lesions, and rarely, condyloma lata (slightly exophytic, papillated lesions at the commissures and genital mucosa). Mucocutaneous manifestations of secondary syphilis usually resolve spontaneously after 3 to 12 weeks.

Tertiary syphilis develops in about one-third of patients with untreated secondary syphilis and may arise after a prolonged latency period. Tertiary syphilis is characterized by the widespread development of localized, destructive granulomas (*gummas*) that develop as a consequence of endarteritis obliterans. Oral gummas arise on the tongue, soft palate, and hard palate and may contribute to scarring and palatal perforation. Another oral finding of tertiary syphilis is syphilitic leukoplakia, which may be associated with increased risk for squamous cell carcinoma. Atrophic glossitis, chronic interstitial glossitis, and syphilitic sialadenitis also develop occasionally.

Rarely, syphilis is associated with erythema multiforme-like lesions. Congenital syphilis can predispose the child to multiple intraoral abnormalities, including a high arched palate, mucous patches, Hutchinson's incisors, Mulberry molars, and commissural rhagades.

Because of the diversity of mucosal manifestations associated with syphilis, differential diagnosis is broad.

DIAGNOSIS

In primary and secondary syphilis, definitive diagnosis can be made by dark-field microscopy and direct fluorescent antibody tests on lesional exudate and tissue. Screening can be performed with the nontreponemal tests, including the Venereal Disease Research Laboratory (VDRL) and Rapid Plasma Reagin (RPR) tests. These become reactive within a week of primary infection and can be used to monitor disease response to therapy. Nontreponemal tests should revert to being negative within 1 year after adequate antimicrobial therapy. Diagnostic specificity is enhanced with treponemal tests, including the *Treponema pallidum* hemagglutination assay (TPHA), *T. pallidum* phytohemagglutination assay (TPPA), microhemagglutination assay for antibody to *T. pallidum* (MHA-TP), and fluorescent treponemal antibody absorbed assay (FTA-Abs). Treponemal tests remain positive indefinitely. Patients with syphilis should also be tested for other sexually transmitted infections, including HIV.

TREATMENT

Treponema pallidum is one of only two main pathogens (along with *S. pyogenes*) that remain uniformly susceptible to penicillin, making this agent the drug of choice. In patients with a true penicillin allergy, the preferred second-line therapy is doxycycline. Ceftriaxone and azithromycin may also have a role in treatment. Treatment failure has been reported in patients with concurrent HIV infection, although this might represent re-infection. Jarisch-Herxheimer reaction, a transient febrile reaction following antibiotic treatment in syphilis, is rare.

Mycobacteria

Mycobacteria are facultative anaerobes that resemble bacteria but lack rigid cell walls. Several species have been implicated in diseases with oral manifestations.

Tuberculosis

Tuberculosis, caused by *Mycobacterium tuberculosis*, is uncommon in the United States but is widespread in many parts of the developing world. In the United States, tuberculosis is seen most commonly in immigrants, homeless individuals, alcoholics, and immunocompromised patients.

CLINICAL PRESENTATION

Oral manifestations of tuberculosis are unusual but may result from dissemination of pulmonary tuberculosis or, rarely, from primary oral inoculation. Nonhealing, granulomatous ulcers covered by a grey-yellow exudate develop on the dorsum of the tongue, palate, or, less commonly, buccal mucosa, and lips. Ulcers are usually accompanied by cervical lymphadenopathy with or without overlying skin breakdown (*scrofula*). Macroglossia may result from granulomatous infiltration of the tongue. Differential diagnosis of intraoral tuberculosis includes sarcoidosis, Wegener's granulomatosis, mucormycosis, squamous cell carcinoma, lethal midline granuloma, systemic mycoses, actinomycosis, eosinophilic ulcer, Crohn's disease, and traumatic ulcer.

DIAGNOSIS

A tuberculin skin test is usually placed as part of the preliminary evaluation. Results may be false positive if the patient has ever been exposed to *M. tuberculosis* and has been treated

successfully or if the patient has been immunized previously with the Bacille Calmette-Guérin (BCG) vaccine. False-negative results may occur if the patient is immunocompromised (a phenomenon known as *anergy*) or has recently been immunized with a live virus vaccine. In patients with positive tuberculin skin tests or with a high pretest probability for tuberculosis, chest radiography and sputum culture should be obtained. Acid-fast bacilli may be seen on tissue biopsy. Definitive diagnosis requires identification of *M. tuberculosis* on culture.

TREATMENT

The American Thoracic Society has developed a treatment algorithm for pulmonary tuberculosis. In the United States, initial therapy for active tuberculosis includes isoniazid, rifampin, ethambutol, and pyrazinamide for 2 months. In some cases, directly observed therapy is important to ensure patient adherence. Smear and culture should be repeated following 2 months of treatment, and results should guide further therapy. Close patient contacts or exposed health-care workers may need to undergo tuberculin skin testing and, if positive, chest radiography and 9 months of isoniazid prophylaxis.

Mycobacterium avium intracellulare

Oral lesions associated with disseminated *Mycobacterium avium intracellulare* (MAI) in a patient with AIDS has been reported. Lesions appeared as granulomatous masses on the hard palate and gingivae.

Leprosy (Hansen disease)

Mycobacterium lepra, the etiologic agent in leprosy, is an obligate intracellular bacillus that grows optimally at a temperature less than 37°C. Leprosy is a chronic systemic granulomatous disease that can affect the mucosa as well as skin, peripheral nerves, and other tissues. Several forms of the disease exist, including tuberculoid (paucibacillary), lepromatous (multibacillary), borderline, and indeterminate leprosy. The form the disease takes in each individual is dependent on the host's immunologic response to infection. A predominantly cell-mediated immune response generally leads to tuberculoid leprosy, whereas a humoral response results in lepromatous leprosy, for example.

CLINICAL PRESENTATION

Oral lesions are usually seen only with lepromatous leprosy and are present in 20% to 60% of cases. Nodules arise on oral surfaces and ultimately become necrotic and ulcerate. This can be highly destructive to the involved tissue and result in disfigurement (Fig. 22.12). Mucosal findings are rare in other forms of leprosy, although papules, erythema, and ulcers have been observed in borderline leprosy. Leprosy develops after an incubation period of many years. Differential diagnosis includes aspergillosis, Wegener's granulomatosis, sarcoidosis, syphilis, lethal midline granuloma, noma, lymphoma, mucormycosis, and squamous cell carcinoma.

DIAGNOSIS

The diagnosis of leprosy can be made clinically. One study found that in the appropriate clinical scenario, the presence of one of the following three signs had a 97% sensitivity for diagnosis: (1) hypopigmented or erythematous patches with definite loss of sensation, (2) thickened peripheral nerves, or (3) acid-fast bacilli on skin smears or biopsy material. Visualization of an inflamed nerve on skin biopsy in a patient with signs or

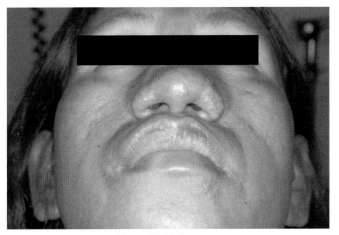

Figure 22.12. Leprosy.

symptoms of leprosy is confirmatory. Lepromin testing assesses delayed-type hypersensitivity to antigens of *M. lepra*, and a positive test indicates brisk cell-mediated immunity (i.e., most consistent with the tuberculoid form).

TREATMENT

For lepromatous (multibacillary) leprosy, a regimen consisting of rifampin, dapsone, and clofazimine is recommended. Rifampin and dapsone without clofazimine should be sufficient for tuberculoid (paucibacillary) cases.

Other Mucosal Infections of Bacterial Origin

Streptococcus

Streptococcus spp., gram-positive cocci that appear in pairs or chains on Gram stain, can be found as part of the normal oral flora or as a pathogen. *Streptococcus viridans*, an important contributor to the normal oral flora, competes with invading bacteria for mucosal adherence sites and secretes bacteriocins. In certain situations of mucosal disruption or host immunocompromise, however, *S. viridians* can migrate from the oral mucosa and cause bacterial endocarditis or sepsis. *S. mutans* is associated with the development of dental caries, and its presence in the mouth is a predictor of future caries. Group A *Streptococcus pyogenes* contains the virulence factor M protein and is the most common cause of acute bacterial pharyngitis.

CLINICAL PRESENTATION

Streptococcal pharyngitis presents with an intensely sore throat, tender anterior cervical lymphadenopathy, and fever. Intraoral findings include petechiae of the soft palate, tonsillar hypertrophy, and tonsillar exudate. Cough and nasal congestion are usually absent, and indeed, their presence lowers the pretest probability of the pharyngitis being attributable to *S. pyogenes* significantly. Streptococcal pharyngitis has been associated with suppurative (i.e. tonsillar exudate, peritonsillar cellulitis or abscess, sinusitis, streptococcal bacteremia) and nonsuppurative (i.e., acute rheumatic fever, acute poststreptococcal glomerulonephritis) postinfectious sequelae. Incubation period for the primary disease is 2 to 4 days.

Scarlet fever results from pyrogenic exotoxin release from Group A β-hemolytic streptococcus (*S. pyogenes*) and presents with high fever, diffuse scarletiniform rash, and erythema of the dorsal tongue papillae ("strawberry tongue"). After the eruption subsides, desquamation may persist for several weeks.

Rarely, balanitis or penile pyoderma may result from streptococcal infection in children via autoinoculation or in adults via oral sex.

DIAGNOSIS

Streptococcal pharyngitis can be diagnosed with the rapid antigen detection test and confirmed by isolation of the organism on throat culture. Serum antistreptolysin O (ASO) antibodies are usually elevated with recent streptococcal infection, but it is not necessary to check ASO antibody levels in uncomplicated acute disease. Scarlet fever is often diagnosed clinically and confirmed by demonstrating acute pharyngeal infection with *S. pyogenes*.

TREATMENT

The treatment of choice for streptococcal pharyngitis is a 10-day course of penicillin. The goal of antimicrobial therapy in streptococcal pharyngitis is to prevent suppurative and certain nonsuppurative complications, such as acute rheumatic fever. The incidence of acute poststreptococcal glomerulonephritis is not affected by antibiotic therapy.

Staphylococcus

Staphylococcus spp. are gram-positive organisms that are found in clusters on Gram's stain. *S. aureus* is a colonizing organism of the nasopharynx and posterior oropharynx and only rarely causes intraoral infection. Intraoral staphylococcal infections occur more commonly in patients with hematologic malignancies.

CLINICAL PRESENTATION

Intraoral abscesses, as well as staphylococcal mucositis and parotitis, may arise rarely as a result of *S. aureus* infection and are accompanied by regional lymphadenopathy. Staphylococcus has also been implicated in angular cheilitis. When the oral cavity is infected with phage group 2 *S. aureus*, the release of epidermolytic toxins A and B can cause staphylococcal scalded skin syndrome.

DIAGNOSIS

Culture is used to identify the organism and determine antibiotic susceptibility patterns of the pathogenic organism.

TREATMENT

Systemic antistaphylococcal antibiotics hasten resolution of intraoral staphylococcal infections. Although only about 5% of *S. aureus* isolates from the oral cavity were methicillin resistant in one recent study, antibiotic selection is best guided by antimicrobial susceptibility testing. Incision and drainage are often necessary to treat abscesses.

Diphtheria

Diphtheria is a rare upper respiratory syndrome that results from production of an exotoxin by *Corynebacterium diphtheriae*. The organism is highly contagious and is transmitted via respiratory droplets or direct mucosal contact with an infected individual. In the United State s, the incidence of disease has declined since the introduction of the diphtheria vaccine in the 1940s.

CLINICAL PRESENTATION

The three phases of upper respiratory infection include (1) catarrhal, (2) paroxysmal, and (3) convalescent phases, with the last phase causing paroxysmal coughing for weeks to months after acute infection. Intraoral manifestations of diphtheria include the development of an adherent white or grey pseudomembrane that coats the posterior oropharynx and bleeds when removed. Diffuse mucosal edema, pharyngeal ulceration, and necrosis may develop in severe disease. If oral lesions and edema extend into the airway, obstruction can result. Paralysis of the soft palate and posterior pharyngeal wall may occur as a consequence of the neurotoxic effects of the *C. diphtheriae* exotoxin. Nasal discharge often accompanies oropharyngeal signs of diphtheria and is associated with the presence of white patches on the nasal septal mucosa. Anterior cervical lymphadenopathy and acute lymphadenitis may accompany intraoral findings. Rarely, the genital mucosa may become infected and cause vulvovaginitis. Previously vaccinated individuals should have a less severe but still prolonged disease course. The presence of the characteristic pharyngeal pseudomembrane on clinical examination differentiates diphtheria from other causes of upper respiratory infection and cough.

DIAGNOSIS

Although organisms may be demonstrated on culture and PCR and fluorescent antibody tests are available, laboratory tests are relatively insensitive for *C. diphtheriae*. Therefore, diphtheria is usually diagnosed clinically and is treated empirically.

TREATMENT

Airway protection is the first goal of therapy in severe disease. Erythromycin, azithromycin, and clarithromycin are equally effective in routine cases. Trimethoprim–sulfamethoxazole may be used as an alternative agent. Prevention is achieved by widespread administration of the diphtheria, tetanus, and acellular pertussis (DTaP) vaccine to infants and children (5 total doses), as well as the adult tetanus and diphtheria (Td) booster every 10 years. The new tetanus, diphtheria, and acellular pertussis (Tdap) vaccine can substitute for one booster dose of Td.

Actinomycosis

Actinomyces spp. are anaerobic or facultative gram-positive rods commonly found in the oral mucosa. Typically, actinomycosis is caused by *A. israelii*, an organism present in the tonsillar crypts and dental calculi.

CLINICAL PRESENTATION

At the site of inoculation, yellow purulent material ("sulfur granules," or colonies of *Actinomyces*) drains from abscesses or sinuses. Generally, *Actinomyces* infects the head and neck (cervicofacial actinomycosis), with the tongue, lips, and buccal mucosa being involved infrequently. Infiltration of the tongue by *A. israelii* can rarely lead to macroglossia. Isolated involvement of the gingiva has also been reported. In severe cases, disease may extend to involve the mandibular or maxillary facial bones. Differential diagnosis includes nocardiosis, staphylococcal infection, tuberculosis, or systemic mycoses.

DIAGNOSIS

Isolation of *Actinomyces israelii* by culture is diagnostic in the appropriate clinical setting. *A. israelii* may also be visualized on histopathologic examination.

TREATMENT

Penicillin is the treatment of choice, while erythromycin or doxycycline are used in patients allergic to penicillin. Surgical debridement may also be required.

Rhinoscleroma

Rhinoscleroma, a chronic granulomatous condition of the nose and upper respiratory tract, is caused by the gram-negative coccobacillus, *Klebsiella rhinoscleromatis*. *K. rhinoscleromatis* is transmitted via inhalation of respiratory droplets. Although endemic in parts of Africa, Central America, and India, rhinoscleroma is relatively rare in the United States. Women are more commonly affected than men, and disease arises in the second and third decades of life.

CLINICAL PRESENTATION

The first symptom associated with rhinoscleroma is rhinitis that evolves into a purulent rhinorrhea. Subsequently, proliferative granulomas erupt in the nasopharynx. Ultimately, these lesions may ulcerate and undergo sclerosis and fibrosis, leading to scarring and, occasionally, stenosis of the nasal passages.

Symptoms include rhinorrhea, nasal obstruction, and epistaxis. Although the nasal cavity is involved in almost every case of rhinoscleroma, lesions may also develop in the larynx, oral cavity, sinuses, or soft tissue of the lip. Rarely, rhinoscleroma can cause upper airway obstruction. Differential diagnosis includes mucosal leishmaniasis, leprosy, lethal midline granuloma, Wegener's granulomatosis, tuberculosis, mucormycosis, and aspergillosis.

DIAGNOSIS

Subepithelial Mikulicz cells may be visualized with cytology or on biopsy with periodic acid-Schiff, Giemsa, Gram, or silver stain. Radiographic imaging of the head with CT or magnetic resonance (MR) imaging delineates the extent of disease involvement.

TREATMENT

Tetracycline, ciprofloxacin, oral rifampicin, and topical rifampicin have been shown to be effective in the treatment of rhinoscleroma. Surgical intervention or laser ablation may also be indicated.

Acute Necrotizing Ulcerative Gingivitis

Also known as "trench mouth," acute necrotizing ulcerative gingivitis (ANUG) is an intraoral infection seen in young people with poor oral hygiene. Implicated organisms include the spirochete *Borrelia vincentii* and other bacteria such as *Bacillus vicentii*, *Bacteroides* spp., and *Selenomonas* spp. Risk factors include psychological stress, smoking, poor oral hygiene, malnutrition, physical debilitation, and immunocompromise.

CLINICAL PRESENTATION

ANUG can present with the sudden onset of fiery red, painful, "punched-out" ulceration at the interdental papillary tips. Ulcers may be covered with a friable grey or yellow pseudomembrane. The disease progresses to involve the interpapillary, lingual, and facial gingiva. Ensuing necrosis may cause substantial tissue destruction. Intraoral findings may be accompanied by constitutional symptoms, such as fever, chills, and malaise. Moreover, patients have a characteristic fetid odor (*fetor oris*) to their breath.

DIAGNOSIS

ANUG is diagnosed clinically. Although various sets of diagnostic criteria have been established, most require a history of gum soreness and bleeding and the presence of blunting, ulceration, and necrosis of the interdental papillae. Foul-smelling breath and pseudomembranous, hemorrhagic ulcerations are supportive findings.

TREATMENT

ANUG is treated with local irrigation and debridement, combined with simultaneous administration of systemic antibiotics, such as metronidazole or penicillin. Treatment of predisposing factors is necessary for cure.

Noma (cancrum oris, gangrenous stomatitis)

Noma is a destructive disease of the hard and soft tissues of the face associated with multiple organisms, such as *Fusobacterium necrophorum*, *Borrelia vincentii*, *Prevotella intermedia*, *Tannerella forsynthesis*, *Porphyromonas gingivalis*, *Bacillus fusiformis*, and *Treponema denticola*. Noma typically affects children younger than 4 years living in developing countries, particularly in sub-Saharan Africa. This condition is associated with malnutrition, overcrowded living conditions, contaminated water supplies, and extreme poverty.

CLINICAL PRESENTATION

Noma starts as ulcerative gingivitis or stomatitis, with gangrenous ulcers that are covered with whitish brown fibrin on the cheeks and lips. The disease progresses rapidly, and the sloughing of necrotic tissues exposes the underlying facial bones and teeth. Associated signs include failure to thrive, salivation, fever, halitosis, anemia, and leukocytosis. Severe disfigurement often results. If left untreated, this disease is associated with a 70% to 90% mortality rate. Differential diagnosis includes lethal midline granuloma, leprosy, squamous cell carcinoma, leukemia, mucormycosis, and aspergillosis.

DIAGNOSIS

Diagnosis is made clinically. Although demonstration of implicated organisms on Gram's stain or tissue culture may be supportive, this is not usually practical.

TREATMENT

Medical therapy should include reversal of dehydration and electrolyte imbalances, as well as administration of antibiotics, such as penicillin or metronidazole. Following the acute phase, surgical debridement and repair may be indicated.

Anthrax

Human anthrax is caused by the gram-positive curved bacillus, *Bacillus anthracis*. Depending on the route of acquisition, anthrax spores may cause cutaneous, intestinal, or respiratory anthrax. In the agricultural setting, anthrax usually results from contact with *B. anthracis* spores on the skin or mucosa. Ingestion of spores, as may occur with the consumption of undercooked herbivore meat in endemic areas, can lead to anthrax of the gastrointestinal tract. Oral anthrax is rare but has been reported. In an outbreak in Northern Thailand, 24 of 52 people who developed anthrax following consumption of undercooked cattle and water buffalo had intraoral manifestations. Anthrax has been of heightened interest in recent years because of the concern regarding its use in bioterrorism, particularly after the outbreaks of inhalation anthrax associated with terrorism in 2001. Inhalation anthrax has not been associated with lesions of the mucous membranes.

CLINICAL PRESENTATION

Mucosal lesions of anthrax resemble those of cutaneous anthrax and arise at the tonsils, hard palate, and posterior oropharynx. These friable, ulcerated lesions undergo necrosis, resulting in black eschars. Mucosal lesions are almost always associated with regional lymphadenopathy. Symptoms include neck swelling, sore throat, hoarseness, and dysphagia. The patient may be otherwise asymptomatic or may have associated symptoms and signs of gastroenteritis, shock, or sepsis. Differential diagnosis includes pyogenic granuloma, Wegener's granulomatosis, syphilis, mucormycosis, and aspergillosis.

DIAGNOSIS

Diagnosis of mucosal anthrax is made by Gram's stain and culture of a lesional smear. The presence of serum antibodies and consistent epidemiologic data are supportive findings.

TREATMENT

Penicillin is the drug of choice in anthrax, although doxycycline and fluoroquinolones can also be used. Airway management is critical when significant oropharyngeal edema is present.

Bacterial vaginosis

The normal flora of the vagina is dominated by lactobacilli, organisms that acidify the vaginal environment with the production of lactic acid. Bacterial vaginosis results when the lactobacillus population is depleted. *Gardnerella (Haemophilus) vaginalis*, a small gram-negative or gram-variable unencapsulated, nonmotile rod that is present in the normal flora of the vagina, is among the organisms that proliferate pathologically in this condition. Though no evidence clearly demonstrates that bacterial vaginosis is transmitted sexually, risk factors for bacterial vaginosis include recent change of sexual partner, frequent douching, and having a female sexual partner.

CLINICAL PRESENTATION

Bacterial vaginosis can cause a stringy, gray-white, vaginal discharge that has a distinctive fishy odor. Some patients report an increase in the volume of vaginal discharge. Disease can also be asymptomatic.

DIAGNOSIS

Bacterial vaginosis is a clinical diagnosis. Amsel's criteria for diagnosis includes the presence of three of the following: (1) visualization of "clue cells" (vaginal squamous epithelial cells with coccobacilli adherent to the cell periphery) on wet prep, (2) positive amine odor test (addition of 10% potassium hydroxide to wet preparation leads to generation of the distinctive amine odor), (3) thin, watery, vaginal discharge, and (4) vaginal pH greater than 4.5. Vaginal culture is not useful, as bacterial vaginosis is due to a polymicrobial overgrowth of organisms usually present in the normal flora.

TREATMENT

Oral metronidazole is the standard treatment for bacterial vaginosis. Women should be advised to avoid alcohol while using this medication because of its disulfiram-like effect. Metronidazole gel and clindamycin cream have similar efficacy as oral metronidazole. Treatment is particularly important in pregnant women, as bacterial vaginosis has been correlated with an increased incidence of preterm labor.

Pseudomonas aeruginosa

Even though *Pseudomonas aeruginosa* thrives in moist environments, infection in the non-respiratory oral and genital mucosa is rare. Necrotizing stomatitis caused by *Pseudomonas aeruginosa* has been described previously in a case series of three patients. Each of these patients were immunocompromised. Authors proposed that these oral lesions represent a mucosal variant of ecthyma gangrenosum.

Table 22.10: Bacterial Organisms That Do Not Usually Cause Disease of the Oral and Genital Mucous Membranes

Aeromonas hydrophila	Klebsiella pneumonia
Bacillus cereus	Legionella pneumophila
Borderella pertussis	Listeria monocytogenes
Borrelia burgdorferi	Pseudomonas aeruginosa
Brucella spp.	Rickettsia spp.
Campylobacter spp.	Salmonella spp.
Clostridium perfringens	Shigella spp.
Escherichia coli	Vibrio spp.
Helicobacter pylori	Yersinia spp.
Hemophilus influenza	

Mycoplasma pneumoniae

Typically a respiratory pathogen, *Mycoplasma pneumoniae* has also been implicated in the development of erythematous vesicles of the oral and genital mucosa, stomatitis, erythema multiforme, and severe erythema multiforme (Stevens-Johnson syndrome). Patients with oropharyngeal involvement from *M. pneumoniae* infection generally have a concurrent infection of the lower respiratory tract.

Tetanus

Tetanus is caused by the tetanospasmin toxin of *Clostridium tetani*, an anaerobic, gram-positive bacillus. Infection results in trismus (*lockjaw, risus sardonicus*) and generalized muscle spasms, followed by apnea and, ultimately, death. A previous report of a patient who developed tetanus without a clear source documented complete disease resolution following dental extraction and gingival debridement. The authors concluded that the source of infection was periodontal.

Bacterial organisms that do not usually cause disease of the oral or genital mucous membranes include (Table 22.10) *Aeromonas hydrophila, Bacillus cereus, Bordetella pertussis, Borrelia burgdorferi, Brucella* spp., *Campylobacter* spp., *Clostridium perfringens, Escherichia coli, Helicobacter pylori, Hemophilus influenza, Klebsiella pneumonia, Legionella pneumophila, Listeria monocytogenes, Pseudomonas aeruginosa, Rickettsia* spp., *Salmonella* spp., *Shigella* spp., *Vibrio* spp., and *Yersinia* spp.

Protozoa

Trichomoniasis

Trichomoniasis results from infection with the sexually transmitted intracellular protozoan, *Trichomonas vaginalis*. Epidemiologic risk factors include harboring other sexually transmitted infections, engaging in sexual activity with a new partner or engaging in sexual activity more frequently than once weekly, and having more than three sexual partners in the preceding month. Trichomoniasis commonly causes vaginitis and urethritis, while oral disease is uncommon.

CLINICAL PRESENTATION

Oral trichomoniasis can present as generalized mucosal inflammation covered with an overlying exudate. Trichomonas vaginitis is symptomatic in most women. Specifically, patients describe dyspareunia, labial pruritus, dysuria, and copious, yellow or green, frothy, odiferous vaginal discharge. On clinical examination, petechiae may be present on the vulva and cervix (*strawberry cervix*). In men, trichomoniasis is usually asymptomatic, although there may be some irritation of the urethra, penile pruritus, or first-void urethral discharge. In both sexes, the involved mucosal surfaces may develop erythematous puncta resulting from local vasodilation and an overlying layer of exudate. Incubation period is 5 to 28 days.

DIAGNOSIS

Trichomonas vaginalis is a highly motile rod that can be seen as a pear-shaped, unicellular organism with two pairs of anterior flagella on wet mount saline preparation. This finding is nonspecific for *T. vaginalis*, however, as other motile trichomonads frequently are present in the mouth or gastrointestinal tract (i.e. *T. tenax* and *T. hominis*, respectively). With trichomonal cervicitis, vaginal pH is typically greater than 4.5 (normal vaginal pH: 4.0).

TREATMENT

The treatment of choice is oral metronidazole, although tinidazole may be used for metronidazole-resistant trichomoniasis. Sexual partners must also be treated.

Leishmaniasis

Leishmaniasis occurs as a result of infection with the protozoan parasite, *Leishmania* spp. The vector is the female sandfly *Phlebotomus* in Old World leishmaniasis and *Lutzomyia* in New World leishmaniasis. Although the patient often reports a recent history of travel to an endemic area, the latency period from infection to the development of clinical manifestations may extend for years.

Leishmaniasis is classified as cutaneous (CL), mucocutaneous (MCL), or visceral (VL). Mucosal lesions are almost exclusively seen in mucocutaneous leishmaniasis, which is caused by *L. braziliensis*. Oral lesions in association with *L. amazonensis* infection also have been documented. Finally, a recent case report describes oral ulcers in a patient with visceral leishmaniasis, although the particular species of *Leishmaniasis* was not reported.

CLINICAL PRESENTATION

Mucosal findings are accompanied by cutaneous signs of leishmaniasis and typically include nonspecific erythematous regions of induration that can become eroded or ulcerated (Fig. 22.13). Mucocutaneous leishmaniasis has a predilection for the nasal septum and larynx, although involvement of the tongue, soft palate, and hard palate may also occur. Nasal septum perforation and significant facial disfigurement may ensue if the patient remains untreated. Differential diagnosis includes paracoccidioidomycosis, histoplasmosis, syphilis, leprosy, Wegener's granulomatosis, tuberculosis, mucormycosis, rhinoscleroma, aspergillosis, systemic mycoses, and nasopharyngeal carcinoma.

DIAGNOSIS

The preferred method of diagnosis is examination of a dermal thin smear obtained from the border of an active lesion. This demonstrates the presence of amastigotes. Organisms also can be isolated with culture. Histopathology reveals a nonspecific granulomatous reaction, and organisms may be seen with

Table 22.11: Protozoal Organisms That Do Not Usually Cause Disease of the Oral and Genital Mucous Membranes

Plasmodium Falciparum

Trypanosoma spp.

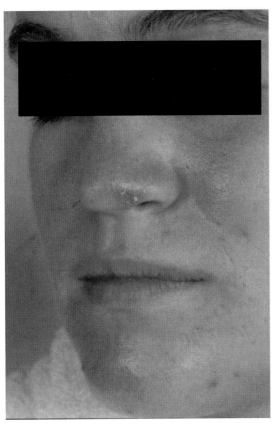

Figure 22.13. Leishmaniasis.

Giemsa stain. Serology and PCR can also be used to confirm diagnosis. A high index of suspicion is required in geographic regions in which leishmaniasis is not endemic.

TREATMENT

Pentavalent antimonies are the standard treatment of mucocutaneous leishmaniasis, although amphotericin B is the drug of choice for advanced disease. Early therapy can lead to an excellent cure rate. A recent study found that itraconazole is not an effective pharmacologic alternative. Disease is prevented in endemic areas with use of netting impregnated with permethrin, protective clothing, and insect repellent.

Protozoal organisms that do not usually cause disease of the oral or genital mucous membranes include (Table 22.11) *Plasmodium falciparum* and *Trypanosoma* spp.

PITFALLS AND MYTHS

One of the most common pitfalls in assessing infections of the mucosal membranes is the failure to fully examine the mucosa. This can be readily overcome by routinely and meticulously examining the oral cavity and genitalia in patients who have signs or symptoms suggestive of mucosal disease. Another common pitfall is to mistake normal clinical findings for pathology. The importance of routine mucosal examination as a means to gain familiarity with normal mucosal anatomy cannot be overemphasized.

Even when a thorough examination is performed, accurate diagnosis of mucosal infections can be challenging, because similarly appearing lesions may result from a variety of insults to these tissues. Therefore, the practitioner should obtain a complete patient history, including constitutional symptoms, travel history, sexual practices, and environmental exposures. This is particularly important in diagnostically challenging cases. Finally, the index of suspicion for atypical disease presentations or unusual opportunistic infections must be raised when evaluating immunocompromised patients.

SUGGESTED READINGS

Bruce AJ, Rogers RS 3rd. Acute oral ulcers. *Dermatol Clin* 2003; 21:1–15.

Bruce AJ, Rogers RS 3rd . Oral manifestations of sexually transmitted diseases. *Clin Dermatol* 2004;22(6):520–527.

Eckert LO. Acute vulvovaginitis. *N Engl J Med* 2006;355(12):1244–1252.

Fiumara NJ. Genital ulcer infections in the female patient and the vaginitides. *Dermatol Clin* 1997;15(2):233–245.

Gerber MA. Diagnosis and treatment of pharyngitis in children. *Ped Clin North Am* 2005;52(3):729–747, vi.

Glick M, Siegel MA. Viral and fungal infections of the oral cavity in immunocompetent patients. *Infect Dis Clin North Am* 1999; 13:817–831.

Grudeva-Popova J, Goranov S. Mucocutaneous infections in hematologic malignancies. *Folia Medica* 1999;41(3):40–44.

Hutton KP, Rogers RS 3rd. Recurrent aphthous stomatitis. *Dermatol Clin* 1987;5:761–768.

Knowles MR, Boucher RC. Mucus clearance as a primary innate defense mechanism for mammalian airways. *J Clin Invest* 2002; 109(5):571–577.

Laskaris G. Oral manifestations of infectious diseases. *Dent Clin North Am* 1996;40(2):395–423.

Laskaris G. *Color atlas of oral disease*. 3rd edition. New York: Thieme Stuttgart, 2003.

Maderazo EG, Jameson JM. Infections and the host. In: Topazian RG, Goldberg MH, Hupp JR, eds. *Oral and maxillofacial infections*. 4th edition. St. Louis: W. B. Saunders, 2002.

McNally MA, Langlais RP. Conditions peculiar to the tongue. *Dermatol Clin* 1996;12:257–272.

Pusey WA. *The History of Dermatology*. Springfield, Illinois: Thomas Books, 1933.

Rogers RS 3rd, Bruce AJ. The tongue in clinical diagnosis. *J Eur Acad Dermatol Venereol* 2004;18:254–259.

Schuster GS. Microbiology of the orofacial region. In: Topazian RG, Goldberg MH, Hupp JR, eds. *Oral and Maxillofacial Infections*. 4th edition. St. Louis: W.B. Saunders, 2002.

Terezhalmy GT, Naylor GD. Disorders affecting the oral cavity. Oral manifestations of selected sexually related conditions. *Dermatol Clin* 1996;14(2):303–317.

VIRUSES

Burd EM. Human papillomavirus and cervical cancer. *Clin Microbiol Rev* 2003;16(1):1–17.

Choukas NC, Toto PD. Condylomata acuminatum of the oral cavity. *Oral Surg Oral Med Oral Pathol* 1982;54:480–485.

Corey L, Spear PG. Infections with herpes simplex viruses (2). *N Engl J Med* 1986;314:749–757.

De Faria, PR, Vargas, PA, Saldiva, PH, Bohm, GM, Mauad, T, de Almeida, OP. Tongue disease in advanced AIDS. *Oral Dis* 2005;11(2):72–80.

Eisen D. The clinical characteristics of intraoral herpes simplex virus infection in 52 immunocompetent patients. *Oral Surg Oral Med Oral Pathol Oral Radiol Endod* 1998;86:432–437.

Garlick JA, Taichman LB. Human papillomavirus infection of the oral mucosa. *Am J Dermatopathol* 1991;13:386–395.

Glick M, Muzyka BC, Lurie D, et al. Oral manifestations associated with HIV-related disease as markers for immune suppression and AIDS. *Oral Surg Oral Med Oral Pathol* 1994;77:344–349.

Greenberg MS. Disorders affecting the oral cavity: HIV-associated lesions. *Dermatol Clin* 1996;14(viii-ix):319–326.

Greenspan D, Greenspan JS. Oral mucosal manifestations of AIDS. *Dermatol Clin* 1987;5:733–737.

Hairston BR, Bruce AJ, Rogers RS 3rd . Viral diseases of the oral mucosa. *Dermatol Clin* 2003;21:17–32.

Jing W, Ismail R: Mucocutaneous manifestations of HIV infection: a retrospective analysis of 145 cases in a Chinese population in Malaysia. *Int J Dermatol* 1999;38:457–463.

Katz J, Guelmann M, Stavropolous M, Heft M. Gingival and other oral manifestations in measles virus infection. *J Clin Periodont* 2003;30(7):665–668.

Leong IT, Fernandes BJ, Mock D. Epstein-Barr virus detection in non-Hodgkin's lymphoma of the oral cavity: an immunocytochemical and in situ hybridization study. *Oral Surg Oral Med Oral Pathol Oral Radiol Endod* 2001;92:184–193.

Lynch DP. Oral manifestations of HIV disease: an update. *Semin Cutan Med Surg* 1997;16:257–264.

Lynch DP. Oral viral infections. *Clin Dermatol* 2000;18:619–628.

Mikala G, Xie J, Berencsi G, Kiss C, Marton I, Domjan G, Valyi-Nagy I. Human herpesvirus 8 in hematologic diseases. *Pathol Oncol Res* 1999;5(1):73–79.

Miller CS. Disorders affecting the oral cavity: viral infections in the immunocompetent patient. *Dermatol Clin* 1996;14:225–241.

Meyrick Thomas RH, Dodd H, Yeo J, et al. Oral acyclovir in the suppression of recurrent non-genital herpes simplex virus infection. *Br J Dermatol* 1985;113:731–735.

Moussavi S. Focal epithelial hyperplasia: report of two cases and review of literature. *J Am Dent Assoc* 1986;113:900–902.

Nahass GT, Goldstein B, Zhu W, Serfling U, Penneys N, Leonardi C. Comparison of Tzanck smear, viral culture, and DNA diagnostic methods in detection of herpes simplex and varicella-zoster infection. *JAMA* 1992;268:2541–2544.

Pielop J, Wood AC, Hsu S. Update on antiviral therapy for herpes simplex virus infection. *Dermatol Ther* 2000;13:235–257.

Rooney J, Bryson Y, Mannix ML, et al. Prevention of ultraviolet-light-induced herpes labialis by sunscreen. *Lancet* 1991; 338:1419–1422.

Rooney JF, Strauss S, Mannix M, et al. Oral acyclovir to suppress frequently recurrent herpes labialis: a double-blind, placebo-controlled trial. *Ann Intern Med* 1993;118:268–272.

Safrin S, Shaw H, Bolan G, et al. Comparison of virus culture and the polymerase chain reaction for diagnosis of mucocutaneous herpes simplex virus infection. *Sex Transm Dis* 1997;24: 176–180.

Samonis G, Mantadakis E, Maraki S. Orofacial viral infections in the immunocompromised host. *Oncol Rep* 2000;7:1389–1394.

Saslow D, Castle PE, Cox JT, Davey DD, Einstein MH, Ferris DG, et al. American Cancer Society Guideline for human papillomavirus (HPV) vaccine use to prevent cervical cancer and its precursors. *CA Cancer J Clin* 2007;57(1):7–28.

Schofer H, Ochsendorf FR, Helm EB, et al. Treatment of oral "hairy" leukoplakia in AIDS patients with vitamin A acid (topically) or acyclovir (systemically). *Dermatologica* 1987;174:150–151.

Scott DA, Coulter WA, Lamey PJ. Oral shedding of herpes simplex virus type I: a review. *J Oral Pathol Med* 1997;26:441–447.

Slots J. Update on human cytomegalovirus in destructive periodontal disease. *Oral Microbiol Immunol* 2004 Aug;19(4):217–223.

Straus SE, Rooney JF, Hallahan C. Acyclovir suppresses subclinical shedding of herpes simplex virus. *Ann Intern Med* 1996;125(9):776.

Swan RH, McDaniel RK, Dreiman BB, et al. Condyloma acuminatum involving the oral mucosa. *Oral Surg Oral Med Oral Pathol* 1981;51:503–508.

Vander Straten MR, Carrasco D, Tyring SK. Treatment of human herpesvirus 8 infections. *Dermatol Ther* 2000;13:277–284.

Whitley RJ, Gnann Jwj. The epidemiology and clinical manifestations of herpes simplex virus infections. In: Roizman B, Whitley RJ, Lopez C, eds. *The human herpesviruses.* New York: Raven Press, 1993.

Wutzler P. Antiviral therapy of herpes simplex and varicella zoster virus infections. *Intervirology* 1997;40:343–56.

FUNGI

Barrak, HA. Hard palate perforation due to mucormycosis: report of four cases. *J Laryngol Otol* 2007; 1–4 (E-pub).

Bingham JS. Vulvo-vaginal candidosis – an overview. *Acta Derm Verereol (Stockh)* 1986;121:39–46.

de Almeida OP, Scully C: Oral lesions in the systemic mycoses. *Curr Opin Dent* 1991;1(4):423–8.

Fotos PG, Lilly JP. Clinical management of oral and perioral candidosis. *Dermatol Clin* 1996;14(2):273–280.

Godoy A, Reichart PA. Oral manifestations of paracoccidioidomycosis: report of 21 cases from Argentina. Mycoses 2003;46:412–417.

Kancherla VS. Mumps resurgence in the United States. *J Allergy Clin Immunol* 2006;118(4):938–941.

Lehner T, Ward RG. Iatrogenic oral candidosis. *Br J Dermatol* 1970;83:161–166.

Lilic D. New perspectives on the immunology of chronic mucocutaneous candidiasis. *Curr Opin Infect Dis* 2002;15:143–147.

Mehrabi M, Bagheri S, Leonard MK Jr, Perciaccante VJ. Mucocutaneous manifestation of cryptococcal infection: report of a case and review of the literature. *J Oral Maxillofac Surg* 2005 Oct;63(10):1543–1549.

Meyer RD. Cutaneous and mucosal manifestations of the deep mycotic infections. *Acta Derm Venereol Suppl* 1986;121:57–72.

Ray TL. Oral candidiasis. *Dermatol Clin* 1987;5(4):651–662.

Rodriguez RA, Konia T. Coccidioidomycosis of the tongue. *Arch Pathol Lab Med* 2005 Jan;129(1):e4–6.

Rosman N. Oropharyngeal and cutaneous candidosis in patients with decreased resistance to infections. *Acta Derm Venereol (Stockh)* 1986;121:47–49.

Scully C, de Almeida OP. Orofacial manifestations of the systemic mycoses. *J Oral Pathol Med* 1992;21(7):289–294.

Sposto MR, Mendes-Giannini M, Moraes R, Branco R, Scully C. Paracoccidioidomycosis manifesting as oral lesions: clinical, cytological and serological investigation. *J Oral Pathol Med* 1994;23(2):85–87.

BACTERIA

Bozbora A, Erbil Y, Berber E, Ozarmagan S, Ozarmagan G. Surgical treatment of granuloma inguinale. *Br J Dermatol* 1998;138(6):1079–1081.

Dalmau J, Alegre M, Roe E, Sambeat M, Alomar A. Nodules on the tongue in an HIV-positive patient. *Scand J Infect Dis* 2006;38(9):822–825.

Enwonwu CO. Noma – the ulcer of extreme poverty. *N Engl J Med* 2006;354(3):221–224.

Enwonwu CO. Noma (orofacial gangrene). *Int J Dermatol* 2005; 44(8):707.

Ferris DG, Litaker MS, Woodward L, Mathis D, Hendrich J. Treatment of bacterial vaginosis: a comparison of oral metronidazole, metronidazole vaginal gel, and clindamycin vaginal cream. *J Fam Pract* 1995;41(5):443–449.

Gregory DS: Pertussis. a disease affecting all ages. *Am Fam Physician* 2006;74(3):382.

Johnson BD, Engel D. Acute necrotizing ulcerative gingivitis: a review of diagnosis, etiology and treatment. *J Periodontol* 1986 Mar;57(3):141–150.

Laskaris, G. PL10 Oral manifestations of orogenital bacterial infections. *Oral Dis* 2006;12(s1):2–3.

Leao JC, Gueiros LA, Porter SR. Oral manifestations of syphilis. *Clinics* 2006;61(2):161–166.

Lenis A, Ruff T, Diaz JA, Ghandour EG. Rhinoscleroma. *South Med J* 1988;81(12):1580–2.

Miller KE. Diagnosis and treatment of C. trachomatis infection. *Am Fam Physician* 2006;73(8):1411–1416.

Roberts A. Bacteria in the mouth. *Dent Update* 2005 Apr;32(3): 134–136,139–140,142.

Scott CM, Flint SR. Oral syphilis – re-emergence of an old disease with oral manifestations. *Int J Oral Maxillofac Surg* 2005;34:58–63.

Sirisanthana T, Brown AE. Anthrax of the gastrointestinal tract. *Emerg Infect Dis* 2002;8(7):649–651.

Sirisanthana T, Navachareon N, Tharavichitkul P, Sirisanthana V, Brown AE. Outbreak of oral-oropharyngeal anthrax: an unusual manifestation of human infection with Bacillus anthracis. *Am J Trop Med Hyg* 1984;33(1):144–150.

Smith AJ, Robertson D, Tang MK, Jackson MS, MacKenzie D, Bagg J. Staphylococcus aureus in the oral cavity: a three-year retrospective analysis of clinical laboratory data. *Br Dent J* 2003;195(12):701–703.

Ulmer A, Fierlbeck G. Oral manifestations of secondary syphilis. *N Engl J Med* 2002;347(21):1677.

Veeranna S, Raghu TY. Oral donovanosis. *Int J STD AIDS* 2002; 13(12):855–856.

Wang J. Bacterial vaginosis. *Prim Care Update Ob Gyns* 2000;7(5):181–185.

PROTOZOA

Forna F, Gulmezoglu AM. Interventions for treating trichomoniasis in women. *Cochrane Database Syst Rev* 2003(2):CD000218.

Motta ACF, Lopes MA, Ito FA, Carlos-Bregni R, de Almeida OP, Roselino AM. Oral leishmaniasis: a clinicopathological study of 11 cases. *Oral Dis Online Early Article* 2006.

PART VI: SPECIAL DISEASE CATEGORIES

23 | INFECTIONS IN SKIN SURGERY

Jean-Michel Amici, Anne-Marie Rogues, and Alain Taïeb

HISTORY

Dermatologic surgery has grown in popularity and stature during the past few decades. Skin surgery is routinely performed by dermatologists and plastic surgeons, mostly using local anaesthesia. Types of skin surgery include, skin biopsy (punch biopsy, shave biopsy, incisional biopsy, and excisional biopsy), excision of the skin lesion, curettage, and cautery, flap, skin grafting, and Mohs microscopically controlled excision (for cancers at high risk of local recurrence). It is common to remove benign tumors. It is even more common to remove malignant tumors such as basal cell carcinoma (BCC), squamous cell carcinoma (SCC), or melanoma. Skin cancer is the most common malignancy in humans and its incidence, especially that of BCC, has increased over the last decades and is still increasing. Left untreated, these lesions may become locally destructive (BCC) and others (SCC and mostly melanoma) have a potential for metastasis. The primary treatment of cutaneous neoplasms is surgical excision, and dermatologists have expanded their practice to include surgical procedures in response to the epidemic of cutaneous tumors related to an increased elderly population worldwide. Besides the treatment of tumors, dermatologic surgery is used for cosmetic purposes, and in emergency cases to drain abscesses or inflamed cysts.

A survey of the American Society for Dermatologic Surgery found that members performed about 3.9 million procedures a year. Of these procedures, skin cancer surgery was the most common with 1.4 million operations. Surgery performed by dermatologists on an outpatient basis under local anesthesia is less costly than other more complex options and has become the treatment of choice for many cutaneous malignancies.

This chapter focuses on infections within the context of conventional excisional surgery excluding facial resurfacing, liposuction, and other cosmetic surgical procedures.

Thus, we will first review the description, frequency, and risk factors for skin infections following dermatologic surgery. And in the second part, we will discuss management and prevention.

EPIDEMIOLOGY OF SKIN SURGERY INFECTIONS

Definition and Classification

Infection after skin surgery is a surgical site infection (SSI) defined by the Centers for Disease Control and Prevention (CDC) as any surgical wound that produces a suppuration within 30 days of the procedure, even in the absence of a positive culture. Inflammation without suppuration is not sufficient to classify the wound as infected. The CDC wound classification correlates four degrees of contamination of wounds with subsequent infection rates (Table 23.1).

Most dermatological procedures are considered "clean" or "clean-contaminated." The Mohs extirpation of cutaneous tumors is more correctly classified as a clean-contaminated procedure. As a consequence, acceptable rates of wound infection for "clean" procedures are thought to range between 1% and 4% or between 5% and 10% for "clean-contaminated" procedures.

A literature search for the incidence of infections in skin surgery produced a very limited number of relevant publications, and studies that have looked at postoperative wound infection rates in dermatologic surgery indicate a lower rate of infection than expected in the CDC classification. Indeed, the frequency of SSI in skin surgery reported in different studies varies between 0.7% and 7.6%. This wide range is explained by different types of wound and patient categories.

One of the first studies was conducted by Whitaker and colleagues, who found an overall infection rate of 0.7% while performing over 3,900 clinic-based dermatologic surgical procedures including Mohs surgery, simple excisions, flaps, grafts, scalp reductions, and hair transplantations. Dettenkofer et al. followed a cohort of 995 patients undergoing surgical procedures in a German university hospital. They reported an infection rate of 7.6% after surgery for BCC. In this study, none of the 163 patients with malignant melanoma acquired an infection after surgery. Regarding Mohs surgery, Futoryan and Grande reported an overall infection rate of 2.4% in 520 cases. Two large prospective studies that reported data on dermatologic surgery proceeding without Mohs micrographic surgery (MMS) in outpatients showed an overall incidence of infections of 1.5% and 1.9%.

In a prospective study assessing the incidence of various complications associated with MMS based on 1,358 procedures for skin cancers, the complication rate was 1.6% with only one wound infection. In the Australian Mohs database which includes 2,673 patients, a total of 11.7% of cases had recipient-site complication, and infection accounted for only 3.5% of all complications (graft hypertrophy: 42.3%, partial graft failure: 27.2%, and graft contraction: 15.3%).

The total incidence of anesthetic, hemorrhagic, and infectious complications in 3,788 surgical procedures performed by a French dermatologist was 5.6% including 2.1% for wound infections. The first signs of clinical infection following procedure appeared a mean of 6.3 days (1–12 days) later.

By far, the most common pathogen isolated in SSIs is *Staphylococcus aureus*. Streptococcal species, *Pseudomonas aeruginosa* and coliform bacteria, are also occasionally encountered,

Table 23.1: Wound Status and Infection Rate

Wound Status	Class		Infection Rate %
Clean	I	Elective incision on non-inflamed tissues using strict aseptic technique	1–4
Clean-contaminated	II	Surgery in contaminated areas (axilla, perineum, mucosal areas)	5–10
Contaminated	III	Major breaks in sterile technique, obviously inflamed skin	6–25
Infected	IV	Frank purulence (Abscess)	>25

especially in selected anatomic sites, such as the perioral area or ear. *Pseudomonas aeruginosa* is known to colonize the auricular canal, and thereby as a result there is a relatively high risk of infection for any wound that involves the auricular cartilage.

Risk factors

Multiple factors play a role in increasing the risk of surgical wound infections. They can be classified into three categories: intrinsic factors that relate to host defenses, an independent category related to the nature of the surgical procedure, and extrinsic factors that are aimed at decreasing the opportunity for bacterial contamination.

Intrinsic factors related to the patient

Aspects of the patients' health may affect a propensity to wound infection. Many preexisting, sometimes coexistent, conditions have been identified in the literature as risk factors for SSIs. These include diabetes mellitus, obesity, smoking, renal failure, malnutrition, corticosteroid use and other immunosuppressant medications, and an immunocompromised status. However, in dermatologic surgery such risk factors have rarely been significantly linked with SSIs.

Smoking may be an important risk factor in undesired outcomes of cutaneous surgery. In a retrospective study that evaluated the effects of cigarette smoking on tissue survival in wounds repaired after Mohs extirpations (916 flaps and full-thickness grafts performed during a 10-year period), heavy smokers (1 or more packs per day) developed tissue necrosis at a rate that was approximately 3-fold higher than that of controls.

Factors related to the nature of the surgical procedure

TYPE OF PROCEDURE AND REPAIR

Regarding the surgical technique, flap surgery has a significantly higher infection incidence than elliptical excision and closure. There is some evidence that more complicated procedures (flaps or skin grafts) are associated with increased infection rates, independent of the size of the excision. However, this should be mitigated by the notion that well-designed flaps and grafts maximize blood supply and minimize ischemia, which can lead to the development of devitalized tissue and the potential for wound infection. In our experience, the incidence of wound infections was higher for excisions with a reconstructive procedure. However, no difference was found in the incidence of infectious complications between two types of simple excision surgical procedures with an overall scar of less than 2 cm or an overall scar greater than 2 cm.

In Mohs surgery, the mean area of the infected defects was twice that of the noninfected group, and procedures performed on the ear were found to have a higher rate of wound infections. Longer procedure duration led to a greater risk of infectious complications which was consistent with other reported surgery practices.

TYPE OF LESION

In an Australian general practice study the histological subtypes, basal cell carcinoma (BCC) (11.4%) and squamous cell carcinoma (SCC) (13.5%), and prevalence of diabetes were independently correlated with wound infection. Those findings were consistent with a study conducted in a specialist dermatology clinic, which suggested that oncologic surgery (excision for skin cancer) is associated with a higher risk of infection. In a recent study concerning 1,400 Mohs procedures, the difference in infection rate between SCC and BCC was statistically significant. It was 2.7% for SCC versus 1.4% for BCC.

LOCATION

Some anatomical areas with moist conditions and increased resident microbial counts, such as the ear or facial region, have a higher risk of developing a wound infection. The study of Futuroyan et al. clearly shows that the infection rate for MMS performed on the ear is significantly higher than on non-ear anatomic sites. In this study, wound infections on the ear occurred in 6 out of 48 patients with an infection rate of 12.5%. Furthermore, there was a significantly higher risk of wound infection when cartilage was involved. The rate was 28.5% versus the 5.9% found in cases where the tumor-free tissue was above the level of the cartilage. This rate is higher than the recent study reported by Campbell, who mentioned a rate of infection of 5.5% in 144 excisions of BCC and SCCs of the auricular area or that of Kaplan and Cook who had no cases of suppurative chondritis in 337 patients who underwent cartilage procedures.

In a French multicenter study reported by our group, the infection rate for procedures performed on the nose or nostril was higher than that found for other anatomical locations whatever the size of the excision. In another study the higher risk of infection for nasal or auricular areas was found to be independent of the type of lesion being excised (benign vs. malignant) or of the complexity of the surgery (skin grafts and local flaps). Other body locations reported to be at a higher risk for wound infection following dermatologic surgery included the lip and the axilla.

Extremities are believed to be at a higher risk of wound infection. Surgery below the knee (n = 448) had an infection incidence of 6.9% (31/448). Multivariate generalized linear modeling conducted on data provided by a prospective study on minor skin excisions in Australian general practice also confirmed increased infectious risk for legs, feet, and thighs (15%).

BLEEDING DURING PROCEDURE

A prospective multivariate analysis of 3,788 surgical skin procedures showed that hemorrhagic complication is an independent factor for SSIs. The control of hemorrhagic complications is an important challenge to prevent SSIs. Maintaining good hemostasis and eliminating "dead space" via the appropriate use of sutures, the use of pressure dressing, and occlusion are significant surgical considerations to help minimize postoperative morbidity.

MANAGEMENT AND PREVENTION

Management of infection after skin surgery

In cases of suspicion of a postoperative wound infection, the wound should be examined in a sterile facility under local anesthesia if required. Some or all sutures are removed and, after the wound is sampled for culture, the wound is washed to remove all debris. The wound can either be packed with sterile gauze or allowed to remain open to heal by second intention. Empirical antibiotics are begun, based on the presumed causal pathogen, and can be adjusted based on the culture susceptibility profiles.

In our experience, most infections after skin surgery were minor superficial suppurations requiring additional antibiotic treatment, in 18 of 79 cases. However, cases of serious infectious complications after dermatologic surgery have been reported: such as toxic shock syndrome and necrotizing fasciitis following excision of a malignant melanoma. Disastrous outcomes such as suppurative chondritis are fortunately exceedingly rare following incisions or manipulation of auricular cartilage.

Aseptic technique

Little is known about the sterile conditions required for this type of surgery and the optimal resources needed are unclear.

The surgical hand scrub serves to remove transient flora and soil from the fingernails and hands. For minor or short-lived procedures, the literature does not support the need for a formal surgical hand scrub, but it is recommended before more lengthy or invasive procedures.

Surgical gloves provide a second line of defense against potential contamination from the hand flora of the surgical team. In dermatologic surgery, gloves become perforated in approximately 11% of procedures, and the wearer recognizes that a perforation has occurred in only 17% of these cases. In this manner, the aseptic barrier between the surgeon's hand and the patient's wound can be unknowingly breached for extended periods of time. The risk of glove perforation in dermatologic surgery is lower than in other specialties and double gloving provides additional protection from perforation but may limit sensitivity and dexterity.

A recent study evaluating infection rates in 1,400 surgical procedures revealed no statistical difference in infection rates when sterile or nonsterile gloves were used for MMS before reconstruction. However, it was a retrospective study and the surgeons involved used sterile gloves for all reconstructions. Recently, in a prospective study, with 3,491 dermatologic surgical procedures, there was a significantly higher risk of infectious complications when no sterile gloves were worn for excisions with a reconstructive procedure, even after controlling other factors, and irrespective of the place where the surgery was performed (private office or hospital setting).

Gowns serve as personal protection but there is no scientific data to show that wearing a sterile gown versus not wearing one affects the incidence of SSIs in skin surgery. Sterile gowns may be considered optional for minor surgical procedures. Face masks were originally designed to limit contamination of the surgical site from microorganisms expelled by operators. They not only protect the surgical wound from airborne contamination but also serve to protect the wearer's mouth and nose from unexpected splashes of blood and bodily fluids. All devices that enter the sterile field must be sterile. Instruments should be steam autoclaved. Sterile drapes serve to protect the surgical site from microorganisms present on the surrounding nonsterile surfaces.

There is no published evidence that dermatologic surgical procedures are riskier when carried out in a private office as opposed to a hospital setting. Hospital theatres are not required for most dermatologic surgery procedures. Further studies have shown that dermatologic surgery can be safely performed in outpatient settings without a significant risk of infection. The data from Cook and Perone confirm that office-based dermatologic surgery involving Mohs surgery and reconstruction is very safe when performed by properly trained physicians. A controlled trial study is needed to confirm that the risk factor for dermatologic surgery procedures carried out in private office as opposed to hospital setting is not different irrespective of the procedure or the type of patients. However, there are sufficient grounds to approach surgery on certain locations or certain patient types with appropriate caution. Kaplan's experience has suggested that the frequency of inflammatory and infectious complications associated with the manipulation of auricular skin and cartilage during reconstructive procedures is minimal when sterile, gentle operative techniques are used.

Surgical site care

Surgical site preparation is a major goal to lower the resident bacterial count as much as possible and limit rebound growth with minimal skin irritation. A preoperative shower with an antiseptic soap has been shown to decrease wound infection rates and may be considered for procedures with large surgical fields. At the time of the surgery, after a thorough cleansing, it is necessary to apply an antiseptic solution appropriate for the location. Heavily colonized areas such as the umbilicus or nasal vestibule should receive close attention. Similar to cardiac surgery, where intranasal mupirocin treatment decreases the rate of *Staphylococcus aureus* surgical site infection, this strategy could be effective in skin surgery. Administration of intranasal mupirocin before surgery is cost saving because health care-associated infections are very expensive.

Hair removal is only indicated if the hair will obscure the surgical field or hinder proper surgical technique. Shaving with a razor in particular should be avoided, because it causes abrasions that compromise skin integrity and allow bacteria to flourish.

Wound dressing is an important part of surgical site care. No single dressing is suitable for all types of wounds. Dressings should perform one or more of the following functions: maintain a moist environment at the wound, absorb excess exudates without leakage to the surface of the dressing, provide thermal insulation and mechanical protection, provide bacterial protection, be nonadherent to the wound and easily removed without trauma, be nontoxic, nonallergic, nonsensitizing, and sterile.

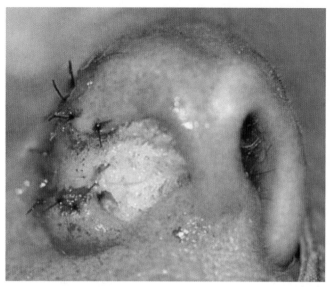

Figure 23.1. Intranasal dressing.

Wound dressing and tape, with or without pressure to encourage hemostasis, are important to help prevent wound infections. Pressure dressings help prevent postoperative hematoma formation. We recommend the use of an intranasal dressing during surgery of the nasal sidewall because this area is particularly susceptible to hemorrhage and infection. Packing done with tulle gauze has three advantages: it acts as a support block to improve the compressive nature of the external dressing, it acts as a nostril conformator and finally, it physically limits colonization of the wound by endonostril bacteria (Fig. 23.1).

Guidelines for managing surgical wounds that are primarily closed (i.e., those with the skin edges re-approximated at the end of the procedure) include instructing the patients to keep their wound dry and covered for 24 to 48 hours. This allows a degree of epithelialization to take place and seals the edges of the wound from bacterial contamination. However, if the dressing becomes soaked with blood or wound exudates before then, a change of dressing is necessary.

Antibiotic prophylaxis

The usage of wound infection prophylaxis in dermatologic surgery varies greatly from surgeon to surgeon, with some studies reporting a widespread usage of antibiotics. Some Mohs surgeons use prophylactic antibiotics in up to 77% of cases. Antibiotic wound infection prophylaxis for dermatologic surgery can be topical (including within the wound itself) and systemic.

In a prospective randomized controlled trial, Dixon et al. demonstrated a lack of efficacy of topical mupirocin in preventing wound infections in skin cancer surgery. A controlled study has compared the incidence of suppurative chondritis after auricular surgery in patients who have received gentamicin ointment versus petrolatum during second-intention healing of auricular wounds after Mohs surgery. There was no statistically significant difference between the two groups of patients in terms of postoperative auricular suppurative chondritis but the data demonstrates a disproportionate number of cases of inflammatory chondritis in patients who used gentamicin ointment. This study, however, was not powered sufficiently to obtain statistical

significance. Regarding inflammatory chondritis, Smack and colleagues noted similar observations in their comparisons of bacitracin and petrolatum. They randomized 922 postsurgical patients into two groups receiving topical therapy and prospectively evaluated infection rates. Overall infection rates in both groups were less than 2% and they were not statistically significant. In addition, several adverse events have been related to topical antibiotic administration, including contact dermatitis, anaphylaxis, and Stevens-Johnson syndrome. We agree that the use of topical antibiotics in dermatologic surgery should be considered only in contaminated or infected class III or IV wounds.

The literature suggests that in the majority of dermatologic surgery procedures, systemic antibiotic prophylaxis is not needed because the overall incidence of infection is low and infections are not severe. During prolonged Mohs procedures, delayed repairs, grafts, takedowns of interpolation flaps, or any procedure that breaches a mucosal surface, the evidence is less clear, and decisions should be made on a case-by-case basis. Additional studies may help clarify the most appropriate indications, and the appropriate patient populations.

It is important to distinguish between antibiotic prophylaxis for wound infection and antibiotic prophylaxis for bacterial endocarditis. The guidelines pertaining to prescription of prophylactic antibiotics to prevent endocarditis during dermatologic surgery appears clear. Manipulation of clinically infected skin is associated with a high incidence (>35%) of bacteremia with organisms known to cause endocarditis. Although, few studies have investigated bacteremia associated with dermatologic surgery procedures, those that do exist seem to indicate that the incidence of bacteremia following dermatologic surgery is low. The bacteremia generally occurs within the first 15 minutes of the procedure and is short lived, with growing organisms not commonly causing endocarditis. The British Society for Dermatological Surgery, in agreement with the British Society for Antimicrobial Chemotherapy, states that antibiotic prophylaxis for endocarditis is not required for routine dermatological surgery procedures (such as punches, shaves, curettage and simple excisions) even in the presence of a preexisting heart lesion. In clean-contaminated skin surgery, antibiotic prophylaxis may be considered in patients with a cardiac lesion because a wound infection may result in bacteremia and subsequent endocarditis. In contaminated, dirty and/or infected classes of wounds the risk of wound infection is even higher. Elective skin surgery should be postponed if possible until the wound infection is treated with therapeutic antibiotics.

PITFALLS AND MYTHS

- Before surgery procedure, detect an already infected tumor and in particular do no forget to scratch the scabs that often cover ulcerated carcinomas (Fig. 23.1). In this case surgery should be delayed and wound infection should be treated with antibiotics.
- In the nasal area take special care because of the high incidence of infection.
- Remember that bleeding needs to be controlled in order to prevent infection because of the strong association between hemorrhagic and infectious complications.

– Standard precautions have to be applied and no touch technique should be used.

– Do not believe that nonsterile gloves are sufficient to perform all procedures. For reconstruction, use systematically sterilized gloves because they are protective against infection occurrence.

– Systematic antibiotic prophylaxis is not necessary because no significant advantage has been reported for the prevention of SSIs.

CONCLUSION

The incidence of infection in skin surgery is low in the vast majority of dermatologic surgery cases. Major determinants of infection are the type of procedure, location, bleeding and intrinsic factors related to the patient. Good operative techniques, including meticulous hemostasis, can reduce the risk of SSIs. Nevertheless, excisions followed by a reconstructive procedure or performed on some anatomical sites such as the nose may require more strict infection control protocols. Further studies are needed to establish optimal guidelines for these kinds of surgery.

SUGGESTED READINGS

Aasi SZ, Leffell DJ. Complications in dermatologic surgery. How safe is safe? *Arch Dermatol* 2003;139: 213–214.

Affleck AG, Birnie AJ, Gee TM, Gee BC. Antibiotic prophylaxis in patients with valvular heart defects undergoing dermatological surgery remains a confusing issue despite apparently clear guidelines. *Clin Exp Dermatol* 2005;30(5):487–489.

Amici JM, Rogues AM, Lashéras A, Gachie JP, Guillot P, Beylot C, Thomas L, Taïeb A. A prospective study of the incidence of complications associated with dermatological surgery. *Br J Dermatol* 2005;153:967–971.

Anaes. Carcinomes basocellulaires. Recommandations pour la pratique clinique 2004. *Ann Dermatol Venereol* 2004;13:680–756.

Bosley ARJ, Bluett NH, Sowden G. Toxic shock syndrome after elective minor dermatological surgery. *B M J* 1993;306:386–387.

Campbell RM, Perlis CS, Fisher E, Gloster HM. Gentamicin ointment versus petrolatum for management of auricular wounds. *Dermatol Surg* 2005;31(6):664–669.

Chang JK, Calligaro KD, Ryan S, Runyan D, Dougherty MJ, Stern JJ. Risk factors associated with infection of lower extremity revascularization: analysis of 365 procedures performed at a teaching hospital. *Ann Vasc Surg* 2003;7:91–96.

Coldiron B. Office surgical incidents: 19 months of Florida data. *Dermatol Surg* 202;28:710–713.

Cook JI, Perone JB. A prospective evaluation of the incidence of complications associated with Mohs micrographic surgery. *Arch Dermatol* 2003;139:143–152.

Dettenkofer M, Wilson C, Ebner W, Norgauer J, Ruden H, Daschner FD. Surveillance of nosocomial infections in dermatology patients in a German university hospital. *Br J Dermatol* 2003;149:620–623.

Dirschka T, Winter K, Kralj N and Hofmann F. Glove perforation in outpatient dermatologic surgery. *Dermatol Surg* 2004;30:1210–1213.

Dixon AJ, Dixon MP, Askew DA, Wilkinson D. Prospective study of wound infections in dermatologic surgery in the absence of prophylactic antibiotics. *Dermatol Surg* 2006;32:819–26.

Finn L, Crook S. Minor surgery in general practice-setting the standards. *J Publi Hlth Med* 1998;20:169–174.

Futoryan T, Grande D. Postoperative wound infection rates in dermatologic surgery. *Dermatol Surg* 1995;21:509–514.

Garner JS, Jarvis WR, Emori TG, Horan TC, Hughes JM. CDC definition for nosocomial infections. *Am J Infect Control* 1988;16:128–140.

Gibbon KL, Bewley AP. Acquired streptococcal necrotizing fasciitis following excision of malignant melanoma. *Br J Dermatol* 1999;141:717–719.

Goldminz D, Bennett RG. Cigarette smoking and flap and full-thickness graft necrosis. *Arch Dermatol* 1991;127:1012–1015.

Gross DJ, Jamison Y, Martin K, Fields M, Dinehart SM. Surgical glove perforation in dermatologic surgery. *J Dermatol Surg Oncol* 1989;15:1226–1228.

Haas AF, Grekin RC. Antibiotic prophylaxis in dermatologic surgery. *J Am Acad Dermatol* 1995; 32:155–176.

Halpern AC, Leyden JJ, Dzubow LM, McGinley KJ. The incidence of bacteremia in skin surgery of the head and neck. *J Am Acad Dermatol* 1988;19:112–116.

Heal C, Buettner P and Browning S. Risk factors for wound infection after minor surgery in general practice. *M J A* 2006;185:255–258.

Heal C, Buettner P, Raasch B, Brownig S, Graham D, Bidgood R, Campbell M, Cruikshank R. Can sutures get wet? Prospective randomised controlled trial of wound management in general practice. *B M J* 2006;332:1053–1056.

Hochberg J, Murray GF. Principles of operative surgery. Antisepsis, technique, sutures and drains. In : Sabiston Jr DC, ed. *Textbook of Surgery*, 14th edition. Philadelphia, WB Saunders; 1991.

Kaplan AL, Cook JL. The incidences of chondritis and perichondritis associated with the surgical manipulation of auricular cartilage. *Dermatol Surg* 2004;30:58–62.

Kimyai-Asadi A, Goldberg LH, Peterson SR, Silapint S, and Jih MH. The incidence of major complications from Mohs micrographic surgery performed in office-based and hospital-based settings. *J Am Acad Dermatol* 2005;53:628–634.

Leibovitch I, Huilgol SC, Richards S, Paver R, Selva D. The Australian Mohs database: short-term recipient-site complications in full-thickness skin grafts. *Dermatol Surg* 2006;32(11):1364–1368.

Malone DL, Genuit T, Tracy JK, Gannon C, Napolitano LM. Surgical site infections: reanalysis of risk factors. *J Surg Res* 2002;103:89–95.

Maragh SL, Otley CC, Roenigk RK, Phillips PK. Antibiotic prophylaxis in dermatologic surgery: updated guidelines. *Dermatol Surg* 2005;31:83–91.

Messingham MJ, Arpey CJ. Update on the use of antibiotics in cutaneous surgery. *Dermatol Surg* 2005;31:1068–1078.

Moiemen NS, Frame JD. Toxic shock syndrome after minor dermatological surgery. *B M J* 1993;306:386–387.

Naimer SA, Trattner A. Are sterile conditions essential for all forms of cutaneous surgery? The case of ritual neonatal circumcision. *J Cutan Med Surg* 2000; 4:177–180.

Nicholson MR, Huesman LA. Controlling the usage of intranasal mupirocin does impact the rate of Staphylococcus aureus deep sternal wound infections in cardiac surgery patients. *Am J Infect Control* 2006;34:44–48.

Rhinehart MB, Murphy MM, Farley MF, Albertini JG. Sterile versus nonsterile gloves during Mohs micrographic surgery: infection rate is not affected. *Dermatol Surg* 2006;32:170–176.

Robinson JK, Hanke CW, Sengelmann RD, DM Siegel; eds. Surgery of the skin: Procedural Dermatology. Philadelphia: Elsevier Mosby, 2005.

Rogues AM, Lashéras A, Amici JM, Guillot P, Beylot C, Taïeb A, Gachie JP. Infection control practices and infectious complications in dermatological surgery. *J Hosp Infection* 2007;65:258–263.

Rudolph R, Miller SH. Reconstruction after Mohs cancer excision. *Clin Plast Surg* 1993;20:157–165.

Salasche SJ. Acute surgical complications: cause, prevention, and treatment. *J Am Acad Dermatol* 1986;15:1163–1185.

Salopek TG, Slade JM, Marghoob AA, Riegel DS, Kopf AW, Friedman RJ. Management of cutaneous malignant melanoma by dermatologists of the American Academy of dermatology. II. Definitive surgery for malignant melanoma. *J Am Acad Dermatol* 1995;33:451–461.

Sebben JE. Survey of sterile technique used by dermatologic surgeons. *J Am Acad Dermatol* 1988;18:1107–1113.

Smack DP, Harrington AC, Dunn C, Howard RS, Szkutnik AJ, Krivda SJ, Caldwell JB, James WD. Infection and allergy incidence in ambulatory surgery patients using white petrolatum versus bacitracin ointment. A randomized controlled trial. *JAMA* 1996; 276:972–977.

Sylaidis P, Wood S, Murray DS. Postoperative infection following clean facial surgery. *Ann Plast Surg* 1997;39:342–346.

Tuleya S. A status report dermatological surgery. *Skin Aging* 2002;10:10.

Wasserberg N, Tulchinski H, Schachter J, Feinmesser M, Gutman H. Sentinel-lymph node biopsy (SLNB) for melanoma is not complication-free. *Eur J Surg Oncol* 200;30:851–856.

Whitaker DC, Grande DJ, Johnson SS. Wound infection rate in dermatologic surgery. *J Dermatol Surg Oncol* 1988;14(5):525–528.

Young LS, Winston LG. Preoperative use of mupirocin for the prevention of healthcare-associated Staphylococcus aureus infections: a cost-effectiveness analysis. *Infect Control Hosp Epidemiol* 2006;27:1304–1312.

Zack L, Remlinger K, Thompson K, Massa MC. The incidence of bacteremia after skin surgery. *J Infect Dis* 1989;159:148–150.

24 | VENEREAL DISEASES

Travis Vandergriff, Mandy Harting, and Ted Rosen

INTRODUCTION

Because many of the most common sexually transmitted diseases (STDs) present with prominent and characteristic skin lesions, dermatologists have historically played a key role in their diagnosis and treatment. Dermatologists continue to contribute in both diagnostic and therapeutic endeavors, often working closely with gynecologists, urologists, infectious disease specialists, and family physicians, and others. Despite improved public awareness and continued diagnostic and therapeutic advances, STDs remain a major source of morbidity and mortality throughout the world. The urgency with which the health-care profession addresses STDs will intensify along with a better understanding of the full impact they have on public health. It has recently become apparent, for example, that the genital ulcers associated with many of the common STDs facilitate the transmission of the human immunodeficiency virus (HIV) and that some STDs (notably herpes progenitalis) may adversely affect the course of HIV infection. Moreover, recent Centers for Disease Control and Prevention (CDC) estimates place the direct health-care costs for STDs at well over $13 billion annually in the United States alone (http://www.cdc.gov/std/stats04/trends2004.htm, accessed May, 2007). The long- and short-term physical and mental health consequences of STDs are indeed extensive, and it is critical that health-care providers remain apprised of current trends in epidemiology, diagnosis, and management of these diseases. The present chapter focuses on the cutaneous manifestations and current diagnostic and therapeutic recommendations for STDs including syphilis, chancroid, lymphogranuloma venereum, granuloma inguinale, gonorrhea, and genital bite wounds. Scabies, pubic lice, genital herpes, and anogenital warts are covered in more detail elsewhere in this book. However, as the latter are commonly transmitted through sexual contact, these disorders will be briefly summarized herein as well.

HISTORY

The origin of syphilis is controversial, but current evidence seems to support the so-called "Columbian theory," which holds that the disease originated in the New World and was imported to Europe by Spanish soldiers returning from exploratory voyages led by Christopher Columbus in the late 15th century. Bony changes characteristic of syphilis, including tibial remodeling and gummatous destruction, have been identified by anthropologists in North and South American skeletal remains dating back more than 8000 years, but no such changes have been identified in skeletons from pre-Columbian Europe. A major epidemic of syphilis swept across Europe in the late 15th and early 16th centuries, and the disease became known as the "great pox" to distinguish it from smallpox. The disease was a source of public embarrassment, and the British and Germans began calling it *morbus gallicus*, or the "French disease." The Russians labeled the disease "Polish sickness" while the Poles impugned the Germans with the term "German sickness," and the Japanese knew the disease by the name of "Chinese ulcer." The disease was later called *lues venerea*, or "venereal pest," but the disease's most well-known name originated from an epic poem written in 1530 by Girolamo Fracastoro, an Italian physician and poet. In his "*Syphilis sive morbus gallicus*" (translated: Syphilis, or the French disease), Fracastoro relates the tale of Syphilis, a shepherd afflicted with the first case of the disease as a punishment for offending the god Apollo. Controversy surrounding the disease again resurfaced in Alabama in 1972 as the infamous Tuskegee Syphilis Study was exposed. This study, in which African-American men with syphilis were intentionally denied treatment so that the natural history of the disease could be studied, ran from 1932 to 1972 and marks a gloomy chapter in the history of modern medicine. The study ultimately led to the development of informed consent protocol and patient rights advocacy.

Chancroid was recognized as a clinical entity distinct from syphilis in the mid 19th century. The term "chancre" was already used popularly to describe the ulcer caused by primary syphilis, and in the 1850s the term "soft chancre" was applied to the ulcer of chancroid. This designation stems from an important distinction: while the syphilitic chancre has an indurated, almost cartilaginous peripheral consistency, the ulcer of chancroid is soft and fleshy. Through the years, the ulcer was also known as *ulcus molle* (soft ulcer) and *chancre mou* (soft chancre). In 1889, the causative bacillus was identified by Augusto Ducrey, an Italian dermatologist who made the discovery after a series of experimental autoinoculations with ulcer material gathered from patients. Clinical descriptions of lymphogranuloma venereum (LGV) date back to the early 19th century, but it was in 1913 that the disease was recognized and described as a unique entity by the French dermatologists Joseph Durand, Maurice Nicolas, and Joseph Favre. In 1925, the German dermatologist Wilhelm Frei developed the Frei test for LGV by intradermally injecting antigens prepared from causative *Chlamydia* species cultured in chick embryos. Because the test lacks specificity it is no longer used today, but Frei's name continues to be linked to LGV. The disease has also been known as tropical bubo, climatic bubo, Frei's disease, and Durand-Nicolas-Favre disease.

Kenneth McLeod, a Scottish professor of surgery, first described granuloma inguinale as "serpiginous ulcer" while seeing patients in Madras in 1882. In 1905, the Irish physician Charles

Donovan described the presence of intracellular microorganisms in ulcer debris. Visualization of these so-called "Donovan bodies" still constitutes an important aspect of diagnosis today. In honor of Dr. Donovan, the disease was designated donovanosis in 1950, and is today known as both donovanosis and GI. Gonorrhea, recognized since ancient times, was named by the Greek physician Galen in the second century. He created the term gonorrhea, literally meaning "flow of seed," after mistakenly identifying the purulent urethral discharge commonly associated with the disease as involuntary flow of semen. For centuries, physicians believed gonorrhea and syphilis to be the same disease. In 1530, Paracelsus declared gonorrhea to be an early stage of syphilis, and it was not until the late 19th century that the two diseases were clinically distinguished. In 1879, Albert Neisser first identified the gonococcus after examining the purulent urethral exudates of patients with gonorrhea. The bacterium was later determined to be the causative agent of the disease.

Scabies has been described by physicians for more than 2500 years and has been referred to in the biblical Old Testament and the writings of Aristotle and Galen. In 1687, the Italian physician Giovan Cosimo Bonomo, in collaboration with a colleague Diacinto Cestoni, isolated the mite from a patient with widespread pruritic papules, identified the mite as the cause of the disease, and published illustrations of the ectoparasite. This significant discovery marked the first microorganism specifically linked to an infectious disease.

Syphilis

A founder of modern medicine, Sir William Osler once stated that "syphilis simulates every other disease. It is the only disease necessary to know." Indeed, the protean manifestations of syphilis have puzzled physicians for centuries and have earned the disease its designation as "the great imitator." Syphilis continues to be the subject of contemporary research, and our current understanding of the disease stems from an interesting and well-documented history.

Epidemiology

Syphilis continues to be one of the world's most common STDs with a worldwide incidence in excess of 12 million cases yearly. The disease is most prevalent in developing countries, where up to 10% of the population has been infected. In the United States, syphilis is historically most common in the South and among young, sexually active African-Americans. Reported cases of syphilis in the United States declined through the 1990s to reach an all-time low in 2000. Since that time, however, the number of reported cases of syphilis has been steadily rising by more than 10% per year and currently stands at an estimated 3 cases per 100,000 population. The recent resurgence of syphilis can be almost completely attributed to cases in men. Since 2000, the incidence of syphilis in men has risen by more than 70%, and the vast majority of these cases occur in men who have sex with men (MSM). Similar alarming trends have been observed in Europe and in Canada. In the United Kingdom, for example, the number of reported cases since 2000 has risen three-fold in women and 25-fold in MSM. One theory suggests that the recent dramatic increase in syphilis among MSM is due to an increase in risky sexual behavior as patients have become less fearful of HIV with the advent of highly active antiretroviral therapy (HAART). The current epidemic of syphilis among MSM now appears to be the dominant obstacle to overcome if syphilis is ever to be eliminated as a major public health concern.

Clinical presentation and diagnosis

Syphilis is caused by the spirochete *Treponema pallidum* and is transmitted through direct sexual contact, as well as transplacentally. Although the clinical manifestations of syphilis have traditionally been divided into three distinct stages, these stages may have significant overlap and serve mostly to simplify our understanding of the disease and classify its presenting signs and symptoms.

The first stage, called *primary syphilis*, is characterized by the chancre, a lesion that develops at the site of inoculation 14 to 21 days after exposure. The chancre begins as a red, painless papule 0.5 to 2 cm in diameter and eventually ulcerates, creating a clean base with indurated, rolled borders and a characteristic "punched-out" appearance (Fig. 24.1). The remarkably painless ulcer may have a slight yellow or gray exudate and may be accompanied by moderate bilateral inguinal adenopathy. When the chancre appears on the penis or scrotum in men or on the vulva or at the vaginal introitus in women, the ulcer is usually readily apparent, and the diagnosis may be made in the primary stage. However, when occurring in the vaginal canal, rectum, or oropharynx, it may go unnoticed by the patient. Occult chancres are common in women and MSM, and in such cases the diagnosis is not typically made until later stages. Regardless of its location, the chancre may last from 3 to 6 weeks and resolves spontaneously without treatment. In untreated patients, the treponemes proliferate and migrate through the lymphatic channels to the bloodstream where they are disseminated throughout the body. Metastatic accumulations of treponemes create the lesions characteristic of the second stage of syphilis.

Secondary syphilis is characterized by many different signs and symptoms, some of which are fairly generic and some of which are quite distinct. It is the litany of possible manifestations of secondary syphilis that have earned the disease its designation as "the great imitator." Because the lesions of secondary syphilis appear 4 to 10 weeks after the development of the primary chancre,

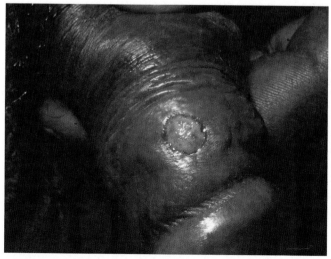

Figure 24.1. Solitary, indurated, "punched-out" erosion (chancre).

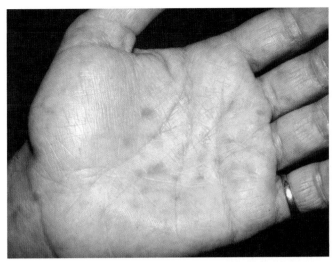

Figure 24.2 . Asymptomatic palmar macules (secondary syphilis).

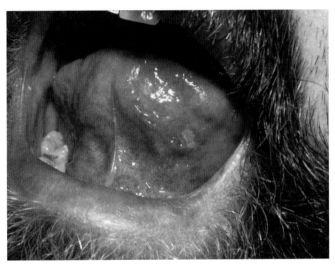

Figure 24.3 . Oral erosion (mucous patch) of secondary syphilis.

with diffuse lymphadenopathy, low-grade fever, malaise, fatigue, myalgias, arthralgias, and weight loss. The signs and symptoms of secondary syphilis also eventually resolve without treatment. Untreated patients enter a stage of latency in which treponemes continue to proliferate while the patient remains asymptomatic.

From the latent state, one-third of untreated patients will ultimately go on to develop late sequelae or tertiary syphilis. This stage begins 3 to 15 years after the initial infection, and complications are responsible for most of the mortality associated with syphilis. Cardiovascular complications include stenosis of the coronary artery, ostia, and aortic root aneurysm, leading to aortic insufficiency. The nervous system is commonly involved in tertiary syphilis, and patients may present with seizures, blindness, altered mental status, focal neurologic deficits, tabes dorsalis, dementia, or psychosis. Persons co-infected with HIV are at increased risk of developing tertiary neurosyphilis. Another characteristic lesion of tertiary syphilis is the gumma, a necrotic granulomatous ulcer with indurated dusky-red serpiginous borders. Gummas occur in hard and soft tissues including skin, cartilage, bone, and brain, and they are often locally destructive.

In its primary stage, syphilis must be distinguished from other causes of genital ulcers, including chancroid, genital herpes, lymphogranuloma venereum, granuloma inguinale, neoplasms, fixed drug eruptions, bullous diseases, and Behçet's disease. A definitive diagnosis of syphilis can be made in the primary stage by identifying treponemes on dark-field microscopy of the ulcer exudate. When performed properly, this technique has very few false-negative results and no false-positive results. Alternatively, the exudate may be tested with direct fluorescent antibody (DFA) assays. Serologic tests may also be used in primary syphilis, but results must be interpreted cautiously. The nontreponemal tests include the rapid plasma reagin (RPR) and the venereal disease research laboratory (VDRL) test, both of which measure antibody to cardiolipin and both of which are equally valid. The treponemal tests, including the fluorescent treponemal antibody absorption test (FTA-ABS) and the microhemagglutination assay for *Treponema pallidum* antibodies (MHA-TP), measure antibodies to specific treponemal proteins. Within 1 week of chancre development, the nontreponemal tests are positive in approximately 85% of patients with primary syphilis but usually yield titers lower than 1:16. Additionally, false-positive results are possible in cases of autoimmune disease, collagen vascular disease, HIV, tuberculosis, pregnancy, rickettsial infection, and bacterial endocarditis. The treponemal tests are positive in 90% of patients with primary syphilis. However, the majority of patients with reactive treponemal assays will continue to have reactive assays for life unless the disease is treated early in the primary stage. Therefore, the specific treponemal assays are of limited use in making a diagnosis of infection, but a negative result may exclude the diagnosis or confirm a false-positive result on nontreponemal tests.

The cutaneous findings of secondary syphilis must be distinguished from primary HIV infection, pityriasis rosea, erythema multiforme, lichen planus, drug eruptions, scabies, and psoriasis among many other diagnoses. In the second stage, serologic tests become more reliable with both treponemal and nontreponemal assays, virtually always yielding positive results. Nontreponemal assays are positive in high titers and often exceed 1:64. A fourfold increase in titer presumptively diagnoses active infection. Additionally, dark-field microscopy may identify spirochetes in

there is some potential for overlap between the two stages. In the modern era, patients who have a persistent chancre during clinically obvious secondary syphilis should be highly suspect of being HIV co-infected. More than 90% of patients with secondary syphilis have skin or mucous membrane involvement. Typically, patients first develop a transient macular erythema on the trunk, which spreads to the shoulders and extremities, sparing the face, palms, and soles. Patients later develop a papulosquamous eruption with a characteristic copper hue. The typically asymptomatic eruption classically involves the palms and soles and may also manifest as shallow erosions on oral mucous membranes. This creates the so-called "mucous patches" (Figs. 24.2 and 24.3). When the eruption involves the scalp, a non-cicatricial, patchy or "moth-eaten" alopecia results. Another characteristic lesion of secondary syphilis is condyloma latum, a smooth, moist, white-gray flat papule occurring in aggregates in intertriginous areas. Condyloma lata often have eroded surfaces oozing a spirochete-rich drainage, making them the most infectious of all lesions of secondary syphilis. Additionally, patients often have generalized symptoms associated with secondary syphilis and may present the exudates from lesions of secondary syphilis. Although it is not necessary for diagnosis, histopathologic evaluation of biopsied tissue reveals a polymorphous cellular infiltrate typically rich in plasma cells, macrophages, and lymphocytes. A positive result on VDRL testing of cerebrospinal fluid is highly specific for tertiary neurosyphilis.

Treatment

As with other STDs, practitioners should review current recommendations from the Centers for Disease Control and Prevention (CDC) when treating patients with syphilis. Parenterally administered penicillin G remains the preferred drug for treating syphilis in all stages. For adults with primary or secondary syphilis, a single intramuscular (IM) dose of 2.4 million units of benzathine penicillin G is the recommended treatment and has been used for more than 50 years to achieve clinical resolution. Children with acquired primary or secondary syphilis should be evaluated for sexual abuse and treated with benzathine penicillin G in a single IM dose of 50,000 units/kg, up to the adult dose of 2.4 million units. Pregnant women with syphilis should be treated with the adult dose of benzathine penicillin G, and pregnant patients allergic to penicillin should be desensitized and treated with penicillin. Non-pregnant patients with penicillin allergy may be treated with doxycycline (100 mg orally twice daily for 14 days) or tetracycline (500 mg orally four times daily for 14 days). Although azithromycin administered in a single oral dose of 2 g may be effective, treatment failure has been reported and justifies caution when using this drug. Similarly, single-dose ceftriaxone remains an unproven alternative to single-dose penicillin for syphilis management.

In the absence of active lesions, as occurs in the latent stage, patients are not contagious to sexual contacts. Therefore, treatment of latent syphilis does not reduce transmission of syphilis to others but benefits the patient by preventing late sequelae. The treatment of latent syphilis may require a different dosing protocol. Patients with latent syphilis who acquired the infection within the past year are considered to have "early latent syphilis" and should be treated with 2.4 million units of benzathine penicillin G in a single IM dose. Patients with latent syphilis of greater than 1 year duration or of unknown duration should be treated with a total of 7.2 million units of benzathine penicillin G, administered in 3 IM doses of 2.4 million units separated by 1 week intervals. All patients with tertiary syphilis should be treated with this same regimen. Pregnant patients with penicillin allergy and latent syphilis should be desensitized and treated with penicillin. Non-pregnant patients with penicillin allergy and early latent syphilis should be treated with the alternative regimens appropriate for primary and secondary syphilis, while patients with late latent syphilis should receive either doxycycline (100 mg orally twice daily for 28 days) or tetracycline (500 mg orally four times daily for 28 days).

All patients should be warned about a possible Jarisch-Herxheimer reaction, an acute febrile reaction occurring within 12 hours of initial treatment. Antipyretic treatment has not been shown to prevent this reaction. Sex partners of patients diagnosed with syphilis should be clinically and serologically evaluated for syphilis and appropriately treated if necessary. Furthermore, persons who have been exposed within the last 90 days preceding the diagnosis of syphilis in a sex partner may have false-negative seroreactivity and should be treated for a presumptive diagnosis of syphilis. Because of the high risk of co-infection, patients diagnosed with syphilis should always be evaluated for other STDs, including HIV. Treatment failure may occur with any regimen, and patients should be clinically and serologically reexamined 6 and 12 months after initial treatment. Patients with persistent clinical signs or symptoms or a sustained four-fold increase in nontreponemal titers should be retreated and reevaluated for HIV infection.

Chancroid

In addition to syphilis, chancroid is a major cause of genital ulcer disease worldwide. While the two diseases share some common features, important differences exist in their epidemiology, clinical presentation, diagnosis, and treatment.

Epidemiology

Because of global irregularities in diagnostic accuracy and reporting practices, the exact incidence of chancroid is unknown. However, some experts suspect that its worldwide incidence may surpass that of syphilis. Chancroid constitutes a major proportion of genital ulcer disease worldwide, especially in areas of chronic endemicity. In parts of sub-Saharan Africa, chancroid is the most common cause of genital ulcer disease, and in India more than half of all genital ulcers are caused by chancroid. Other endemic locales include the Caribbean basin and southern Asia. In the United States and other developed countries, chancroid occurs in discrete and sporadic outbreaks in restricted geographic areas. In the United States, most reported cases occur in New York, South Carolina, and Texas, and the number of cases has been steadily declining from nearly 5,000 in 1987 to just 143 in 1999. Most recent CDC statistics suggest that chancroid is becoming exceedingly rare in the United States. Many of the prior outbreaks affected mostly African-American and Hispanic heterosexuals with a male to female ratio ranging from 3:1 to 25:1. Commercial sex workers appear to be important vectors of transmission, and outbreaks have also been associated with crack cocaine use.

Clinical presentation and diagnosis

Chancroid is caused by *Haemophilus ducreyi*, a gram-negative facultative anaerobic coccobacillus. The bacterium enters the skin through epidermal microabrasions created during intercourse. Four to 7 days later, a tender erythematous papule or pustule develops at the site of inoculation, although this incubation period may be longer in patients with concomitant HIV infection. Within days, the papule or pustule erodes and forms a deep, painful ulceration with central necrosis. The ulcer is characteristically tender, soft, and friable with ragged undermined margins. There is often a foul-smelling yellow or gray exudate and surrounding erythema. The ulcer occurs in men most commonly on the prepuce and shaft of the penis, while ulcers in women tend to occur on the labia and fourchette. Extragenital chancroid is rare. One-half of patients go on to develop painful unilateral or bilateral inguinal lymphadenopathy within one to two weeks (Fig. 24.4). Affected lymph nodes may become matted or fluctuant, eventually rupturing and forming suppurative sinus

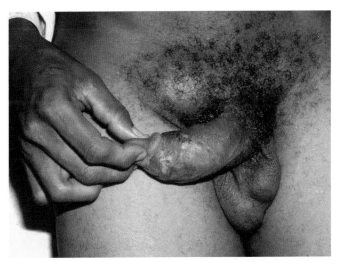

Figure 24.4 . Several painful ulcerations and marked adenopathy of chancroid.

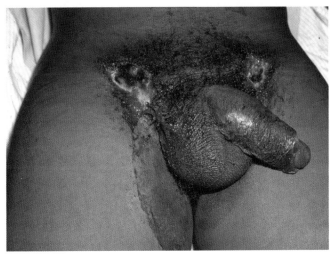

Figure 24.5. Ruptured inguinal lymph nodes of late chancroid.

tracts (Fig. 24.5). Because of the propensity of chancroidal ulcers to autoinoculate adjacent skin, multiple opposing ulcerations or "kissing lesions" are not uncommon. Untreated infections typically resolve spontaneously within 3 months, but potential complications include phimosis, local tissue destruction, and fistulae formation.

Less common clinical presentations of chancroid have also been described. In transient chancroid, the ulcer resolves in 4 to 6 days and suppurative inguinal adenopathy develops weeks later. Follicular chancroid is characterized by ulcerations of the pilar apparatus in hair-bearing areas. In giant chancroid, multiple small ulcerations coalesce to form a single ulcer with the potential for severe local destruction of tissue. Finally, phagedenic chancroid results in widespread necrosis and soft tissue destruction of the genitals and perineum.

Laboratory techniques for the diagnosis of chancroid are imperfect and not uniformly available. Gram's stain of the ulcer debris may show the classic "school of fish" pattern of pleomorphic gram-negative coccobacilli in parallel chains or clusters. A definitive diagnosis requires the isolation of *H. ducreyi* on

gonococcal culture media with high humidity and low oxygen tension. However, even in experienced laboratories the sensitivity of this technique is less than 80%. Nucleic acid amplification tests developed for research laboratories are the most sensitive and specific diagnostic assays but are not commercially available for routine diagnosis. Because of the suboptimal diagnostic modalities available to physicians, the diagnosis of chancroid is, in practice, largely clinical. According to CDC recommendations, a likely diagnosis of chancroid can be made if all of the following criteria are met: (a) the patient has one or more painful genital ulcers; (b) the patient has no evidence of *T. pallidum* infection by dark-field examination of ulcer exudate or by a serologic test for syphilis performed at least 7 days after onset of ulcers; (c) the clinical presentation, appearance of genital ulcers and, if present, regional lymphadenopathy are typical for chancroid; and (d) a test (viral culture-PCR) for HSV performed on the ulcer exudate is negative.

Treatment

Current recommendations made by the CDC direct physicians to treat patients with chancroid with one of the following medications: azithromycin (1 g orally in a single dose), ceftriaxone (a single 250 mg IM dose), ciprofloxacin (500 mg orally twice daily for 3 days), or erythromycin (500 mg orally three times daily for 7 days). Both azithromycin and ceftriaxone offer the benefit of single-dose therapy, eliminating potential problems of medication noncompliance.

Patients diagnosed with chancroid should be tested for other STDs, including syphilis and HIV. In the United States, up to 10% of patients with chancroid also have concomitant syphilis. Patients should also be clinically reexamined 3 to 7 days after beginning treatment. Failure to observe objective improvement in the ulcer within 1 week of appropriate therapy suggests unsuccessful treatment. In these cases the treating physician must consider whether the diagnosis of chancroid is correct, or if the patient has another, confounding concomitant STD including HIV, or if the specific *H. ducreyi* isolate is resistant to the chosen medication. Suppurative lymph nodes heal more slowly than primary ulcers and usually require needle aspiration or surgical drainage to allow for complete resolution.

Lymphogranuloma venereum

Included in the differential diagnosis of genital ulcer disease is lymphogranuloma venereum (LGV), a disease that has recently received considerable and renewed attention in the literature due to its reappearance in developed countries around the world.

Epidemiology

Lymphogranuloma venereum (LGV) is caused by *Chlamydia trachomatis* serovars L1, L2, or L3 and has classically been a disease of tropical and subtropical climates. Areas of endemicity include India, Southeast Asia, South America, sub-Saharan Africa, and the Caribbean basin. Even in these areas, LGV is a relatively uncommon cause of genital ulcers, accounting for less than 10% of cases. In 2003, the first cases of LGV in Europe were documented in the Netherlands. Since then, outbreaks have been reported in Belgium, Germany, France, the United Kingdom, Sweden, and the United States, with virtually all cases occurring in MSM and presenting as proctitis rather than as genital ulcers. In 2004, 27 cases of LGV were reported to the CDC. Gene amplification techniques have identified the L2b strain of *C. trachomatis* as the common variant in recent outbreaks in industrialized countries. Additionally, these techniques have also determined that the L2b strain has been present in the United States since 1981. LGV has been underdiagnosed in the United States in past decades, and recent cases probably represent the discovery of a slow but ongoing epidemic rather than a new outbreak.

Clinical presentation and diagnosis

LGV classically presents in three stages. First, after an incubation period of 3 to 30 days, a small painless papule or herpetiform ulcer develops at the site of inoculation. The primary ulcer resolves without treatment after 2 to 6 weeks and most often goes unnoticed by the patient. The second stage of the disease is known as the inguinal syndrome, and it is at this stage that most patients present for medical evaluation. LGV is predominantly a disease of the lymphatic tissue, and in the second stage, the nodes draining the site of inoculation enlarge and develop necrotic abscesses (Fig. 24.6). Painful, enlarged regional lymph nodes may develop into fluctuant buboes, which ultimately rupture in one-third of patients. In men, adenopathy often involves the inguinal and femoral nodes. Prominent unilateral or bilateral inflammation of these nodes around the inguinal ligament create the so-called "groove sign," a finding considered to be pathognomonic for LGV. In women, however, only 20% to 30% of patients develop inguinal adenopathy. More commonly, the deep iliac and perirectal nodes are involved as they drain the vaginal canal, cervix, rectum, and urethra. Systemic symptoms including fever, malaise, and arthralgia may be present in the second stage. Rare systemic complications have also been reported during the second stage and include pneumonitis, hepatitis, aseptic meningitis, and ocular inflammatory disease. The third stage is known as the genitoanorectal stage and tends to affect mostly women and MSM. The continued presence of bacteria in regional lymphatic channels leads to chronic inflammation, resulting in lymphedema, ulceration, scarring, strictures, and

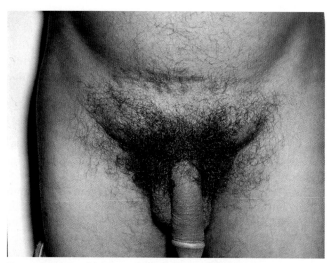

Figure 24.6. Painful, bilateral adenopathy without an erosive lesion (LGV).

fistulae formation. Patients develop proctocolitis, perirectal abscesses, and lymphorroids. They may present with complaints of purulent or mucoid anal discharge, rectal bleeding, constipation, or tenesmus. Genital elephantiasis also occurs and is known as "esthiomene" in women and as "saxophone penis" in men. Nearly all cases of LGV recently diagnosed in Europe and the United States have presented in the second and third stages with signs and symptoms of proctocolitis rather than genital ulcers or inguinal lymphadenopathy.

The diagnosis of LGV is based primarily on clinical findings, nonspecific laboratory techniques, and the exclusion of other diagnoses. The U.S. Food and Drug Administration (FDA) has approved the use of nucleic acid amplification tests for genital and lymph node specimens. These tests are nonspecific chlamydial assays and are not currently approved for use on rectal specimens. The CDC has recently announced that clinicians with patients whose symptoms are suggestive of LGV may send rectal swabs to CDC laboratories to be tested with LGV-specific genotyping techniques that are not commercially available. In the absence of specific testing, the CDC recommends that patients with likely LGV based on clinical findings be treated for this presumptive diagnosis.

Treatment

Doxycycline is the preferred treatment of LGV and should be orally administered at a dose of 100 mg twice daily for 21 days. Alternatively, patients may receive erythromycin 500 mg orally four times daily for 21 days. Pregnant and lactating women should receive erythromycin rather than doxycycline. Although treatment cures infection, tissue scarring due to chronic inflammation may not be reversible. Furthermore, buboes may require needle aspiration or surgical drainage to achieve resolution. Patients diagnosed with LGV should be evaluated for other STDs including HIV. In one series, 84% of patients with LGV in the United States had concomitant HIV infection.

Granuloma inguinale

Like LGV, granuloma inguinale (GI) is a cause of genital ulcer disease, which infrequently occurs outside of endemic areas. Nonetheless, cases are reported in industrialized countries, and clinicians should be aware of this diagnosis when differentiating genital ulcers.

Epidemiology

The causative agent of GI is the intracellular gram-negative rod *Klebsiella granulomatis* (formerly known as *Donovania granulomatis* and *Calymmatobacterium granulomatis*). The disease is endemic in India, Southeast Asia, South Africa, the Caribbean basin, Brazil, Papua New Guinea, and aboriginal Australia. The largest epidemic occurred in an area of Papua New Guinea from 1922 to 1952, where 10,000 cases were documented among a population of 15,000 people. Aggressive public health campaigns have dramatically reduced the incidence of GI in northern Australia. Less than ten cases are reported annually in the United States, and most of these are related to international travel. Men are infected two to six times more often than women, and infection rates peak in the third decade of life.

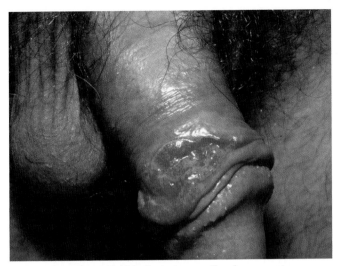

Figure 24.7. Friable deep ulcer typifies donovanosis.

Clinical presentation and diagnosis

The exact incubation period of GI is unknown and may last up to 1 year, but most patients develop clinical evidence of the disease within 2 to 6 weeks of exposure to *K. granulomatis*. Ulcerogranulomatous disease, the most common presentation, begins as single or multiple subcutaneous nodules that develop at the site of inoculation. These nodules enlarge and erode, becoming painless ulcers with clean bases and sharply demarcated rolled margins. The ulcer bases are classically described as "beefy red" and consist of friable granulation tissue, which bleeds readily when touched (Fig. 24.7). Ulcers occur most commonly on the coronal sulcus in men and on the labia minora in women. However, 6% of ulcers are extragenital and have been reported to occur on the oropharynx, nose, neck, and chest. True inguinal lymphadenopathy does not develop in the absence of bacterial superinfection. Rather, subcutaneous edema and granulomas lead to inguinal enlargement in 10% of patients. These pseudobuboes may ulcerate or form abscesses. Less common clinical presentations of GI include hypertrophic or verrucous ulcers, necrotic ulcers, and cicatricial GI, which is characterized by extensive fibrosis and sclerosis. Constitutional symptoms are not typically associated with GI, but severe local complications have been reported and include genital elephantiasis, urethral and vaginal stenosis, and autoamputation of the penis. Untreated lesions have no tendency to resolve and can be quite destructive as they progress. Additionally, squamous cell carcinoma develops in 0.25% of cases and involvement of the cervix can lead to fatal hemorrhage during childbirth.

The differential diagnosis of GI includes other causes of genital ulcers, such as syphilis, chancroid, LGV, genital herpes, carcinoma, and amebiasis. *K. granulomatis* is difficult to isolate on culture media. Therefore, routine clinical diagnosis of GI is made by visualizing Donovan bodies in a crush preparation of granulation tissue obtained from the ulcer base. The tissue is obtained by scraping or punch biopsy. It is then stained with Wright's, Giemsa, Warthin-Starry, or other stains. These stains reveal the fine cytological detail that is necessary for diagnosis. Ultrathin tissue samples may be optimal for disclosing the characteristic Donovon bodies. Donovan bodies appear as bipolar

safety pin–shaped rods located within mononuclear cells and are the actual infecting bacteria engulfed by macrophages and monocytes.

Treatment

Few studies have been conducted to determine optimal treatment for GI, but the traditionally preferred treatment is with doxycycline (100 mg orally twice daily for at least 3 weeks or until lesions have healed). However, there is now a relatively high risk of therapeutic failure when utilizing tetracycline derivatives in the management of GI, especially in cases encountered in North America. Alternative medications include trimethoprim–sulfamethoxazole (one 160 mg/800 mg tablet orally twice daily for at least 3 weeks), ciprofloxacin (750 mg orally twice daily for at least 3 weeks), erythromycin (500 mg orally four times daily for at least 3 weeks), or azithromycin (1 g orally once weekly for at least 3 weeks). TMP-SMX is probably the best alternative drug and may actually be the drug of choice for current American cases. Treatment should continue for at least 3 weeks or until all lesions have healed.

Gonorrhea

Gonorrhea remains an extremely common STD in the United States and worldwide, and while most cases produce signs and symptoms restricted to the urogenital tract, prominent cutaneous manifestations may develop in local infection sites (e.g., Bartholin's or Skene's glands) or when the infection disseminates.

Epidemiology

Gonorrhea, caused by the gram-negative intracellular diplococcus *Neisseria gonorrhoeae*, is quite common, with an estimated worldwide incidence of 60 million cases annually. In the United States alone, more than 600,000 new cases occur each year. The disease incidence peaked in the 1960s and 1970s and declined steadily through the late 1990s. However, since 1997, the incidence has again been on the rise, with an increase of 7% from 1997 to 2001. The disease is especially prevalent in African-Americans, Hispanic adolescents, prisoners, commercial sex workers, MSM, and patients with HIV. In one study, 15% of MSM presenting to an STD clinic had evidence of gonorrheal infections, with the pharynx being the most common site.

Clinical presentation and diagnosis

After an incubation period of 1 day to 2 weeks, patients infected with *N. gonorrhoeae* may develop signs and symptoms of inflammation at the site of primary inoculation. Common presenting complaints include pharyngitis, urethritis, intense burning or painful dysuria, profuse, purulent urethral discharge, and pelvic pain. (Fig. 24.8) However, up to one-half of patients will have completely asymptomatic infections. Occasionally, primary cutaneous lesions develop. If the inoculation is from sexual contact, a genital pustule or tender furuncle may appear. In cases of traumatic inoculation, abscesses or pustules may also occur. The primary lesions of the skin are uncommon and tend to go unnoticed. The most prominent cutaneous manifestations occur when the gonococcal infection disseminates widely. Disseminated

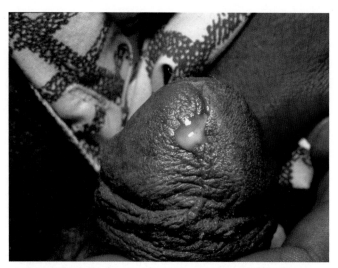

Figure 24.8 . Profuse purulent gonococcal urethral discharge.

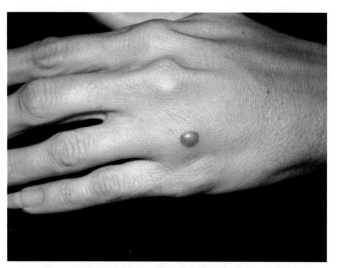

Figure 24.9. Distal hemorrhagic bulla (gonococcemia).

gonoccocal infection (DGI) develops in 1% to 3% of cases and usually occurs in young healthy patients with asymptomatic genital, rectal, or oropharyngeal infection. Other risk factors for the development of DGI include hereditary defects in the terminal complement pathway and hypocomplementemia due to lupus erythematosus.

Two distinct clinical presentations exist and may occur concomitantly in cases of DGI. The septic arthritis syndrome is characterized by fever and inflammation of one or more joints with pain, swelling, erythema, and decreased range of motion. The tenosynovitis-arthritis-dermatitis syndrome occurs in 60% of cases of DGI. Patients develop tenderness and erythema over tendons and their bony insertion sites. Additionally, a migratory arthralgia or arthritis involving appendicular joints occurs and typically affects less than three joints. The characteristic skin lesions of DGI begin as erythematous macules and progress to form tender necrotic pustules or hemorrhagic bullae (Fig. 24.9). The pustules usually occur on the dorsal aspect of distal extremities near the joints of the wrists, hands, and ankles. These pustules result from bacterial embolization followed by microabscess formation. Typically, there is a paucity of lesions present.

In symptomatic male patients, a Gram's stain of the urethral discharge is virtually always positive and diagnostic of gonorrhea. However, Gram's stains of oropharyngeal, rectal, or endocervical specimens lack the appropriate sensitivity and specificity for diagnosis. In cases of DGI, blood cultures and specimens from pustules rarely yield positive results. Culture or gene amplification techniques are recommended for diagnosis in these cases. Therefore, the diagnosis of DGI should be made based on clinical findings and isolation of *N. gonorrhoeae* from the primary site of infection. Culture of *N. gonorrhoeae* offers the additional benefit of determining antimicrobial susceptibility and allowing for appropriate therapy.

Treatment

Due to the ongoing development of drug resistance in strains of *N. gonorrhoeae*, the CDC has made frequent updates to its recommendations for therapy of gonorrhea. Currently, only cephalosporins are recommended for first-line therapy of gonorrhea. High levels of fluoroquinolone resistance have eliminated these drugs from the treatment algorithm. Patients with uncomplicated infections of the urethra, rectum, or cervix may be treated with ceftriaxone (125 mg IM in a single dose) or cefixime (400 mg orally in a single dose). Patients with cephalosporin allergy should be treated with spectinomycin (2 g IM in a single dose). The management of DGI requires more aggressive treatment. Patients should be hospitalized and monitored for complications such as bacterial endocarditis, meningitis, or perihepatitis. These cases should be managed with parenteral antibiotics. The recommended regimen is with ceftriaxone (1 g IM or IV every 24 hours) and alternatives include cefotaxime (1 g IV every 8 hours) and ceftizoxime (1 g every 8 hours). Treatment with IV antibiotics should continue for 24 to 48 hours after clinical improvement begins, at which point the patient may be switched to cefotaxime (400 mg orally twice daily) for a total of at least 1 week of antibiotic therapy. Cephalosporin allergic patients should receive spectinomycin (2 g IM every 12 hours) for the same duration of therapy. Patients diagnosed with gonorrhea should be evaluated for other STDs including chlamydia, syphilis, and HIV.

Genital Bite Wounds

Without a doubt, genital bite wounds and resultant complications are underreported and underdiagnosed. Patients with genital bite wounds often seek medical care late in the course of disease, if at all, and presentation is delayed because of patient embarrassment and attempts at self-treatment. The subject receives very little attention in the medical literature, and consequently clinicians have few resources for diagnostic or therapeutic recommendations.

Traumatic orogenital contact occurs frequently and is not restricted to any demographic group. The exact incidence of genital bite wounds is unknown, but it is estimated that more than 1% of emergency center visits are related to bite injuries. The clinical presentation of a patient with a genital wound is dependent on the amount of time that has elapsed since the injury and the severity of the injury. Patients may present with painful, superficially to deeply necrotic laceration or ulceration of the external genitalia (Fig. 24.10). Although most genital wounds are superficial, the loose subcutaneous tissue of the perineum

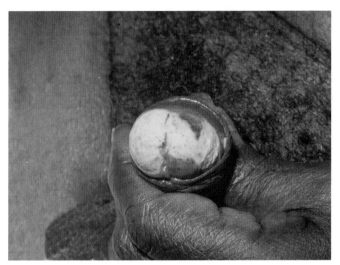

Figure 24.10 . Rapidly progressive, painful necrosis due to *Eikenella Corrodens*.

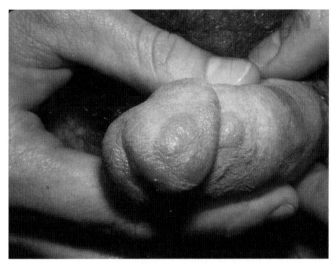

Figure 24.11. Pruritic nodules on glans typifies scabies.

facilitates the spread of microorganisms and creates the potential for severe complications including rapidly advancing cellulitis, balanoposthitis, Fournier's gangrene, abscess formation, lymphangitis, and sepsis. The most important complication of genital bite wounds is the risk of infection with oropharyngeal flora. Infections are nearly always polymicrobial and often involve *Eikenella corrodens* and various oral anaerobes. Patients presenting later in the course of disease usually have some form of advanced complication. Particularly, aggressive orogenital contact can also result in disfigurement and may ultimately lead to sexual dysfunction, urethral strictures, and fistulae formation. Additionally, transmission of diseases such as syphilis, viral hepatitis, tetanus, tuberculosis, and HIV has been reported to occur through human bites.

Wounds should be cultured for both aerobic and anaerobic bacteria. If a genital ulcer is present, additional assessment with dark-field microscopy and viral culture is warranted. Genital wounds should be cleansed by copious irrigation with a bactericidal and virucidal solution such as 1% povidone-iodine. Because of the high risk of infection, genital bite wounds should not be closed primarily. There are no standardized or evidence-based recommendations for treatment of genital bite wounds in the medical literature. However, empiric antibiotic therapy should cover for potential pathogens such as gram-positive cocci and gram-negative rods, especially *Eikenella corrodens*. No guidelines have been established, but successful treatment has been reported with amoxicillin-clavulanic acid (500 mg/125 mg twice daily for 14 days). Alternatives may include second generation cephalosporins (e.g. cefuroxime) or combination therapy with dicloxacillin and penicillin. Antibiotic therapy should ultimately be adjusted according to antimicrobial sensitivity results obtained from wound cultures whenever feasible.

Scabies

To this day, scabies maintains a worldwide distribution but is most prevalent in areas of endemicity including India, South Africa, Brazil, Central America, and aboriginal Australia. While estimates place the global incidence at 300 million cases annually,

or 5% of the world population, scabies may affect up to one-half of the population in isolated areas of endemicity. The disease is caused by the mite *Sarcoptes scabiei var hominis*, an obligate human ectoparasite transmitted by direct skin-to-skin contact. The prolonged and intimate contact that occurs during sexual activity makes it an especially important mode of transmission as dislodged mites use heat and odor as guides to find new hosts. General risk factors for transmission include low socioeconomic status, poor nutrition, and poor hygiene. Risk factors specific to sexual transmission include multiple sexual partners and MSM.

The female mites lay eggs in the stratum granulosum, and the hatched larvae later dig burrows while enzymatically digesting the skin and consuming the debris for nutrition. A host hypersensitivity response to mite saliva, eggs, and feces leads to sensitization and ultimately pruritus, a clinical hallmark of scabies infection. The pruritus classically worsens at night and spares the head and neck in adults. Physical examination of the patient may reveal erythematous papules or the pathognomonic scabietic burrows, which prominently involve the interdigital spaces, the flexural aspect of the wrists, the umbilicus, the glans and shaft of the penis, and the nipple-areolar zone (Fig. 24.11). While the common form of infection involves only 10 to 15 mites per host, other clinical variants of scabies may involve many more mites. Immunocompromised or malnourished patients are especially susceptible to crusted or Norwegian scabies with more than one million mites infecting the host. In this variant, heavily crusted and often fissured pruritic patches are characteristic. Fissures may predispose to eventual bacterial septicemia.

The diagnosis of scabies is unequivocal when the clinician visualizes the mite, its eggs, or its feces. The so-called "scabies preparation" is performed by coating a blade in mineral oil and scraping a suspected burrow. The debris is transferred to a slide and microscopically examined for evidence of mite infection. Alternatively, dermoscopy of burrows is equally as sensitive but less specific for identifying the presence of mites, eggs, or feces. Patients diagnosed with scabies should be treated with 5% permethrin cream applied to the entire body from the neck down and thoroughly washed after 8 to 14 hours. Alternatively, patients may receive a dose of ivermectin (200 mcg/kg orally once and repeated in two weeks). Although topical lindane may also be used, the potential for neurotoxicity (even without abuse, such as over-zealous application or ingestion) restricts its place to second- or third-line therapy. There are no standard recommendations for treatment of crusted scabies, but some recommend combination therapy with a topical scabicide and oral ivermectin. All patients with scabies should wash clothing and bed sheets in hot water. Fumigation of the home environment is not necessary.

Pubic Lice

Public lice, like the other ectoparasites, have infested human hosts for millennia. Paleoarcheologists have discovered pubic lice in mummified human remains dating back 2000 years in both Europe and South America. Today the pubic louse has a worldwide distribution and is most common in MSM, patients aged 15 to 25, and in patients of lower socioeconomic status. The pubic louse is almost always transmitted by sexual contact. There is a 95% transmission rate when an individual has sexual contacts with an infected person.

Because pubic lice is not a reportable disease, the exact incidence of the disease is not known, but some estimates place the number at 3 million cases (or 1% of the population) in the United States annually. The pubic or crab louse, *Pthirus pubis*, is a one mm ectoparasite visible to the naked eye. The louse attaches to hair of the pubis and adjacent areas, including the abdomen, buttocks, thigh, and perineum. (Fig. 24.12) The lice are capable of migrating up to 10 cm daily, and are thus occasionally found in the hair of the chest and eyelashes. Rarely is the face or scalp involved with infestation by the pubic louse. Infested patients may be asymptomatic or complain of pruritus or erythema. Physical examination reveals the lice and their nits attached to coarse pubic hairs. The lice are usually abundant, and the diagnosis of pediculosis pubis is made when the lice are visually identified. Additionally, maculae ceruleae, or blue-gray macules due to deep dermal hemosiderin, can be observed at sites of louse bites. Rarely, patients develop pediculid, which is an id reaction to pediculosis that resembles a viral exanthem.

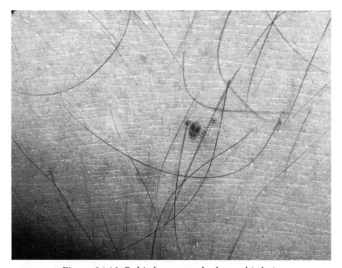

Figure 24.12. Pubic louse attached to pubic hair.

The CDC recommends that patients with pubic lice be treated with 1% permethrin cream applied to affected areas and rinsed away after 10 minutes. Alternative treatment regimens include 0.5% malathion lotion applied to affected areas and washed away after 8 to 12 hours. Patients preferring oral therapy can receive ivermectin (250 mcg/kg orally once, repeated in 2 weeks). Clinicians should remind patients using topical treatment to apply the medication to all perineal areas as well as the pubis. Pediculocides should not be applied near the eyes. Patients with eyelash involvement should apply an occlusive eyelid ointment or petroleum jelly to the eyelid margins twice daily for 10 days. Alternatively, ophthalmologic pilocarpine preparations may prove to be selectively neurotoxic to the lice while safe for use around the human host's eye. Finally, bed sheets and clothing should be washed in hot water, but household fumigation is not necessary.

Genital Herpes

Genital herpes is a chronic and life-long viral infection, which has become the most prevalent cause of genital ulcer disease in the United States and other developed countries. The disease is caused by the herpes simplex virus (HSV), an enveloped double-stranded DNA virus. There are two variants of HSV, named HSV-1 and HSV-2, and both are capable of causing genital herpes. Traditionally, HSV-1 is associated with labial herpes and HSV-2 is associated with genital herpes infections. While historically most cases of genital herpes are due to HSV-2, HSV-1 is emerging as an important cause of genital herpes and now is responsible for up to 30% of cases.

Genital herpes is one of the most common STDs, and approximately less than 20% of Americans above the age of 12 nationwide are currently infected with HSV-2 based on recent seroprevalence studies. In densely populated urban areas and inner cities, the prevalence exceeds 50%. Risk factors for the acquisition of genital herpes include multiple sex partners, lower socioeconomic status, African-American or Hispanic ethnicity, and female gender. The virus is transmitted through direct contact with an infected person. The most efficient transmission occurs with symptomatic lesions shedding high viral loads, but transmission can also occur in asymptomatic patients continually shedding the virus in smaller numbers. In fact, more than 70% of genital herpes infections are transmitted by patients unaware of their own infection and resultant asymptomatic shedding status.

After a postexposure incubation period of 2 days to 2 weeks, primary genital herpes develops and is characterized by widespread vesicles on the genitalia accompanied by regional lymphadenopathy and dysuria. The vesicles resolve without treatment and the virus migrates to the sensory nerve ganglia where it remains for the lifetime of the patient. During times of dormancy, the patient is asymptomatic but continues to shed the virus at unpredictable intervals. Reactivation of the virus leads to overt recurrent outbreaks. The outbreaks tend to begin with a 3- to 4-day prodrome of pruritus, pain, tingling, and burning. Small edematous grouped papules appear on the genitalia and progress to thin-walled vesicles and ulcers. The vesicles and ulcers form soft crusts, which eventually dry and heal over, and the virus resumes a period of latency. Patients with HSV-1 infection average one recurrence annually, while patients with HSV-2 infection have four or more recurrences each year. Triggers for viral reactivation include sunlight, emotional stress, extremes of temperature, concurrent infections, menstruation, and skin trauma (as in sexual contact).

The clinical diagnosis of genital herpes lacks sensitivity and specificity, so specific laboratory analyses are required for the diagnosis. Because the prognosis differs between HSV-1 and HSV-2, the identification of the exact viral type responsible for infection is an important aspect of diagnosis. Specimens from genital ulcers may be cultured or tested with gene amplification assays to determine the presence of HSV-1 or HSV-2. Additionally, type-specific serologic assays can be used to test for antibodies to HSV-1 and HSV-2. Because HSV-2 is almost exclusively acquired through sexual contact, the presence of antibodies to HSV-2 is diagnostic of genital herpes. However, because HSV-1 may cause either labial or genital herpes, the presence of antibodies to HSV-1 should be interpreted more cautiously. Current serologic assays demonstrate well in excess of 90% sensitivity and specificity. However, they may be subject to some delay in seroconversion following initial contact. Currently, there is no serological test that can determine when the disease was acquired.

The first episode of genital herpes should be treated with acyclovir (400 mg orally three times daily for 7 to 10 days, or 200 mg orally five times daily for 7 to 10 days), valacyclovir (1 g orally twice daily for 7 to 10 days), or famciclovir (250 mg orally three times daily for 7 to 10 days). In patients with frequent recurrences, suppressive therapy reduces outbreaks and improves quality of life. These patients should be treated with acyclovir (400 mg orally twice daily), valacyclovir (500 mg to 1 g orally once daily), or famciclovir (250 mg orally twice daily). In the past, patients with infrequent outbreaks may have preferred episodic treatment; however, more recent data suggests that due to asymptomatic shedding, chronic suppressive therapy may be recommended to all infected patients to decrease transmission to their susceptible sexual partners. In the only small head-to-head comparison, valacyclovir outperformed famciclovir in terms of efficiency of suppression.

Anogenital Warts

Anogenital warts, or condyloma accuminata, are caused by the human papilloma virus (HPV). There are more than 100 serotypes of HPV, and 30 types are capable of infecting the anogenital region. Genital HPV infection is very common, and infections are usually self-limited and may be completely asymptomatic. It is estimated that 75% of adults of reproductive age have been infected at least once with sexually transmitted HPV, and there are more than 5 million new infections annually in the United States alone. Most infections go unnoticed by the patient and ultimately resolve without treatment. In fact, only about 1% of adults have clinical evidence of anogenital warts.

HPV types 6 and 11 are the most common causes of anogenital warts, although many more types are capable of causing condylomata. Other serotypes, most notably types 16, 18, 31, and 45 are associated with anogenital dysplasia and squamous cell carcinoma. In fact, nearly all cervical neoplasia and anogenital carcinomas are related to HPV infection. Anogenital warts are not considered to have malignant potential, but HPV types 6 and

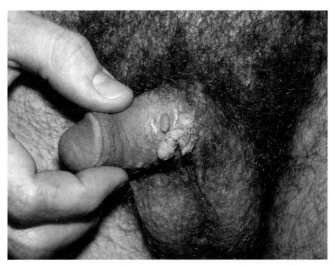

Figure 24.13. Large cauliflower-like, verrucous mass (venereal warts).

11 have been associated with the Buschke-Lowenstein tumor, a slow-growing but locally destructive verrucous carcinoma.

Anogenital warts appear as fleshy verrucous papules, either individual or coalesced into clusters. They may also have a filiform or pedunculated appearance, and confluent warts can form large cauliflower-like lesions of the anogenital zone (Fig. 24.13). Although the warts occur most often on the fourchette in women and on the glans or subprepuce in men, they may appear anywhere where sexual contact has been made. The diagnosis of condyloma is made by clinical inspection and identification of the warts. Histopathological evaluation of biopsied lesions can confirm the diagnosis, revealing papillomatosis and koilocytes. Serologic testing is not recommended for use in the routine diagnosis of anogenital warts.

Untreated genital warts resolve because of cell-mediated immunity in less than one-third of patients. Treatment is recommended to prevent an increase in the size and number of warts and to reduce the likelihood of transmission to sex partners. Treatment options are many, and the chosen regimen should be based on patient preferences and available resources. For warts of the external genitalia, the CDC recommends the use of 0.5% podofilox solution (Condylox) or imiquimod 5% cream (Aldara). Condylox is applied twice daily to warts for 3 days, followed by 4 days of no therapy, with up to four cycles of repetition as necessary. Aldara is applied once daily to warts for 3 weeks at a time, and up to 16 weeks total. Physicians can also apply podophyllin 10% resin or trichloracetic acid 80% solution to the warts in the office setting. Alternatively, the clinician may use cryotherapy, curettage, electrodessication, or excision to destroy the warts. For warts of the vaginal canal, anus, or urethral meatus, the CDC recommends destruction with liquid nitrogen cryotherapy. Use of these options is discussed in detail elsewhere in this text.

PITFALLS AND MYTHS

Syphilis

Because syphilis has been considered the prototypical STD for centuries, public awareness is higher than with other STDs.

However, with increased public awareness comes a significant amount of misinformation, and the advances in telecommunications and Internet technology have only facilitated dissemination of this misinformation. Practitioners should anticipate some of the common misconceptions their patients may hold regarding syphilis. First, it is common for patients to believe that syphilis has been eradicated. The recent global increases in incidence and the surge of new cases in MSM disprove this belief. Additionally, patients may assume that if they were infected with syphilis they would be aware of the infection. While it is true that most chancres in heterosexual men occur on the penis or scrotum and are readily apparent, women and MSM often have occult chancres and present at later stages of the disease. Finally, patients may believe that having syphilis once provides lasting immunity against future infection. In fact, no immunity is developed after infection by *T. pallidum* and patients are subject to future re-infection. The specific treponemal antibodies measured in the FTA-ABS and MHA-TP assays provide no protective immunity.

Chancroid

Because of the dramatic decline in reported cases of chancroid in the United States in recent years, both patients and physicians may believe the disease to have been eliminated. However, sporadic outbreaks continue to occur, and the disease remains quite common worldwide. Just as patients may believe that a prior case of syphilis offers protective immunity to future infection, they may also believe repeat infection with chancroid to be impossible. Neither natural nor experimental infection with chancroid appears to protect against future infections. However, repeated experimental inoculation in a swine model has led to a moderate degree of humoral immunity and diminished severity of future infections. While these results are not immediately applicable to human patients, researchers hope to eventually develop a vaccine that may confer at least partial resistance to infection with *H. ducreyi*. This is especially likely since a putative etiopathogenic factor has been recently characterized (cytolethal distending factor).

Lymphogranuloma Venereum

Because LGV is endemic to tropical climates and was heretofore underrecognized in the United States, both physicians and patients may be unaware of LGV as a cause of genital ulcers and proctocolitis. Physicians should consider LGV when differentiating possible causes of genital ulcers, lymphadenopathy, and proctocolitis, especially in MSM and patients with HIV.

Granuloma Inguinale

Like LGV, GI is a very rare source of genital ulcers in the United States. Many clinicians may not consider the diagnosis routinely. However, with the ease of international travel, GI is certainly a diagnostic possibility both in the United States and abroad.

Gonorrhea

The common symptoms of gonorrhea, including urethritis and urethral discharge, are well known among the public. Some patients may describe their symptoms as "the clap," a slang term

referring to gonorrhea and originating from the Old French *clapoir* (venereal sore) and *clapier* (brothel). However, the potentially fatal complications of DGI are not well known and the disease may be underrecognized. Furthermore, patients with DGI typically do not have symptoms of primary infections, so physicians must complete comprehensive histories and physical examinations in patients with widespread pustular and necrotic eruptions or septic arthritis to ensure proper diagnosis and management.

SUGGESTED READINGS

Baughn RE, Musher DM. Secondary syphilitic lesions. *Clin Microbiol Rev* 2005;18:205–216.

Bong CT, Bauer ME, Spinola SM. Haemophilus ducreyi: clinical features, epidemiology, and prospects for disease control. *Microbes Infect* 2002;4:1141–1148.

Brown TJ, Yen-Moore A, Tyring SK. An overview of sexually transmitted diseases. Part I. *J Am Acad Dermatol* 1999;41:511–532.

Brown TJ, Yen-Moore A, Tyring SK. An overview of sexually transmitted diseases. Part II. *J Am Acad Dermatol.* 1999;41:661–677.

Buntin DM, Rosen T, Lesher JL Jr., et al. Sexually transmitted diseases: bacterial infections. *J Am Acad Dermatol* 1991;25:287–299.

Centers for Disease Control and Prevention. Sexually transmitted diseases treatment guidelines, 2006. MMWR 2006;55(No. RR-11).

Centers for Disease Control and Prevention. Trends in Reportable Sexually Transmitted Diseases in the United States, 2005. Available online at http://www.cdc.gov/std/stats/trends2005.htm.

Centers for Disease Control and Prevention. Updated recommended treatment regimens for gonococcal infections and associated conditions. 2007. Available online at http://www.cdc.gov/std/treatment/2006/updated-regimens.htm.

Chosidow O. Clinical practices. Scabies. *N Engl J Med* 2006;354:1718–1727.

Cole LE, Toffer KL, Fulcher RA, et al. A humoral immune response confers protection against Haemophilus ducreyi infection. *Infect Immun* 2003;71:6971–6977.

Corey A, Wald L, Patel R, et al. Once daily valacyclovir to reduce the risk of transmission of genital herpes. *N Engl J Med.* 2004;350:67–8.

de Vries HJ, Fennema JS, Morre SA. Lymphogranuloma venereum among men having sex with men; what have we learned so far? *Sex Transm Infect* 2006;82:344.

Dupuy A, Dehen L, Bourrat E, et al. Accuracy of standard dermoscopy for diagnosing scabies. *J Am Acad Dermatol* 2007;56:53–62.

Ghosn SH, Kibbi AG. Cutaneous gonococcal infections. *Clin Dermatol* 2004;22:476–480.

Golden MR, Marra CM, Holmes KK. Update on syphilis: resurgence of an old problem. *JAMA* 2003;290:1510–1514.

Griego RD, Rosen T, Orengo IF, et al. Dog, cat, and human bites: a review. *J Am Acad Dermatol* 1995;33:1019–1029.

Hampton T. Lymphogranuloma venereum targeted: those at risk identified; diagnostic test developed. *JAMA* 2006;295:2592.

Hart CA, Rao SK. Donovanosis. *J Med Microbiol* 1999;48:707–709.

Hart G. Donovanosis. *Clin Infect Dis* 1997;25:24–30.

Hengge UR, Currie BJ, Jager G, et al. Scabies: a ubiquitous neglected skin disease. *Lancet Infect Dis* 2006;6:769–779.

Herring A, Richens J. Lymphogranuloma venereum. *Sex Transm Infect* 2006; 82(Suppl 4):iv23–5.

Heukelbach J, Feldmeier H. Scabies. *Lancet* 2006;367:1767–1774.

Hutchinson CM, Hook EW 3rd, Shepherd M, et al. Altered clinical presentation of early syphilis in patients with human immunodeficiency virus infection. *Ann Intern Med* 1994;121:94–100.

Ison CA, Dillon JA, Tapsall JW. The epidemiology of global antibiotic resistance among Neisseria gonorrhoeae and Haemophilus ducreyi. *Lancet* 1998;351 Suppl 3:8–11.

Jones C, Rosen T, Clarridge J, et al. Chancroid: results from an outbreak in Houston, Texas. *South Med J* 1990;83:1384–89.

Jones CC, Rosen T. Cultural diagnosis of chancroid. *Arch Dermatol.* 1991;127:1823–7.

Joseph AK, Rosen T. Laboratory techniques used in the diagnosis of chancroid, granuloma inguinale, and lymphogranuloma. *Dermatol Clin* 1994;12:1–8.

Ko CJ, Elston DM. Pediculosis. *J Am Acad Dermatol* 2004;50:1–12.

Kumar N, Doug B, Jenkins C. Pubic lice effectively treated with Pilogel. *Eye* 2003;17:538–9.

Lewis DA. Chancroid: clinical manifestations, diagnosis, and management. *Sex Transm Infect* 2003;79:68–71.

Lupi O, Madkan V, Tyring SK. Tropical dermatology: bacterial tropical diseases. *J Am Acad Dermatol* 2006;54:559–578.

Mehrany K, Kist JM, O'Connor WJ, et al. Disseminated gonococcemia. *Int J Dermatol* 2003;42:208–209.

Moorthy TT, Lee CT, Kim KB, et al. Ceftriaxone for treatment of primary syphilis in men: a preliminary study. *Sex Transm Dis* 1987;14:116–118.

Morris SR, Klausner JD, Buchbinder SP, et al. Prevalence and incidence of pharyngeal gonorrhea in a longitudinal sample of men who have sex with men: the EXPLORE study. *Clin Infect Dis* 2006;43:1284–1289.

O'Farrell N. Donovanosis. *Sex Transm Infect.* 2002;78:452–457.

Patterson K, Olsen B, Thomas C, et al. Development of a rapid immunodiagnostic test for Haemophilus ducreyi. *J Clin Microbiol* 2002;40:3694–3702.

Peterman TA, Furness BW. The resurgence of syphilis among men who have sex with men. *Curr Opin Infect Dis* 2007;20:54–59.

Ramos-e-Silva M. Giovan Cosimo Bonomo (1663–1696): discoverer of the etiology of scabies. *Int J Dermatol* 1998;37:625–630.

Rick FM, Rocha GC, Dittmar K, et al. Crab louse infestation in pre-Columbian America. *J Parasitol* 2002;88:1266–1267.

Rompalo AM. Can syphilis be eradicated from the world? *Curr Opin Infect Dis* 2001;14:41–44.

Rosen T, Conrad N. Genital ulcer caused by human bite to the penis. *Sex Transm Dis* 1999;26:527–530.

Rosen T, Tchen JA, Ramsdell W, et al. Granuloma inguinale. *J Am Acad Dermatol* 1984;11:433–7.

Rosen T. Unusual presentations of gonorrhea. *J Am Acad Dermatol* 1982;6:369–72.

Rosen T. Penile ulcer from traumatic orogenital contact. *Dermatol Online J* 2005;11:18.

Rothschild BM. History of syphilis. *Clin Infect Dis* 2005;40:1454–1463.

Sehgal VN, Srivastava G. Chancroid: contemporary appraisal. *Int J Dermatol* 2003;42:182–190.

Smith JL, Bayles DO. The contribution of cytolethal distending toxin to bacterial pathogenesis. *Crit Rev Microbiol* 2006;32:227–48.

Varela JA, Otero L, Espinosa E, et al. Phthirus pubis in a sexually transmitted diseases unit: a study of 14 years. *Sex Transm Dis* 2003;30:292–296.

Wald A, Selke S, Warren T, et al. Comparative efficacy of famciclovir and valacyclovir for suppression of recurrent genital herpes and viral shedding. *Sex Transm Dis* 2006;33:529–33.

Wolf JS Jr, Gomez R, McAninch JW. Human bites to the penis. *J Urol* 1992;147:1265–1267.

Xu F, Sternberg MR, Kottiri BJ, et al. Trends in herpes simplex virus type 1 and type 2 seroprevalence in the United States. *JAMA* 2006;296:964–73.

Zeltser R, Kurban AK. Syphilis. *Clin Dermatol* 2004;22:461–468.

25 | LIFE-THREATENING SKIN INFECTIONS: SKIN SIGNS OF IMPORTANT BACTERIAL INFECTIOUS DISEASES

Lisa A. Drage

An important group of bacterial infectious diseases are life-threatening conditions that require immediate intervention and treatment. Appropriate diagnosis and management of this group of severe bacterial infections can be expedited by recognition of their distinctive cutaneous findings. The clinical manifestations, diagnosis, and management of meningococcal disease, Rocky Mountain spotted fever (RMSF), Staphylococcal toxic shock syndrome, and Streptococcal toxic shock syndrome will be highlighted herein with emphasis being placed on their cutaneous signs.

HISTORY

Reports of illnesses resembling meningococcal disease date back to the 1500s. The description reported by Vieusseux in 1805 is considered the first identification of the disease, and the causative organism was first isolated by Weichselbaum in 1887. Today, meningococcal disease remains a feared cause of significant morbidity and mortality throughout the world.

Rocky Mountain spotted fever (RMSF) was first described in Boise, Idaho, by Marshall Wood, an Army Physician in 1896. More than 100 years have elapsed since Howard T. Ricketts first identified the pathogen and demonstrated its transmission by Montana ticks. Four years after his classic investigation, Ricketts died at the age of 40 of epidemic typhus while investigating that disease in Mexico City.

Toxic Shock Syndrome (TSS) was first described in 1978 by Todd and associates as a complication of infection by *Staphylococcus aureus*. An early association was made between TSS and concomitant tampon usage in menstruating women. The sudden increase in TSS in the early 1980s was temporally related to the introduction of these super absorbent tampons, which were subsequently withdrawn from the market. A case definition of Staphylococcal TSS was first published in 1982.

Severe invasive Group A Streptococcal infections reemerged in the mid-1980s after a period of low streptococcal morbidity and mortality in the mid-20th century. Prominent media coverage of the dramatic outbreaks of "flesh-eating bacteria" in the 1990s raised public awareness of the potential serious nature of these infections.

** The author has no conflict of interest to disclose. There were no funding sources for this work.

MENINGOCOCCAL DISEASE

Acute meningococcemia and meningococcal meningitis are caused by *Neisseria meningitidis,* a distinctive encapsulated gram-negative diplococcus. Ten percent to twenty percent of healthy people are nasopharyngeal carriers of this organism and the percentage of carriers increases in crowded conditions, such as military settings or college dormitories. Most often, nasopharyngeal colonization imparts protective antibodies and immunity to the disease. Factors that increase colonization such as crowding, viral upper respiratory infection, and active or passive smoking are associated with an increased risk of transmission of meningococcal disease. Meningococcal disease is not highly contagious, and transmission is via direct contact with large droplet respiratory secretions or saliva, so very close contact is needed. The disease occurs most commonly in people who lack protective antibodies and have newly acquired *N. meningitidis.* Although the highest rate of meningococcal disease occurs during the late winter and spring months in patients younger than 5 years, more than half of cases occur in people aged 18 or older. Students newly arrived to college who live in dormitories have a moderately increased risk for meningococcal disease.

The mortality rate of meningococcal disease ranges from 10% to 14%. Substantial sequelae occur in 11% to 19% of survivors and include neurologic damage, hearing loss, and limb loss associated with disseminated intravascular coagulation (purpura fulminans). Improved patient outcomes depend heavily on early recognition and prompt use of appropriate antibiotics and supportive measures. Recognition of the skin findings associated with meningococcal disease can aid in early diagnosis.

Clinical Manifestations

Invasive meningococcal disease is infamous for its rapidly evolving, dramatic signs and symptoms; yet it begins with nonspecific findings of fever, headache, nausea, vomiting, and myalgias. Altered consciousness, severe headache, and nuchal rigidity signal meningitis. Children are often markedly lethargic. Skin lesions are a common and early sign that offers an important clue to this rapidly progressive disease. The majority of patients with meningococcemia present with a rash. Classically, the rash appears as petechiae scattered over the trunk and extremities and quickly evolves into purpura with distinctive gun metal gray centers and geographic or angular borders (Fig. 25.1). However, the initial skin findings may be macular, papular, or urticarial. A thorough skin examination is important as some patients present with only a few petechiae or purpura. Clusters of petechiae may occur at

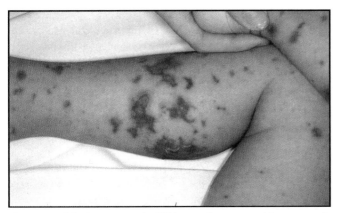

Figure 25.1. Meningococcemia. Widespread purpura with gun metal grey centers and geographic borders.

sites of pressure such as the site of a blood pressure cuff or elastic bands of the socks. Adults with meningococcal disease are less likely than children to have the classic skin findings. Fulminant meningococcal disease (Waterhouse-Friderichsen syndrome) can be complicated by purpura fulminans – generalized ecchymoses and hemorrhagic bullae that are cutaneous manifestations of disseminated intravascular coagulation. This dramatic scenario may be accompanied by ischemia of the digits or limbs with resultant necrosis or autoamputation and death.

Diagnosis

Meningococcal disease should be suspected in an acutely ill patient, especially a child or young adult, presenting with a petechial eruption in the setting of fever, headache, and myalgias. While the gold standard of diagnosis is Gram's stain and culture of the blood or cerebrospinal fluid, microbiologic testing of skin lesions can help with a definitive diagnosis. Gram's stain of smears from active skin lesions may demonstrate the characteristic gram-negative diplococcus in up to 70% of cases. Gram's stain and culture of a biopsy from an active skin lesion may be positive for *N. Meningitidis* even after the blood and CSF fluid have been rendered sterile by antibiotics. PCR techniques may also be helpful in diagnosing the disease.

Management

Early treatment is the highest priority in any suspected case of meningococcal disease. Appropriate antibiotic therapy should not be forestalled while awaiting transfer or hospitalization of a patient. Prehospital antibiotic treatment is advocated. Initial empiric therapy is based on the most common bacteria causing meningitis or sepsis based on the patient's age, clinical setting, and local patterns of antimicrobial susceptibility. After the results of cultures and susceptibility testing are available, antimicrobial therapy should be modified for optimal treatment. Adjunctive dexamethasone therapy may be instituted in carefully selected patients with meningitis. Aggressive supportive care and monitoring in an intensive care setting is necessary with an emphasis on restoration of circulation, correction of DIC, and prevention of hypoxia.

Chemoprophylaxis with rifampin (non-pregnant adults and children) or ciprofloxacin (non-pregnant adults) or intramuscular ceftriaxone is offered to close contacts of documented cases (household members, childcare contacts and hospital personnel

with secretion exposure). In the United States, most cases of invasive meningococcal disease are caused by serogroups B, C, and Y, each of which accounts for approximately one-third of cases. While there is no current vaccine for serogroup B, a new meningococcal conjugate vaccine A, C, Y, and W-135 (Menactra, Sanofi Pasteur) is available and currently recommended for children aged 11 to 12, teens entering high school, and college freshman in dormitories. Vaccination is also recommended for outbreak or epidemic settings, patients with a terminal complement pathway deficiency, patients with anatomic or functional asplenia, travelers to hyperendemic areas (sub-Saharan Africa, or Saudi Arabia), and military recruits.

Since catastrophic outbreaks occur in college, school, and day-care settings, meningococcal infections can cause community panic. Prevention of meningococcal disease by vaccination is the best control strategy. Institution of new vaccine recommendations may help to minimize the disease; however, there is still no vaccine available to prevent the most common cause of meningococcal disease in young children, serogroup B. This situation makes prompt recognition and treatment of patients with suspected meningococcal disease essential in preventing mortality and associated morbidities.

ROCKY MOUNTAIN SPOTTED FEVER

Rocky Mountain spotted fever (RMSF) is a tick-borne zoonoses caused by *Rickettsia rickettsii*, an obligate intracellular coccobacillus. This organism is maintained in a natural cycle involving mammals and ixodid (hard-bodied) ticks. Transmission to humans occurs through the bite of infected ticks. The most common tick vectors include *Dermacentor variabilis* (American dog tick) in the eastern, central, and pacific coastal United States and *Dermacentor andersoni* (Rocky Mountain wood tick) in the western United States. Other tick species such as *Rhipicephalus sanguineus* (Brown dog tick) and *Amblyomma Cajennense* (Cayenne tick) cause RMSF in Arizona and Texas, respectively.

From an epidemiologic standpoint, the term Rocky Mountain spotted fever is deceiving. While first described in the Bitter Root valley of Montana, most cases are currently centered in the south-eastern and south-central United States. More than half of RMSF cases are from five states: North Carolina, South Carolina, Tennessee, Oklahoma, and Arkansas. The disease, however, has been reported in all states of the contiguous United States except Vermont and Maine and due to modern travel patterns, the disease could be encountered in patents from any of the 50 states.

Rocky Mountain spotted fever is a seasonal disease reflecting the activity levels of the vectors, reservoirs, and humans that increase exposure to the disease. Most cases occur during the spring and summer months when ticks are most active and human–tick contacts are most likely to occur. Ninety percent of cases occur between April and September. Outdoor workers, recreationalists, and young children are most frequently affected by RMSF. In the past, young children were the most common victims, but recent surveillance data has shown that adults aged 40 to 64 had the highest reported incidence of RMSF. Mortality rates range from 5% in treated cases to 20% in untreated cases. Outcomes thus depend heavily on prompt recognition of the disease and early initiation of specific antibiotic therapy. The skin manifestations of RMSF may be a helpful clue to making a life-saving diagnosis.

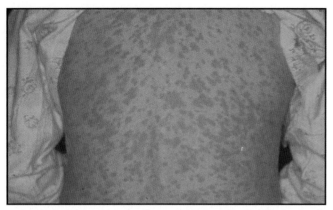

Figure 25.2. Rocky Mountain Spotted Fever. Although the rash demonstrates centripetal spread, it may be generalized when first viewed. (*From Mayo Clinic Proceedings with permission*)

Clinical manifestations

Fever, chills, malaise, myalgia, and severe headaches are the most common initial features of Rocky Mountain spotted fever and resemble the nonspecific findings of other infectious diseases. Nausea, vomiting, and abdominal pain may be striking symptoms seen in a subset of patients with RMSF. Most patients visit a physician during the first 2 to 4 days of the illness, before the development of the petechial (spotted) rash that is the hallmark of the disease. This presents a formidable challenge to the physician who must diagnose the disease early in the clinical course when antibiotic treatment is most effective.

The dermatologic findings provide clues that lead to consideration of the diagnosis and can help "rule out" other exanthemata. Classically, the rash of RMSF begins on day 4 of the illness (range: 1–15 days) on the wrists and ankles. It then spreads to the palms and soles and subsequently involves the proximal extremities and trunk (Fig. 25.2). This classic centripetal spread is a hallmark of RMSF. However, most patients do not discern this pattern and health-care providers may first see the patient when the rash has generalized (Fig. 25.2). Initially the exanthem presents with small pink or red macules that blanch with pressure and evolves into petechia and purpura. Periorbital and peripheral edema and conjunctivitis may also be present. Calf pain and tenderness has been reported in the literature. Gangrenous areas may develop on the fingers, toes, ears, scrotum, and vulvar areas. Involvement of the scrotum and vulva has been heralded as a diagnostic clue, albeit a late one. The classic rash is absent in up to 20% of RMSF patients. In addition, the skin finding may be difficult to appreciate in patients with deeply pigmented skin or late development in the disease course. Rocky Mountain "spotless" fever is a recognized presentation that is associated with a higher fatality rate.

Diagnosis

During the early stages of RMSF, rapid laboratory confirmation is not available to guide acute therapeutic decisions. Diagnosis is based on the recognition of the epidemiologic clues and clinical findings of: fever, headache, and rash in a person with a known or potential exposure to a tick bite. A history of tick bite, travel to an endemic area, or recent outdoor activity should be sought from the patient. Similar illness in a family member, coworker, or even a family pet may provide an important clue. Household clusters of disease have been reported and dogs may develop RMSF alongside human family members. Unfortunately, the "classic" triad of fever, rash, and a history of a tick bite is elicited in only 60% to 70% of patients on initial examination.

Laboratory clues to the disease may include a left-shift in the WBC, thrombocytopenia, elevated hepatic transaminases, and hyponatremia. Although serologic tests are confirmatory, they are not helpful in guiding immediate therapeutic decisions. Early in the course of the disease, the serologic tests will be negative and it is only after 2 to 3 weeks when the acute and convalescent serum samples can be compared for a rising IgG and IgM level (a four-fold or greater increase in antibody titer) that the diagnosis of RMSF is confirmed. Direct immunofluorescence testing of a skin biopsy can be helpful in the acute setting; however, while 100% specific, it is only 70% sensitive and is not widely or immediately available. Immunohistochemical (IHC) staining may also be used to document presence of the organism in a skin biopsy or other tissue. Polymerase chain reaction (PCR) testing of a skin biopsy is a rapid method for evaluation of RMSF but is only available in limited venues (Centers for Disease Control and Prevention [CDC], certain state public health laboratories, a few research and commercial labs) and has a low sensitivity. *Rickettsia rickettsii*, an obligate intracellular coccobacillus, may only be isolated using cell culture techniques in laboratories equipped to handle Biosafety Level-3 agents; thus culture is rarely used for diagnosis. Owing to sensitivity or time issues surrounding these complex diagnostic tests, they are used primarily in a confirmatory role and the initial treatment decisions for RMSF are based primarily on clinical and epidemiologic evidence.

Management

Early treatment is of the highest priority in a suspected case of Rocky Mountain spotted fever. Empiric antibiotic treatment should be initiated when clinical and epidemiologic clues even suggest RMSF. Doxycycline (oral or intravenous) is the drug of choice for adults and children with Rocky Mountain spotted fever. The American Academy of Pediatrics Committee on Infectious Diseases has endorsed the use of doxycycline for treatment of presumed or confirmed cases of RMSF in children of all ages given the life-threatening nature of the disease and the negligible risk for tooth staining with a limited course of treatment. Chloramphenicol is typically the preferred treatment for RMSF during pregnancy; however, the use of tetracycline might be warranted during pregnancy in life-threatening situations where the clinical suspicion of RMSF is high. Supportive care may be needed for severely ill patients. Of importance, typical "broad-spectrum" antibiotic coverage will not treat RMSF. Empiric treatment should be initiated when clinical and epidemiologic clues even suggest RMSF. Failure to consider the diagnosis of RMSF and institute early effective antibiotic treatment can be a fatal error.

STAPHYLOCOCCAL TOXIC SHOCK SYNDROME

Staphylococcal toxic shock syndrome (TSS) is caused by infection or colonization with the common skin pathogen,

Staphylococcus aureus. A toxin-mediated disease; menstrual toxic shock syndrome is caused by the superantigen exotoxin toxic shock syndrome toxin-1 (TSST-1). In this multisystem disease, superantigens overactivate the human immune system to release various cytokines that cause the clinical features of TSS such as fever, capillary leak, and rash.

Nowadays, nonmenstrual toxic shock syndrome is more common than menstrual TSS and can occur in anyone, male or female, young or old. Nonmenstrual toxic shock syndrome settings include post-influenza, postpartum, postsurgical, nasal packing or stent use, barrier contraceptive use, localized infections (cellulitis, burns, abscess, hidradenitis suppurativa, wounds), and postviral upper respiratory infection. Nonmenstrual TSS is mediated by TSST-1 (50%) or by staphylococcal exotoxin B or C (up to 50%). The mortality rate for menstrual TSS has dropped to 5%, but remains higher for nonmenstrual cases, possibly because of the delay in making a definitive diagnosis.

With the emergence of community-acquired methicillin-resistant *S. aureus* (CA-MRSA), an increase in high toxin-producing strains capable of causing TSS is occurring. In addition, "new" clinical patterns such as purpura fulminans and necrotizing fasciitis in association with *S. aureus* are emerging.

Clinical Manifestations

The prodromal features of staphylococcal TSS include fever, malaise, myalgias, nausea, vomiting, diarrhea, and prominent confusion. The cutaneous signs can be quite striking and typically include a "sunburn-like" diffuse or patchy macular erythroderma with perineal accentuation. A scarlatiniform eruption with flexural accentuation may also be present. Desquamation follows in 5 to 14 days and is prominent on the hands, feet, and perineal areas (Fig. 25.3). As it occurs during the convalescent phase, it is generally not a helpful skin sign in the acute stage of the illness. Conjunctiva injection, mucosal hyperemia (oral and genital), and strawberry tongue are helpful clinical clues, especially in deeply pigmented patients in whom the erythroderma may be subtle or overlooked. Less common findings include edema of the hands and feet, petechia, and the late loss of hair and nails. Purpura fulminans, most commonly associated with meningococcal disease, has been reported in association with CA-MRSA and toxic shock syndrome. Necrotizing fasciitis in association with CA-MRSA

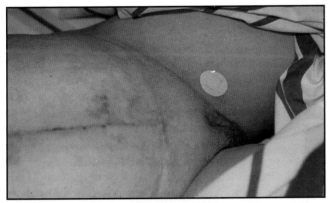

Figure 25.3. Staphylococcal Toxic Shock Syndrome. Desquamative erythroderma in the groin and perineal area.

is an emerging clinical entity requiring urgent surgical and medical therapy.

Diagnosis

Formal diagnostic criteria for TSS have been developed and include fever, desquamative erythroderma, and hypotension within a setting of multiple organ system involvement. The multisystem involvement (three or more systems) may include gastrointestinal, hepatic, musculoskeletal, renal, cardiopulmonary, CNS, metabolic findings, and mucosal hyperemia. TSS is a diagnosis of exclusion and other causes of sepsis must be "ruled out." Milder cases of TSS do occur and may not fulfill all of the criteria of the case definition. Severe sepsis associated with CA-MRSA may or may not present with the emblematic desquamating erythroderma of "classical" TSS and may not fulfil the diagnostic criteria for TSS.

As a toxin-mediated disease, *Staphylococcus aureus* is rarely isolated from TSS blood cultures. A thorough search to identify the potential sources of infection includes a close examination of the skin surface to identify any wounds or abscesses. The classic signs of localized infection at a wound or surgical site such as erythema, tenderness, and purulence may be absent, making clinical diagnosis challenging. Cultures must be obtained from all mucous membranes (vaginal, oropharyngeal, and conjunctival) as well as from blood and urine. All wounds and surgical sites should be cultured and considered possible sources of infection even without signs of local infection. Toxins may be identified by antibody reactivity or PCR.

Management

Treatment of staphylococcal TSS includes the identification and removal of the source of the *Staphylococcus aureus*, initiation of effective anti-staphylococcal antibiotic coverage, and supportive care. Examples of removal of the source of infection may include incision and drainage of an access, surgical debridement of a wound site, or the removal of nasal packing or tampon. With the emergence of CA-MRSA, initial treatment of an infection should be based on the antibiotic resistance patterns in the community.

Vancomycin is included for empirical coverage of severe infections. Additional therapies to consider include intravenous immunoglobulin to neutralize circulating toxins and clindamycin, which may help reduce the actual toxin production. Aggressive management of the hypovolemia associated with capillary leak, vasodilation and fluid loss is a mainstay of therapy. Patients may require vast amounts of fluid replacement.

Primary prevention of TSS is via education about the early signs and symptoms of TSS, risk factors, and limited use of high-absorbency tampons. Up to 30% of women diagnosed with menstrual TSS relapse during subsequent menses. Tampons and barrier contraceptives should be avoided in women who do not have documented seroconversion after the acute illness.

STREPTOCOCCAL TOXIC SHOCK SYNDROME

Streptococcal toxic shock syndrome (STSS) is caused by infection with Group A β-hemolytic streptococcus (*Streptococcus pyogenes),* the same organism that causes strep throat and simple skin infections. However, the strains leading to STSS possess virulence properties that lead to severe and life-threatening disease. STSS is typically encountered in the setting of invasive soft tissue infection. Cellulitis, necrotizing fasciitis, or myonecrosis is present in 80% of cases. However, it is also seen in association with streptococcal pharyngitis, pneumonia, septic arthritis, endophthalmitis, peritonitis, meningitis, and sinusitis. Cases have been encountered where there is no obvious evidence of a strep infection but only a history of blunt trauma or muscle strain – hematogenous spread from a pharyngeal source to the site of muscle or soft tissue injury has been hypothesized. Most cases of STSS occur sporadically with only occasional clusters reported in nursing homes, health-care workers, or family members.

In cases associated with a soft tissue infection, a portal of entry is often discernible such as surgical excision, laceration, burn site, varicella lesion, childbirth trauma, decubitus ulcer, or an insect bite. Comorbidities such as diabetes mellitus, peripheral arterial disease, obesity, alcohol abuse, human immunodeficiency virus (HIV), or recent varicella-zoster virus (VZV) may be present, but many patients are healthy, immunocompetent, and are in the 20- to 50-year age range. The mortality for STSS has been reported as 30% to 60% despite aggressive modern treatments.

Special features of the streptococcal bacterium make the syndrome more deadly. M-1 and M-3 surface proteins increase adherence to tissue, possess antiphagocytic properties that blunt the immune response, and induce capillary leak. Streptococcal pyrogenic exotoxins function as superantigens. They bypass and amplify the conventional immune response, interacting nonspecifically with T-cells to activate a large segment of the T-cell population and trigger a massive cytokine release. The cytokines cause the fever, hypotension, rash, and tissue injury of the toxic shock syndrome. Host factors, such as lack of past exposure to virulent bacteria and possession of specific HLA class II haplotypes that determine the magnitude of the cytokine response, predispose to invasive Group A streptococcal disease. Interplay between the bacterial virulence factors and host factors allow this severe and life-threatening form of streptococcal infection to develop.

Clinical Manifestation

Streptococcal toxic shock syndrome often occurs in a young, previously healthy person who seeks medical care because of the abrupt onset of fever, hypotension, and skin findings accompanied by severe, localized pain. Pain is the most common initial symptom and is typically localized to an extremity and is disproportionate to the examination findings. The pain may be so out of proportion to the clinical signs that physicians may suspect that the patient is displaying malingering or drug-seeking behavior. Twenty percent of patients have an influenza-like prodrome with fever, chills, myalgias, nausea, vomiting, and diarrhea. While fever is the most common presenting sign of STSS, confusion is present in over half of patients and may manifest as combativeness. In 80% of patients, STSS is accompanied by clinical signs of soft tissue infection, which in 70% of patients, will progress to necrotizing fasciitis or myositis.

The initial skin signs of STSS may be subtle, and a thorough examination of the skin is needed to look for portals of entry and

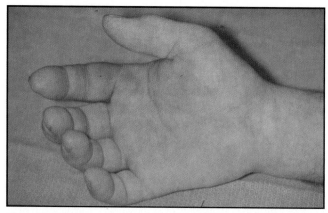

Figure 25.4. Streptococcal Toxic Shock Syndrome. Necrotizing fasciitis. Dusky, violaceous erythema, edema and tenderness. A bulla developed between the first and second finger webspace.

evidence of a soft tissue infection such as tenderness, localized swelling, or erythema. The disease progresses at an alarming rate with the development of red/purple discoloration, dusky blue pigment, and distinctive violaceous vesicles or bullae. These are ominous signs of necrotizing fasciitis or myonecrosis (Fig. 25.4). The evolving area may also develop decreased sensation. The crepitance noted in a patient with a polymicrobial or anerobic infection is not prominent in patients with streptococcal necrotizing fasciitis. Desquamating erythroderma is noted in only 10% of patients with STSS.

Diagnosis

A clinical case definition for STSS is established and includes the isolation of Group A Streptococcus from a normally sterile site, hypotension, and multisystem involvement. Involvement of two or more organ systems is required and may include a generalized erythematous rash that may desquamate, soft tissue necrosis, renal impairment, coagulopathy, liver involvement, and acute respiratory distress syndrome. An intraoperative Gram's stain, culture, and biopsy are helpful in making a definitive diagnosis. The presence of gram-positive cocci in pairs and/or in chains supports the diagnosis of streptococcus. As opposed to staphylococcal toxic shock syndrome, 60% of patients with STSS will have bacteremia and positive blood cultures. Magnetic resonance imaging, muscle compartment pressure monitoring, and creatine kinase levels can be used to help diagnose, monitor, and predict necrotizing fasciitis or myonecrosis.

Management

The management of STSS in association with necrotizing fasciitis or myonecrosis relies on both surgical and medical intervention. Early surgical involvement with aggressive exploration and debridement of soft tissue infection is the standard of care. While small retrospective studies have shown successful medical management with high-dose IV immunoglobulin and antibiotics in patients too unstable for aggressive surgical treatment, early surgical consultation and action is the mainstay of therapy. Early surgical exploration facilitates the definitive diagnosis through acquisition of Gram stains, tissue cultures, and biopsies.

A series of surgical reexplorations with repeated debridements or amputation may be necessary to remove necrotic tissue. Empiric treatment includes broad-spectrum antibiotic coverage until the results of cultures and sensitivities return, intravenous immunoglobulin to help neutralize circulating toxins, and clindamycin to decrease toxin synthesis. Aggressive supportive care is necessary and extensive reconstructive surgery and rehabilitation is part of a long-term rehabilitation plan.

PITFALLS AND MYTHS

Meningococcal Disease
- Misdiagnosing meningococcal disease as "viral exanthem" in a child
- Failing to recognize the signs and symptoms of meningococcus in an adult (especially a college-age student)
- Failing to identify risk factors for meningococcal disease: patients with a terminal complement pathway deficiency, patients with anatomic or functional asplenia, military recruits, travelers to hyperendemic areas (sub-Saharan Africa, or Saudi Arabia), and college-age students in dormitory settings
- Failing to recognize the early skin signs of meningococcal disease
- Neglecting to perform a complete skin examination and missing the key clue in patients who present with only a few petechiae
- Delaying initiation of antibiotic treatment while awaiting blood culture, imaging tests, or transfer to a hospital
- Failing to treat upon clinical suspicion

Rocky Mountain Spotted Fever
- Failing to obtain a history that elicits exposure to ticks, tick habitats, or concurrent illness in household pets or family members
- Discounting the diagnosis when there is no history of a tick bite
- Waiting for the petechial rash ("spots") to develop on the palms/soles before making a diagnosis
- Failing to consider RMSF in the differential diagnosis of a generalized petechial rash
- Excluding the diagnosis of RMSF because of geography
- Misdiagnosing as gastroenteritis due to significant nausea and vomiting
- Failing to treat upon clinical suspicion
- Failing to treat with an appropriate antimicrobial agent (doxycycline)
- Failing to use doxycycline in children suspected of having RMSF

Staphylococcal Toxic Shock Syndrome
- Failing to recognize the disease in men
- Failing to recognize "nonmenstrual" cases
- Missing the early skin signs of the disease, thus delaying diagnosis and treatment
- Waiting for desquamation, a late skin finding
- Not identifying and treating/removing the source of infection
- Overlooking the erythroderma in dark-skinned patients
- Failing to recognize the high recurrence rate in menstrual staphylococcal TSS
- Decreasing the level of vigilance for cases of staphylococcal TSS

Streptococcal Toxic Shock Syndrome
- Failing to recognize the early skin signs of the disease
- Overlooking "portals of entry" for the streptococcal pathogen
- Misdiagnosing as gout or a musculoskeletal disease
- Ascribing the patient's severe pain (out of proportion to the exam findings) to "drug-seeking" behavior or malingering
- Difficulty in differentiating cellulitis from necrotizing fasciitis
- Failing to involve surgical consultation early in the disease course
- Delaying surgical intervention or relying on medical management when surgical treatment is the mainstay of effective therapy

SUGGESTED READINGS

Ade PV, Montgomery CP, Husain AN, et al. Staphylococcus aureus sepsis and the Waterhouse-Friderichsen syndrome in children. N Engl J Med 2005;353:1245–1251.

Bilukha OO, Rosenstein N. Prevention and control of meningococcal disease. Recommendations of the Advisory Committee on Immunization Practices (ACIP). MMWR Recomm Rep 2005 27;54(RR-7):1–21.

Bisno AL, Brito MO, Collins CM. Molecular basis of group A streptococcal virulence. Lancet Infect Dis 2003;3:191–200.

Bisno AL, Stevens DL. Streptococcal infections of skin and soft tissues. N Engl J Med 1996;334:240–245.

Bruce MG, Rosenstein, NE, Capparella JM, Shutts KA, Perkins, BA, Collins M. Risk factors for meningococcal disease in college students. JAMA 2001;286:688–693.

Buckingham SC, Marshall GS, Schutze GE, Woods CR, Jackson MA, Patterson LE, Jacobs RF; Tick-borne Infections in Children Study Group. Clinical and laboratory features, hospital course, and outcome of Rocky Mountain spotted fever in children. J Pediatr 2007;150(2):180–184.

Center for Disease Control and Prevention. Fatal cases of Rocky Mountain spotted fever in family clusters – three states, 2003. MMWR 2004:53(19);407–410.

Drage LA. Life-threatening rashes: dermatologic signs of four infectious diseases. Mayo Clin Proc 1999;74:68–72.

Gardner, P. Prevention of meningococcal disease. N Engl J Med 2006;355:1466–73.

Kirkland KB, Wilkinson WE, Sexton DJ. Therapeutic delay and mortality in cases of Rocky Mountain spotted fever. Clin Infect Dis 1995;20:1118–1121.

Kowalski TJ, Berbari EF, Osmon DR. Epidemiology, treatment and prevention of community-acquired methicillin-resistant Staphylococcus aureus infections. Mayo Clin Proc 2005;80:1201–1207.

Kravitz GR, Dries DJ, Peterson, ML Schlievert PM. Purpura Fulminans due to Staphylococcus aureus. Clin Inf Dis 2005;40:941–947.

Manders SM. Toxin-mediated streptococcal and staphylococcal disease. J Am Acad Dermatol 1998;39:383–398.

Masters EJ, Olson GS, Weiner SJ, Paddock CD. Rocky Mountain spotted fever: a clinician's dilemma. Arch Intern Med 2003;163:769–774.

McGinly-Smith DE, Tsao SS. Dermatoses from ticks. *J Am Acad Dermatol* 2003;49:363–92.

Miller LG, Perdreau-Remington F, Rieg G, Sherherbano M, Perlroth J, Bayer AS, Tang AW, Phung TO, Spellberg B. Necrotizing fasciitis caused by community-associate methicillin-resistant *Staphylococcus aureus* in Los Angeles. *N Engl J Med* 2005;352:1445–1453.

Murray RJ. Recognition and management of *Staphylococcus aureus* toxin-mediated disease. *Int Med Journal* 2005;35:S106–119.

Norrby-Teglund A, Muller MP, Megeer A, Gan BS, Guru V, Bohnen J, Thulin P, Low DE. Successful management of severe group A streptococcal soft tissue infections using an aggressive medical regimen including intravenous polyspecific immunoglobulin together with a conservative surgical approach. *Scan J infect Dis* 2005;37:166–172.

Rosenstein NE, Perkins BA, Stephens DS, Popovic T, Hughes, JM. Meningococcal Disease. *N Engl J Med.* 2001;344:1378–1388.

Spach DH, Liles WC, Campbell GL, et al. Tick-borne diseases in the United States. *N Engl J Med* 1993;329:936–947.

Stephens DS. Conquering the Meningococcus. *Fems Microbiol Rev* 2007;31:3–14.

Stephens DS, Zimmer SM. Pathogenesis, therapy and prevention of meningococcal sepsis. *Curr infect dis rep* 2002;4:377–386.

Stevens DL. The toxic shock syndromes. *Infect Dis Clin North Am* 1996;10:727–46.

Stevens DL. Streptococcal toxic shock syndrome associated with necrotizing fasciitis. *Annu Rev Med* 2000;51:271–288.

Tickborne Rickettsial Diseases Working Group; CDC. Diagnosis and management of tickborne rickettsial diseases: Rocky Mountain spotted fever, ehrlichioses, and anaplasmosis – United States: a practical guide for physicians and other health-care and public health professionals. *MMWR Recomm Rep* 2006;55(RR-4):1–27.

van de Beek D, de Gans J, Tunkel AR, Wijdicks EF. Community-acquired bacterial meningitis in adults. *N Engl J Med* 2006 Jan 5;354(1):44–53.

Vinh DC, Embil JM. Severe skin and soft tissue infections and associated critical illness. *Curr Inf Dis Rep* 2006;8:375–383.

Walker DH. Rocky Mountain spotted fever: a seasonal alert. *Clin Inf Dis* 1995;20:1111–1117.

Welch SB, Nadel S. Treatment of Meningococcal infection. *Arch Dis Child* 2003;88:608–614.

Index

abscesses, 17, 189. *See also* carbuncles; furuncles
acanthamebiasis, in HIV infection, 193–194
Acanthamoeba spp., 121
Acanthaster planci (crown of thorns) starfish, 173
acellular pertussis (DTaP) vaccination, 294
acetaminophen, for HSV 1 and 2 infections, 277
Acinetobacter baumannii, 189
Ackerman, A. Bernard, 6
acne miliaris necrotica, 262
Acquired Immune Deficiency Syndrome (AIDS). *See also* HIV-related skin infections; Kaposi's sarcoma (KS)
    acid-fast bacilli in, 72
    anergy, presence of, in, 4
    coccidioidomycosis and, 144
    cryptococcus with, 111
    cutaneous tuberculosis with, 73
    diabetes and, 8
    disseminated histoplasmosis (DH) and, 104
    esophageal infections with, 221
    historical background, of, 185
    Mycobacterium avium intracellulare with, 292
    pbmycosis with, 108
    progressive vaccinia and, 23
    pulmonary tuberculosis in, 60
    systemic tropical mycoses and, 96
    tuberculosis and, 60
Acremonium spp., 113, 270–272
actinias, reactions to, 169–171
Actinomadura madurae grains, 97, 156
Actinomyces, 3
Actinomyces israelii, 294
actinomycosis, 294
acute disseminated miliary tuberculosis (tuberculosis cutis miliaris acuta generalisata), 67
acute exanthem, 145
    of HIV infection
        cytomegalovirus, 187
        Epstein-Barr virus, 187
        herpes simplex virus (types 1 and 2), 186
        human herpes virus 8, 188–189
        pox virus, 187
        varicella-zoster virus, 186–187
acute febrile neutrophilic dermatosis (Sweet's syndrome), 146

acute infections, primary signs of, 8
acute miliary cutaneous tuberculosis, 60, 74
acute necrotizing ulcerative gingivitis, 294–295
acute paronychial infections, 268–269
acyclovir
    for congenital herpes simplex, 30
    for genital herpes, 319
    for hand-foot-and-mouth disease, 282
    for herpes simplex virus, 200, 277
    for herpes virus B, 34
    for herpes zoster, 31
    for HSV-1/HSV-2, 29
    oral, for HSV, 186
    for oral hairy leukoplakia, 187, 279
    for suspected neonatal HSV, 225
    for varicella zoster virus, 31, 201
    for VZV, 187
Aedes aegypti mosquito, 92, 95, 151, 152
African Americans
    and lepromatous leprosy, 77
    and pediculosis, 230
    and pseudofolliculitis barbae, 216
    and tinea capitis, 43
agent formulary for topical therapy, 11
albendazole
    for cysticercosis, 129
    for echinococcosis, 129
    for enterobiasis, 128
    for filariasis, 124
    for loiasis, 124
    for mansonelliasis, 128
    for onchocercosis, 176
    for trichinellosis, 128
Alcyonidrium gelatinosum bryozoans, 175
Alcyonidrium hirsutum bryozoans, 175
Alcyonidrium topsenti bryozoans, 175
algae/Bryozoans and aquatic dermatoses
    algae, 174
    Bryozoans, 175
    protothecosis, 174–175
allopurinol, for Old World CL, 144
allylamine, for tinea unguium (onychomycosis), 52
Almeida, Floriano de, 151
Alternaria spp., 113, 270
aluminum acetate (Burrow's solution), for impetigo, 261–262
Amblyomma americanum (lone star tick), 215
Amblyomma Cajennense (Cayenne tick), 323
American Society for Dermatologic Surgery survey, 303

American Thoracic Society, 292
American trypanosomiasis, 123
amikacin with tetracycline, for protothecosis, 175
aminoglycosides
    for ecthyma gangrenosum, 215
    for nocardiosis, 198
amitriptyline for post-herpetic neuralgia, 31
amorolfine
    nail lacquers, for tinea unguium, 219
    topical, for tinea unguium, 236
amoxicillin
    complications from, 33, 278–279
    for genital bite wounds, 317
    for Lyme disease, 215
    for perianal streptococcal dermatitis, 212
amphotericin B
    for candidiasis, 191
    for chromoblastomycoses, 156
    for coccidioidomycosis, 148
    for cryptococcosis, 112
    for cutaneous cryptococcus, 191
    for entomophthoromycosis, 111
    with 5-fluorocytosine
        for aspergillosis/cryptococcosis/ candidiasis, 114
    for histoplasmosis, 192
    IV, for protothecosis, 175
    for leishmaniasis, 297
    liposomal, for mucormycosis, 110
    for mycetoma, 157
    for Old World CL PVA failures, 143
    for paracoccidioidomycosis, 109
        intravenous, 159
    for penicilliosis, 193
    for rhinosporidiosis, 104
    for sporotrichosis, 102
amyloidosis (primary) and Hansen's disease, 78
Anaerobic streptococci, 250
Anaplasma phagocytophilum, 215
Ancylostoma braziliensis (hookworm of dogs and cats), 125, 127, 176
Ancylostoma caninum, 125, 176
Anemonia sulcata actinia, 168–170
anergic leishmaniasis, 151
angular cheilitis (perleche), 221
anogenital disease
    bowenoid papulosis, 26
    condyloma acuminatum, 26
    verrucous carcinoma, 26–27
anogenital warts, 319

anopheline (malaria-carrying) mosquitos, 95
anthrax, 295
Anthraxin test, 4
antibiotics. *See* individual antibiotics
anticonvulsants. *See* carbamazepine;
    gabapentin; pregabalin
antifungal medications. *See also* fluconazole;
    griseofulvin; itraconazole;
    ketoconazole; terbinafine
    for pityriasis versicolor (PV), 52–53
    for seborrheic dermatitis/pityriasis
        capitis, 256
    for tinea capitis, 51
    for tinea corporis/cruris/faciei, 50–51
    for tinea pedis/manuum, 47–50
    for tinea unguium (onychomycosis),
        51–52
antifungal shampoos, 51, 217, 218, 256, 258
antihistamines
    for folliculitis, 189
    for mite symptom control, 231
    for pediculosis capitis itch control, 260
antimalarials, for ENL treatment, 84
anti-retroviral therapy
    for acute exanthem, 186
    for hairy leukoplakia, 279
    for KS, 34
Aphrodite aculeata polychaete, 176
Apophysomyces elegans, 109
aquatic dermatoses from biotic organisms
    from algae/Bryozoans
        algae, 174
        Bryozoans, 175
        protothecosis, 174–175
    from aquatic bacteria
        erysipeloid, 179
        mycobacterium marinum, 178–179
    from aquatic worms
        cercariae, 175
        contact with bait, 176
        leeches, 176
        nematodes, 176–177
        onchocercosis, 175–176
        polychaetes, 176
    from arthropods, 174
    from coelenterates, 167–172
        actinia reactions, 169–171
        jellyfish reactions, 168–169
        physaliae/corals/hydroid reactions,
          172
        sea bather's eruptions, 171–172
    from echinoderms
        sea urchins, 172–173
        starfish, 173–174
    from fish, 177–178
    historical background, 167
    from mollusks, 174
    from sponges, 174
aquatic worms and aquatic dermatoses
    cercariae, 175
    contact with bait, 176
    leeches, 176
    nematodes, 176–177
    onchocercosis, 175–176
    polychaetes, 176

arboviruses. *See* arthropod-borne infections
Argentinian hemorrhagic fever, 153
Aristotle
    on contagiousness of phthisis, 59
    on parasites, 117
arthropod-borne infections. *See also* Chagas'
    disease; Dengue fever; ectoparasite
    infestation; mouse-borne diseases;
    sandfly-borne diseases; tick-borne
    diseases; Yellow fever
    diagnosis, 93–94
    epidemiology, 93
    general information, 92
    historical background, 92–93
    pitfalls and myths, 95
    therapy, 94–95
arthropods, lesions from, 174
Asians
    and lepromatous leprosy, 77
    syphilis rates in pregnant women, 222
aspergillosis, 7, 47, 109, 192, 206, 207
    clinical presentation, 288
    diagnosis, 288
    at hospital sites, 206
    invasive, in AIDS, 192
    in mucormycosis, 287
    in transplant patients, 264
    treatment, 288
Aspergillus spp., 270–272
asymmetry (as sign of acute infection), 8
athletes, skin infections in
    atypical mycobacteria (swimming pool
        granuloma), 244
    bacterial infections
        folliculitis, 239
        furunculosis, 238–239
        gram negative hot tub folliculitis, 240
        green foot, 240
        hot foot syndrome, 240
        impetigo, 238
        pitted keratolysis, 239–240
        tropical ulcers, 240
    fungal infections
        tinea corporis gladiatorum, 243–244
        tinea pedis, 243
    historical background, 238
    parasites (cutaneous larvae migrans), 244
    viral infections
        herpes simplex
          activation, 240
          skin-to-skin transmission, 240–241
        molluscum contagiosum, 241–242
        verruca, 242
atopic dermatitis, 21, 114, 193, 225
atovaquone, for tularemia, 95
atypical mycobacterioses, 6
    classification, 88–89
        Mycobacterium avium complex, 89
        Mycobacterium chelonae-
          Mycobacterium abscessus
          complex, 89
        Mycobacterium fortuitum complex, 89
        Mycobacterium kansasii, 88
        Mycobacterium marinum, 67, 88
        Mycobacterium scrofulaceum, 64, 74, 89

    clinical presentation, 89–90
    diagnosis, 90
    historical background, 88
    pitfalls and myths, 90–91
    therapy, 90
autoimmune polyendocrinopathy-
    candidiasis-ectodermal dystrophy
    (APECED) syndrome, 222
Ayurveda, 59
azidothymidine (AZT), for HIV, 185, 284
azithromycin
    for bacillary angiomatosis, 189–190,
        198
    for cat-scratch disease, 215
    for chancroid, 313
    for diphtheria, 294
    for granuloma inguinale, 315
    for syphilis, 312
    for tularemia, 95
azoles
    for coccidioidomycosis, 148, 192
    for Old World CL, 143
    for pityriasis versicolor, 53
    for tinea unguium (onychomycosis), 52
    topical, for erythrasma, 249

B. dermatitides, 7
babesiosis, 92
bacillary angiomatosis (BA)
    in HIV, 189–190
    in transplant recipients, 197–198
Bacillus anthracis, 295
Bacillus Calmette-Guerin (BCG), 60, 67
    vaccinations of against TB, 4, 62, 65,
        72–73
bacillus Calmette-Guerin (BCG)
    vaccinations, 4
Bacillus vincentii, 294
bacterial infections in athletes
    folliculitis, 239
    furunculosis, 238–239
    gram negative hot tub folliculitis, 240
    green foot, 240
    hot foot syndrome, 240
    impetigo, 238
    pitted keratolysis, 239–240
    tropical ulcers, 240
bacterial infections in elderly patients
    cellulitis/erysipelas, 234
    herpes zoster, 235
    impetigo/folliculitis/furunculosis,
        234–235
    necrotizing fascitis, 235
bacterial infections of the scalp
    eosinophilic pustular folliculitis, 261
    erysipelas/scalp cellulitis, 262
    folliculitis, 260
    impetigo, 261–262
    staphylococcal folliculitis, 260–261
bacterial infections related to HIV
    bacillary angiomatosis, 189–190
    folliculitis, 189
    impetigo, abscesses, cellulitis, necrotizing
        fascitis, 189
    mycobacterial infections, 189

bacterial infections related to mucous
membranes
actinomycosis, 294
acute necrotizing ulcerative gingivitis,
294–295
anthrax, 295
bacterial vaginosis, 295
diphtheria, 293–294
mycoplasma pneumoniae, 296
noma (cancrum oris/gangrenous
stomatitis), 295
pseudomonas aeruginosa, 295
rhinoscleroma, 294
staphylococcus, 293
streptococcus, 293
tetanus, 296
bacterial uSSSIs. See uncomplicated skin and
skin structure infections (uSSSIs)
bacterial vaginosis, 295
bacterial/viral disease in transplant recipients
bacillary angiomatosis, 197
B-hemolytic streptococcus, 196–197
gram-negative bacilli (GNB), 197
historical background, 195
necrotizing fasciitis, 197
nocardiosis, 198
Staphylococcus aureus, 195–196
vibrio vulnificus, 197
Bacteroides, 250
Baker-Rosenbach's erysipeloid, 179
Balamuthia mandrillaris, 121
Barmah Forest virus (BFV), 152–153
Bartonella, 4, 197
Bartonella henselae, 189, 197, 215
Bartonella quintana, 92, 189, 197
basal cell carcinoma (BCC), 303
Basidiobolus haptosporus, 110
Basidiobolus ranarum, 110
Bayle, Gaspard Laurent, 59
Bazin, Ernest, 69. *See also* erythema
induratum of Bazin
bedbugs, 232
benzathine penicillin
for endemic treponematoses, 216
for scarlet fever, 212
for syphilis, 190, 312
congenital, 223
benznidazole
for American trypanosomiasis, 123
for Chagas' disease, 160
benzocaine preparations, for HSV, 277
benzoyl peroxide, 20, 21
benzyl benzoate
for demodicidosis, 260
for scabies, 193, 260
betadine, for impetigo, 261–262
bifonazole
for pityriasis versicolor, 53
with urea, for tinea unguium
(onychomycosis), 219
Bipolaris, 113
black piedra, 154, 258
black superficial onychomycosis (BSO),
271–272
black-dot tinea capitis, 257

Blastomyces dermatitidis, 105
blastomycosis. *See also*
chromoblastomycosis; North
American blastomycosis;
paracoccidioidomycosis (South
American blastomycosis)
chromomycosis (*see*
chromoblastomycosis)
clinical presentation, 289
diagnosis, 289
differentiation from
lupus vulgaris, 63, 74
warty tuberculosis, 65
in HIV infection, 193
keloidal blastomycosis, 102, 157
in mucous membrane infections, 289
oral itraconazole for, 47
bleomycin injections, for verrucae vulgaris/
condyloma acuminatum, 203
blister beetles, 232
blistering dactylitis, in children, 212
Bolivian hemorrhagic fever, 153
borderline lepromatous (BL) disease, 79, 83
borderline tuberculoid (BT) leprosy, 78, 83
Borrelia, 4
Borrelia burgdorferi, 215
Borrelia vincentii, 294
bowenoid papulosis, 26
breasts, tuberculosis of, 72
British Society for Antimicrobial
Chemotherapy, 306
British Society for Dermatological
Surgery, 306
Brucella, 3
Brugia malayi, 123
Brugia timori, 123
bryozoans and dermatitis, 175
bullous impetigo, 195, 211
Bunostomum phlebotomum, 125
Burkitt lymphoma, 187, 279
Buruli ulcer, 7
Burulin intradermal reaction, 4
Butcher's warts, 26
butenafine
for tinea corporis/cruris/faciei, 50
for tinea pedis/manuum, 47

C. immitis, 7
C. neoformans, 7
Calymmatobacterium granulomatis, 314
Calymmatobacterium granulomatis Gram-
negative rod, 151, 190
CA-MRSA. See community-acquired
methicillin resistant *Staphylococcus
aureus* (CA-MRSA)
cancer patients and skin infections
cutaneous infections
bacterial infections, 207
fungal infections, 207
viral infections, 207
diagnosis, 206
epidemiology, 206
historical background, 206
malignant infections
angiosarcoma, 209

breast cancer, inflammatory, 208–209
cancers metastatic to skin, 210
keratoacanthoma, 209–210
lethal midline granuloma, 209
leukemia cutis, 208
lymphoma, 208
squamous cell cancer, 209
Stewart-Treves syndrome, 209
verrucous carcinoma, 209
therapy principles for cutaneous
infections, 208
Candida, 3
Candida albicans, 191, 235, 246, 271, 272, 286
Candida dubliniensis, 191
Candida glabrata, 191
Candida krusei, 191
Candida parapsilosis, 191, 271
Candida tropicalis, 191
candidal onychomycosis, 221, 236
candidiasis
in children, 220–221
in diabetes mellitus, 246–247
in elderly patients, 235–236
in HIV infection, 191
Candidin test, 4
Capnocytophaga, cat and dog bites from, 19
Capnocytophaga canimorsus, 19, 112
carbamazepine, for post-herpetic neuralgia, 31
carbapenems (newer generation), for MRSA
strains, 20
carbaryl, for pediculosis capitis, 259
carbuncles, 17. *See also* furuncles
in diabetes mellitus, 248–249
in folliculitis, 234, 260
S. aureus as causative, 19
treatment of, 20
carpal tunnel syndrome and Hansen's
disease, 78
cat and dog bites, *Pasteurella* spp. as
causative, 19
caterpillars and moths, 232
cat-scratch disease, 6, 92, 215
Caucasians, and lepromatous leprosy, 77
cefixime, for gonorrhea, 315–316
cefoperazone sodium, for necrotizing
fasciitis, 213
ceftriaxone
for chancroid, 313
for erysipeloid, 214
for gonorrhea, 315–316
intramuscular, for meningococcal
disease, 323
for nocardiosis, 198
for syphilis, 190
cefuroxime
for genital bite wounds, 317
for Lyme disease, 215
cellulitis, 17–18
in diabetes mellitus, 249
in elderly patients, 234
in HIV, 189
of lower extremity, pitfalls and myths, 21
S. aureus/S. pyogenes as causative, 19
in scalp infections, 262
treatment of, 20

Centers for Disease Control and Prevention
  on arthropod-borne diseases
    risk factors, 93
    treatment, 94–95
  on treatment for cutaneous TB, 73
cephalopods, dermatoses from, 174
cephalosporin
  for cellulitis/erysipelas, 234
  for erysipelas, 20
  for folliculitis keloidalis, 262
  for genital bite wounds, 317
  for gonorrhea, 316
  for *S. aureus*, 196
cercarial dermatitis (swimmer's itch), 130,
  175
Cercopithecus aethiops (green monkeys), 153
Cerqueira, Alexandre, 150
cestodes, 128–130
  coenurosis, 129–130
  cysticercosis, 129
  echinococcosis, 129
  sparganosis, 129
Chagas, Carlos, 159
Chagas' disease, 123. *See also* American
  trypanosomiasis
  diagnosis, 160
  treatment, 160
chancroid, 309, 312–313
chemical peels, for pseudofolliculitis barbae,
  216
chemotherapy
  for Burkitt lymphoma, 279
  for cervical intraepithelial neoplasms, 281
  for chromomycosis, 100
  for cutaneous tuberculosis, 73
  for KS, 34, 202
  pre-bone marrow transplant, 264
  skin infections after, 206
    candidiasis, 221
    ecthyma gangrenosum, 214
    oral mucositis, 275
chickenpox, 30, 186, 200, 235
Chironex fleckeri jellyfish, 169
Chiropsalmus quadrigatus jellyfish, 169
Chlamydia, 4
Chlamydia trachomatis, 191, 313
chloramphenicol, for Rocky Mountain
  spotted fever, 324
chlorhexidine
  for impetigo, 261–262
  for *S. aureus* in transplant recipients, 196
  for skin colonization issues, 21
chromoblastomycosis, 6, 7, 98–100
  differentiation from warty tuberculosis,
    65
  genera differences, 99–100
  treatment, 100
chronic granulomatous disease, 74
chronic hepatitis C virus (HCV), 37
chronic mucocutaneous candidiasis (CMC),
  221–222
chronic paronychial infections, 269
chronic traumatic lymphedema of the hands,
  from sea urchins, 173
Chrysops spp3, 124

ciclopirox
  for piedra, 259
  for tinea corporis/cruris/faciei, 50
  for tinea pedis/manuum, 47, 47–50, 236
  for tinea unguium (onychomycosis), 219,
    236
  topical, for pityriasis versicolor, 53
  (topical), for white piedra, 154
ciclopirox olamine (1%), for tinea pedis/
  manuum, 47
ciclopirox shampoo, 256
cidofovir
  for condyloma acuminata, 188
  for herpes simplex virus, 200
cimetidine, for verrucae vulgaris/condyloma
  acuminatum, 203
ciprofloxacin
  for cat-scratch disease, 215
  for chancroid, 313
  for erysipeloid, 214
  for granuloma inguinale, 315
  for rhinoscleroma, 294
Cladophialophora carrionii, 98–99
cladosporiosis. *See* chromoblastomycosis
Cladosporium carrionii dematieous fungus,
  156
clarithromycin
  for atypical mycobacteria, 244
  for atypical mycobacterioses, 90
  for bacillary angiomatous, 189–190
  for diphtheria, 294
clindamycin
  for acne miliaris necrotica, 262, 262
  for bacterial vaginosis, 295
  for erythrasma, 214
  for necrotizing fasciitis, 213
  oral, for nasal carriage issues, 21
  for perianal streptococcal dermatitis, 212
  for pitted keratolysis, 214
  with rifampicin, for scalp cellulitis, 263
  topical, 20
  for tularemia, 95
clofazimine
  for leprosy, 293
  for lobomycosis, 103, 158
  for multibacillary disease, 84
clotrimazole
  for erythrasma, 249
  for pityriasis versicolor, 53
  for tinea corporis/cruris/faciei, 50
  for tinea pedis/manuum, 47
  for tinea unguium (onychomycosis), 219
cloxacillin, for carbuncles, 249
cnidocytes (of coelenterates), 167–168
Coccidioides immitis, 104
Coccidioidin test, 4
coccidioidomycosis and the skin
  acute exanthem, 145
  diagnosis, 144–145
  disseminated infection, 147
  epidemiology, 144
  erythema multiforme-like eruptions,
    145–146
  erythema nodosum, 145
  historical background, 144

  in HIV infection, 192
  interstitial granulomatous dermatitis,
    146–147
  pitfalls and myths, 148
  primary cutaneous coccidioidomycosis,
    147–148
  serologic testing, 148
  Sweet's syndrome, 146
  treatment, 148
coelenterates
  and aquatic dermatoses, 167–172
    actinia reactions, 169–171
    jellyfish reactions, 168–169
    physaliae/corals/hydroid reactions,
      172
    sea bather's eruptions, 171–172
  description of actions, 167–168
coenurosis, 129–130
colchicine, for ENL treatment, 84
color (as sign of acute infection), 8
Colorado tick fever, 92
common warts (verruca vulgaris), 25,
  203, 280
community-acquired methicillin resistant
  Staphylococcus aureus (CA-MRSA),
  19, 211, 238, 262
  S. aureus colonization from, 21
  treatment of, 20
complement fixation (CF) test, 4
complications
  measles/rubeola, 36
Condylactis aurantiaca actinia, 170
condyloma acuminatum (genital warts), 203
  clinical manifestations, 26
  preventative therapies, 26
  treatment, 26
congenital cytomegalovirus, 33
congenital HSV, 30
congenital indifference to pain and Hansen's
  disease, 78
  cytomegalovirus, 224
  neonatal HSV, 224–225
  parvovirus B19, 225
  rubella, 223–224
  syphilis, 222–223
  varicella zoster, 225
congenital rubella syndrome, 37
conidiobolomycosis, 110
Conidiobolus coronatus, 110
Conidiobolus incongruens, 111
Conus aulicus shell, 174
Conus geographus shell, 174
Conus gloria maris shell, 174
corals, reactions to, 172
corticosteroids
  for folliculitis, 189
  for folliculitis keloidalis, 262
  for scalp cellulitis, 263
  for tinea capitis, 217
  for trichinellosis, 128
Corynebacterium diphtheriae, 293
Corynebacterium minutissimum, 214, 249
co-trimoxazole, for entomophthoromycosis,
  111
cowpox, 24

Coxsackie A-16. *See* hand, foot, and mouth disease
creatinine phosphokinase, for differentiation of necrotizing fascitis, 8, 213
crotamiton
    for demodicidosis, 260
    for scabies, 260
crusted (ecthymatous) zoster, 186
cryotherapy
    for anogenital warts, 319
    for chromoblastomycoses, 156
    for condyloma acuminata, 188
    for genital warts, 319
    for KS, 202
    for lobomycosis, 103
    for molluscum contagiosum, 187
    for Old World CL, 143
    for verruca, 228
    for verrucae vulgaris/condyloma acuminatum, 203, 228
cryptococcal meningitis, 47, 111
cryptococcosis, 96, 111–112, 187
    clinical presentation, 287
    diagnosis, 112, 287–288
    in HIV infection, 191
    treatment, 112, 114, 288
    vs. molluscum contagiosum, 187
Cryptococcus, 4
Culex mosquito, 152
Cunnigham, D. D., 135
Cunninghmaella bertholletiae, 109
curettage
    for anogenital warts, 319
    for genital warts, 319
    for molluscum contagiosum, 23, 187
    for verrucae vulgaris/condyloma acuminatum, 203
Curvularia, 113
cutaneous infections (possibly) indicative of underlying cancer
    fungal infections
        aspergillosis, 207
        Rhizopus/Mucor spp/saprophytes, 207
        S. Aureus of streptococcal cellulitis, 207
        therapy principles, 208
    viral infections
        herpes simplex, 207
        herpes zoster, 207
        warts, 207
cutaneous larva migrans, 124–125
cutaneous pneumocystosis, 187
cutaneous tuberculosis
    classification, 62
    clinical features
        acute disseminated miliary tuberculosis, 60, 67
        erythema induratum of Bazin, 69–70
        erythema nodosum, 70, 75
        lichen scrofulosorum, 68–69
        lichen scrofulosorum (LS), 75
        lupus vulgaris, 60, 62–64, 74
        orificial tuberculosis, 60, 67–68, 74–75
        papulonecrotic tuberculids, 68, 75
        primary inoculation tuberculosis, 67
        scrofuloderma, 60, 64

        tuberculids, 68
        tuberculosis gumma, 68, 74
        tuberculosis verrucosa cutis, 60, 65, 74
        tuberculous chancre, 60
    diagnosis, 61–62, 73–74
    general information, 59–60
    histopathology, 70–71
    historical background, 59
    HIV with, 59, 72
    pathogenesis, 60–61
    pitfalls and myths of, 73–75
    systemic involvement, 71–72
    treatments, 73
Cyclops, 124–125, 129
cyclosporine, with fluconazole, 47
cysticercosis, 129
cytomegalovirus (CMV), 33
    in children, 224
    diagnosis, 33
    in HIV infection, 187
    in mucous membrane infections, 279
    in transplantation recipients, 201–202
    treatment, 33

da Fonseca Filho, Olympia, 151
Dakin's solution, for skin colonization issues, 21
dapsone
    for leprosy, 293
    for multibacillary disease, 84
    for Old World CL, 144
    for paucibacillary disease, 84
daptomycin, for MRSA strains, 20
Dasypus novemcinctus, 106
DEET (N,N-diethyl-3-methylbenzamide)
    mosquito repellant, 95
    for deterrence of sandflies, 137
    for prevention of cercarial dermatitis, 130
Demodex brevis mite, 260
Demodex folliculorum mite, 260
demodicidosis, 193, 260
demodicidosis (of the scalp), 260
Dengue fever, 92, 95, 151–152
    cutaneous features, 151–152
    treatment, 152
dental pastes, for HSV, 277
depilatory creams, for pseudofolliculitis barbae, 216
Dermacentor andersoni (Rocky Mountain wood tick), 323
Dermacentor variabilis (American dog tick), 323
dermatophyte onychomycosis (of fingernails/ toenails), 47, 47, 52
dermatophytosis, 42, 53, 191, 249, 256. *See also* tinea capitis
dermatoses, aquatic (from biotic organisms)
    from algae/Bryozoans
        algae, 174
        Bryozoans, 175
        protothecosis, 174–175
    from aquatic bacteria
        erysipeloid, 179
        mycobacterium marinum, 178–179
    from aquatic worms

        cercariae, 175
        contact with bait, 176
        leeches, 176
        nematodes, 176–177
        onchocercosis, 175–176
        polychaetes, 176
    from arthropods, 174
    from coelenterates, 167–172
        actinia reactions, 169–171
        jellyfish reactions, 168–169
        physaliae/corals/hydroid reactions, 172
        sea bather's eruptions, 171–172
    from echinoderms
        sea urchins, 172–173
        starfish, 173–174
    from fish, 177–178
    from mollusks, 174
desert infections, Eastern hemisphere
    Old World cutaneous leishmaniasis, 117–118
        clinical presentation, 138–140
        diagnosis, 140–141
        epidemiology, 135–136
        historical background, 135
        patient follow-up, 144
        prevention, 137–138
        transmission (sandfly vector/ *Leishmania* lifecycle), 136–137
        treatment, 141–144
desert infections, Western hemisphere
    coccidioidomycosis and the skin
        acute exanthem, 145
        diagnosis, 144–145
        disseminated infection, 147
        epidemiology, 144
        erythema multiforme-like eruptions, 145–146
        erythema nodosum, 145
        historical background, 144
        interstitial granulomatous dermatitis, 146–147
        pitfalls and myths, 148
        primary cutaneous coccidioidomycosis, 147–148
        serologic testing, 148
        Sweet's syndrome, 146
        treatment, 148
desipramine, for post-herpetic neuralgia, 31
Dharmendra lepromin antigen, 4
diabetes mellitus, skin infections
    cutaneous infections
        candida, 246–247
        carbuncles, 248–249
        cellulitis, 249
        erysipelas, 249
        erythrasma, 249
        furuncles, 248
    dermatophyte fungal infections, 247–248
    diagnosis, 246
    epidemiology, 246
    historical background, 246
    life threatening infections
        Fournier's gangrene, 251
        malignant otitis externa, 251

diabetes mellitus, skin infections (cont.)
  necrotizing fascitis, 250
  rhinocerebral mucormycosis, 251
  predisposition to, 8
  S. aureus colonization from, 21
  terbinafine for, 47
  therapy for, 252
diabetic ketoacidosis, 110, 251, 286
diabetic neuropathy and Hansen's disease, 78
diaper dermatitis (monilial diaper
  dermatitis), 221
Dick's test, 4
diethylcarbamazine (DEC)
  for filariasis, 124
  for loiasis, 124
  for onchocerciasis, 124
diffuse cutaneous leishmaniasis, 4
diloxanide, for enteric amebiasis, 121
diphenhydramine elixir with Maalox, for
  HSV, 277
diphtheria, 293–294
diphtheria vaccination, 294
directly observed therapy (DOTS), 73, 292
dissecting cellulitis (of the scalp), 262–263
disseminated herpes-zoster, 186
disseminated histoplasmosis (DH), 104
disseminated infection, 147
distal subungual onychomycosis, 236
distal/lateral subungual onychomycosis, 270
DNA microarray technology (DNA chip
  technology), 6
DNA viruses. *See also* herpes virus, various
  presentations
  hepadnaviruses, 35 (*See also* hepatitis B)
  human papillomavirus (HPV)
    anogenital disease
      bowenoid papulosis, 26
      condyloma acuminatum, 26
      verrucous carcinoma, 26–27
    nongenital cutaneous diseases
      Butcher's warts, 26
      common warts (verruca
        vulgaris), 25
      epidermodysplasia verruciformis
        (EV), 25–26
      flat warts (verrucae plana), 25
      palmoplantar warts (myrmecia),
        25
    nongenital mucosal disease
      oral focal hyperplasia (Heck
        disease), 27
  in mucous membrane infections
    cytomegalovirus, 279
    Epstein-Barr virus, 278–279
    HSV-1 and HSV-2, 276–278
    human papilloma virus, 280–281
    Kaposi's sarcoma, 280
    molluscum contagiosum, 281
    parvovirus B19, 281
    roseola infantum, 279–280
    varicella zoster (HSV-3), 278
  parvoviruses, 34–35
  pox viruses
    cowpox, 24

Molluscum Contagiosum (MCV), 23
  monkey pox, 24
  smallpox, 23
docosanol (10%) cream, for herpes labialis,
  277
Donovan, C., 135
Donovania granulomatis, 314
doxycycline
  for acne miliaris necrotica, 262
  for actinomycosis, 294
  for anthrax, 295
  for atypical mycobacterioses, 90
  for bacillary angiomatosis, 189–190, 198
  for cat-scratch disease, 215
  for ehrlichiosis, 215
  for endemic treponematoses, 216
  for granuloma inguinale, 191, 315
  for Lyme disease, 215
  for Lyme disease/rickettsial diseases, 95
  for lymphogranuloma venereum, 191,
    314
  for Rocky Mountain spotted fever, 324
  for syphilis, 312
  for tick-borne disease, 95
  for *vibrio vulnificus*, 197
dracunculiasis, 124–125
Dracunculus medinensis, 124–125
Dyptera Order of insects (vectors), 161

Ebola virus, 153, 284
EBV-associated large cell lymphoma, 187
echinococcosis, 129
Echinococcosis granulosus, 129
Echinococcosis multilocularis, 129
Echinococcosis vogeli, 129
echinoderms and aquatic dermatoses
  from fish, 177–178
  sea urchins, 172–173
  starfish, 173–174
econazole
  for tinea corporis/cruris/faciei, 50
  for tinea pedis/manuum, 47
ecthyma, 18, 24, 229
  in children, 211
  diagnosis, 20
  S. aureus/*S. pyogenes* causative for,
    19, 197
  similarity to mucormycosis, 109
  in varicella zoster virus, 186, 200
ecthyma gangrenosum, 109, 197, 214–215,
  295
ecthymatous (crusted) zoster, 186
ectoparasite infestation, 92
Edwardsiella lineata anemone, 171–172
eflornithine
  for pseudofolliculitis barbae, 216
  for trypanosomiasis, 123
Ehrlichia chaffeensis, 215
ehrlichiosis, 92
Eikenella corrodens, 317
elderly people, skin infections in
  bacterial infections
    cellulitis/erysipelas, 234
    herpes zoster, 235

impetigo/folliculitis/furunculosis,
  234–235
  necrotizing fascitis, 235
  fungal infections
    candidiasis, 235–236
    onychomycosis, 236
    tinea pedis/manum, 236–237
  historical background, 233–234
Electra pilosa bryozoan, 175
electric razor shaving, for pseudofolliculitis
  barbae, 216
electrocautery
  for Butcher's warts, 26
  for common warts, 25
  for condyloma acuminata, 26, 188
  for genital warts, 319
  for lupus nodules, 73
  for oral florid papillomatosis, 281
electrodesiccation
  for anogenital warts, 319
  for molluscum contagiosum, 187
  for oral florid papillomatosis, 281
emetine hydrochloride, for enteric amebiasis,
  121
endemic treponematoses, in children,
  215–216
Entamoeba histolytica, 121
enteric amebiasis, 121
Enterobacteriaceae, 19
enterobiasis, 128
Enterovirus 71. *See* hand, foot, and mouth
  disease
Enteroviruses
  hand, foot, and mouth disease, 35–36,
    281–282
  hepatovirus/hepatitis A, 36
  herpangina, 36, 276, 282–283
Entomophthorales (Zygomycosis), 109–110
entomophthoromycosis, 110–111
eosinophilic pustular folliculitis (EPF), 216,
  261
epidermodysplasia verruciformis (EV),
  25–26, 228
epithelioid cell granulomas, 74
Epstein-Barr virus (EBV)
  clinical manifestations, 32
  in HIV infection, 187
  lethal midline granuloma association, 209
  in mucous membrane infections, 278–279
  in transplantation recipients, 201
  treatment, 33
equine encephalitis, 92
erosion (as sign of acute infection), 8
erosive pustular dermatosis (of the scalp), 263
erysipelas, 18
  in diabetes mellitus, 249
  in elderly patients, 234
  pitfalls and myths of, 21
  S. pyogenes as causative, 19
  in scalp infections, 262
  treatment of, 20
erysipeloid (Baker-Rosenbach's
  erysipeloid), 179
  in children, 214

Erysipelothrix rhusiopathiae, 179, 214
erythema induratum of Bazin, 69–70
erythema infectiosum. *See* parvovirus B19
erythema multiforme-like eruptions,
        145–146
erythema nodosum (EN), 70, 75, 145
erythema nodosum leprosum (ENL), 81
erythrasma
        in children, 214
        clindamycin for, 214
        from *Corynebacterium minutissimum,* 214
        in diabetes mellitus, 249
        Whitfield's ointment for, 214
erythromycin
        for actinomycosis, 294
        for bacillary angiomatosis, 189–190, 198
        for cat-scratch disease, 215
        for chancroid, 313
        for diphtheria, 294
        for endemic treponematoses, 216
        for erythrasma, 249
        for granuloma inguinale, 315
        for pitted keratolysis, 214
        for scarlet fever, 212
erythromycin-clindamycin double disk
        testing, 20
ethambutol
        for cutaneous TB treatment, 73
        for pulmonary tuberculosis, 292
Exophiala, 113
Exophiala jeanselmei, 113
extrapulmonary paragonimiasis, 131
extrapulmonary tuberculosis, 5, 59

famciclovir
        for congenital herpes simplex, 30
        for genital herpes, 319
        for herpes simplex virus, 200, 277
        for herpes zoster, 31, 264
        for HSV-1/HSV-2, 250
        for varicella zoster virus, 31, 201
        for VZV, 187
Fasciola gigantica, 127, 130
Fasciola hepatica, 127, 130
fascioliasis, 130
fetal toxoplasmosis, 222
Fibula nolitangere touch me not
        sponge, 174
filariasis, 123–124, 150
Filoviridae virus, 153
fingernail onychomycosis, 51
Finsen, Niels, 59
fish and aquatic dermatoses, 177–178
5-fluorocytosine
        with amphotericin B
                for aspergillosis/cryptococcosis/
                        candidiasis, 114
        for chromoblastomycoses, 156
5-fluorouracil injectable gel
        for condyloma acuminata, 188
        for oral florid papillomatosis, 281
        flat warts (verrucae plana), 25
        treatment, 25
Flaviviridae genus, 151, 152

flaviviruses. *See* Dengue fever; hepatitis C
        virus
flea-borne diseases, 231–232
fluconazole
        for *Balamuthia mandrillaris,* 122
        for coccidioidomycosis, 192
        for cryptococcosis, 112
        for cutaneous cryptococcus, 191
        for entomophthoromycosis, 111
        with 5-fluorocytosine, for candidiasis/
                cryptococcosis, 114
        for pityriasis versicolor, 53
        for sporotrichosis, 102
        for tinea capitis, 217, 258
fluconazole (oral)
        adverse effects, 47
        for candidiasis, 191
        for cryptococcal meningitis, 47
        for dermatophyte fungal infections, 248
        for old world leishmaniasis, 120, 143
        for onychomycosis, 191
        for oropharyngeal/esophageal
                candidiasis, 47
        for pityriasis versicolor, 53
        for tinea capitis, 51
        for tinea corporis/cruris/faciei, 50–51
        for tinea unguium (onychomycosis), 52
        for vaginal candidiasis, 47, 248
flucytosine
        for *Balamuthia mandrillaris,* 122
        for cryptococcosis, 112
Fluorescent In Situ Hybridization (FISH), 5
fluoroquinolones
        for anthrax, 295
        for CA-MRSA, 20
        for cellulitis/erysipelas, 234
        for malignant otitis externa, 251
        for nocardiosis, 198
follicular zoster, 186
folliculitis, 17
        in AIDS/HIV, 186, 189
        in athletes, 239
        carbuncles in, 234
        in elderly patients, 234–235
        eosinophilic pustular folliculitis, 261
        in HIV, 189
        hot tub folliculitis, 19, 240
        pitfalls and myths of, 21
        in scalp infections, 260
                eosinophilic pustular (EPF), 261
                staphylococcal, 260–261
        therapies for, 20
folliculitis decalvans, 262–263
folliculitis keloidalis (acne keloidalis), 262
Fonsecaea compacta dematiaceus fungus,
        98–99, 156
Fonsecaea pedrosoi dematiaceus fungus,
        98–99, 156
Fonseca's disease. *See* chromoblastomycosis
foscarnet
        for CMV, 187
        for herpes simplex virus, 200
        for HSV (in acyclovir-resistant patients),
                186

Foshay test, 4
Fournier's gangrene, 8
        in diabetes mellitus, 251
        treatment, 252
free living amebas, 121–122
Frei's test, 4
fulminant meningococcal disease
        (Waterhouse-Friderichsen
        syndrome), 323
fungal infections (common)
        diagnostic procedures, 43–44
        epidemiology, 42–43
        historical background, 42
        pitfalls and myths, 53
        therapy, 44 (*See also* antifungal
                medications)
fungal infections (deep)
        general information, 96
        historical background, 96
        opportunistic cutaneous infections, 114
        pitfalls and myths, 114–116
        subcutaneous mycosis
                chromomycosis, 98–100
                mycetoma, 97–98
                rhinosporidiosis, 103–104
                sporotrichosis, 100–102, 193
        systemic mycosis
                blastomycosis (North American),
                        105–106, 193
                cryptococcosis, 111–112, 192
                entomophthoromycosis, 110–111
                histoplasmosis, 104–105
                hyalohyphomycosis, 113–114
                mucormycosis, 109–110
                paracoccidioidomycosis (S.A.
                        blastomycosis), 106–109, 192
                        chronic form (adult type), 107–108
                        residual/sequel form, 108–109
                phaeohyphomycosis, 112–113
                zygomycosis, 109
fungal infections in athletes
        tinea corporis gladiatorum, 243–244
        tinea pedis, 243
fungal infections in children, 216–221
        candidiasis, 220–221
        piedra, 220
        tinea capitis, 217–218
        tinea cruris, 218
        tinea faceii, 218
        tinea imbricata (tokelau), 219
        tinea incognito, 218
        tinea nigra, 220
        tinea unguium (onychomycosis),
                218–219
fungal infections in elderly patients
        candidiasis, 235–236
        onychomycosis, 236
        tinea pedis/manum, 236–237
fungal infections in mucous membrane
        infections
        chronic mucocutaneous candidiasis, 286
        endemic mycoses, 288–290
                blastomycosis, 289
                coccidioidomycosis, 289–290

fungal infections in mucous membrane
infections (cont.)
histoplasmosis, 288–289
paracoccidioidomycosis, 289
nonendemic mycoses, 286–288
aspergillosis, 288
disseminated candidiasis, 286
mucormycosis, 286–287
superficial mycoses/*Candida* spp., 284–286
fungal infections of HIV infection
aspergillosis, 192
blastomycosis/sporotrichosis, 193
candidiasis, 191
coccidiomycosis, 192
cryptococcus, 191
dermatophytosis, 191
histoplasmosis, 191–192
paracoccidiomycosis, 192
penicilliosis, 192–193
pneumocystosis, 191
fungal infections of the nail unit, 269–273
combined variants of onychomycosis,
272–273
distal/lateral subungual onychomycosis,
270
mid-plate onychomycosis, 272
proximal subungual onychomycosis, 270
relapse of onychomycosis, 273
total dystrophic onychomycosis, 272
white/black superficial onychomycosis,
271–272
fungal infections of the scalp
piedra, 258–259
pityriasis amiantacea, 256
pityriasis capitis, 255–256
seborrheic dermatitis, 255–256
tinea capitis, 256–258
fungating granulomas, 67
fungi
dematieous fungi
Cladosporium carrionii, 156
Fonsecaea compacta, 156
Fonsecaea pedrosoi, 156
Phialophora verrucosa, 156
Rhinocladiella aquaspersa, 98–99, 156
dimorphic fungi
Paracoccidioides brasiliensis, 106–109,
158–159
Sporothrix schenckii, 155, 155
Hortaea werneckii, 154
Lacazia loboi, 102, 157
furuncles, 17. *See also* carbuncles
in diabetes mellitus, 248
S. aureus as causative, 19
treatment, 20
furunculosis
in athletes, 238–239
in elderly patients, 234–235
in mycobacterium fortuitum complex, 89
Fusarium spp., 113, 270, 271–272
fusidic acid, for scalp cellulitis, 263

gabapentin
for herpes zoster, 235
for post-herpetic neuralgia, 31

Galen, on treatment of ulcerations, 59
ganciclovir (oral), for CMV, 187, 202
Gardnerella (Haemophilus) vaginalis, 295
genital bite wounds, 316–317
genital herpes, 318–319
in AIDS patients, 186
from HSV-2, 27, 276
genital ulcers, 3, 275
genital warts (condyloma acuminatum), 203
clinical manifestations, 26
preventative therapies, 26
treatment, 26
gentamicin antibiotic ointment, for Old
World CL, 143–143
Germ Theory paradigm, 275
gingival stomatitis, 27
gingivitis, acute necrotizing ulcerative,
294–295
Glucantime® (meglumine antimonate), for
Old World CL, 143
glycopeptides, for cellulitis/erysipelas, 234
gnathostomiasis, 126–127
Gnathostomiasis americanum, 126
Gnathostomiasis binucleatum, 126
Gnathostomiasis doloresi, 126
Gnathostomiasis miyasaki, 126
Gnathostomiasis procyonis, 126
Gnathostomiasis spinigerum, 126
Gnathostomiasis turgidum, 126
gonococcal infection, 3
gonorrhea, 315–316
clinical presentation/diagnosis,
315–316, 320
epidemiology, 315
historical background, 310
with HIV, 284
treatment, 316
gram-negative bacteria (in children)
cat-scratch disease, 215
ecthyma gangrenosum, 214–215
ehrlichiosis, 215
gram-positive bacteria (in children)
blistering dactylitis, 212
ecthyma, 211
erysipeloid, 214
erythrasma, 214
impetigo, 211
necrotizing fascitis, 213
orbital/periorbital cellulitis, 213
perianal streptococcal dermatitis, 212
pitted keratolysis, 214
scarlet fever, 212
trichomycosis axillaris, 214
granuloma annulare, 78
granuloma annulare vs. Hansen's disease
lesions, 78
granulomas
from *Aphrodite aculeata* ("sea mouse"), 176
candidal, 222
categories, 6
epithelioid, 74, 83
fungating, 67
lymphocytes in, 61
necrotizing, 141
pelvic/peritoneal, 128

pyogenic granulomata, 189, 197
from sea urchins, 173, 180
tuberculoid, 6, 7, 62, 70
granulomatous diseases, 2
entomophthorales infections, 111
fish tank/swimming pool granulomas, 88,
178, 244
granuloma inguinale (donovanosis), 3, 6,
190–191
granulomatous dermatitis, 114
granulomatous meningo-encephalitis,
121
interstitial granulomatous dermatitis,
146–147
lethal midline granulomas, 122, 209, 287
lymphogranuloma venereum (LGV),
191
Majocchi's disease, 191, 234
mycetoma, 97–98
pbmycosis, 106
Wegner's granulomatosis, 164
green foot, in athletes, 240
griseofulvin (oral), 47
for tinea capitis, 51, 217, 258
for tinea imbricata (tokelau), 219
group A b-hemolytic streptococci (GABHS)
blistering dactylitis from, 212
ecthyma from, 211
impetigo from, 211
perianal streptococcal dermatitis from,
212
scarlet fever from, 212
gyrate erythema, 78

H. capsulatum, 7
Haemagogus, 152
Haemophilus ducreyi, 312, 313
Haemophilus influenza, 19, 213
hair-cutting (treatment)
for black piedra, 154
for white piedra, 154
HA-MRSA. See hospital associated
methicillin resistant *Staphylococcus
aureus*
hand, foot, and mouth disease, 35–36,
283–284
Hansen, Gerhard Henrik Armauer, 76
Hansen's disease (leprosy). *See also*
borderline lepromatous (BL) disease;
borderline tuberculoid (BT) leprosy;
lepromatous leprosy (LL)
clinical findings/classification criteria
Ridley-Jopling (classification), 78–80,
83
WHO (classification), 76, 80
epidemiology/microbiology/
transmission, 76–77
historical background, 76
hypersensitivity reactions, 80–82
immunology/pathogenicity, 77
laboratory tests, 82–83
pathology, 83–84
pitfalls/myths about, 86–87
treatment/therapy, 84–86
Hapalochlaena maculosa octopus, 174

helminths, 123–131
  cestodes, 128–130
    coenurosis, 129–130
    cysticercosis, 129
    echinococcosis, 129
    sparganosis, 129
  nematodes, 123–128
    cutaneous larva migrans, 124–125
    dracunculiasis, 124–125
    enterobiasis, 128
    filariasis, 123–124
    gnathostomiasis, 126–127
    loiasis, 124
    mansonelliasis, 128
    onchocerciasis, 124
    trichinellosis, 127–128
  trematodes, 130–131
    fascioliasis, 130
    paragonimiasis, 131
    schistosomiasis, 130
b-hemolytic Group A streptococci, 250
hemorrhagic fevers, 92, 151, 153. See also
    South American hemorrhagic fevers
hepatitis A virus (HAV), 36
hepatitis B virus (HBV), 35
  clinical manifestations, 35
  diagnosis, 35
  treatment, 35
hepatitis C virus (HCV), 37
  clinical manifestations, 37
  treatment, 37
Hermodice carunculata polychaetes, 176
herpangina, 36, 276, 282–283
herpes labialis, 27, 240, 276
herpes simplex virus (HSV)
  in athletes
    activation, 240
    skin-to-skin transmission, 240–241
  chronic ulcerative, 30
  generalized acute mucocutaneous, 30
  in immunosuppressed patients, 29–30
  in scalp infections, 264
  systemic, 30
herpes simplex virus 1 (HSV-1)
  clinical manifestations, 27
  diagnosis, 27
  in HIV infection, 186
  in mucous membrane infections, 276–278
  in transplantation recipients, 199–200
  treatments, 29
  viral properties, 27
herpes simplex virus 2 (HSV-2)
  clinical manifestations, 29
  in HIV infection, 186
  in mucous membrane infections, 276–278
  in transplantation recipients, 199–200
  treatments, 29
  viral properties, 29
herpes virus, various presentations of
  chickenpox, 30
  congenital HSV, 30
  cytomegalovirus (HHV-5), 33
  Epstein-Barr virus (HHV-4), 31–32
  human herpes virus 7, 33
  in-utero infections

congenital varicella syndrome, 30
    infantile zoster, 31
    neonatal varicella, 31
  Kaposi sarcoma (HHV-8), 33–34
  roseola infantum (HHV-6), 33
  treatment, 30
  varicella zoster (HHV-3), 30
  zoster (shingles), 31–32
herpes virus B (herpes simiae), 34
herpes zoster virus (HSV), 3, 30, 207
  in AIDS patients, 186
  diagnosis, 31
  in elderly patients, 235
  pediatric manifestations
    eczema herpeticum, 225–226
    gingivostomatitis, 225
    herpes gladiatorum, 226–227
    herpetic whitlow, 226
  in scalp infections, 264
  treatment, 31
  vaccination for, 31, 235
herpetic folliculitis, in AIDS patients, 186
herpetic whitlow, 186, 226
HHV 4. See Epstein-Barr virus (EBV)
HHV-8. See Kaposi's sarcoma (KS)
highly active antiretroviral therapy
    (HAART)
  causative for varicella zoster virus, 186
  for folliculitis, 189
  for HIV, 185, 310
  for oral hairy leukoplakia, 187
  for penicilliosis, 193
Hippocrates, 275
histoid leprosy, 80
Histoplasma, 3
Histoplasma capsulatum, 104
Histoplasmin test, 4
histoplasmosis, 104–105
  diagnosis, 104
  in HIV infection, 191–192
  in mucous membrane infections,
      288–289
  oral itraconazole for, 47
  treatment, 104–105
  vs. molluscum contagiosum, 187
historical background
  of AIDS, 185
  of arthropod-borne infections, 92–93
  of athlete skin infections, 238
  of atypical mycobacterioses, 88
  of bacterial/viral disease in transplant
      recipients, 195
  of cancer patients and skin infections,
      206
  of common bacterial infections, 18–19
  of common fungal infections, 42
  of cutaneous tuberculosis, 59
  of HIV-related skin infections, 185
  of Kaposi sarcoma, 185
  of life-threatening skin infections, 322
  management principles, 8
  of mucous membrane infections, 275
  of Old World cutaneous leishmaniasis,
      135
  of parasitology, 117

of pediatric skin infections, 211
  of sexually transmitted diseases, 309–310
  of skin surgery-related infections, 303
History of Animals (Aristotle), 117
HIV-related skin infections. See also sexually
    transmitted diseases (STDs) and HIV
    skin infections
  acute exanthem
    cytomegalovirus, 187
    Epstein-Barr virus, 187
    herpes simplex virus (types 1
        and 2), 186
    human herpes virus 8, 188–189
    pox virus, 187
    varicella-zoster virus, 186–187
  bacterial infections
    bacillary angiomatosis, 189–190
    folliculitis, 189
    impetigo, abscesses, cellulitis,
        necrotizing fascitis, 189
    mycobacterial infections, 189
  co-infections
    cutaneous lesions of histoplasmosis,
        104
    cutaneous tuberculosis, 59, 72
    with Mycobacterium leprae, 83
  diagnosis, 38
  fungal infections
    aspergillosis, 192
    blastomycosis/sporotrichosis, 193
    candidiasis, 191
    coccidiomycosis, 192
    cryptococcus, 191
    dermatophytosis, 191
    histoplasmosis, 191–192
    paracoccidiomycosis, 192
    penicilliosis, 192–193
    pneumocystosis, 191
  historical background, 185
  mucous membrane infections, 284
  parasitic/ectoparasitic infections
    acanthamebiasis, 193–194
    demodicidosis, 193
    leishmaniasis, 194
    scabies, 193
  from sexually transmitted diseases
      (STDs)
    granuloma inguinale (donovanosis),
        190–191
    lymphogranuloma venereum (LGV),
        191
    syphilis, 190
HLA-DQ1 association with lepromatous
    leprosy, 77
Horta, Parreiras, 151
Hortaea werneckii fungus, 154
hospital associated methicillin resistant
    Staphylococcus aureus
    (HA-MRSA), 19
hospital gangrene. See necrotizing fascitis
hot-tub folliculitis, 19, 20, 240, 261
human African trypanosomiasis (sleeping
    sickness), 122–123
human granulocytic anaplasmosis (HGA),
    215

human herpes virus 3 (HHV-3). *See* varicella zoster virus
human herpes virus 4 (HHV-4). *See* Epstein-Barr virus
human herpes virus 5 (HHV-5). *See* cytomegalovirus
human herpes virus 6 (HHV-6). *See* roseola infantum
human herpes virus 7 (HHV-7), 33
human herpes virus 8 (HHV-8). *See* Kaposi's sarcoma
human monocytic ehrlichiosis (HME), 215
human papillomavirus (HPV)
  anogenital disease
    bowenoid papulosis, 26
    condyloma acuminatum, 26, 188
    verrucous carcinoma, 26–27
  in HIV infection, 187–188
  low risk/high risk subtypes, 188
  in mucous membrane infections, 280–281
  nongenital cutaneous diseases
    Butcher's warts, 26
    common warts (verruca vulgaris), 25
    epidermodysplasia verruciformis (EV), 25–26
    flat warts (verrucae plana), 25
    palmoplantar warts (myrmecia), 25
  nongenital mucosal disease
    oral focal hyperplasia (Heck disease), 27
  in transplantation recipients, 203
Hutchinson, Jonathan, 59
hyalohyphomycosis, 113–114
  causative agents, 113
  treatment, 113–114
hydroids, reactions to, 172
hyperbaric oxygenation, 9
hyperglycemia control for diabetes skin infections, 249, 251, 252
hyper-IgE syndrome, 222
hyperimmune globulin, for South American hemorrhagic fevers, 153

IgG immunoglobulin, 9
IL-8 cytokine association with lepromatous leprosy, 77
IL-12 cytokine association with lepromatous leprosy, 77
imidazoles
  for localized *Candida,* 286
  for piedra, 259
imipenem, for nocardiosis, 198
imiquimod (topical)
  for condyloma acuminata, 188
  for molluscum contagiosum, 187
  for Old World CL, 144
  for verrucae vulgaris/condyloma acuminatum, 203
immune reconstitution inflammatory syndrome (IRIS), 186
immunoglobulin (IV)
  for staphylococcal TSS, 325
  for streptococcal TSS, 326
impetigo, 18
  in athletes, 238

in children, 211
diagnosis, 20
in elderly patients, 234–235
in HIV, 189
S. aureus/S. pyogenes causative for, 19
in scalp infections, 261–262
treatment, 20
In Situ Hybridization (ISH), 5
Indians, and lepromatous leprosy, 77
Indo-Aryans, 59
induration (as sign of acute infection), 8
infections diseases, diagnostic techniques
  culture, 3
  intradermal reactions, 3–4
  molecular biology, 5–6
  sample collection, 2
  serology, 4–5
  skin biopsy, 6–7
  smears, 2–3
infestations of children, 230–232
  bedbugs, 232
  blister beetles, 232
  caterpillars and moths, 232
  fleas, 231–232
  mites, 230–231
  papular urticaria, 231
  pediculosis, 230
  scorpions, 231
  spiders, 231
  stinging insects, 232
insect repellants. *See* DEET (N,N-diethyl-3-methylbenzamide) mosquito repellant
interferon a
  for condyloma acuminata, 188
  for hepatitis B, 35
  for KS, 34
interstitial granulomatous dermatitis, 146–147
intradermal reactions, 3–4
intraepidermal abscesses (in chromomycosis), 99
intralesional interferon
  for KS, 280
  for verrucae vulgaris/condyloma acuminatum, 203
intralesional vinblastine, for KS, 34, 280
in-utero herpes infections
  congenital varicella syndrome, 30
  infantile zoster, 31
  neonatal varicella, 31
isoniazid
  for cutaneous TB treatment, 73
  for pulmonary tuberculosis, 292
isotretinoin
  for erosive pustular dermatosis of scalp, 263
  for scalp cellulitis, 263
Ito Reenstierna test, 4
itraconazole
  for candidiasis, 191
  for coccidioidomycosis, 192
  for cutaneous cryptococcus, 191
  for entomophthoromycosis, 111
  for histoplasmosis, 192
  for hyalohyphomycosis, 113

  for lobomycosis, 158
  for mycetoma, 157
  for Old World CL, 143
  for onychomycosis, 191
  for paracoccidioidomycosis, 109, 159
  for protothecosis, 175
  for tinea capitis, 217, 258
itraconazole (oral), 47
  adverse effects, 47
  for North American blastomycosis, 105–106
  for penicilliosis, 193
  for pityriasis versicolor, 53
  for sporotrichosis, 102
  for tinea capitis, 51, 51
  for tinea corporis/cruris/faciei, 50–51
  for tinea pedis/manuum, 47–50
  for tinea unguium (onychomycosis), 52, 236
  for toenail onychomycosis, 52
itraconazole (topical), for tinea nigra, 154–155
ivermectin
  for demodicidosis, 260
  with doxycycline for onchocerciasis, 124
  for filariasis, 124
  for gnathostomiasis, 127
  for loiasis, 124
  for mansonelliasis, 128
  for onchocerciasis, 124
  for onchocercosis, 176
  for scabies, 193, 260, 317–318
Ixodes pacificus, 215
Ixodes scapularis, 215

jellyfish, reactions to, 168–169
Jones, Joseph, 8
Jorge Lobo's disease. *See* keloidal blastomycosis

K. rhinoscleromatis, 7, 7
Kaposi's sarcoma (KS), 5, 33–34
  clinical manifestations, 33
  diagnosis, 34
  historical background, 185
  in HIV infection, 188–189
  in mucous membrane infections, 280
  in transplantation recipients, 202
  treatment, 34
Katayama syndrome, 130
keloidal blastomycosis, 102, 157
ketoconazole
  for entomophthoromycosis, 111
  for Old World CL, 143
  for paracoccidioidomycosis, 109
  for pityriasis versicolor, 53
  for tinea capitis, 51, 258
  for tinea corporis/cruris/faciei, 50
  for tinea pedis/manuum, 47
ketoconazole (oral), 47
  adverse effects, 47
  for dermatophyte fungal infections, 248
  for North American blastomycosis, 105–106
  for pityriasis versicolor, 53
  for protothecosis, 175

ketoconazole (shampoo), 256
  for tinea capitis, 217, 218
  for tinea corporis gladiatorum, 244
ketoconazole (topical)
  for tinea nigra, 154–155
  for tinea pedis/manuum, 47–50, 236
  for white piedra, 154
Klebsiella pneumoniae, 19
Koch, Robert, 59
KOH preparations, 2–3

L. loboi (lobomycosis), 3, 7
Lacazia loboi fungus, 102, 157
Laennec, Rene, 59
larva currens, 126
larva migrans cutanea, 176–177
laser treatment
  for Bowenoid papulosis, 26
  for condyloma acuminata, 188
  for folliculitis keloidalis, 262
  for oral florid papillomatosis, 281
  for pseudofolliculitis barbae, 216
  for rhinoscleroma, 294
  for verrucae vulgaris/condyloma
    acuminatum, 203, 228
Lassa fever, 153
Latruncula magnifica red sponge, 174
Laws of Manu, 59
Leão, Arêa, 151
leeches, reactions to, 176
Legionella, 4
Leishman, W. B., 135
Leishmania aethiopica, 117–118
Leishmania amazonensis, 119, 161
Leishmania braziliensis (viannia), 117, 120,
    150, 160–161
Leishmania chagasi, 119
Leishmania donovani, 117, 119
Leishmania guyanensis, 161
Leishmania infantum, 117–118, 119
Leishmania major, 117–118
Leishmania mexicana, 117
Leishmania panamensis, 120
Leishmania peruviana, 117
Leishmania tropica, 117
leishmaniasis, 92, 117–121. *See also* anergic
    leishmaniasis; mucocutaneous/
    tegmental leishmaniasis; Old World
    cutaneous leishmaniasis
  classifications
    cutaneous leishmaniasis, 117
    diffuse cutaneous, 4
    lupus leishmaniasis, 74
    mucocutaneous leishmaniasis, 119
    new world leishmaniasis, 118–121
    old World leishmaniasis, 117–118
  clinical manifestations, 161, 296
  diagnosis, 120
  in HIV infection, 194
  in Texas, borne by sandflies, 92
  treatment, 120–121
  vacuolated histiocytes with
    lymphoplasmacytic infiltrate
    in, 6
  visceral, 4

Leishmanin test (Montenegro test), 4
lepromatous leprosy (LL), 4, 7, 77, 79
  histopathology, 83
  HLA-DQ1 association, 77
  Lucio's phenomenon in, 82
  oral lesions in, 292
  resemblance to disseminated
    coccidioidomycosis, 147
Lepromin test, 4
leprosy. *See* Hansen's disease
Leptospira, 4
Letterer-Siwe syndrome, 74
lichen scrofulosorum (LS), 68–69, 75
lidocaine (topical)
  for herpes zoster, 235
  for HSV, 277
  for oral infections, 275, 277
  for post-herpetic neuralgia, 31
life-threatening skin infections
  historical background, 322
  meningococcal disease, 322–323
  Rocky Mountain spotted fever, 92,
    323–324
  staphylococcal toxic shock syndrome,
    324–325
  streptococcal toxic shock syndrome,
    325–327
ligase based method (of PCR), 5
lindane
  for demodicidosis, 260
  for pediculosis capitis, 259
  for scabies, 260
  topical, for scabies, 317–318
linear streaking along lymphatics (as sign of
    acute infection), 8
linezolid
  for impetigo/folliculitis/furunculosis,
    235–234
  for MRSA strains, 20
  for nocardiosis, 198
  for *S. aureus*, 196
Linuche unguiculata jellyfish, 171–172
Loa loa, 124
Lobo, Jorge, 102, 151
lobomycosis, 102–103, 151
  diagnosis, 103
  treatment, 103
loiasis, 124
lower extremity cellulitis, pitfalls and
    myths, 21
Lucio's phenomenon, 82, 84, 85
lupoid rosacea, 74
lupus leishmaniasis, 74
lupus vulgaris, 59, 62–64, 74, 78
Lutz, Adolpho, 151
Lutzomyia genera, 117
Lyme disease, 92, 95, 215
lymphadenopathy (as sign of acute
    infection), 8
lymphogranuloma venereum (LGV), 309,
    313–314
Lyngbya majuscola seaweed, 174

macrolides
  for atypical mycobacterioses, 90

for *Balamuthia mandrillaris*, 122
  for perianal streptococcal dermatitis, 212
Madurella mycetomatis grains, 156
Majocchi's granuloma, 191
malaria, 92, 93, 95, 150
Malassezia globosa yeast, 256
Malassezia restricta yeast, 256
malathion
  for pediculosis capitis, 259
  for public lice, 318
malignant otitis externa, 251
malignant skin infections
  angiosarcoma, 209
  breast cancer, inflammatory, 208–209
  cancers metastatic to skin, 210
  keratoacanthoma, 209–210
  lethal midline granuloma, 209
  leukemia cutis, 208
  lymphoma, 208
  squamous cell cancer, 209
  Stewart-Treves syndrome, 209
  verrucous carcinoma, 209
management principles
  clinical diagnosis, 8
  historical background, 8
  laboratory diagnosis, 8
  myths/pitfalls, 9–13
  treatment, 8–9
Mansonella ozzardi, 128
Mansonella perstans, 128
Mansonella streptocerca, 128
mansonelliasis, 128
Mantoux test, 4
maprotiline, for post-herpetic neuralgia,
    31
Marburg/Ebola virus, 153
Masters of the Salerno School of Medicine,
    59
Mastomys natalensis rodent, 153
measles/rubeola, 36–37
  clinical manifestations, 36
  diagnosis, 37
  in mucous membrane infections, 283
  ProQuad vaccine for, 278
  treatment, 37
mebendazole
  for dracunculiasis, 125
  for enterobiasis, 128
  for trichinellosis, 128
melarsoprol, for trypanosomiasis, 123
Meleney's ulcer, 8
meningococcal conjugate
    vaccine A, C, Y, W-135, 323
meningococcal disease
  clinical manifestations, 322–323
  diagnosis, 323
  management, 323
  pitfalls and myths, 327
meningoencephalitis, 152, 152
methicillin, introduction of, 19
methicillin resistant *Staphylococcus aureus*
    (MRSA), 19, 20, 189, 195, 238, 262
methicillin sensitive *Staphylococcus aureus*
    (MSSA), 19, 195
N-methylglucamine, for leishmaniasis, 164

methylprednisolone, for post-herpetic
    neuralgia, 31
metronidazole
    for acute necrotizing ulcerative
        gingivitis, 295
    for bacterial vaginosis, 295
    for demodicidosis, 260
    for dracunculiasis, 125
    IV/oral, for enteric amebiasis, 121
    for noma, 295
    for trichomoniasis, 296
miconazole
    for erythrasma, 249
    for hyalohyphomycosis, 113
    for pityriasis versicolor, 53
    for tinea corporis/cruris/faciei, 50
    for tinea pedis/manuum, 47
    topical, for tinea nigra, 154–155
miconazole nitrate 1%, for tinea pedis/
    manuum, 47
microbial paronychial infections, 268
Microciona prolifera sponge, 174
Micrococcus (Kytococcus) sedentarius, 214
Micrococcus spp., 189
Microsporum audouinii, 256
Microsporum canis, 256
Microsporum distortum, 256
mid-plate onychomycosis, 272
Miller's nodules (Paravaccinia)
    clinical manifestations, 24
    diagnosis, 24
    treatment, 24
miltefosine, for Old World CL, 144
minocycline. *See also* ROM therapy
    for atypical mycobacteria, 244
    for *mycobacterium marinum,* 179
    for nocardiosis, 198
Mitsuda lepromin antigen, 4
MMR (measles, mumps, rubella)
    vaccination, 283
Moh's surgery, 303, 305
molecular biology, 5–6
molluscum contagiosum virus (MCV),
    7, 23
    in athletes, 241–242
    in children, 228–229
    clinical manifestations, 23
    in HIV infection, 187
    in mucous membrane infections, 281
    in transplantation recipients, 202–203
    treatment, 23
mollusks and aquatic dermatoses, 174
monkeypox, in children, 229
Montenegro, João, 151
Montenegro test (Leishmanin test), 4
Mosquito Magnet (mosquito trap), 95
mosquito vectors
    of Barmah Forest virus, 153
    of mucocutaneous/tegmental
        leishmaniasis, 161
    of West Nile virus, 152
    of Yellow fever, 152
moths and caterpillars, 232
mouse-borne diseases, 92

mouth rinses with topical anesthetic agents,
    for HSV 1/2 infections, 277
MRSA. See methicillin resistant
    Staphylococcus aureus
mucocutaneous/tegmental leishmaniasis,
    160–164
    clinical manifestations, 161–164
    diagnosis, 164
    mosquito vectors, 161
    transmission, 161
    treatment, 164
Mucorales (Zygomycosis), 109
mucormycosis, 7, 109–110. *See also*
    rhinocerebral mucormycosis
    clinical patterns, 109, 287
    diagnosis, 287
    treatment, 110, 287
mucous membrane infections
    bacterial infections, other
        actinomycosis, 294
        acute necrotizing ulcerative gingivitis,
            294–295
        anthrax, 295
        bacterial vaginosis, 295
        diphtheria, 293–294
        mycoplasma pneumoniae, 296
        noma (cancrum oris/gangrenous
            stomatitis), 295
        pseudomonas aeruginosa, 295
        rhinoscleroma, 294
        staphylococcus, 293
        streptococcus, 293
        tetanus, 296
    DNA viruses
        Epstein-Barr virus, 278–279
        human papilloma virus,
            280–281
        human simplex 1 and 2,
            276–278
        Kaposi's sarcoma, 280
        molluscum contagiosum, 281
        parvovirus B19, 281
        roseola infantum, 279–280
        varicella zoster, 278
    fungal infections
        chronic mucocutaneous candidiasis,
            286
        endemic mycoses, 288–290
            blastomycosis, 289
            coccidioidomycosis, 289–290
            histoplasmosis, 288–289
            paracoccidioidomycosis, 289
        nonendemic mycoses, 286–288
            aspergillosis, 288
            disseminated candidiasis, 286
            mucormycosis, 286–287
        superficial mycoses/*Candida* spp.,
            284–286
    historical background, 275
    mycobacterial infections
        leprosy, 292–293
        mycobacterium avium intracellulare,
            292
        tuberculosis, 292

protozoa
    leishmaniasis, 296–297
    trichomoniasis, 296
RNA retroviruses, 284
    HIV, 284
    human T-lymphotropic virus, 284
RNA viruses, 281–284
    hand-foot-and-mouth disease, 281–282
    herpangina, 282–283
    measles, 283
    mumps, 283
    rubella, 283–284
sexually transmitted bacterial infections
    spirochetes, 291
    syphilis, 291–292
mumps
    in mucous membrane infections, 283
    ProQuad vaccine for, 278
mupirocin (topical)
    for folliculitis, 20, 239
    for impetigo, 20, 211
    for nasal carriage, 21
    for *S. aureus* in transplant recipients, 196
mycetoma, 97–98, 156–157
Mycobacterium abscessus, 3
Mycobacterium africanum, 60
Mycobacterium avium complex, 89, 292
Mycobacterium avium-intracellulare
    lymphadenitis, 64, 74
Mycobacterium bovis, 60, 64. *See also*
    scrofuloderma
Mycobacterium chelonae, 3
*Mycobacterium chelonae-Mycobacterium
    abscessus complex,* 89
Mycobacterium fortuitum, 3
Mycobacterium fortuitum complex, 89
Mycobacterium kansasii, 4, 88
Mycobacterium leprae, 3, 4, 5, 7, 60, 76,
    292–293. *See also* Hansen's disease
Mycobacterium marinum, 7, 67, 88, 173,
    178–179
Mycobacterium microti, 60
Mycobacterium scrofulaceum, 4, 64, 74, 89
Mycobacterium tuberculosis, 3, 4, 6, 7, 60, 61.
    See also cutaneous tuberculosis
    causative for tuberculosis, 292
    classification, 62
    diagnosis, 61–62
    histopathology, 70–71
    HIV and, 72
    PCR for, 189
Mycobacterium ulcerans, 3–5, 7
mycoplasma pneumoniae, 296
Mycosel anaerobes, 3

Naegleria spp., 121
naftifine hydrochloride 1%, for tinea pedis/
    manuum, 47
nail unit infections
    fungal infections, 269–273
        combined variants of onychomycosis,
            272–273
        distal/lateral subungual
            onychomycosis, 270

mid-plate onychomycosis, 272
    proximal subungual onychomycosis, 270
    relapse of onychomycosis, 273
    total dystrophic onychomycosis, 272
    white/black superficial onychomycosis, 271–272
  historical background, 268
  paronychial infections
    acute, 268–269
    chronic, 269
    microbial, 268
  pitfalls and myths, 273
  structure of nail unit, 268
necrosis (as sign of acute infection), 8
necrosis lipoidica vs. Hansen's disease lesions, 78
necrotizing fascitis, 8
  in children, 213
  in diabetes mellitus, 250
  differentiation of via creatinine phosphokinase, 8
  in elderly patients, 235
  in HIV, 189
  HIV infection and, 189
  medication for
    cefoperazone sodium, 213
    clindamycin for, 213
    creatinine phosphokinase, 213
  in transplant recipients, 197
Neisseria gonorrhoeae, 2, 315, 316
Neisseria meningitidis, 4, 322, 322
nematocysts of coelenterates, 168
nematodes, 123–128
  and aquatic dermatoses, 176–177
  cutaneous larva migrans, 124–125
  dracunculiasis, 124–125
  enterobiasis, 128
  filariasis, 123–124
  gnathostomiasis, 126–127
  loiasis, 124
  mansonelliasis, 128
  onchocerciasis, 124
  trichinellosis, 127–128
new world leishmaniasis, 118–121
nifurtimox
  for American trypanosomiasis, 123
  for Chagas' disease, 160
N-methylglucamine, for leishmaniasis, 164
nocardia, 2, 198, 264
Nocardia asteroides, 198
Nocardia brasiliensis, 97, 156
nocturnal pruritus, 260
noma (cancrum oris/gangrenous stomatitis), 295
non-bullous impetigo, 211
nongenital cutaneous diseases
  Butcher's warts, 26
  common warts (verruca vulgaris), 25
  epidermodysplasia verruciformis (EV), 25–26
  flat warts (verrucae plana), 25
  palmoplantar warts (myrmecia), 25

nonsteroidal anti-inflammatory drugs (NSAIDs)
  association with gangrene, 8
  for ENL treatment, 84
  for HSV 1 and 2 infections, 277
  for HSV infection, 277
  for multibacillary/paucibacillary disease, 84
North American blastomycosis, 6, 105–106
  diagnosis, 105
  treatment, 105–106
Nucleic Acid Sequence-based Amplification (NASBA), 5
nucleoside reverse transcriptase inhibitors (NRTIs), 38

Occult amigdalitis paracoccidioica, 107
Ochlerotatus mosquito, 152, 153
Octopus vulgaris, 174
olamine (topical)
  for tinea pedis/manuum, 47
  for white piedra, 154
Old World cutaneous leishmaniasis (CL), 117–118
  clinical presentation, 138–140
  diagnosis, 140–141
  epidemiology, 135–136
  historical background, 135
  patient follow-up, 144
  prevention, 137–138
  transmission: sandfly vector/*Leishmania* lifecycle, 136–137
  treatment, 141–144
Onchocerca skin test, 4
Onchocerca volvulus, 124, 175
onchocerciasis, 123, 124, 175–176
onychomycosis. *See also* tinea unguium
  dermatophyte onychomycosis, 47, 52
  distal subungual onychomycosis, 236
  distal/lateral subungual, 270
  mid-plate, 272
  proximal subungual, 270
  relapse of, 273
  total dystrophic, 272
  white/black superficial, 271–272
opiates, for herpes zoster, 235
oral hairy leukoplakia (OHL), 187
orbital cellulitis, 213, 287
orf virus, 81.10
organomegaly, 130
orificial tuberculosis, 67–68, 74–75
oropharyngeal candida (thrush), 221
oropharyngeal/esophageal candidiasis, 47
otitis externa (malignant), 246, 251–252
oxygen therapy, for Dengue fever, 152

P. braziliensis (South American blastomycosis). *See* paracoccidioidomycosis
Paecilomyces spp., 113
PAIR ((percutaneous aspiration, infusion of scolicidal agents, respiration)) procedure, 129
palmoplantar warts (myrmecia), 25

Panstrongylus megistus parasite, 160
papular urticaria, 231
papulonecrotic tuberculids, 68, 75
Paracentrotus lividus sea anemone, 172
paracoccidioidomycosis (South American blastomycosis), 6, 106–109, 158–159
  acute/subacute form (childhood/juvenile type), 106–107
  chronic form (adult type), 107–108
  clinical manifestations, 106, 158
  diagnosis, 108, 158–159
  discovery of, 151
  in HIV infection, 192
  in mucous membrane infections, 289–290
  residual/sequel form, 108–109
  treatment, 108–109, 159
paragonimiasis, 131. *See also* extrapulmonary paragonimiasis; scrotal paragonimiasis
Paragonimiasis westermani, 131
Paramyxoviridae virus, 153
parasitic infections of the scalp
  demodicidosis, 260
  pediculosis capitis, 259–260
  scabies, 260
parasitology
  helminths, 123–131
    cestodes, 128–130
    nematodes, 123–128
    trematodes, 130–131
  historical background, 117
  pitfalls and myths, 131
  protozoa
    enteric amebiasis, 121
    free living amebas, 121–122
    leishmaniasis, 117 (*see also* leishmaniasis)
    trypanosomiasis, 122–123
parenteral penicillin, for congenital syphilis, 223
Parinaud's oculoglandular syndrome, 215
PARK2 promoter region, association with Hansen's disease, 77
paromomycin (topical), for Old World CL, 143
paronychial infections of the nail unit
  acute, 268–269
  chronic, 269
  microbial, 268
parvovirus B19, 35
  clinical manifestations, 34
  diagnosis, 35
  in mucous membrane infections, 281
  treatment, 35
paucibacillary disease treatment guidelines (WHO), 84
pbmycosis. *See* paracoccidioidomycosis (South American blastomycosis)
PCR. See polymerase chain reaction (PCR)
pediatric infestations, 230–232
  bedbugs, 232
  blister beetles, 232
  caterpillars and moths, 232

pediatric infestations (cont.)
fleas, 231–232
mites, 230–231
papular urticaria, 231
pediculosis, 230
scorpions, 231
spiders, 231
stinging insects, 232
pediatric periorbital cellulitis, 19
pediatric skin infections
clinical infections
angular cheilitis (perleche), 221
chronic mucocutaneous candidiasis
(CMC), 221–222
chronic paronychia, 221
congenital candidiasis, 221
diaper dermatitis (monilial diaper
dermatitis), 221
invasive fungal dermatitis, 221
oropharyngeal candida (thrush), 221
spontaneous intestinal perforation, 221
systemic candidiasis, 221
congenital infections, 222–225
cytomegalovirus, 224
neonatal HSV, 225
parvovirus B19, 225
rubella, 223–224
syphilis, 222–223
varicella zoster, 225
eosinophilic pustula folliculitis, 216
fungal infections, 216–221
dermatophytes
candidiasis, 220–221
piedra, 220
tinea capitis, 217–218
tinea cruris, 218
tinea faceii, 218
tinea imbricata (tokelau), 219
tinea incognito, 218
tinea nigra, 220
tinea unguium (onychomycosis),
218–219
gram-negative bacteria, 214–215
cat-scratch disease, 215
ecthyma gangrenosum, 214–215
ehrlichiosis, 215
gram-positive bacteria, 211–214
blistering dactylitis, 212
ecthyma, 211
erysipeloid, 214
erythrasma, 214
impetigo, 211
necrotizing fascitis, 213
orbital/periorbital cellulitis, 213
perianal streptococcal dermatitis, 212
pitted keratolysis, 214
scarlet fever, 212
trichomycosis axillaris, 214
historical background, 211
infestations, 230–232
bedbugs, 232
blister beetles, 232
caterpillars and moths, 232
fleas, 231–232
mites, 230–231

papular urticaria, 231
pediculosis, 230
scorpions, 231
spiders, 231
stinging insects, 232
pseudofolliculitis barbae, 216
spirochetes, 215–216
endemic treponematoses, 215–216
Lyme disease, 215
viral diseases
HSV manifestations
eczema herpeticum, 225–226
gingivostomatitis, 225
herpes gladiatorum, 226–227
herpetic whitlow, 226
molluscum and poxviridae, 228–229
monkeypox, 229
vaccinia and variola, 229–230
verruca, 227–228
pediatric streptococcal dermatitis, 212
pediculosis, 154, 230
pediculosis capitis (of the scalp), 259–260
Pediculosis humanus capitis parasite, 259
pediculosis pubis, 318
Pedroso and Lane's mycosis. *See*
chromoblastomycosis
peginterferon a for hepatitis C virus, 37
pegylated interferon + ribavirin for hepatitis
C virus, 37
Pelagia noctiluca jellyfish, 168
Pelodera strongyloides, 125
penciclovir, for herpes labialis, 277
penicillin
for actinomycosis, 294
for acute necrotizing ulcerative
gingivitis, 295
for anthrax, 295
anti-pseudomonal, for ecthyma
gangrenosum, 215
for cellulitis/erysipelas, 234
for erysipeloid, 214
for folliculitis keloidalis, 262
for impetigo/folliculitis/furunculosis,
235–234
introduction of, 18
with metronidazole
for Fournier's gangrene, 252
for necrotizing fascitis, 252
for noma, 295
for perianal streptococcal dermatitis, 212
for *S. pyogenes* caused erysipelas, 20
for scarlet fever, 212
for streptococcal pharyngitis, 293
penicillin G, for syphilis, 223, 312
penicilliosis, in HIV infection, 192–193
Penicillium marneffei infection, 187
Penicillium spp., 113, 187
pentamidine
for *Balamuthia mandrillaris,* 122
for enteric amebiasis, 121
for trypanosomiasis, 123
pentavalent antimonials, for leishmaniasis,
164, 297
Pentostam® (sodium stibogluconate), for Old
World CL, 121, 143, 164

pentoxifylline, for ENL treatment, 84
perianal streptococcal dermatitis, in
children, 212
periorbital cellulitis, in children, 213
peripheral neuropathies, from Hansen's
disease, 76
perleche (angular cheilitis), 221
permethrin (topical)
for demodicidosis, 260
for pediculosis capitis, 259
for public lice, 318
for scabies, 193, 260
phaeohyphomycosis, 112–113
Phialophora verrucosa, 98–99, 113, 156
phlebotominae insects (vectors), 161
Phlebotomus papatasi, 136
Phlebotomus sandfly, 117, 136–137.
See also Old World cutaneous
leishmaniasis (CL)
Phlebotomus sergenti, 136
photodynamic therapy, for Old World CL,
144
Physalia physalis physaliae (Portuguese man-
of-war), 172
Physalia utriculus physaliae, 172
physaliae, reactions to, 172
picornaviruses
Enteroviruses
hand, foot, and mouth disease, 35–36
hepatovirus: hepatitis A, 36
herpangina, 36
Piedra hortae, 258
piedra nigra, 151, 220
Piedraia hortai, 151
pilocarpine preparations
for leprosy diagnosis, 79
for pubic lice, 318
Pirquet test, 4
pitfalls and myths
of arthropod-borne infections, 95
of athletic skin infections, 244
of atypical mycobacterioses, 90–91
of cancer-related skin infections, 208
of common fungal infections, 53
of cutaneous tuberculosis, 73–75
of deep fungal infections, 114–116
of diabetic skin infections, 251
of elderly patient skin infections, 237
of erysipelas, 21
of folliculitis, 21
of Hansen's disease, 86–87
of HIV-related skin infections, 90–91
of lower extremity cellulitis, 21
of marine biotic agents, 179–181
of meningococcal disease, 327
of mucous membrane infections, 297
of nail unit infections, 273
of parasitology, 131
of pediatric skin infections, 232
of Rocky Mountain spotted fever, 327
of scalp infections, 264–265
of sexually transmitted disease, 319–320
of skin infections, 9–13
of staphylococcal toxic shock syndrome,
327

of surgical skin infections, 306–307
of tropical infections, 164–165
of viral skin infections, 38
pitted keratolysis
in athletes, 239–240
in children, 214
pityriasis amiantacea (of the scalp), 256
pityriasis capitis (of the scalp), 255–256
pityriasis lichenoides et varioliformis acuta
(PLEVA), 74
pityriasis versicolor (PV), antifungal
medications for, 52–53
PLEVA. See pityriasis lichenoides et
varioliformis acuta (PLEVA)
Pliny the Elder, on tuberculosis, 59
Pneumocystis carinii pneumonia, 185
pneumocystosis
cutaneous, 187
in HIV infection, 191
podophyllin (topical)
for molluscum contagiosum, 187
for oral hairy leukoplakia, 187
podophyllotoxin solution (or resin)
for anogenital warts, 319
for condyloma acuminata, 188
for oral florid papillomatosis, 281
for oral hairy leukoplakia, 279
for verrucae vulgaris/condyloma
acuminatum, 203
polychaetes, dermatitis from, 176
polymerase chain reaction (PCR), 5, 7, 38
posaconazole, 110, 287
potassium iodide (KI)
for entomophthoromycosis, 111
for sporotrichosis, 102
povidone iodine shampoo, for tinea
capitis, 51
pox viruses
Molluscum Contagiosum (MCV), 23
orthopox
cowpox, 24
monkey pox, 24
smallpox, 23
vaccinia, 24
parapox
Miller's nodules (Paravaccinia), 24
orf, 24
PPD-Y intradermal reaction, 4
praziquantel
for cysticercosis, 129
for fasciolasis, 130
for paragonimiasis, 131
pregabalin, for post-herpetic neuralgia, 31
primary cutaneous coccidioidomycosis,
147–148
primary inoculation tuberculosis
(tuberculosus chancre), 67
progressive hypertrophic familial neuropathy
and Hansen's disease, 78
Propionibacterium acnes, 262
ProQuad vaccine, for measles/mumps/
varicella, 278
Prototheca green seaweed mutant, 174
Prototheca wickerhamii, 174
prototothecosis infection, 174–175

protozoa. *See also* individual *Leishmania*
species
Chagas' disease, 159–160
enteric amebiasis, 121
free living amebas, 121–122
leishmaniasis, 117. *See also* leishmaniasis
mucocutaneous/tegmental leishmaniasis,
160–164
in mucous membrane infections
leishmaniasis, 296–297
trichomoniasis, 296
trypanosomiasis, 122–123
American trypanosomiasis, 123
human African trypanosomiasis,
122–123
proximal subungual onychomycosis (PSO),
236, 270
Pseudallescheria boydii, 113
pseudoepitheliomatous hyperplasia (in
chromomycosis), 99, 114
pseudolymphoma of the skin, 74
Pseudomonas aeruginosa, 19, 189, 214–215,
251, 295, 303
psoriasis
guttate psoriasis, 211, 212
impetigo infections from, 261
mimicking of
by lupus vulgaris, 74
by onychomycosis, 53
nail dystrophy from, 236
pityriasis amiantacea from, 256
vs. Hansen's disease lesions, 78
pubic lice, 318
Public Health Service (PHS) paucibacillary
disease treatment guidelines, 84
pulmonary tuberculosis, 5
pustulation (as sign of acute infection), 8
pyrazinamide
for cutaneous TB treatment, 73
for pulmonary tuberculosis, 292
pyrethrin extracts, for pediculosis capitis,
259
pyrithione zinc shampoo, 256

quinine, for tularemia, 95
quinolones
for atypical mycobacterioses, 90
for cellulitis/erysipelas, 234
quinupristin/dalfopristin, for MRSA
strains, 20

Rabello, Francisco, 151
ravuconazole, for mucormycosis, 110
recalcitrant cutaneous dermatophyte, 47
"reinfection" tuberculosis, 60
relapsing fever, 92
repellants for insects. *See* DEET (N,N-
diethyl-3-methylbenzamide)
mosquito repellant
retapamulin ointment, for impetigo, 20
retinoids (topical)
for Bowenoid papulosis, 26
for KS, 34
for molluscum contagiosum, 229, 264
for pseudofolliculitis barbae, 216

for verrucae vulgaris/condyloma
acuminatum, 203, 228
Rhabdoviridae virus, 153
rhinocerebral mucormycosis, 251
Rhinocladiella aquaspersa dematieous
fungus, 98–99, 156
rhinophycomycosis, 110
rhinoscleroma, 294
rhinosporidiosis, 103–104
Rhinosporidium seeberi, 103
Rhipicephalus sanguineus (Brown dog tick),
323
Rhizomucor pusillus, 109
Rhizopodiformis, 109
Rhizopus arrhizus (oryzae), 109
Rhizopus microsporus var., 109
Rhodnius prolixus parasite, 160
ribavirin
for chronic HCV, 37
for South American hemorrhagic fevers,
153
Rickettsia rickettsii, 323
rickettsial disease, 92, 95, 311
Ridley-Jopling classification of Hansen's
disease, 78–80, 83
rifampicin
for CA-MRSA, 20
with clindamycin, for scalp cellulitis, 263
for cutaneous TB treatment, 73
for multibacillary disease, 84
for nasal carriage issues, 21
for Old World CL, 144
for paucibacillary disease, 84
for rhinoscleroma, 294
rifampin
for actinomycetoma management, 98
for atypical mycobacteria, 244
for cat-scratch disease, 215
for cutaneous tuberculosis, 73
for ehrlichiosis, 215
for leprosy, 293
for meningococcal disease, 323
for multibacillary disease, 84
for pulmonary tuberculosis, 292
Rig Veda, 59
RNA retroviruses in mucous membrane
infections
HIV, 284
human T-lymphotropic virus, 284
RNA viruses
flaviviruses: hepatitis C, 37
in mucous membrane infections, 281–284
hand-foot-and-mouth disease,
281–282
herpangina, 282–283
measles, 283
mumps, 283
rubella, 283–284
paramyxoviruses: rubeola/measles, 36–37
picornaviruses
enteroviruses
hand, foot, and mouth disease,
35–36
hepatovirus: hepatitis A, 36
herpangina, 36

RNA viruses (cont.)
retroviruses: HIV, 37–38
togaviruses: rubella (German measles), 37
Rocky Mountain spotted fever (RMSF), 92, 323–324
clinical manifestations, 324
diagnosis, 324
historical background, 322
management, 324
Roger of Palermo, 275
Rokintansky, Carl, 59
ROM therapy (rifampin 600 mg, ofloxacin 400 mg, minocycline 100 mg), 84
roseola infantum (HHV 6), 33
bone marrow transplant patients and, 33
clinical manifestations, 33
diagnosis, 33
HIV and, 33
in mucous membrane infections, 279–280
treatment, 33
rubella (German measles), 37
clinical manifestations, 37
congenital, 223–224
diagnosis, 37
treatment, 37
rubeola (measles), 36–37
clinical manifestations, 36
diagnosis, 37
in mucous membrane infections, 283
ProQuad vaccine for, 278
treatment, 37
Rudolph, Max, 151

Saksenaea vasiformis, 109
salicylates, 277, 278
salicylic acid
for Butcher's warts, 26
for common warts, 25
for tinea nigra, 154–155
for verruca, 228
for verruca vulgaris/condyloma acuminatum, 25, 203
sandfly-borne diseases, 92, 136–137, 137. See also Old World cutaneous leishmaniasis
Sappinia diploidea, 121
sarcoidal granulomas, 6
Sarcoptes scabiei var. hominis, 260, 317
scabies, 317–318
causative agents, 193
diagnosis, 2
in HIV infection, 193
vs. onchocerciasis, 124
scalp infections
bacterial infections
eosinophilic pustular folliculitis, 261
erysipelas/scalp cellulitis, 262
folliculitis, 260
impetigo, 261–262
staphylococcal folliculitis, 260–261
fungal infections
piedra, 258–259
pityriasis amiantacea, 256

pityriasis capitis, 255–256
seborrheic dermatitis, 255–256
historical background, 255
from intrauterine fetal monitoring devices, 262
parasitic infections
demodicidosis, 260
pediculosis capitis, 259–260
scabies, 260
pitfalls and myths, 264–265
postoperative infections, 262
with presumed bacterial etiology
acne miliaris necrotica, 262
dissecting cellulitis, 262–263
erosive pustular dermatosis, 263
folliculitis decalvans, 262–263
folliculitis keloidalis (acne keloidalis), 262
scalp anatomy, 255
in transplant patients, 264
unusual infections
mycobacterial infection, 264
syphilis, 263–264
viral infections
herpes viral infections, 264
molluscum contagiosum, 264
warts, 264
Scedosporium apiospermum, 113
Schistosoma hematobium, 130
Schistosoma japonicum, 130
Schistosoma mansoni, 130
schistosomal dermatitis. See cercarial dermatitis (swimmer's itch)
schistosomiasis, 130, 150
Scopulariopsis brevicaulis, 219, 236, 270, 271
Scopulariopsis spp., 113
scorpions, 231
Scrofulin intradermal reaction, 4
scrofuloderma, 59, 64, 74
scrotal paragonimiasis, 131
Scytalidium dimidiatum, 272
sea bather's eruption, 171–172
sea urchins, reactions to, 172–173
seborrheic dermatitis, 255–256
secondary syphilis, 74
selenium sulfide
for piedra, 259
for tinea capitis, 51, 217
selenium sulfide shampoos, 51, 217, 256
sexually transmitted diseases (STDs) and HIV skin infections
anogenital warts, 319
chancroid, 309, 312–313
genital bite wounds, 316–317
genital herpes, 318–319
gonorrhea, 310, 315–316
granuloma inguinale (donovanosis), 190–191, 309, 314–315
historical background, 309–310
lymphogranuloma venereum (LGV), 191, 309, 313–314
pubic lice, 318
scabies, 317–318
syphilis, 190, 309, 310–312 (see also syphilis)

Silva, Flaviano, 151
skin surgical site infections (SSIs)
definition/classification, 303–304
historical background, 303
intrinsic risk factors, 304
management/prevention
antibiotic prophylaxis, 306
aseptic technique, 305
surgical site care, 305–306
procedure-related risk factors
bleeding during procedure, 304–305
location, 304
type of lesion, 304
type of procedure and repair, 304
"Slapped Cheeks." See parvovirus B19
sleeping sickness. See human African trypanosomiasis (sleeping sickness)
smallpox virus
clinical manifestations, 23
vaccination for, 23, 229
sodium stibogluconate (Pentostam˙), for leishmaniasis, 121, 143, 164
South American blastomycosis (P. braziliensis). See paracoccidioidomycosis (South American blastomycosis)
South American hemorrhagic fevers, 153
sparganosis, 129
spectinomycin, for gonorrhea, 315–316
Spherulin test, 4
spiders, 231
spirochetes (in children)
endemic treponematoses, 215–216
Lyme disease, 215
Spirometra spp., 129
sponges and aquatic dermatoses, 174
Sporothrix schenckii dimorphic fungus, 155
sporotrichosis, 6, 64, 100–102
cutaneous forms, 100–101
diagnosis, 101–102, 155
extra-cutaneous forms, 101
treatment, 102
zoonotic transmission, 155
Sporotrichum, 7
squamous cell carcinoma (SCC)
anogenital, 187
from chronic sun exposure, 203
differentiation from tuberculosis, 65
epidermoid, 99
lesion excision, 303
oral, 280
PS as suggestive of, 114
subungual, 209
squamous cell carcinoma in situ (SCCIS), 203
staphylococcal scalded skin syndrome (SSSS), 196, 212–213
staphylococcal scarlet fever, 196
staphylococcal toxic shock syndrome, 19, 324–325
clinical manifestations, 325
diagnosis, 325
historical background, 322
management, 325
pitfalls and myths, 327

staphylococcus, 293
Staphylococcus aureus, 18
    blistering dactylitis from, 212
    carbuncles caused by, 19
    cellulitis from, 249
    conditions predisposing to colonization, 21
    ecthyma caused by, 19
    folliculitis from, 189, 234
    furunculosis from, 234
    impetigo from, 19, 211, 234, 238
    orbital/periorbital cellulitis from, 213
    perianal streptococcal dermatitis from, 212
    SSSS from, 212
    staphylococcal TSS from, 322, 325
    surgical skin infections from, 303
    in transplant recipients, 195–196
Staphylococcus epidermis, 189, 212
Staphylococcus pneumoniae, 196, 213
starfish, reactions to, 173
Steven-Johnson syndrome, 45, 185, 258
Stichodactyla gigantea anemone, 170
stinging insects, 232
streptococcal toxic shock syndrome, 19, 325–327
    clinical manifestations, 326
    diagnosis, 326
    historical background, 322
    management, 326–327
    pitfalls and myths, 327
Streptococcus aureus, 250, 262
Streptococcus mutans, 293
streptococcus pharyngitis, 293
Streptococcus pyogenes, 18, 250, 262, 293, 325–326
    ecthyma caused by, 19
    erysipelas caused by, 19
    impetigo caused by, 19
    orbital/periorbital cellulitis from, 213
Streptococcus viridians, 293
Streptomyces somaliensis, 97
streptomycin
    for actinomycetomas, 98
    for tularemia, 95
Strongyloides stercoralis, 125, 126
subcutaneous phaeohyphomycosis, 113
subcutaneous/deep mycoses
    chromoblastomycosis, 98–100, 156 (*see also* chromoblastomycosis)
    lobomycosis, 151, 157 (*see also* lobomycosis)
    mycetoma, 97–98, 156–157
    paracoccidioidomycosis, 158–159 (*see also* paracoccidioidomycosis)
    rhinosporidiosis, 103–104
    sporotrichosis, 100–102, 155–156 (*see also* sporotrichosis)
subungual proximal superficial onychomycosis, 191
sulconazole nitrate 1%, for tinea pedis/manuum, 47
sulfadiazine
    for *Balamuthia mandrillaris,* 122
    for congenital toxoplasmosis, 222

sulfamethoxazole-trimethoprim (SMZ-TMP), for paracoccidioidomycosis, 108, 159
sulfur preparations, for scabies, 260
sulfur shampoos, 256
sunscreen
    on lips, for herpes labialis, 240, 277
    for warts, 203
superficial mycoses
    black piedra, 154
    piedra nigra, 151
    tinea nigra, 154–155
    white piedra, 153–154
suppurative granulomas, 6
suppurative/granulomatous inflammatory infiltrate (in chromomycosis), 99
suramin, for trypanosomiasis, 123
surgical excision
    for anogenital warts, 319
    for chromoblastomycoses, 156
    for coenurosis, 130
    for condyloma acuminata, 188
    for echinococcosis, 129
    for genital warts, 319
    for KS, 202
    for lobomycosis, 103
    for mucormycosis, 110
    for oral florid papillomatosis, 281
    for prototDhecosis, 175
    for rhinosporidiosis, 104
    of solitary KS lesions, 34
Sweet's syndrome (acute febrile neutrophilic dermatosis), 146
swimmers itch. *See* cercarial dermatitis
sympathetic nerve blockade, for post-herpetic neuralgia, 31
syphilis, 190, 275, 309, 310–312
    clinical manifestations, 310
    and secondary/tertiary hair loss, 263–264
systemic corticosteroids
    for candidal infection, 284
    for Lucio's phenomenon, 85
    for Sweet's syndrome, 146
systemic mycosis
    blastomycosis (North American), 105–106
    chronic form (adult type), 107–108
    cryptococcosis, 111–112
    entomophthoromycosis, 110–111
    histoplasmosis, 104–105
    hyalohyphomycosis, 113–114
    mucormycosis, 109–110
    paracoccidioidomycosis (S.A. blastomycosis), 106–109
        chronic form (adult type), 107–108
        residual/sequel form, 108–109
    phaeohyphomycosis, 112–113
    residual/sequel form, 108–109
    zygomycosis, 109

T. pallidum, 3, 216, 292, 313, 320
tacrolimus (topical), for erosive pustular dermatosis of scalp, 263
Taenia crassiceps, 129

Taenia multiceps, 129
Taenia serialis, 129
tar shampoos, 256, 256
Tedania anhelans sponge, 174
Tedania ignis fire sponge, 174
tegmental leishmaniasis. *See* mucocutaneous/tegmental leishmaniasis
teicoplanin, for MRSA strains, 20
telogen effluvium, 256
tenderness (as sign of acute infection), 8
terbinafine (oral)
    for adult dermatophyte onychomycosis, 47
    adverse effects, 47
    for black piedra, 259
    for diabetes mellitus, 47
    for entomophthoromycosis, 111
    mycological cure rates in dermatophyte onychomycosis, 52
    for onychomycosis, 191, 236
    for sporotrichosis, 102
    for tinea capitis, 51, 51, 217, 258
    for tinea corporis/cruris/faciei, 50–51
    for tinea imbricata (tokelau), 219
    for tinea pedis/manuum, 47–50
    for tinea unguium, 52, 191, 236, 237
    for transplant patients, 47
terbinafine (solution, cream, gel, spray), for pityriasis versicolor, 53
tertiary syphilis, 74
tetanus, 294, 296, 317
tetanus, diphtheria, acellular (DTaP) vaccine, 294
tetanus vaccination, 294
tetracyclines
    for acne miliaris necrotica, 262
    for atypical mycobacterioses, 90
    for CA-MRSA, 20
    for endemic treponematoses, 216
    for folliculitis keloidalis, 262
    for rhinoscleroma, 294
    for syphilis, 312
thermocoagulation, for condyloma acuminata, 188
ThermoMed™ device, for Old World CL, 142–143
thrush (oropharyngeal candida)
    in children, 221
    in elderly people, 235
tick-borne diseases, 92
tigecycline, for MRSA strains, 20
Tilbury, William, 59
tinea capitis. *See also* dermatophytosis
    antifungal medications for, 51
    black-dot tinea capitis, 257
    in children, 217–218
    oral vs. topical medication, 45
    of the scalp, 256–258
Tinea corporis, 191
tinea corporis/cruris/faciei, 50–51, 78
tinea cruris, in children, 218
tinea imbricata (tokelau), in children, 219
tinea incognita, 2, 218
tinea nigra, 154–155, 220

tinea pedis/manuum, 47–50, 236–237
Tinea rubrum, 191
tinea unguium, 42, 51–52
 antifungal medications for, 51–52
 in children, 218–219
 in elderly patients, 236
 mimicking by other conditions, 53
 North American prevalence, 42
 oral vs. topical therapy, 45
 subtypes of, 236
 white onychomycosis, 2
tinidazole
 for enteric amebiasis, 121
 for trichomoniasis, 296
toenail onychomycosis, 51, 52
togaviruses. *See* rubella (German measles)
toll-like receptor-(TLR)-2 association with
 lepromatous leprosy, 77
tolnaftate solution, for tinea unguium
 (onychomycosis), 219
topical clindamycin, 20, 214
topical mupirocin
 for localized impetigo, 20
 for nasal carriage issues, 21, 196
topical therapy, agent formulary/guidelines,
 11
total dystrophic onychomycosis, 272
toxic shock syndrome (TSS), 196, 305.
  See also staphylococcal toxic shock
  syndrome; streptococcal toxic shock
  syndrome
Transcription Mediated Amplification
 (TMA), 5
transplant recipients, bacterial/viral diseases
 bacillary angiomatosis, 197
 B-hemolytic streptococcus, 196–197
 gram-negative bacilli (GNB), 197
 historical background, 195
 necrotizing fascitis, 197
 nocardiosis, 198
 Staphylococcus aureus, 195–196
 vibrio vulnificus, 197
transplantation-related viral disease
 cytomegalovirus, 201–202
 Epstein-Barr virus, 201
 herpes simplex virus, 1 and 2, 199–200
 Herpetoviridae (human herpes viruses),
  199
 human herpes virus-8, 202
 human papilloma virus, 203
 molluscum contagiosum, 202–203
 varicella-zoster virus, 200–201
trematodes, 130–131
 fasciolasis, 130
 paragonimiasis, 131
 schistosomiasis, 130
treponemal serology test, 4
tretinoin (topical), for molluscum
 contagiosum, 187
Triamota infestans arthropod, 160
Trichinella britovi, 127
Trichinella murrelli, 127
Trichinella native, 127
Trichinella nelsoni, 127
Trichinella papuae, 127

Trichinella pseudospiralis, 127
Trichinella solium, 128
Trichinella spiralis, 127
trichinellosis, 127–128
 diagnosis, 128
 treatment, 128
trichloroacetic acid (80%)
 for anogenital warts, 319
 for Butcher's warts, 26
 for common warts, 25
 for condyloma acuminata, 26, 188
 for molluscum contagiosum, 23
Trichoderma spp., 113
trichomycosis axillaris, in children, 214
Trichophytin test, 4
Trichophyton mentagrophytes, 243, 257–258
Trichophyton rubrum, 243, 270–271
Trichophyton schoenleinii, 256, 258
Trichophyton soudanense, 272
Trichophyton tonsurans, 256–258
Trichophyton verrucosum, 257–258
Trichophyton violaceum, 256, 272
Trichosporon asahii, 112, 258
Trichosporon asteroides, 258
Trichosporon beigelii yeast, 153
Trichosporon cutaneum, 258
Trichosporon inkin, 258
Trichosporon interdigitale, 271
Trichosporon mucoides, 258
Trichosporon ovoides, 258
triclabendazole, for fasciolasis, 130
triclosan, for skin colonization issues, 21
tricyclic antidepressants
 for herpes zoster, 235
 for post-herpetic neuralgia, 31
trifluridine, for herpes simplex virus, 200
trimethoprim/sulfamethoxazole
 (TMP-SMX)
 for atypical mycobacterioses, 90
 for CA-MRSA, 20
 for cat-scratch disease, 215
 for granuloma inguinale, 191, 315
 for nocardiosis, 198
tropical infections
 in athletes (ulcers), 240
 general information, 150
 historical background, 150–151
 pitfalls and myths, 164–165
 protozoa
  Chagas' disease, 159–160
  mucocutaneous/tegmental
   leishmaniasis, 160–164
 subcutaneous/deep mycoses
  chromoblastomycoses, 156 (*see also*
   chromoblastomycosis)
  lobomycosis, 151, 157–158 (*see also*
   lobomycosis)
  mycetoma, 97–98, 156–157
  paracoccidioidomycosis, 158–159 (*see
   also* paracoccidioidomycosis)
  sporotrichosis, 155 (*see also*
   sporotrichosis)
 superficial mycoses
  black piedra, 154
  piedra nigra, 151

  tinea nigra, 154–155
  white piedra, 153–154
 viruses
  Barmah Forest virus (BFV), 152–153
  Dengue fever, 92, 95, 151–152
  hemorrhagic fevers, 151
  Lassa fever, 153
  Marburg/Ebola virus, 153
  South American hemorrhagic fevers,
   153
  West Nile virus (WNV), 152
  Yellow fever, 152
Trypanosoma cruzi parasite, 159
Trypanosomatidae family, 161, 117. *See also*
 Leishmania entries
trypanosomiasis, 92, 122–123, 150
 American trypanosomiasis, 123
 human African trypanosomiasis,
  122–123
Trypanosomiasis brucei gambiense, 122
Trypanosomiasis brucei rhodesiense, 122
Trypanosomiasis cruzi, 122
tuberculids, 68
Tuberculin test (PPD/purified protein
 derivative), 4
tuberculoid granulomas, 6, 7, 62, 70. *See also*
 leishmaniasis; sporotrichosis
tuberculosis. *See* cutaneous tuberculosis;
 extrapulmonary tuberculosis;
 Mycobacterium tuberculosis
tuberculosis (TT) leprosy, 79
tuberculosis chancre (primary inoculation
 tuberculosis), 67
tuberculosis cutis miliaris acuta generalisata
 (acute disseminated miliary
 tuberculosis), 67
tuberculosis gumma, 68, 74
tuberculosis of the breast, 72
tuberculosis verrucosa cutis (warty
 tuberculosis), 60, 65, 74, 78
 vs. Hansen's disease lesions, 78
tuberculous lymphadenitis with lupus
 vulgaris, 63
tularemia, 67, 74, 92
tumor necrosis factor A (TNFA) association
 with lepromatous leprosy, 77

ulceration (as sign of acute infection), 8
Uncinaria stenocephala, 125, 176
uncomplicated skin and skin structure
 infections (uSSSIs). *See also*
 *Staphylococcus aureus; Streptococcus
 pyogenes*
 abscesses/carbuncles/furuncles, 17
 cellulitis, 17–18
 diagnosis of, 20
 ecthyma, 18
 epidemiology of, 19–20
 erysipelas, 18
 folliculitis, 17
 historical background, 18–19
 impetigo, 18
 therapies for, 20–21
unilateral regional lymphadenopathy, 74
urethral secretions, 2

uSSSIs. See uncomplicated skin and skin structure infections

vaccinations
   for Argentinian hemorrhagic fevers, 153
   Bacillus Calmette-Guerin (BCG), 4, 62, 65, 72–73
   for diphtheria, 294
   measles, 37
   for measles, mumps, rubella (MMR), 278, 283
   meningococcal conjugate vaccine A, C, Y, W-135, 323
   smallpox virus, 23, 229
   varicella zoster virus, 31–32, 201
   for Yellow fever, 152
vaccinia
   in children, 229–230
   clinical manifestations, 24
   treatment, 24
vaginal candidiasis, 47, 248, 252
valacyclovir
   for congenital herpes simplex, 30
   for genital herpes, 319
   for herpes simplex virus, 200, 277
   for herpes zoster, 31, 235, 264
   for HSV, 186
   for HSV-1/HSV-2, 29
   for oral hairy leukoplakia, 187
   for varicella zoster virus, 31, 201
valganciclovir, for CMV, 33, 187, 202, 279
vancomycin
   for cellulitis/erysipelas, 234
   for impetigo/folliculitis/furunculosis, 234–235
   for MRSA strains, 20
   for *S. aureus*, 196
   for staphylococcal TSS, 325
varicella zoster virus (HHV-3), 5, 30
   in acute exanthem of HIV infection, 186–187
   children's treatment, 31
   in mucous membrane infections, 278
   neonatal varicella, 31
   in transplantation recipients, 200–201

vasculitic appearance (as sign of acute infection), 8
Vedic scriptures, 59
verrucous carcinoma
   treatment, 27
   types of
      epithelioma cuniculatum, 26–27
      giant condyloma of Buschke and Lowenstein, 27
      oral florid papillomatosis, 27
verrucous zoster, 186
vesiculation (as sign of acute infection), 8
Viana, Gaspar, 150, 160–161
Villemin, Jean Antoine, 59
vinblastine, for KS, 34, 202, 280
viral disease in transplantation
   cytomegalovirus, 201–202
   Epstein-Barr virus, 201
   herpes simplex virus, 1 and 2, 199–200
   herpetoviridae (human herpes viruses), 199
   human herpes virus-8, 202
   human papilloma virus, 203
   molluscum contagiosum, 202–203
   varicella-zoster virus, 200–201
viral encephalitis, 92
viral hemorrhagic fevers, 92
viral infections in athletes
   herpes simplex
      activation, 240
      skin-to-skin transmission, 240–241
   molluscum contagiosum, 241–242
   verruca, 242
Virchow, Rudolph, 59, 59
visceral leishmaniasis, 4
Vitamin A
   for measles, 37
   topical, for oral hairy leukoplakia, 279
volume expanders, for Dengue fever, 152
voriconazole
   with amphotericin B, for hyalohyphomycosis, 113–114
   for aspergillosis, 288

Wangiella dermatitidis, 98–99, 113
warmth (as sign of acute infection), 8

warts. *See* Butcher's warts; common warts (verruca vulgaris); condyloma acuminatum (genital warts); flat warts (verrucae plana); palmoplantar warts (myrmecia)
warty tuberculosis (tuberculosis verrucosa cutis), 60, 65, 74
Waterhouse-Friderichsen syndrome (fulminant meningococcal disease), 323
West Nile virus (WNV), 92, 152
   clinical manifestations, 152
   diagnosis/treatment, 152
   mosquito vectors, 152
white piedra, 153–154, 220, 258
white superficial onychomycosis (WSO), 236, 271–272
Whitfield's ointment
   for erythrasma, 214
   for tinea imbricata (tokelau), 219
Willan, Robert (British Dermatology founder), 59
World Health Organization (WHO)
   classification of Hansen's disease, 76, 80
   hepatitis C estimates, 37
   leishmaniasis data
      mucocutaneous/tegmental leishmaniasis, 160
      Old World cutaneous leishmaniasis, 135–136
   paucibacillary disease treatment guidelines, 84
   TB infection estimates, 59
Wuchereria bancrofti, 123

Yellow fever, 151, 152
   clinical findings, 152
   diagnosis, 152
   mosquito vectors, 152
   treatment, 152

zinc pyrithione, for tinea capitis, 51
zinc sulfate, for Old World CL, 144
zoonosis infection, 126, 161. *See also* American trypanosomiasis; leishmaniasis
zygomycosis, 96, 103, 109, 209